TRADITIONAL CHINESE VETERINARY MEDICINE

Fundamental Principles

TRADITIONAL CHINESE VETERINARY MEDICINE
Fundamental Principles

Huisheng Xie, DVM, PhD
Vanessa Preast, DVM

Copyright © 2007 by Chi Institute

Book design: Huisheng Xie and Vanessa Preast
Illustration, page layout: Vanessa Preast
Cover design: Stewart J. Thomas
Printer: Tianjin Jincai Arts Printing Co., Ltd.
Tianjin, China

Xie, Huisheng
Traditional Chinese Veterinary Medicine, Volume 1: Fundamental Principles

First Edition
Library of Congress Control Number: 2007935274
Includes appendices, indexes, and bibliographical references
ISBN-13: 978-0-9720045-1-0
ISBN-10: 0-9720045-0-5

Chi Institute
9700 West Hwy 318 6
Reddick, Florida 32686, USA
1-800-891-198

Printed in Tianjin, China
Third printing, Oct 2007

TRADITIONAL CHINESE VETERINARY MEDICINE

Fundamental Principles

Huisheng Xie, DVM, PhD, MS

Vanessa Preast, DVM

PREFACE

This text *Traditional Chinese Veterinary Medicine-Fundamental Principles* is a collaborative work that has developed into an update and expansion of the text *Traditional Chinese Veterinary Medicine* published in 1994 by Dr. Huisheng Xie. This volume intends to clarify the basic principles and foundations of Traditional Chinese Veterinary Medicine (TCVM).

We have created this text for several reasons. First, Traditional Chinese Veterinary Medicine has been used to treat animals for thousands of years in China. Only in recent history have practices such as acupuncture and herbal therapy come into use in the Western world. The majority of the literature about these traditional techniques is written in Chinese and is inaccessible to most Westerners. Because of the paucity of texts in the English language regarding these techniques, we hope this text will fill some gaps in the current knowledge. This is especially true of the basic philosophies and principles of traditional medicine for which English-language information is quite deficient. For this reason, we dedicate the entire first volume to the underlying principles of Traditional Chinese Veterinary Medicine.

Second, we wish to create a book which would be a relevant, functional resource for veterinarians and students who wish to apply these principles. For this reason, we intend to present the material in a practical manner and to illustrate these principles with case examples and questions at the end of the chapters. In addition, the final chapter of this book consists of numerous, lengthy case studies with descriptions and explanations of all the findings and treatments. It is our hope that this will promote understanding of how one may apply these principles to clinical cases.

Third, creating a new edition of *Traditional Chinese Veterinary Medicine* provided us an opportunity to clarify the text, to add additional detail, and to alter the appearance of the book. We hope that the diagrams and illustrations in this text will further enhance readers' understanding. Much of the new information in this book had not been available in the original edition. Readers familiar with the first edition will also note that we avoided detailed discussions of herbal formulas and acupuncture techniques in this book. These topics will be discussed in subsequent volumes.

We sincerely appreciate the efforts of all who have helped to make this book possible. Special thanks to Drs. Robert Spiegel and Bruce Ferguson for proofreading the manuscript and to Mr. Li Hongfan for coordinating with the press. Thanks also to family and friends for their patience, encouragement and support.

HUISHENG XIE
VANESSA PREAST

ABOUT THE AUTHORS

Huisheng Xie received his Doctor of Veterinary Medicine at the Sichuan College of Animal Science and Veterinary Medicine in Sichuan, China in 1983. Dr. Xie became an assistant and staff veterinarian in the College of Veterinary Medicine of the Beijing Agricultural University from 1983 to 1987. In 1988, he received his Master of Veterinary Science in Veterinary Acupuncture. From 1988 to 1994, he was an Assistant and Associate Professor in the Beijing Agricultural University College of Veterinary Medicine. In 1992, he also received advanced training in human acupuncture at the Beijing College of Traditional Chinese Medicine and the National Academy of Traditional Chinese Medicine. In 1999, he received his Ph.D. from the University of Florida for his investigation of the mechanisms of pain control in horses using acupuncture. Currently, he serves as the Complementary and Alternative Veterinary Medicine Clinician in the Veterinary Medical Teaching Hospital at the University of Florida. In 1998, Dr. Xie founded the Chi Institute in Reddick, Florida to train veterinarians in Chinese acupuncture and herbal medicine.

Dr. Xie's academic accomplishments in China include Achievement Awards from the Ministry of Agriculture, the National Science and Technology Committee and the Beijing Agricultural University. He has been invited to talk about veterinary acupuncture and herbal medicine all over the United States, Japan, Mexico and Europe. He is also the author of eight books and 35 scientific papers. His English-language textbook, *Traditional Chinese Veterinary Medicine,* was published in 1994 and has been used for TCVM training programs in China, Europe and the United States.

Vanessa Preast received her Doctor of Veterinary Medicine from the University of Florida. As a graduate of the Chi Institute, she has become certified in small animal acupuncture. She practiced integrative medicine in small animal practice.

NOTICE

This book is written for use by veterinarians who practice Traditional Chinese Veterinary Medicine (TCVM). It is a guide to the general principles behind this medical system, and it is not intended to be a substitute for sound medical education. Veterinarians are strongly advised to seek a comprehensive TCVM training program before using acupuncture or herbal medicine. There are several certification programs in the United States that are available to veterinarians. Nonveterinarians are cautioned against practicing medicine on animals, unless permitted by law. Untrained or inadequately-trained individuals are unable to accurately assess a patient's health status and make appropriate recommendations.

Traditional Chinese Veterinary Medicine, as with any other medical system, is an ever-changing field. In addition, much of the information in this book is based on clinical observations, as opposed to controlled studies. The publisher, editor, and authors make no warrant as to results of acupuncture or other treatments described in this book. Medical practitioners should be aware of the standard safety precautions and make appropriate changes in therapies as new research becomes available and as clinical experience grows. Any person administering medical therapy is responsible for using his or her professional skill and experience to determine the best treatment for the patient and to assure that the benefits of this treatment justifies the associated risk. Thus, the information within this book should not be construed as specific instructions for individual patients, and readers should use clinical judgment in deciding when and if the acupuncture procedures described should be applied. The authors cannot be responsible for misuse or misapplication of the material in this work.

While every effort has been made to ensure the accuracy of information contained herein, the publisher, editor, and authors are not legally responsible for errors or omissions. Readers are advised to check the product information currently provided by the manufacturer of each drug or formula to be administered to be certain that changes have not been made in the recommended dose or in the contraindications for administration.

TABLE OF CONTENTS

CHAPTER SEVEN
Diagnostic Methods

INTRODUCTION

Knowing others is wisdom;
Knowing the self is enlightenment.
Mastering others requires force;
Mastering the self needs strength.

He who knows he has enough is rich.
Perseverance is a sign of will power.
He who stays where he is endures.
To die but not to perish is to be eternally present.

– Lao Tsu, "Thirty-Three" of *Tao Te Ching*

Traditional Chinese Veterinary Medicine (TCVM), although relatively new to the Western world, is a medical system that has been used to treat animals in China for thousands of years. This system developed as prehistoric people tried to understand domestic animal disease and each subsequent generation has added their knowledge and discoveries to those of the previous generation up through present day. As such, TCVM continues to change and grow as new information is incorporated into the system. Thus, even though many of the therapeutic techniques were developed through the trials and observations of ancient Chinese people, TCVM is not immune to adaptations from other cultures and to advances in technology. For example, ancient Chinese techniques are combined with modern medical practice through the use of sterile, single-use filiform acupuncture needles, hypodermic needles with syringes, electrical current or laser-light to stimulate acupoints. The scientific research of recent history has also added to the ever-growing understanding of this medical system.

Today, the practice of TCVM in the Western world differs from its Chinese origins. First, most of the acupoints and Meridian lines used by Western veterinarians are transposed from humans. The ancient texts describing many of the classical Meridian lines and charts were lost long ago; however, some ancient books describing the acupoint locations were preserved and are still used today. This has inspired some discussion about the actual location of the Meridian lines and points in species with fewer digits or more ribs than humans. The energetic significance of some of these points is also called into question when one considers a human biped compared to a quadruped animal that has all four limbs touching the ground. Second, veterinary acupuncture in China was primarily used for agriculturally important species such as cattle, pigs and horses. In Western society, dogs, cats and birds have great significance as companions, so the understanding of acupuncture in these species has grown greatly in recent history. Third, many of the ancient techniques have been modified to fit Western perceptions and medical practice. For example, the needles commonly used today are very thin, solid and sterile. The traditional tools were large, non-sterile needles of various shapes and sizes. Last, Western practitioners may combine TCVM with a variety of other medical techniques such as chiropractics, Western herbal medicine and homeopathy. These modifications are not inherently good or bad but are merely part of the system's continued development.

Traditional Chinese Veterinary Medicine may initially be quite foreign to Western-trained minds. To some, it may seem that the principles of TCVM and Western Veterinary Medicine (WVM) are separated by a great abyss. Bridging that gulf is largely an individual mental process, but readers of this text have already made the first steps towards understanding through their interest and willingness to accept new ideas.

These medical systems are not mutually exclusive. Each has aspects that place them on opposite ends of the spectrum, but there is a large area of overlap between them. This common ground provides some familiarity for those new to TCVM concepts. It does, however, make accurate simplification and categorization of the systems difficult for teaching purposes. Bearing this in mind, realize that the complexities of medical systems are learned through experience, and this text provides only a framework to build upon.

Learning TCVM requires a shift in perspective. In general, Western medicine believes in control while traditional Chinese medicine believes in balance; WVM is more mechanistic while TCVM is more energetic. Western medical practitioners are very familiar with analyzing a disease process to discover its specific, fundamental, physical cause whether this is an infectious agent, an enzymatic defect or a toxic insult. By fully understanding the functions of the physical body all the way down to a cellular or molecular level, one can target the abnormality and better control the disease process. On the other hand, TCVM practitioners recognize disease as an imbalance in the body. They understand that the body is an integrated, energetic structure, and that disturbance of energy flow creates disease in the whole organism. When a disease Pattern is identified, one can restore balance and health by helping the body regulate itself.

Both systems rely on medical history and physical examination to make a diagnosis or identify a Pattern. Western medicine adds in diagnostic tests such as bloodwork or radiographs. The diagnostic tests of TCVM include palpation of the pulse and the *shu* points. In both cases, an experienced clinician interprets the findings and chooses an appropriate therapeutic regimen. A Western veterinarian may recommend surgery or reach for antibiotics, steroids or other pharmaceuticals. A TCVM practitioner may recommend herbs, acupuncture or special management practices as therapy.

Generally, the goals of TCVM and WVM are the same; both hope to promote health and to prevent disease. They are merely two different ways of viewing the world, and each system has its own strengths and weaknesses. Western medicine deals well with acute diseases and has advanced surgical techniques. TCVM can be beneficial for chronic diseases, especially those that Western medicine can only control but not cure. Due to the more individual nature of TCVM, Western medicine can better handle herd health problems. Although Western veterinarians promote disease prevention through yearly physical exams and vaccines, TCVM is very beneficial for identification of potential problems and preventing disease through dietary modification or preventative therapies. In addition, when veterinarians practice traditional Chinese medical techniques such as *Tai Qi Quan* or *Qi Gong*, they are able to remain centered and to better assist their patients. The therapeutics of TCVM can avoid some of the deleterious side effects of the Western drugs, but the Western drugs act much more quickly. Thus, through integration of the two systems, one may take advantage of the strengths of each while minimizing the weaknesses. Practitioners who are able to bridge the mental gap between Eastern and Western medicine may find that this combination brings better results than either one alone.

CHAPTER ONE

YIN AND YANG

Under heaven all can see beauty as beauty only
because there is ugliness.
All can know good as good only because there is evil.

Therefore having and not having arise together.
Difficult and easy complement each other.
Long and short contrast each other;
High and low rest upon each other;
Voice and sound harmonize each other;
Front and back follow one another.

— Lao Tsu, "Two" of *Tao Te Ching*

Yin-Yang and the Five Elements are two philosophical views originating in ancient China. These were initially developed in order to understand and interpret natural phenomena. These principles were applied in the field of Chinese Medicine some time between the Spring and Autumn Period (722-481 B.C.) and the Warring States Period (403-221 B.C.). Yin-Yang and the Five Elements promoted the development of two theoretical systems: Traditional Chinese Medicine (TCM) and Traditional Chinese Veterinary Medicine (TCVM). Yin-Yang and Five Elements represent the conceptual foundation of each system and have guided clinical work up to the present.

The Concept of Yin-Yang

The earliest reference to Yin and Yang is probably in *Yi Jing* (*Book of Changes*) which dates back to about 700 B.C. In this book, Yin and Yang are respectively represented by a broken line (— —) and an unbroken line (———). By combining the broken and unbroken lines into pairs, four diagrams are formed. These represent utmost Yin, utmost Yang, Yang within Yin and Yin within Yang (Figure 1.1). The addition of another broken or unbroken line to these four diagrams forms the eight trigrams. In this case, various combinations of the three lines form eight different characters (Figure 1.2). These trigrams can also be paired to compose the sixty-four hexagrams (Figure 1.3). The hexagrams symbolize all possible phenomena in the universe.

For example, each of the three example hexagrams illustrated in Figure 1.3 has a different meaning. 1) The *Tai* diagram represents the harmony between Yin and Yang. Yin lies in the upper part and Yang lies in the lower part. Yin descends to nourish Yang, and Yang rises to support Yin. 2) The *Weiji* diagram represents the disconnection between Water (Kidney) and Fire (Heart). The Fire goes up while Water descends, thus Fire and Water fail to connect and support each other. 3) The *Xiaoguo* diagram represents Cold or Yang Deficiency. Yang is surrounded by too much Yin (Cold).

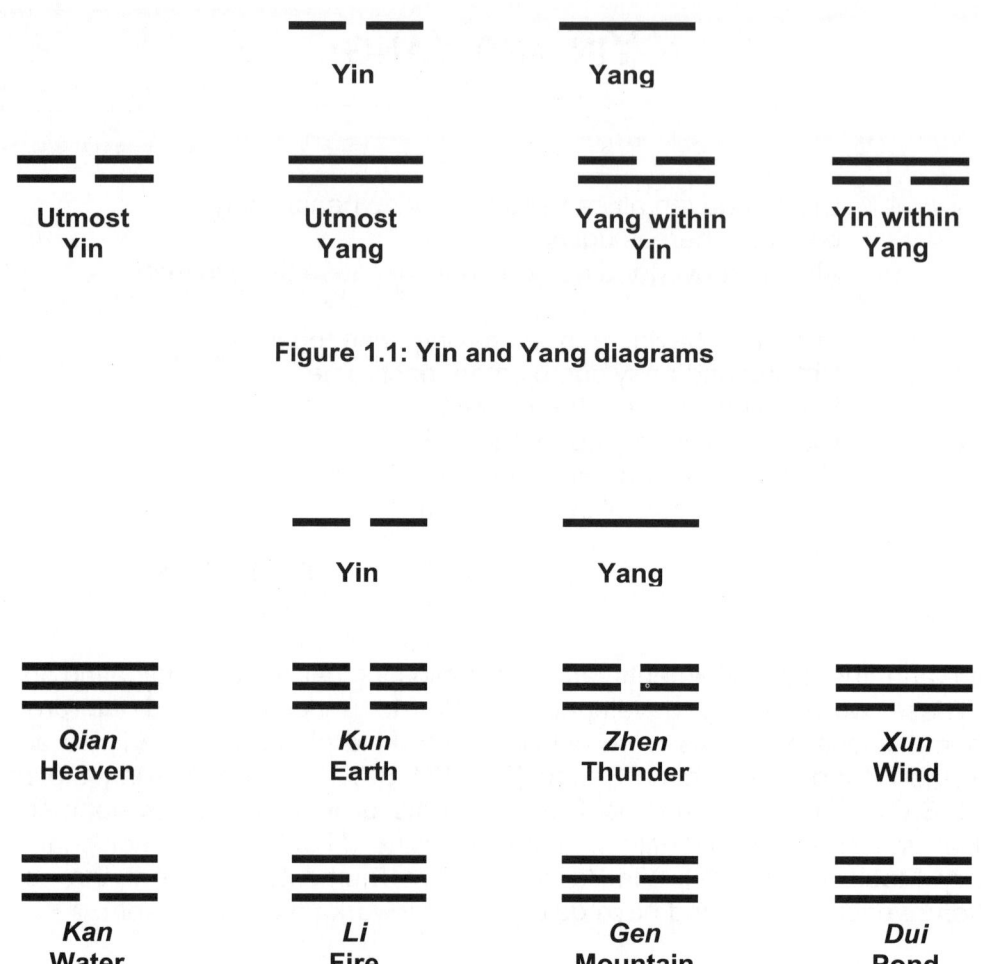

Figure 1.1: Yin and Yang diagrams

Figure 1.2: The Eight Trigrams

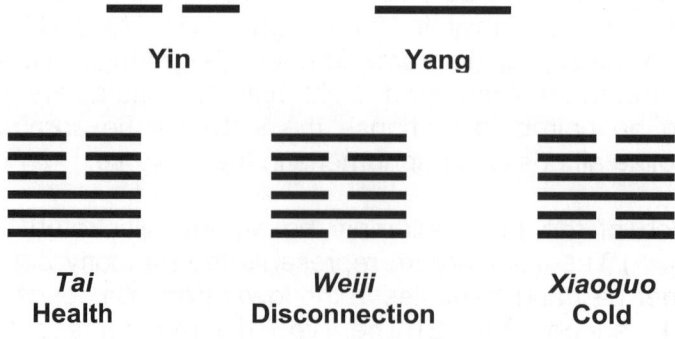

Figure 1.3: An example of three hexagrams

The Yin-Yang principles are derived, in part, from observation of the cyclical alternation between day and night. Day belongs to Yang and night belongs to Yin. Similarly, light and activity relate to Yang, as darkness and rest relate to Yin. The continuous interchange between two alternate poles observed for every circumstance can be described in terms of Yin and Yang. Light, Sun, Brightness, Activity, Heat, and Strength correspond to Yang while Darkness, Moon, Dimness, Rest, Cold, Weakness correspond to Yin. From this perspective, Yin and Yang are two stages of a cyclical movement or phenomenon; thus, Yin and Yang are representative names for dual opposites and interdependent aspects of everything in the universe. Chapter five of the book *Su Wen* (*Plain Questions*) pointed out that "Yin and Yang are the laws of heaven and earth, the great framework of everything, the parents of change, the root and beginning of life and death." According to *Su Wen*, all natural events and states of being are rooted in Yin and Yang, and they can be analyzed by the theory of Yin and Yang.

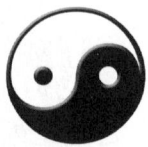

Tai Ji

The symbol above is traditionally used to represent the interrelationship of Yin and Yang. One can think of Yin and Yang as a way of trying to understand the events of the universe by organizing phenomena into distinct categories. It is at once extremely simple and staggeringly complex.

Basically, all conceivable entities or events are broken down into two opposite aspects. Many concepts may even lose their meaning without a comparison to their opposites. For example, what is heat without cold? How do we recognize dark without light? Yin and Yang are opposite sides of the same coin; they are inseparable. Like a bar magnet, no matter how it is divided, there will always be a North and South pole, a Yang and a Yin. Keep cutting and you get smaller and smaller pieces, each with a North and South pole. Any Yin or Yang aspect can be further broken down into other Yin and Yang qualities. Our world is full of endless shades of grey. Summer may be considered Yang, but there is still nighttime (Yin) as well as daytime (Yang) throughout the summer months. What about a cool summer day compared to a hot summer day? What about an eclipse of the Sun? Similarly, Yin becomes Yang and Yang becomes Yin in an endless cycle of transformation and generation. Day turns to night and back to day again.

The circle can represent the universe divided equally into Yin (black) and Yang (white). The division is not straight; but rather, Yin and Yang merge and continuously cycle with each other. Each controls and transforms into the other while carefully maintaining balance. The small circles within Yin and Yang represent the seeds of Yang within Yin and Yin within Yang. Yin and Yang compose and divide all things; yet, they cycle unceasingly in a state of eternal transformation.

The theory of Yin and Yang is a conceptual framework. It is a means to generalize any two opposite principles, which may be observed in all related phenomena within the natural world. In this way, Yin-Yang may be used to explain animal physiology and pathology and to guide clinical diagnosis and treatment. Yin and Yang represent not only two separate phenomena with opposing natures, but also two different and opposite aspects within the same phenomenon. Generally speaking, one may compare the different properties of everything in the universe, as shown in Table 1.1 and Figure 1.4.

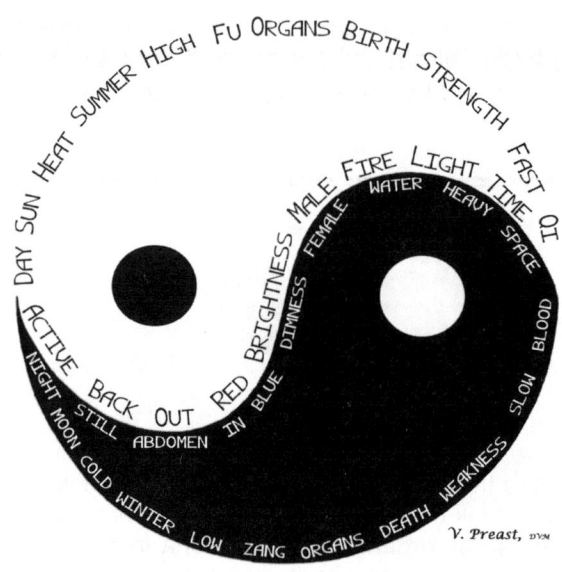

Figure 1.4: A Pictorial view of the Yin-Yang aspects of Phenomenon

The Yin-Yang nature of a phenomenon or event is not absolute; it is relative. This relative nature of Yin-Yang includes two meanings. First, under certain conditions, Yang may change into Yin. For instance, the day (Yang) turns into night (Yin), and vice versa. Second, any phenomenon or thing can be infinitely divided into its Yin and Yang aspects thus reflecting its own inner relationship, which may be Yang within Yin or Yin within Yang. For example, day is Yang, while night is Yin. Each day and night, however, can be further classified as follows: morning is Yang within Yang, afternoon Yin within Yang, the first half of night Yin within Yin, and the second half of the night Yang within Yin. In an animal, the back belongs to Yang, but the thorax and abdomen belong to Yin. The front half of back is Yang within Yang while the second half is Yin within Yang. The thorax is Yang within Yin while the abdomen is Yin within Yin. The front limb is Yang while the rear limb belongs to Yin. The body surface (the Exterior) belongs to Yang, but the internal organs (the Interior) are Yin.

Yin-Yang theory maintains that everything is essentially composed of two opposing, yet complementary pairs of opposites. Yin-Yang theory can extend to TCVM physiology, pathology, pharmaceutics, diagnosis and treatment with acupuncture or herbs.

Table 1.1: Comparison of Yin and Yang

Parameter	Yang	Yin
Time of Day	Day	Night
Heavenly Body	Sun	Moon
Light	Brightness	Dimness
Position	Movement / Activity	Stillness / Rest
Temperature	Heat	Cold
Season	Summer	Winter
Color	Red (Light)	Blue (Dark)
Weight	Light	Heavy
Catalyst	Fire	Water
Speed	Fast	Slow
Elements	O, K, P	Na, Ca
Building	Outside / Roof	Inside / Bottom
Vibration	Short wave	Long Wave
Gender	Male	Female
Biological	Vegetable	Animal
Food	Salad	Cereals
Nerve	Sympathetic	Parasympathetic
Birth/death	Birth	Death
Physical Condition	Health	Illness
Attitude	Active / Positive / Excited	Gentle / Negative / Depressed
Tendency	Expansion	Contraction
Direction	Ascend / Forward / Outward	Descent / Backward / Inward
Structure	Time	Space
Fitness	Strength	Weakness
Space	Heaven	Earth
Shape	Round	Flat
Compass Direction	East / South	West / North
Body	Back	Abdomen
Qi / Blood	Qi	Blood
Taste	Pungent / Bitter	Salty / Sweet
Organs	*Fu* Organs Large Intestine, LI Bladder, BL Gall Bladder, GB Stomach, ST Small Intestine, SI Triple Heater, TH	*Zang* Organs Lung, LU Kidney, KID Liver, LIV Spleen, SP Heart, HT Pericardium, PC

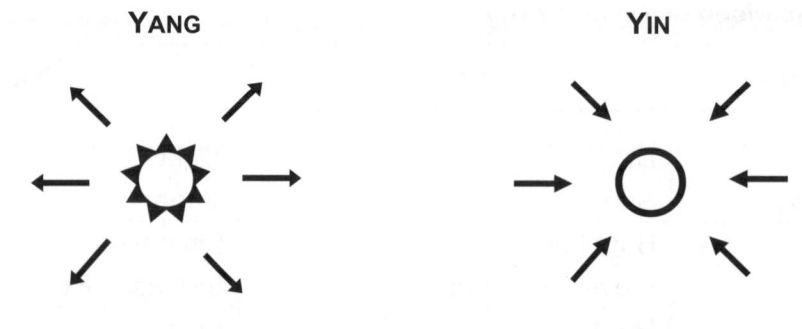

Energy goes out from a center   Energy comes into a center

Figure 1.5: The Energy relationship with Yin and Yang

In summary, anything that relates to activity, brightness or function and whose direction goes or tends to go upwards and outwards belongs to Yang. On the other hand, anything that relates to inactivity, darkness or structure and whose direction goes or tends to go downwards and inwards belongs to Yin.

Five Principles of Yin-Yang

1. Everything in the universe has two opposite aspects: Yin and Yang

Male •——• Female
Warm •——• Cold
Morning •——• Afternoon
Left •——• Right

2. Any Yin-Yang division can be further divided into Yin and Yang aspects.

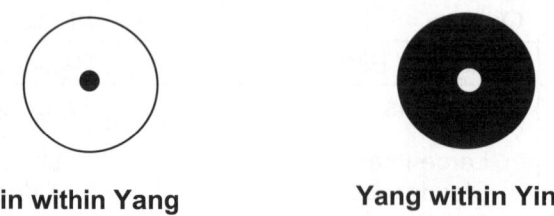

Yin within Yang   **Yang within Yin**

Day (Yang):   Morning (Yang)   → Yang within Yang
                     Afternoon (Yin)   → Yin within Yang

Night (Yin):   1st half of night   → Yin within Yin
                     2nd half of the night → Yang within Yin

Back (Yang):   Upper back   → Yang within Yang
                     Lower back   → Yin within Yang

Abdomen (Yin): Upper abdomen → Yin within yang
                     Lower abdomen → Yin within Yin

3. Yin and Yang control each other

Everything in the universe has two opposite aspects, Yin and Yang, which struggle with and control each other. For example, Heat (Yang) and Cold (Yin) are two opposite aspects. Heat may dispel Cold, but Cold may lower a high temperature (Heat). Thus, the Yin or Yang aspect within any phenomenon will restrict the other through opposition. Under normal conditions in the animal body, a relative physiological balance is maintained through the mutual opposition of Yin and Yang.

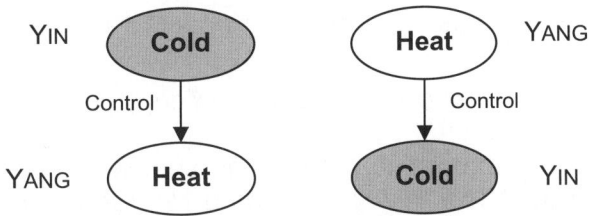

However, the opposition of Yin and Yang is relative, not absolute. Nothing is totally Yin or completely Yang. Everything contains the seed of its opposite aspect. Because everything that is associated with Yin or Yang is relative to something else, the opposition of Yin-Yang must be relative as well. Therefore, strictly speaking, it is wrong to say that something is always Yang or always Yin. For instance, activity pertains to Yang insofar as stillness pertains to Yin.

4. Yin and Yang mutually create each other

Although Yin and Yang oppose each other, they are also interdependent. The existence of one of the two opposites, Yin or Yang, depends upon the existence of the other. Neither of them can exist in isolation. There is no Yang without Yin, and there is no Yin without Yang. There is no meaning of Heat (Yang) without Cold (Yin). There is no meaning of upward movement (Yang) without downward movement (Yin). The existence of either Yin or Yang is mandatory for the other's existence.

Neither of Yin and Yang can exist without the other. Moreover, they support each other. For instance, nutrient substances of the animal body correspond to Yin while the functional activities correspond to Yang. Therefore, the production of Yin needs the activities of Yang and vice versa.

Yin and Yang co-exist in a constant and dynamic state in which one rises while the other declines. Yin and Yang are not fixed. Instead, they exist in a state of continuous mutual consumption and support. For example, the production of various functional activities (Yang) of the animal body will necessarily consume a certain amount of nutrient substances (Yin). This process is called "consumption of Yin leads to gaining of Yang". On the other hand, the production of various nutrient substances (Yin) will necessarily consume a certain amount of energy (Yang). This process is called the "consumption of Yang leads to the gaining of Yin".

The mutual creation of Yin and Yang is also called "the Ebb-Rise relation". Under normal conditions, the Ebb-Rise relation of Yin and Yang is in a state of relative balance. This balance is maintained by continuous adjustment of the relative Yin and Yang levels. However, if this relationship goes beyond normal physiological limits, the relative balance of Yin and Yang will not be maintained. This results in a Deficiency or Excess of either Yin or Yang as well as the development of disease.

"Consumption of Yin leads to growth of Yang"

Consumption of nutrients (Yin)

⇩

Functional activities (Yang)

In this case, nutrients or Yin is used to provide the supplies needed for the activities or Yang Functions of the body. The Yin is consumed to produce Yang. For example, an animal's body uses the stored glycogen to provide energy for running.

"Consumption of Yang leads to growth of Yin"

Consumption of energy (Yang)

⇩

Nutrient substances (Yin)

In this case, energy or Yang is expended to form nutrients or Yin. The Yang is consumed to produce Yin. For example, it requires energy for the body to create and store the glycogen.

Because Yin and Yang are related in this manner, deficiency or excess of one can lead to an imbalance in the other.

Yang Deficiency ⇨ Yin Deficiency

Yin Deficiency ⇨ Yang Deficiency

5. Yin and Yang may transform into each other in certain circumstances

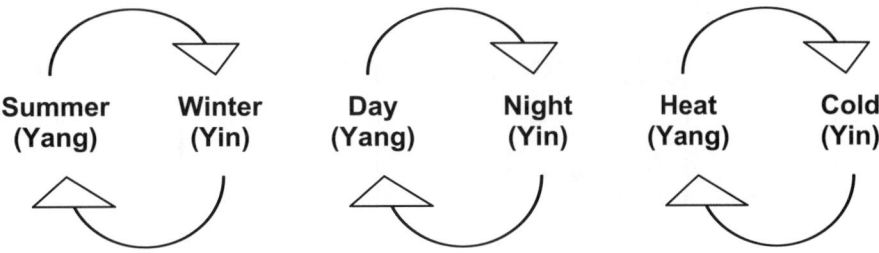

Yin and Yang transform into each other as the seasons, with their temperature changes, flow into one another. Each transition from day to night is a transformation from Yang to Yin and back again.

Yin and Yang are not static. Under certain circumstances, they may mutually transform into each other. Yin may change into Yang and vice versa. This change does not happen at random; instead, it occurs only at a certain stage of development. Summer changes into winter, day changes into night, heat changes into cold. If the Ebb-Rise of Yin and Yang is a process of quantitative change; then, inter-transformation is a process of qualitative change.

For example, a patient with an acute febrile disease has a high fever, a rapid respiratory rate, a red tongue and a fast pulse, which is considered Yang (Excess Heat). Long-term Excess Heat tends to consume body fluids and damage Qi, leading to Cold signs (Yin). After a persistent high fever, severe Cold symptoms may appear. This is a process of Yang transforming into Yin. If proper emergency treatment is given in time, the Yang Qi will be resuscitated and the Cold symptoms may disappear. This process is the transformation of Yang from Yin.

Clinical Application of the Yin-Yang Theory

PHYSIOLOGICAL ASPECTS

Within the theory of Yin-Yang, the various physiological functional activities of the animal body belong to Yang, while the various nutrient substances correspond to Yin. The functional activities depend on the support of the nutrient substances, and these activities act concurrently as the motive force for the production of nutrient substances. In this circumstance, Yin and Yang within the animal body are mutually supportive. They perform together protecting the body from invasion by pathogenic factors including bacteria and viruses, and they maintain a relative balance within the body thus resulting in disease prevention. The goal of the TCVM practitioner, when providing animal health care, is to achieve and maintain the balanced state.

Balance of Yin and Yang (Harmony)
When there is Balance, there is Health and Homeostasis.

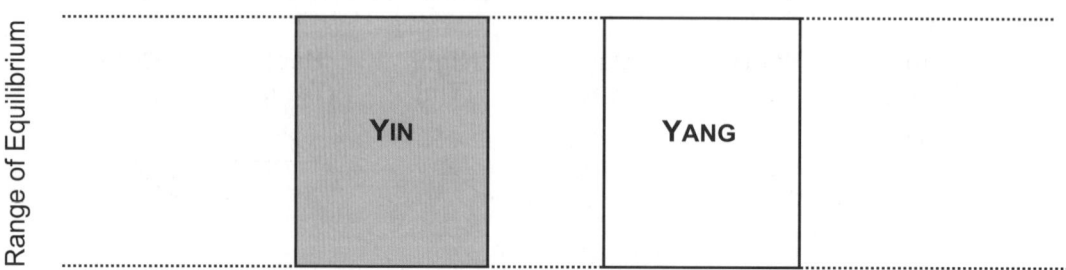

Figure 1.6: Illustration of Yin and Yang in the Normal (Balanced) state

This harmony or balanced state of an animal depends on three pairs of forces. The first is the balance between the universe and the animal itself. The second is the balance between the individual animal and the other animals in the environment, including the humans of the household. The third is the balance between the various organ systems within the animal body. For example, a castrated male Himalayan cat named "Newton" lives together with his human guardian, Mary, and three other cats in a South Florida home. Newton's health depends upon his status at the three different levels:

- How well Newton self-adjusts to the hot, humid weather or how Mary helps Newton to adjust.

- How well Newton gets along with Mary and the other three cats. Do the individuals live in peace and harmony or do they fight with each other?

- Whether or not Newton's own body systems are in balance.

Thus, it is on three levels that a body must maintain balance in order to remain healthy. There is balance between the body and the external elements or the environmental forces. There is emotional or social balance between individuals in contact with each other. There is balance within the body itself among the internal processes.

PATHOLOGICAL ASPECTS

The theory of Yin-Yang is also applied to explain pathological changes. According to Traditional Chinese Veterinary Medicine, no disease occurs if Yin and Yang maintain a relative balance. Disease occurs when there is loss of the balance between Yin and Yang, as with the excess or deficiency of either Yin or Yang due to pathogenic factors. The pathogenic factors can be also classified into two types: Yin and Yang. There are four possible states of imbalance between Yin and Yang: Excess of Yin, Excess of Yang, Weakness of Yin and Weakness of Yang.

Imbalance of Yin and Yang (Disharmony)
When there is not balance, there is illness and disease.

1. Yang Excess (Excess Heat)

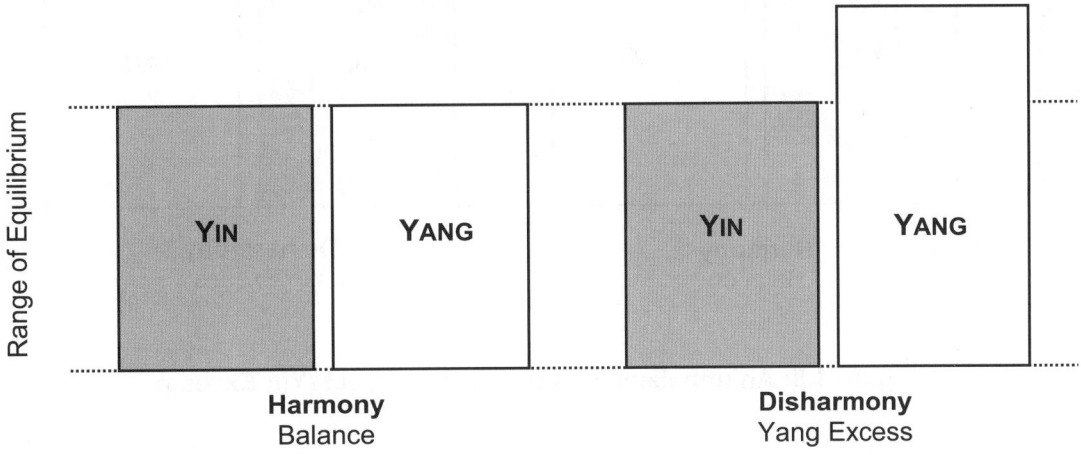

Figure 1.7: An unbalanced state—Excess Heat (Yang Excess)

In this unbalanced state, Yang is greater than normal. The cooling properties of Yin are unable to counteract the warming properties of Yang, so an Excess Heat condition appears. The treatment principle is to clear the Heat or sedate the Yang.

TCVM Diagnosis: Excess Heat or Yang Excess

Treatment Principle: Clear Heat (Sedate Yang)

Treatment: Herb: Coptis *Huang Lian*
                         Acupoint: GV-14

2. Yin Excess (Excess Cold)

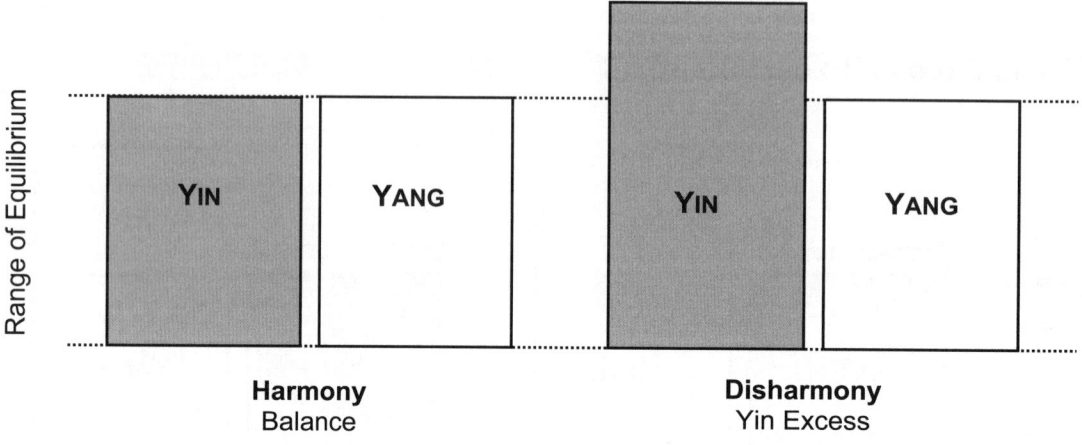

Figure 1.8: An unbalanced state—Excess Cold (Yin Excess)

In this unbalanced state, Yin is greater than normal. The cooling properties of Yin overwhelm the warming properties of Yang, so an Excess Cold condition appears. The treatment principle is to clear the Cold or sedate the Yin.

TCVM Diagnosis: Excess Cold or Yin Excess

Treatment Principle: Clear Cold (Sedate Yin)

Treatment: Herb: Cinnamon *Rou Gui*
                      Acupoint: GV-4

3. Yang Deficiency (Deficient Cold)

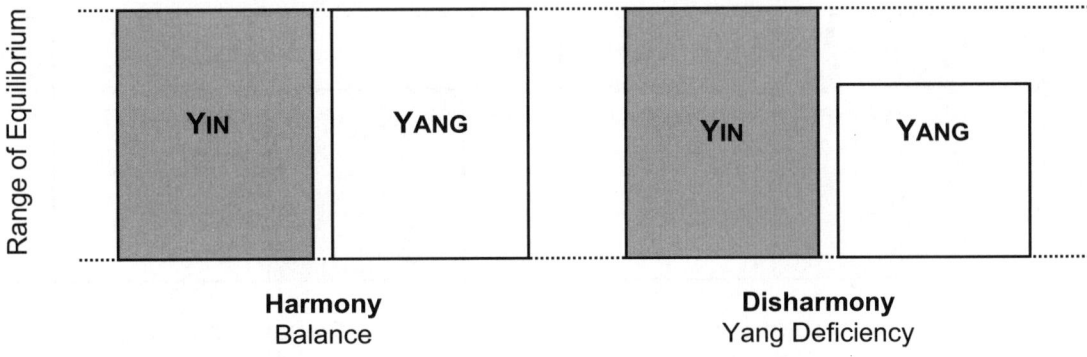

Figure 1.9: An unbalanced state—Deficient Cold (Yang Deficiency)

In this unbalanced state, Yin is at the normal level, but Yang is lower than normal. The warming properties of Yang are insufficient to equalize the cooling properties of Yin, so a cold condition appears. However, the coldness is caused by the Deficiency of Yang. In order to treat this condition, it is necessary to tonify Yang.

TCVM Diagnosis: Yang Deficiency or Deficient Cold

Treatment Principle: Tonify Yang

Treatment: Herb: Morinda *Ba Ji Tian*
                     Acupoint: Moxa at *Bai Hui*

4. Yin Deficiency (Deficient Heat)

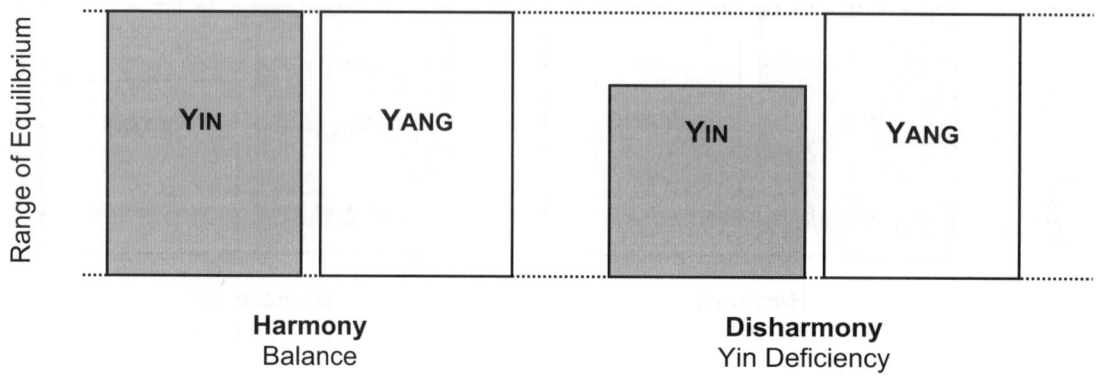

Figure 1.10: An unbalanced state—Deficient Heat (Yin Deficiency)

In this unbalanced state, Yang is at the normal level, but Yin is lower than normal. The cooling properties of Yin are insufficient to equalize the warming properties of Yang, so a Heat condition appears. The Heat is caused by the weakness of Yin. Because Yin is deficient, it is necessary to focus on the nourishment of Yin.

TCVM Diagnosis:	Yin Deficiency or Deficient Heat
Treatment Principle:	Nourish Yin
Treatment:	Herb: Rehmannia *Shu Di Huang* Acupoint: KID-3

HERBOLOGICAL ASPECTS

The theory of Yin-Yang can be applied to the properties and tastes of herbs. If the herb has traits of warmth and Heat, it is associated with Yang. The Yang herbs are designed to treat coldness (Yin diseases). For example, dry Ginger *Gan Jiang* is hot and is considered a Yang herbal medicine. It is commonly used for coldness of the stomach (abdominal pain, vomiting, and abdominal discomfort).

Cooling herbs, however, are associated with Yin. The Yin herbal medicines are used for the treatment of Heat (Yang diseases). For example, Coptis *Huang Lian* is very cold and is considered a Yin herbal medicine. It is commonly used for Large Intestine Heat conditions (bloody diarrhea or inflammatory bowel disease).

Type of Herb	Nature / Property	Indication
Yang Herb	Hot / Warm	Yin Excess, Cold
Yin Herb	Cold / Cool	Yang Excess, Heat

YIN-YANG AS A GUIDE TO CLINICAL DIAGNOSIS AND TREATMENT

Imbalance between Yin and Yang is the root cause for disease occurrence and development. If the Pattern of Yin and the Pattern of Yang are grasped, the correct diagnosis can be made regardless of how complicated or changeable the clinical signs of an animal disease may appear. Yin-Yang is the basis for the Pattern Identification according to the Eight Principles (Yin, Yang, Interior, Exterior, Cold, Heat, Deficiency and Excess). For this diagnostic system, Yin is associated with Interior, Cold and Deficiency Patterns, and Yang is associated with Exterior, Heat and Excess Patterns.

Because a disease occurs due to excessive or inadequate amounts of Yin or Yang, the basic treatment principles are to dispel the Excess and to tonify the Deficiency. In this way, one adjusts the Yin-Yang and allows Yin and Yang to maintain balance once again. For instance, herbs with Cold properties should be used for an Excessive Heat Pattern. Herbs that enhance Yin should be used for a Deficient Yin Pattern.

Table 1.2: Clinical Signs and Treatment of Yin and Yang Patterns

	Patterns	Signs	Treatment
Yang	Excess Heat (Yang Excess)	• Acute onset • Short course • Young age • No general weakness • Hyperactive • High fever • Red or purple tongue • Strong, fast pulse	Clear Heat Sedate Yang GV-14, LI-4, LI-11 Coptis *Huang Lian*
	Deficiency Heat (Yin Deficiency)	• Chronic onset • Long course • Older animal • General weakness • Thirsty • Lower degree of fever • Restless or anxiety • Prefers cool • Red and dry tongue • Thready and fast pulse	Nourish Yin Clear Heat KID-3 Rehmannia *Shu Di Huang*
Yin	Excess Cold (Yin Excess)	• Acute onset • Short course • Young age • No general weakness • Pain • Swelling or edema • Loose stool • Pale or purple tongue • Strong and slow pulse	Clear Cold Moxa at GV-4 Dry Ginger *Gan Jiang*
	Deficiency Cold (Yang Deficient)	• Chronic onset • Long course • Older animal • Coldness at extremities • Edema, Loose stool, • Urinary incontinence • Chronic back pain/weakness • Weakness of the rear limbs • Infertility • Pale tongue • Weak and deep pulse	Warm and tonify Yang Moxa at *Bai Hui* Morinda *Ba Ji Tian*

YIN-YANG AS A GUIDE TO PREVENTION

The best medical care for animals is disease prevention. In TCVM, disease is prevented by maintaining the Yin-Yang balance or by making adjustments to the body based upon the animal's constitution. In general, the active, outgoing, younger animals are Yang. Yang animals tend to have Yang disease including Excess Heat (Yang Excess) or False Heat (Yin Deficiency). In order to keep the Yin-Yang balance for Yang animals, provide a cool environment during Yang weather (summer) and give foods that are cooler in nature, such as fish or bananas.

The quiet, shy and elder animals are Yin. These Yin animals tend to have Yin disease including Excess Cold (Yin Excess) or False Cold (Yang Deficiency). Providing a warmer environment in Yin weather (winter) and feeding warm foods such as chicken, ginger, and garlic can help keep the Yin animal in balance.

	IDENTIFICATION	Yang Animals	Yin Animals
Individual Traits	Activity Level:	Hyperactive	Quiet
	Personality:	Outgoing	Shy
	Preferred Climate:	Cool	Heat
	Age:	Younger	Older

	MODIFICATION	Yang Animals	Yin Animals
Environment	Climate adjustment:	Cooling place Shade Air Conditioning Northern climate Fans and misting	Warming place Sunbathing Heaters Southern climate Blankets
Small Animal Diet	Dietary adjustment:	Cooler diets Fish Turkey Banana Tofu Brown rice Wheat Duck Egg Celery Kelp Spinach Broccoli	Warmer diets Mutton Deer Meat Chicken White rice Oats Citrus Ginger Garlic Pepper Chicken Liver Squash Pumpkin
Equine Diet	Dietary adjustment:	Cooler diets Buckwheat Barley Wheat Bran	Warmer diets Oats Ginger Garlic Onion

Case Examples

Case 1.1

Signalment: A six year old Thoroughbred gelding

Primary Complaint: Photic headshaking unresponsive to conventional therapy

History and Exam:

He is a show hunter for an amateur rider and is a nice, graceful horse. He is fairly sturdy in body type for a thoroughbred. He is active and friendly; he likes attention and loves treats.

The problem is triggered by sunlight. He is fine while in a barn, but he headshakes severely when outdoors in the daylight. At these times, he displays the typical photic type of head flip. When he is turned out at night, he acts normally. No physical problems were noted (including eye problems) other than the photic headshaking. There appears to be little paraesthesia associated with this problem. According to the owner, he will sometimes rub the end of his nose on things when he is in the sunlight. The non-pigmented snip end of his nose will get a little pink (vasodilatation).

His tongue appears red, and the pulse is forceful. His coat is glossy, and his appetite is good. All else is within normal limits.

Case 1.1 Assessment:

This is a "Yang" horse because he is active, likes attention, and looks strong. It is a Yang disease or Excess Heat Condition because the major clinical signs (headshaking triggered by sunlight, forceful pulse and red tongue) are characteristics of Yang.

The treatment strategy is to balance Yin and Yang by clearing the Excess Yang (Excess Heat). The acupuncture points LI-4 and GV-14 (to clear general Heat) and the Chinese herb Coptis *Huang Lian* (to clear Excess Heat) can be used.

Case 1.2

Signalment: A seventeen year old, white Andalusian gelding

Primary Complaint: Cough and Phlegm when beginning work

History and Exam:

He is a tall, quiet and independent horse. He prefers to stay alone and likes warm weather. He caught several respiratory infections with a high fever and cough over the past three years. Now, he has recovered from the infection, but he has an occasional cough and gags up phlegm when he starts work. He continues to have this problem with mucus in his throat. He coughs when he starts to work then seems better. Overall, he does not like work (exercise intolerance).

His tongue is pale, very moist with white foam. He has a white, thin nasal discharge. His pulses are deficient.

Case 1.2 Assessment:

This is a Yin disease*, specifically a Yang Deficiency Pattern, as evidenced by the chronic cough (three year duration), wet tongue, weak pulse, exercise intolerance, and old age (17 years). The treatment strategy is to balance Yin and Yang by enhancing Yang. The acupuncture points GV-4 and CV-17 and herbal medicine *Bu Fei San* (Lung Tonic Powder) are recommended for this case.

* There are two types of Yin diseases: 1) Yin Excess (Excess Cold) and 2) Deficiency Cold (caused by Yang Deficiency).

Case 1.3

Signalment: A seven year old, female spayed Labrador Retriever

Primary Complaint: Separation anxiety

History and Physical Findings:

From a Western perspective, the dog has all the signs of separation anxiety. Acupuncture treatment did not help much. She has also been on the herbal formula *Long Dan Xie Gan Wan* for signs of Liver Stagnation.

Her tongue is slightly red and dry and her gums are tacky. Her eyes are red. Her pulses are thready and fast.

Case 1.3 Assessment:

This is a Yin Deficiency Pattern (Deficient Heat), specifically a Heart Yin Deficiency pattern. The Yin Deficiency can be determined from the red, dry tongue (Heat signs) and the thready and fast pulse. The association with the Heart is based on the major complaint of separation anxiety because this is due to a Shen (Spirit or Mind) disturbance. Of the five Yin organs, the Heart is the one that houses the Shen. Separation anxiety and other behavior problems are mostly related to the Heart. The treatment strategy is to balance Yin and Yang by enhancing Yin. The acupuncture points *An Shen*, HT-7, *Da Feng Men*, and KID-3 as well as the herbal formula Shen Calmer (Modified *Tian Wan Bu Xin Dan*) are recommended for this case.

Case 1.4

Signalment: A thirteen year old female spayed American Eskimo dog

Problem List:

1. Cushing's disease which has been treated with Mitotane for the past four years

2. Seizures which began last month and clustered about once a week.

3. Hypothyroidism

4. Generalized stiffness with weak hind end. There is no limping, but the dog's gait is very stiff. The dog takes three to four steps then huffs and puffs and lies down.

5. Generalized lethargy, weakness, lack of energy.

Physical Findings:

- Pulse is thin and fast
- Ravenous appetite and thirst
- Bilateral cataracts
- Deafness
- Panting constantly
- Poor teeth and gums

- Rose colored thin ocular discharge
- Stool dark brown and foul smelling
- Chronic urinary incontinence, all day, all the time
- Draining pressure sore on left hip
- Pot-bellied with muscle wasting
- Tongue is pink with thin coating

Case 1.4 Assessment:

This can be considered a Deficient Heat (Yin Deficiency) condition with a Qi Deficiency and Internal Wind. The old age, weakness, urinary incontinence and lethargy indicate Qi Deficiency. The fast pulse, thirst, ravenous appetite, constant panting and foul smelling stool can indicate Heat. Seizures are caused by Internal Wind.

The treatment strategy is to use acupuncture to balance Yin and Yang by enhancing Yin and clearing the Wind. In addition, acupuncture can be used for the stiffness while using Chinese Herbal medicine for the internal organ problems. Acupuncture points such as GB-20, LIV-3 and GV-20 may be beneficial for the seizures (Wind). The points KID-3 and SP-6 may be beneficial for Yin. Two herbal formulas may be beneficial: *Tian Ma Gou Teng Yin* for Internal Wind and *Suo Quan Wan* for incontinence and Kidney Qi Deficiency.

Case 1.5

Signalment: An eight year old, male Labrador Retriever dog

Primary Complaint: Crying at night

History and Physical Findings:

This dog has a history of severe hip dysplasia and arthritis; however, the owner does not notice any lameness or stiffness. The owner's main concern is the dog's tendency to cry during the night. This has been occurring for two years and typically happens at 1:00 to 3:00 in the morning. The dog will go back to sleep if the owner gets up and sits with him.

The dog's tongue is purple-pink with very fine central cracks. The pulses are stronger on left than right, and they are thready or wiry. The dog is sensitive at BL-18 to BL-21.

Case 1.5 Assessment:

The TCVM pattern is Heart/Liver Yin Deficiency with Kidney Yang Deficiency. Because the crying occurs at night, this is associated with Yin. The crying itself indicates a disturbance of the dog's Shen (consciousness or Mind) which often relates to the Heart. The time (1 am to 3 am) and the sensitivity at BL-18 and BL-19 are associated with the Liver. The very fine centrally located cracks on the tongue indicate a Yin Deficiency as well. The weaker pulse on the right side and the purple tongue indicate a Yang Deficiency. Because the Kidney is associated with bone, the hip dysplasia in this dog indicates a Kidney problem.

Initially, the treatment should focus on the Heart and Liver Yin Deficiency as the major complaints are crying at night. The usual treatment strategy is to treat the major complaint(s) first and then treat other underlying deficiencies. The treatment period for Heart Yin Deficiency may last one to four months. The acupuncture points HT-7, PC-6, BL-15, BL-18, BL-23, KID-3, and *An Shen* may be beneficial. In addition, *Yi Guan Jian* and Shen Calmer (Modified *Tian Wan Bu Xin Dan*) are two recommended herbal medicines which nourish Yin and calm the Mind.

Subsequent treatment should focus on the Kidney Yang Deficiency. This treatment may require two to five months. Depending upon the character and appearance of the pulse and tongue, Loranthus Powder (to tonify Yang) and *Sang Zhi San* (to resolve Bi syndrome including hip dysplasia and arthritis) are the herbal medications that may be used. Loranthus Powder is the modified *Ba Ji San*. The acupuncture points GV-3, GV-4 and *Bai Hui* may be used as well.

Case 1.6

Signalment: An eight year old, neutered male Bichon Frise

Primary Complaint: Acute cardiovascular collapse

History and Physical Findings:

The dog presented with acute cardiovascular collapse following a dog attack by two Jack Russell Terriers. The patient suffered multiple deep and superficial bite wounds on the face, neck and caudal extremities. There were many wounds on the inner and outer thighs of both hind legs as well as some bruises on the caudal abdomen. There were no penetrating wounds to the abdomen.

The patient was hypothermic with a temperature of 99.4 °F. Initially, he was stabilized with oxygen and intravenous fluids. In addition, he received Solu-Delta-Cortef®, Baytril®, and Penicillin. His wounds were flushed with copious amounts of saline solution, and he was given Torbugesic® for pain management. He improved slowly with treatment, but temperature regulation was still a problem. He continued to remain hypothermic.

Bloodwork revealed azotemia, low glucose, elevated alanine aminotransferase (ALT) levels and an elevated packed cell volume. Radiographs showed no chest involvement; however, soft tissue trauma of the neck muscles was evident. In addition, a large, radioopaque bladder stone was observed.

Case 1.6 Assessment:

Yang is warm. When Yang is deficient in the body, it almost always results in signs of coldness or hypothermia. The two most important organs to keep the body warm are Kidney and Heart. Thus, the TCVM pattern of this case is a Heart and Kidney Yang Deficiency. Traditional Chinese Veterinary Medicine can be used in combination with the conventional Western treatments to assist the patient's recovery. The herbal medication *Si Ni Tang* may be beneficial; however, it should not be used for longer than two weeks. Also, the acupoints *Bai Hui*, GV-4, and *Shen Shu* may be used to tonify Yang. Moxibustion techniques can help provide some extra warming effect as well.

Case 1.7

Signalment: A thirteen year old female cat

Primary Complaint: Constipation

History and Physical Findings:

This cat frequently experiences severe constipation. She occasionally becomes extremely painful, and she requires emergency care to manually evacuate the feces. Her medications include daily Cisapride and every other day Laxatone®. Her feces are very dry and without mucus. She has some halitosis. Her thirst, urination, and temperature preferences do not differ from that of the other household cats. Her tongue is red and dry, and her pulse is fast and thready.

Case 1.7 Assessment:

The major function of Large Intestine (LI) is to excrete feces. Difficulty in defecation can be due to either a Yin Deficiency (fails to moisten the LI and leads to constipation) or a Qi Deficiency (LI Qi is too weak to excrete feces). Very dry feces, a dry, red tongue and a fast, thready pulse indicate Yin Deficiency. Painful defecation, constipation and halitosis indicate Qi Stagnation. The TCVM pattern is Large Intestine Yin Deficiency and Qi Stagnation.

In her case, several recommendations may be helpful. Her diet should be high in fiber. The herbal medication *Ma Zi Ren Wan* may be given for one to three months to moisten the Large Intestine and to move the Stagnation. The suggested acupuncture points include ST-37, ST-25, GV-1, and BL-21. In addition, the owner can massage the acupoints CV-12 and CV-8 for ten minutes twice daily.

Self Test

Of the following pairs, choose which one belongs to Yang.

Question 1.1: Fire (a) or Water (b)
Question 1.2: 10 a.m. (a) or 10 p.m. (b)
Question 1.3: Mare (a) or Stallion (b)
Question 1.4: Winter (a) or Summer (b)
Question 1.5: East (a) or West (b)

Of the following pairs, choose which one belongs to Yin.

Question 1.6: Function (a) or Structure (b)
Question 1.7: Fast (a) or Slow (b)
Question 1.8: Head (a) or Tail (b)
Question 1.9: Interior (a) or Exterior (b)
Question 1.10: Left eye (a) or Right eye (b)

Question 1.11: If the Yin-Yang equilibrium is destroyed by Excess Heat, what is the proper treatment principle to restore the Yin-Yang balance?

a. Clear Excess Heat
b. Tonify Excess Heat
c. Tonify Yang
d. Clear Excess Yin

Question 1.12: If Yin is deficient, what is the treatment principle?

a. Clear Excess Yin
b. Clear Excess Heat
c. Tonify Yang
d. Tonify Yin

Question 1.13: Jumper, a 10-month old castrated male cat, is an outdoor-indoor cat. He enjoys running, climbing trees, and jumping from high places. He is also a good hunter, catching small creatures such as dragonflies and lizards. He likes attention, and he always walks with his human guardian. His whole body feels hot. He drinks a lot, but he does not have any endocrine disorders. What type of animal is Jumper?

a. Yin
b. Yang

Question 1.14: What is the best type of food for Jumper?

a. Yang
b. Yin

CHAPTER TWO

FIVE ELEMENT THEORY

When the minds of the people are closed and wisdom is locked out they remain tied to disease. Yet their feelings and desires should be investigated and made known, their wishes and ideas should be followed; and then it becomes apparent that those who have attained spirit and energy are flourishing and prosperous, while those perish who lose their spirit and energy.

– Huang Ti, *Nei Ching Su Wen*

The Five Elements, also known as *Wu Xing*, the five activities, or the five principles in action, refer to the five categories in the natural world: Metal, Water, Wood, Fire and Earth. These are the indispensable and fundamental elements that constitute the universe. Enhancing, inhibiting and restraining relationships exist between them. Also, these elements are in constant motion and change. In Traditional Chinese Veterinary Medicine, the properties and the mutual relationships of the Five Elements are used to explore and illustrate the basis of medical problems.

The Five Element theory was first formed in China around the time of the Yin and Zhou Dynasties (16th century B.C. to 221 B.C.). Later, it was adopted into medical practice, thus becoming a founding theory of Traditional Chinese Veterinary Medicine. The Five Element principles can describe the nature of the Zang-Fu organs, the inter-relationships between the organs and the relationship between the animal body and the natural world. Thus, the theory of Five Elements, together with the theory of Yin-Yang, serves to guide clinical diagnosis and treatment.

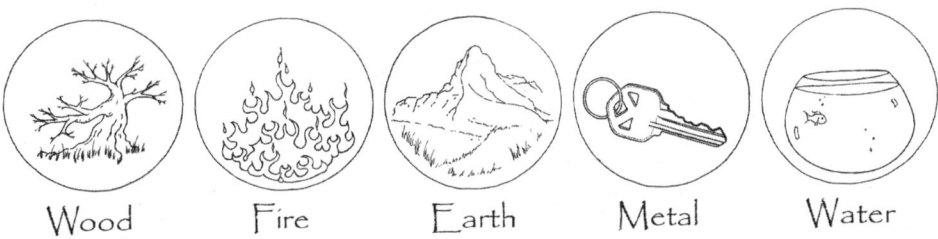

Wood   Fire   Earth   Metal   Water

Table 2.1: Comparison of the Five Element characteristics

	Wood	**Fire**	**Earth**	**Metal**	**Water**
Season	Spring	Summer	Late Summer	Fall	Winter
Climate	Wind	Heat	Damp	Dryness	Cold
Direction	East	South	Center	West	North
Color	Green	Red	Yellow	White	Gray / Black
Flavor	Sour	Bitter	Sweet	Pungent	Salty
Sound	Shouting	Laughter	Singing	Weeping	Groaning
Emotion	Anger Irritation	Joy Fright	Preoccupation Worry	Grief Sadness	Fear Terror
Growth	Germination	Growth	Transformation	Reaping	Storing
Zang Organs	Liver	Heart Pericardium	Spleen	Lung	Kidney
Fu Organs	Gall Bladder	Small Intestine Triple Heater	Stomach	Large Intestine	Bladder
Orifice	Eyes	Tongue	Mouth	Nose	Ears
Sense	Vision	Speech	Taste	Smell	Hearing
Tissue	Tendons Ligaments	Vascular system	Muscles	Skin Hair Coat	Bones
Functions	Purification	Circulation	Digestion	Respiration	Elimination
Exterior	Nails	Complexion	Lips	Skin Pores	Head Hair
Secretion	Tears	Sweat	Saliva	Nasal Fluid	Urine
Body Action	Spasms Tantrums	Mania Depression	Spitting Vomiting	Coughing Wheezing	Trembling Shivering
Body Odor	Rancid	Scorched	Fragrant	Rotten	Putrid
Weakness	Looking	Walking	Sitting	Lying	Standing
Tongue Part	Sides	Tip	Center	Mid-tip	Rear

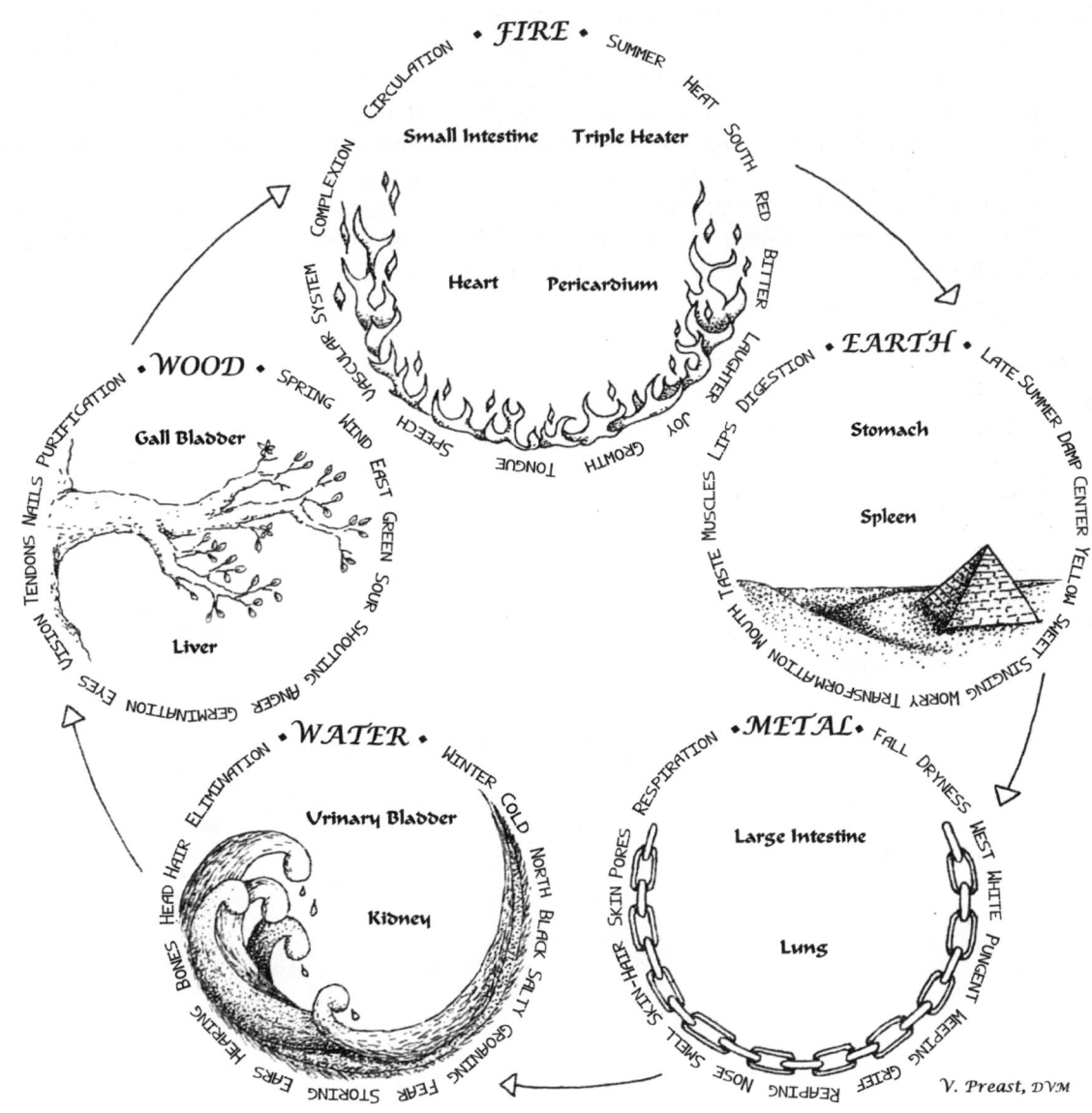

Figure 2.1: The characteristics of the Five Elements

Two Physiological Cycles of the Five Elements

Each of the five internal organs and sense organs pertains to one of the Five Elements. The Five Elements' properties serve as an analogy to explain some of the physiological functions of the five Zang or five Fu organs.

There are two physiological cycles of the Five Element Theory: the inter-promoting and the inter-inhibiting relationships. These explain the interconnections among the five Zang organs or the five Fu organs as well as the connections between Zang and Fu. As discussed in Chapter 4, the Zang-Fu is the collective term for internal organs, which include five major Yin organs (Heart, Lung, Spleen Liver, Kidney) and five major Yang organs (Small Intestines, Triple Heater, Large Intestine, Gallbladder, Bladder). For instance, the Kidney promotes the Liver, which in turn promotes the Heart; therefore, the Liver is the mother of the Heart and the child of the Kidney. On the other hand, each of the five Zang organs or the five Fu organs inhibits another thus maintaining a relative balance among the organs. For instance, the Liver inhibits the Spleen, and the Spleen promotes the Lung, which then inhibits the Liver. The Heart Fire promotes the Spleen, while the Kidney Water inhibits the Heart Fire. The inter-promoting and inter-inhibiting relationships among the five Zang organs are shown in Figure 2.2.

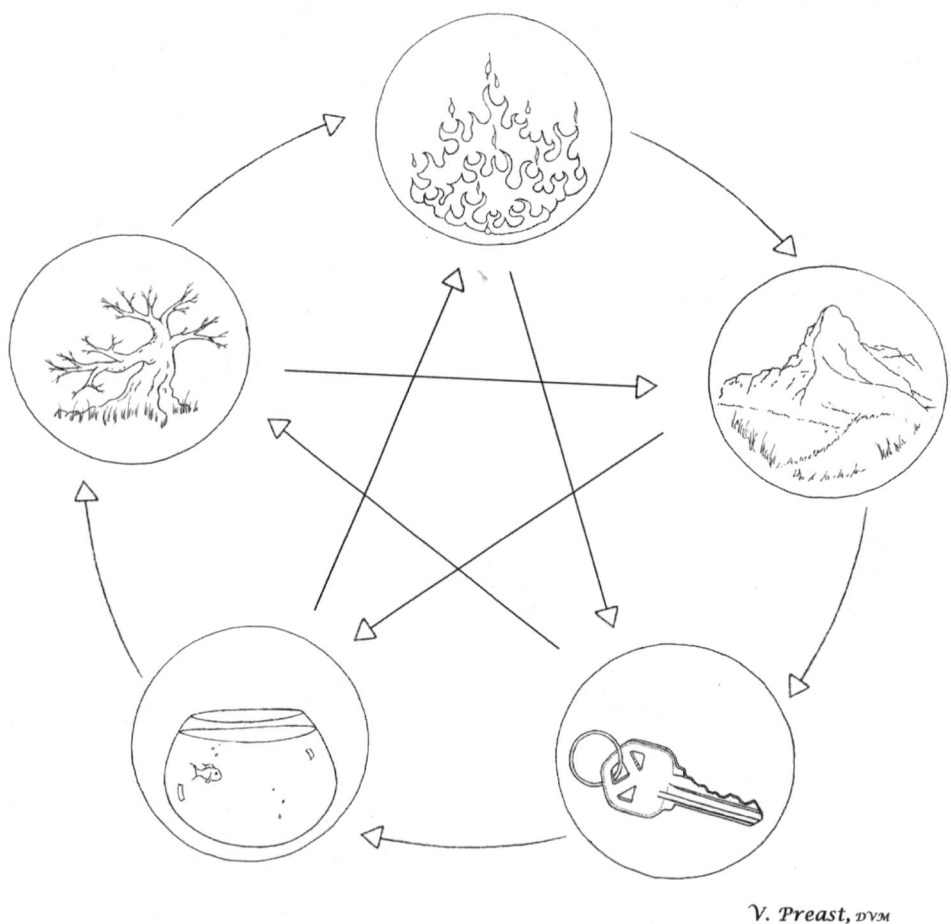

V. Preast, DVM

Figure 2.2: The interactions of the Five Elements

The outer circle of arrows represents the inter-promoting relationship in which each element supports the next. The crossing arrows in the center represent the inter-inhibiting relationship in which each element can restrain another.

THE INTER-PROMOTING CYCLE: *SHENG* CYCLE

Wood ⇨ Fire ⇨ Earth ⇨ Metal ⇨ Water ⇨ Wood

This sequence of elements illustrates how each Element promotes, nurtures, or generates another. For any element, the previous element in the series is the "mother" of the element. Similarly, any element next in the series is the "child" or "son" of the previous element.

Wood promotes Fire:	Wood is the mother of Fire Fire is the child of Wood
Fire promotes Earth:	Fire is the mother of Earth Earth is the child of Fire
Earth promotes Metal:	Earth is the mother of Metal Metal is the child of Earth
Metal promotes Water:	Metal is the mother of Water Water is the child of Metal
Water promotes Wood:	Water is the mother of Wood Wood is the child of Water

THE INTER-RESTRAINING CYCLE: *KE* CYCLE

Wood → Earth → Water → Fire → Metal → Wood

This sequence of elements illustrates how each Element restrains and controls another. For any element, the previous element in this "*Ke* Cycle" series is the "grandparent" of that element. Similarly, any element next in this "*Ke* Cycle" series is the "grandchild" of the previous element. It is the job of the grandparent to control the grandchild. In this way the elements keep each other in check and maintain the balance.

THE *SHENG* AND *KE* CYCLES KEEPING THE BODY IN BALANCE

Together, these cycles form a feedback system that helps to keep everything functioning at the proper level. When one element acts upon another, whether to replenish or to drain the next, the connection between the elements will eventually cause a reaction upon the original element. This prevents one element from acting too severely upon another and causing an imbalance within the system.

Wood restrains Earth (Ke cycle), but at the same time the Earth promotes the Metal which then restrains the Wood. In this instance, the Metal makes sure that the Wood does not restrain the Earth too excessively.

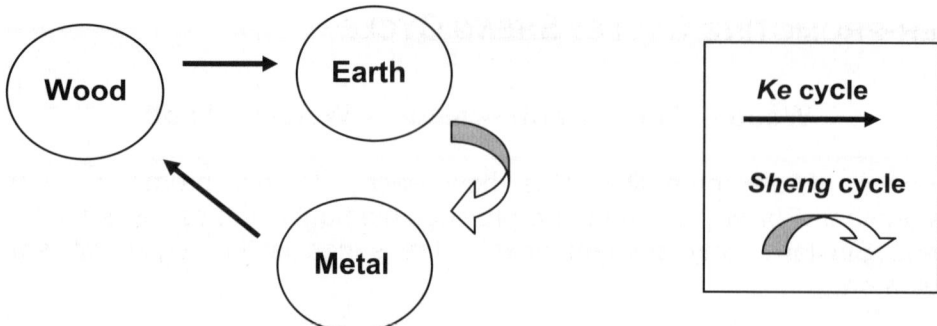

Metal restrains Wood (Ke cycle) to prevent an Excess of Wood, but Wood promotes the Fire which then restrains the Metal. Thus, the Fire restrains the Metal to make sure that it does not restrain the Wood too much.

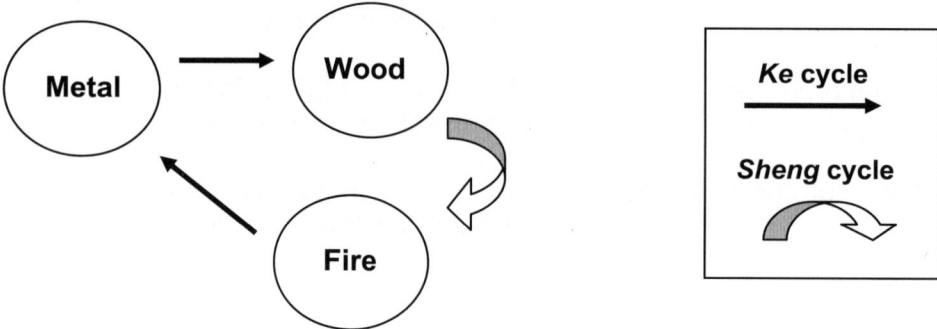

Fire restrains Metal (Ke cycle), but Metal promotes the Water which simultaneously restrains the Fire. In this way, the Fire is unable to restrain Metal too excessively.

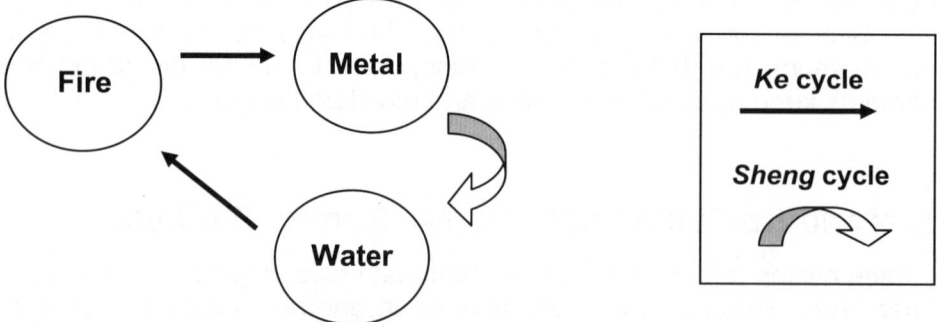

Water restrains Fire (Ke cycle), but Fire promotes the Earth which simultaneously restrains the Water. The Earth prevents the Water from restraining the Fire too much.

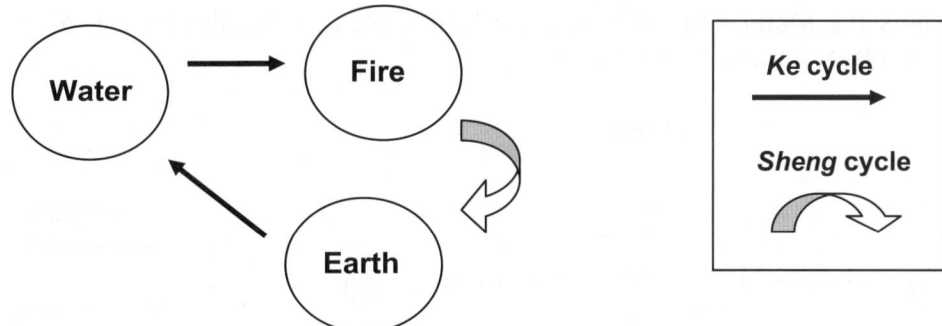

Earth restrains Water (Ke cycle), but Water promotes the Wood which simultaneously restrains the Earth. The Wood prevents excessive restraint of the Water by the Earth.

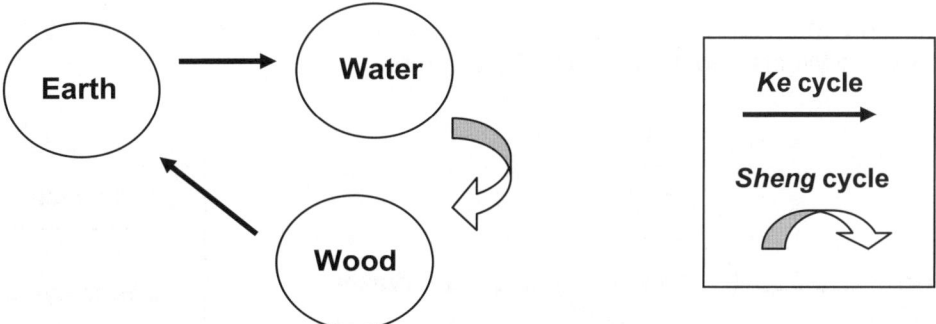

THE SHENG AND KE CYCLES FORMING A NETWORK WITHIN THE BODY

The Sheng and Ke Cycles ensure that each element is connected with the other four elements. Consequently, a network is established within the universe and the body. No element is immune to the forces from the other elements.

For example, Wood restrains (Ke Cycle) the Earth and promotes (Sheng cycle) the Fire. At the same time, the Wood is restrained by the Metal and is promoted by the Water.

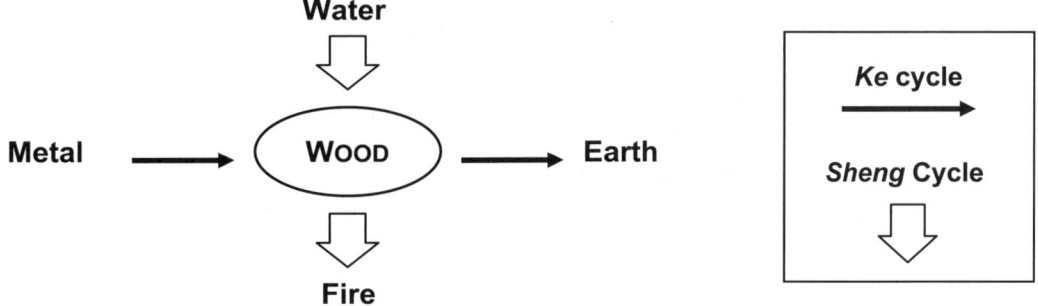

Fire Restrains the Metal and promotes the Earth. Meanwhile, the Fire is restrained by the Water and is promoted by the Wood.

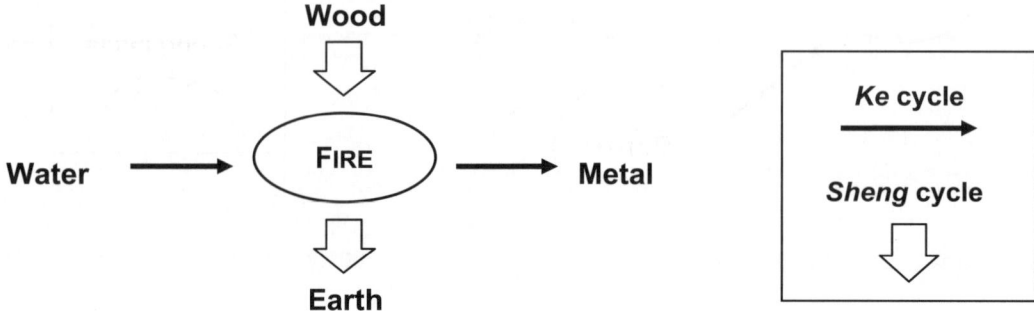

Earth Restrains the Water and promotes the Metal. At the same time, the Earth is restrained by the Wood and is promoted by the Fire.

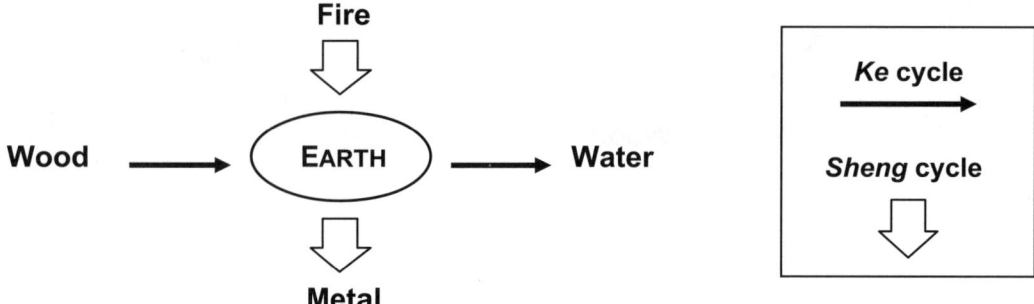

Metal Restrains the Wood and promotes the Water. At the same time, the Metal is restrained by the Fire and is promoted by the Earth.

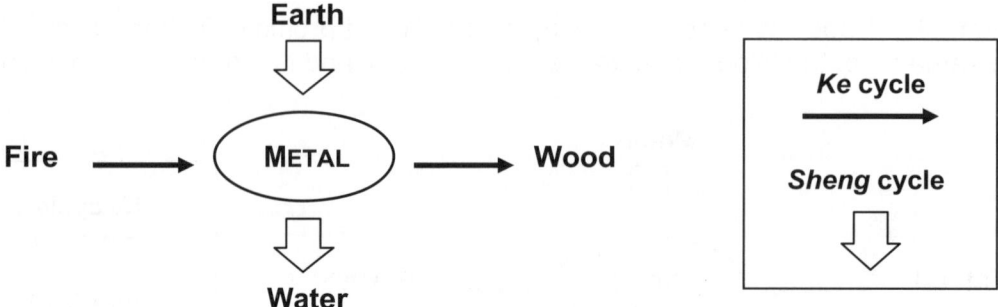

Water Restrains the Fire and promotes the Wood. At the same time, the Water is restrained by the Earth and is promoted by the Metal.

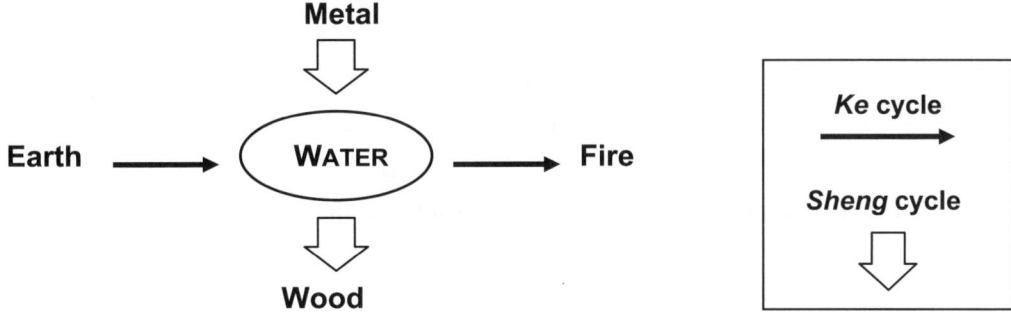

Four Pathological Cycles of the Five Elements

A disease occurs as a pathological manifestation of a Zang-Fu organ and related tissue dysfunction. This may be due to a number of factors. The animal body is an organic whole; there are inter-promoting and inter-inhibiting relationships among the Zang-Fu organs. Disease occurs when the Five Element inter-promoting and inter-inhibiting relationships go out of control thus becoming excessive or deficient. There are four basic pathological cycles: Mother Element to Child Element, Child Element to Mother Element; Overwhelming Cycle and Insulting Cycle.

THE MOTHER ELEMENT (ORGAN) AFFECTS THE SON ELEMENT (ORGAN)

In this case, an imbalance follows along the same route of the promoting cycle; however, the mother element transmits problems to her child instead of nourishment. For instance, a Liver problem will transmit to the Heart. When Liver Blood is deficient, the Liver fails to nourish the Heart. This affects the Heart Blood thus resulting in a Deficiency of Heart Blood. Similarly, Spleen problems can transmit to the Lung. If the Spleen's function of transformation and transportation is impaired, pathogenic phlegm will be formed and will remain in the Lung thus causing a Lung problem.

Example 1:   Liver problems transmitted to the Heart (Wood → Fire)

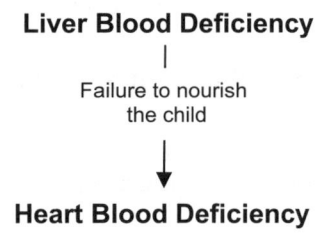

Example 2:   Spleen problems transmitted to the Lung (Earth → Metal)

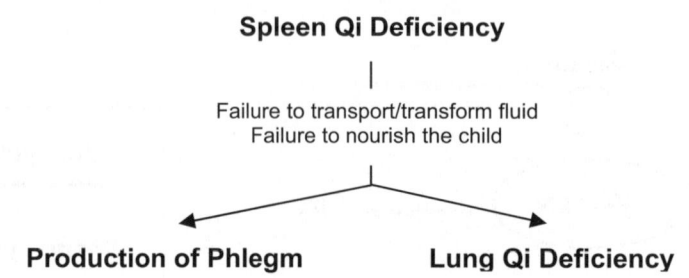

THE SON ELEMENT AFFECTS THE MOTHER ELEMENT

In this case, an imbalance follows along a reverse path of the Sheng cycle; problems with the child are transferred to the parent. For example, a Spleen problem will transmit to the Heart. The Spleen is the original supplier of Qi and Blood, which are important for the Heart. When the Spleen does not make enough Blood, a Deficiency of Heart Blood may occur.

Example: Spleen problems transmitted to the Heart (Earth → Fire)

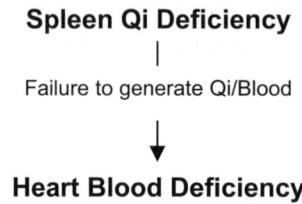

THE OVERWHELMING CYCLE: CHENG CYCLE

Wood → Earth → Water → Fire → Metal → Wood

In this case, an imbalance follows along the same route of the Ke cycle; each element excessively restrains another beyond the normal extent. This usually occurs when an element is in Excess. This is the most common pathological condition seen in practice.

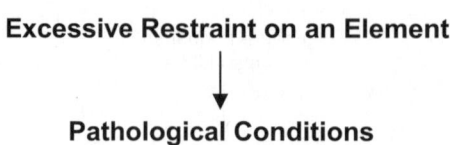

Example 1: Excessive Wood

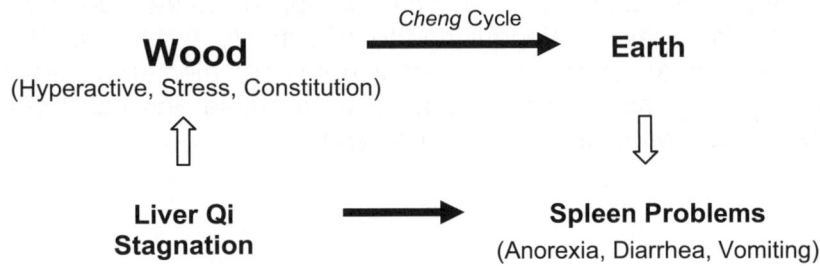

Example 2: Excessive Fire

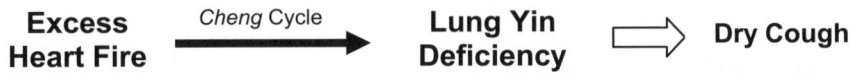

THE INSULTING CYCLE: RU CYCLE

Wood ≻ Metal ≻ Fire ≻ Water ≻ Earth ≻ Wood

In this case, an imbalance follows along the opposite route of the Ke cycle; each element can insult the one that normally restrains it. This reversal of the Ke cycle usually occurs when the balance is broken, especially when one Element is insufficient.

Example 1: Excessive Metal (Lung) or Deficient Fire (Heart)

Lung Problem   *Ru* (Insulting Cycle)   **Impaired Heart Qi**
(Cough, Phlegm)   ──────────────────────▶   **Circulation**

Example 2: Excessive Wood (Liver) or Deficient Metal (Lung)

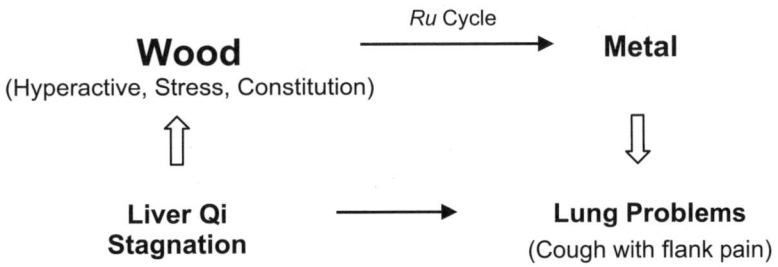

The Five Constitutional Types of Animals

The principles of the Five Element Theory can be applied to the personal characteristics of individuals. This is a way of categorizing the personality and disease tendencies of an animal. By comparing an animal to its most dominant elemental personality type, a TCVM practitioner can understand the patient as a whole and can better address the imbalances associated with that constitutional type.

WOOD TYPE

Personal Characteristics:

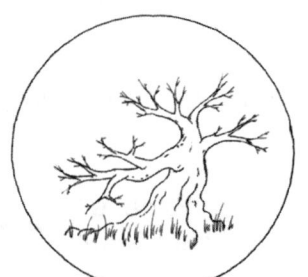

- Dominant behavior or attitude
- Quick, fast movements
- Enjoys or skilled with running or moving
- Impatient
- Easily becomes angry or loses temper
- Alert and responds quickly to stimuli
- Good at adapting to changing conditions
- Good diplomat (human)
- Quickly forms ideas, but then changes his/her mind
- Narrow-minded and intolerant to different ideas

Physical Characteristics:

- Thin body, either tall or short
- Big eyes
- Pulse: Wiry (String-taut)
- Performance: Good, but variable. Sometime good; sometimes bad
- Hooves and tendons are strong and healthy
- Runs like the wind. Quick and nimble movement
- Good type for the racetrack

Disease Predispositions:

- Hypertension
- Stroke
- Allergy
- Depression (Liver Stagnation)
- Hysteria
- Neurosis

Life Span:

Short (a little bit longer than the Fire type)

TCVM Health Suggestion

In TCVM, the Liver (Wood organ) is considered as "Yang function" and "Yin body". Yang function means that the Liver acts upward and outward and has little tolerance for depression. Even a small amount of stress, depression or Stagnation will devastate or strain the Liver function. Thus, foods that have harmonizing or regulating properties are very important to Liver function. Yin body refers to the Liver Yin and the Liver Blood, which are the major sources of nourishment for the tendons, hooves and eyes. The herbal medicine *Xiao Yao San* is recommended to maintain a balanced Liver. The recommended foods include chicken liver or pork liver, green vegetables (mustard greens, spinach, cabbage), carrots, and citrus fruits.

FIRE TYPE

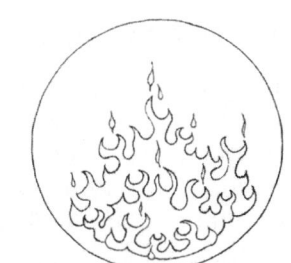

Personal Characteristics:

- Easily excited
- Extroverted
- Love to be loved
- Tends to be the center of party
- Loves and is skilled at fostering a social life
- Difficult to calm down
- Sharp mental activities
- Inventor. Suddenly conceives good ideas
- Persuasive. Skilled at inspiring others
- Proficient in competition or fighting
- Aggressively peruses ambitions
- Arrogant attitude
- Exaggerates. (Making a mountain out of a molehill; blowing things out of proportion)

Physical Characteristics:

- Strong body
- Small head
- Small, but bright, shining eyes
- Red face (human)
- Prominent blood vessels
- Pulse: Fast or Full
- Runs very fast, but easily fatigued
- Good for short-distance racing

Disease Predispositions:

- Cardiovascular Disease
- Chest pain
- Arteriosclerosis
- Stroke
- Separation anxiety
- Restlessness
- Sudden Death

Life Span:

Very short

TCVM Health Suggestion:

The Heart belongs to Fire. Yang is often excessive, and Yin is often deficient; the fire (Heat) easily becomes excessive and damages Yin. A Heart Yin tonic is very important to maintain the functions of the Heart energy system. The herbal formula Shen Calmer (Modified *Tian Wan Bu Xin Dan*) is recommended to help balance the Heart. Diet recommendations include foods such as pork heart, fish, brown rice, wheat and vegetables such as spinach, broccoli, celery and mushrooms.

EARTH TYPE

Personal Characteristics:

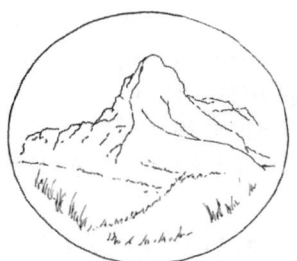

- Honest and kind
- Takes care of others (A good type for a mare)
- Generous and modest
- Laid back
- Humble
- Speaks and walks neither fast nor slow
- Easily satisfied
- Holds oneself aloof from the world
- Slow response to a stimulus
- Good worker, but a little slow

Physical Characteristics:

- Short but sturdy body
- Prominent musculature
- Big head
- Brown hair-coat on the head (Yellow face in humans)
- Thick lips and big nose
- Pulse: Slow

Disease Predispositions:

- Chronic gastrointestinal problems. Diarrhea. Colic.
- Edema
- Obesity

Life Span:

Long

TCVM Health Suggestion:

The Spleen belongs to the Earth. The Spleen is the dominant organ system for Earth type animals. Like the Earth's characteristics, the Spleen consistently works very hard. There are no complaints until a big problem develops. The Spleen deserves special attention and careful medication because the Spleen, as the source of energy, muscular strength, and defending force, is important to the whole body.

The major natural challenge to the Spleen is "Damp". Damp may originate from food, drink, weather changes and the environment. In addition, the collection of damaged cells/tissues or abnormal (mutated) cells within the body is considered Damp or Yin production. The Spleen Qi and Wei Qi are associated with the body's ability to identify abnormal tissue. If the function of the Spleen diminishes, the Damp will not be identified. Damp is thick, sticky and difficult to move. If it is allowed to remain in place for long periods of time, cancerous growths may develop.

According to TCVM herbal theory, plants with "dryness" properties, such as Atractylodes *Cang Zhu*, will support the Spleen because that herb can dry up the "Damp". In addition, the Spleen (Earth) requires Fire because Fire is the mother of Earth. Therefore, all herbs supporting the Spleen should also have the property of "Fire"; they should be warm or hot herbs. This is probably why those who live in humid areas (Damp) prefer hot, spicy foods (Fire).

It is also important to understand that the Spleen is located in the middle-jiao (Middle-Burner) where it dominates the Qi flow (Qi-Ji). The two major directions of Qi flow are upward and downward. All the beneficial substances, nutrients and energy, should be transported upward to the Lung, then to the whole body. All the useless materials (metabolic by-products) and the harmful substances (toxins) should go downward to large intestines for excretion from the body. Thus, a good herbal prescription for Spleen should contain ingredients that maintain this up-down relationship of Qi flow. The Herbal formula *Ping Wei San* may be used. The recommended foods include rumen, lamb, chicken, ginger, garlic, and sweet potato.

METAL TYPE

Personal Characteristics:

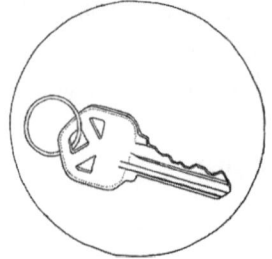

- Foresight and sagacity (good vision)
- Broad-minded
- Good organizer
- A leader in a group
- Always follow the rules
- Righteous
- Holds oneself aloof
- Confident and consistent
- Haughty or vain

Physical Characteristics:

- Broad forehead
- Big and wide nose
- Broad chest
- Good hair coat

Disease Predispositions:

- Respiratory problems. Cough. Asthma. Nasal congestion
- Diabetes
- Constipation

Life-span:

Long

TCVM Health Suggestion:

In TCVM, the Lung (Metal organ) functions primarily to control breathing and to regulate the respiratory system. The Lung is a delicate organ. Dryness and Heat can easily damage the Lung Yin, which holds and supports the Lung Qi. Lung Yin damage (Lung Yin Deficiency) causes malfunction of respiratory activities (Lung Qi) and results in asthma or cough.

The Lung is located at the top of the Three-Burner (Sanjiao, Triple Heaters). It distributes Ying-Qi (nutrients) down to the entire body. This inspiratory direction (descending) of the Lung Qi flow should be downward as well. The expiratory direction (ascending) of the Lung Qi should be upwards. This is the reason why the Lung dominates the ascending and descending Qi flow. In the case of dyspnea or asthma, it is caused by damage of the Lung Qi's descending or ascending direction. The TCVM treatment strategy for the Lung is as follows: 1) use a Yin tonic herb to moisten and nourish the Lung Yin, 2) restore the downward direction of the Lung's Qi flow. The herbal medicine *Bai He Gu Jin Tang* may be used. The recommended foods include eggs, duck, barley, tofu and rice.

WATER TYPE

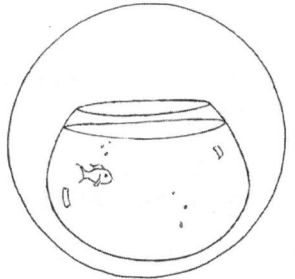

Personal Characteristics:

- Introverted
- Terrified or fearful about everything
- Quiet, but a good observer
- Skilled at planning and scheming
- Good advisor or supervisor
- Prefers deep thought
- Willing to live alone
- Very consistent, but slow when doing something
- Sinister or insidious if evil
- Fear biter

Physical Characteristics:

- Thin, middle sized body
- Black hair on the head
- Deep, big eyes and big ears
- Cold intolerance. Prefers to stay in a warm area
- Pulse: Deep
- Not a favorable type for a stallion

Disease Predispositions:

- Edema
- Infertility
- Back pain
- Urinary infections
- Diarrhea at dawn
- Depression

Life Span:

Very long

TCVM Health Suggestion:

The Kidney (Water organ) dominates reproduction and supplies vital force (Ming-Men Fire, or Kidney Yang). Coldness is the natural enemy of the Kidney. Herbs with warm or hot properties, which eliminate coldness, can help the Kidney.

The Kidney stores the Essence (Jing), which influences the animal's growth, development and reproduction. Therapy for the Kidney should maintain the balance between Kidney Yang (Ming-Men Fire) and Kidney Jing. The herbal formula Epimedium Powder (*Sheng Jing San*) is recommended. The food recommendation includes pork kidney, eggs, duck, mussels, sweet potato, and black beans.

The Five Elements in Diagnosis

The Five Element Theory may be used with the Four Diagnostic Techniques to examine the clinical findings and to elucidate the Patterns of disease according to the nature of the Five Elements.

COLOR OF THE MOUTH OR TONGUE

One of the most important diagnostic parameters is the color of an animal's tongue or mouth. There are five abnormal colors that may indicate an imbalance in the associated Element and its organs.

- A purple, blue, or lavender indicates an imbalance in Wood, which may be due to Stagnation of Liver-Qi.

- A red color indicates an imbalance in Fire, which may be due to an Excess of Heart-Fire.

- A yellow color may indicate an imbalance in Earth, which may be due to a Deficiency of Spleen-Qi.

- A white color may indicate an imbalance in Metal, which may be due to a Deficiency of Lung-Qi.

- A dark color may indicate an imbalance in Water, which may be due to a Deficiency of Kidney Yin.

However, the above diagnostic method is just one possible indication. Because a disease is complex, every symptom should be systematically analyzed before determining the diagnosis.

TISSUES

Pathological changes of the tissues can be used as a diagnostic tool. These changes may indicate an imbalance of a certain organ according to the Five Element associations.

Tendon, ligament disorders may indicate a Liver Yin Deficiency. A problem with blood vessels may indicate a Heart disharmony. Muscle atrophy may indicate a Spleen Qi Deficiency. Dry hair and skin may indicate a Lung Yin Deficiency. Degenerative bone diseases may indicate a Kidney Qi or Kidney Yin Deficiency.

SENSE ORGANS

A problem with one of the five sense organs may reflect an imbalance of the associated internal organ. For example, red and painful eyes often reflect a Liver problem. A tongue problem may indicate a Heart imbalance. A mouth and lip problem may be related to the Spleen. If the nose is troubled by heat, dryness or sneezing, there may be a Lung problem. Deafness may be related to a Deficiency of the Kidney.

Three Treatment Strategies of the Five Element Theory

TONIFY (*BU*) THE MOTHER FOR DEFICIENCY

If an organ is deficient, its mother organ should be tonified. In a case with a Deficiency of Lung Qi, the treatment should involve tonification of Spleen Qi. Because the mother element nourishes the child element, stimulation of the mother will provide more support for a weak child.

CLEAR (*XIE*) THE SON FOR EXCESS

This method is called *Xie* in Chinese. *Xie* can be also translated as clear, reduce or sedate. If an organ is in Excess, the child organ should be sedated. In a case with a Liver Fire Flaring-Up Pattern, the treatment principle may be to reduce the Heart and to eliminate the Fire. By stimulating the child organ, the child organ can draw some of the Excess away from the parent.

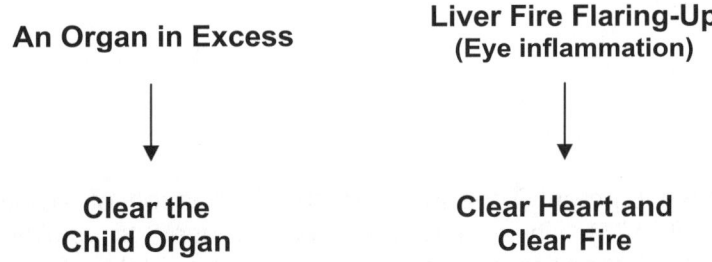

An Organ in Excess

Liver Fire Flaring-Up
(Eye inflammation)

Clear the
Child Organ

Clear Heart and
Clear Fire

STRENGTHEN THE "GRANDCHILD" ELEMENT FOR PREVENTION

It is a common clinical practice to determine the principle of treatment according to the pathological influence among the Zang-Fu organs in the Five Element cycle. When there is disharmony between the Liver and Spleen, the principle of treatment should include methods that promote the Spleen and clear the Liver because Stagnation of Liver Qi over-acts on the Spleen.

If one organ is in Excess, it is beneficial to strengthen its "grandchild" organ (the element that directly follows the child element). An excessive element can over-act (*Cheng*) upon its grandchild organ, thus strengthening the grandchild organ in the Cheng cycle will provide a protective function for that organ.

- If the Liver has problems, strengthen the Spleen for prevention.
- If the Spleen has problems, strengthen the Kidney.
- If there are Heart problems, strengthen the Lung.
- If the Lung has problems, strengthen the Liver.
- If there are Kidney problems, strengthen the Heart.

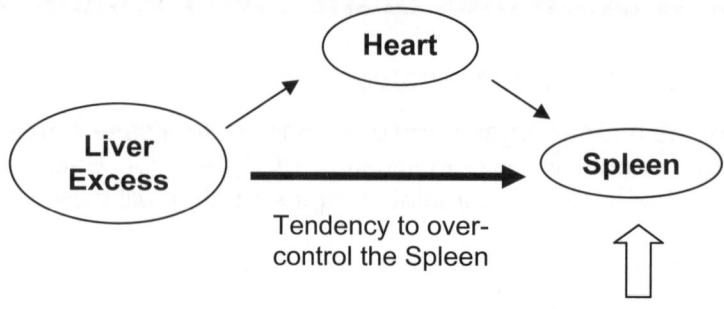

When Liver is Excessive, it tends to over-control (*Cheng*) Spleen. For prevention, Spleen should be reinforced before the signs of Spleen Deficiency occur.

Conclusions

The Yin-Yang and Five Element Theories form the foundation of Traditional Chinese Veterinary Medicine (TCVM). These two theories are used to explain physiological activities and pathological changes and to provide a basic guideline for clinical practice. They are interdependent and cannot be entirely separated during clinical evaluation. For a horse with high fever, the Yin-Yang Theory should be used to determine if it is an Excess Pattern (Yang) or Deficient Pattern (Yin), and the Five Element Theory should be used to determine which organs are affected. Both theories, however, are limited by the historical development of ancient Chinese society. They may be incomplete and need to be complemented with modern, advanced scientific research and clinical experience.

Summary of Normal Five Element Physiology

Inter-Promoting Relationship
Sheng Cycle

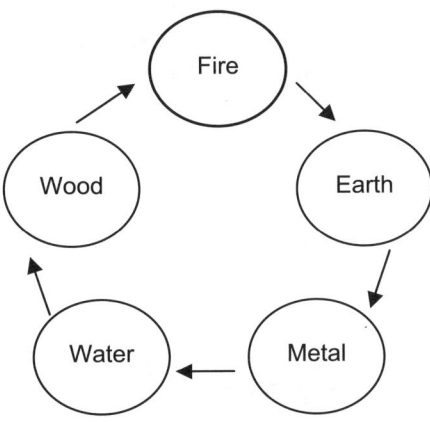

This cycle is the normal generative cycle found in the five-element system. It is a "parent-child" relationship in which one element nourishes the following element. Fire promotes Earth, which promotes Metal, which promotes Water, which promotes Wood, which promotes Fire. In other words, Fire is the "mother" of Earth but is also the "son" of Wood. In this way, each element serves as both a parent and a child to the surrounding elements in the cycle.

It is possible to imagine this sequence in nature with one element promoting and flowing into the next. The river Water nourishes a young seedling, which becomes a great Wood tree. A forest Fire burns the tree and the ash nourishes the Earth's soil. This Earth is mined for Metal ore. Metal tools are used to discover and collect Water; and the Water flows into the river that nourishes the tree.

Inter-Inhibiting Relationship
Ke Cycle

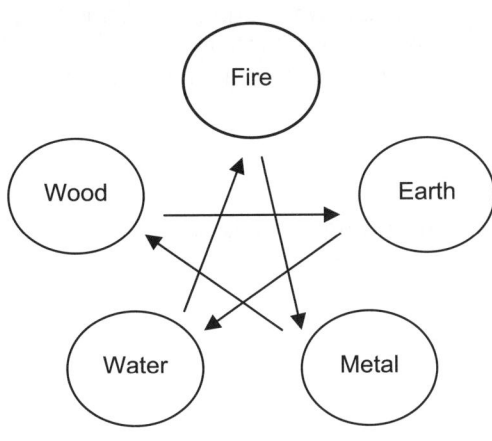

This cycle is the normal control cycle found in the five-element system. It is a restraining relationship between the elements. The elements involved can be called the "grandparent" and the "grandchild". The "grandparent" is the element that is one ahead of the "parent" element, and it is involved in controlling the activity of the "grandchild" element. Water inhibits Fire; Fire inhibits Metal; Metal inhibits Wood; Wood inhibits Earth; and Earth inhibits Water.

Once again an analogy can be used to illustrate the restraining effects that each element can have on another. Fire melts Metal ore and allows it to be shaped. A Metal saw is used to harvest trees for Wood. The Wood is used to mold the Earth into a dam. The dam restrains the flow of Water in a reservoir. The Water collected is used to extinguish the Fire.

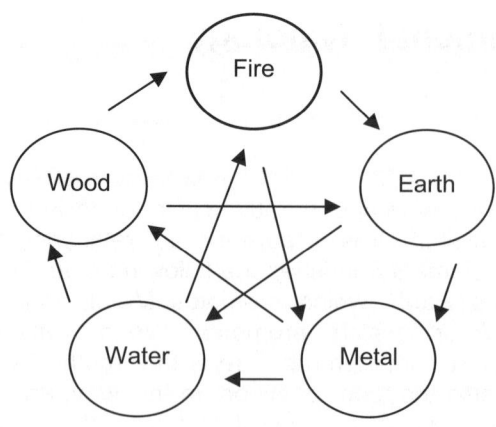

Normal Five Element Interactions

Together these two cycles create balance among the elements. When the elements are cooperating normally through this system of inhibition and promotion, there should be no Excess or Deficiency. When there is Excess or Deficiency of any of the elements, there is an abnormality within one or both of the cycles. In a normal situation, the cycle would work to feed back upon the original element and maintain it at its balanced state. For example, Water inhibits Fire, but then Fire promotes Earth, which inhibits Water.

Summary of Abnormal Five Element Physiology

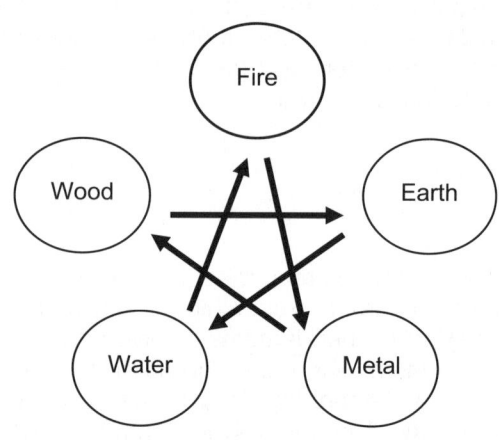

Over-Acting Relationship
Cheng Cycle

This cycle occurs as a pathologic form of the *Ke* cycle when the balance of the normal *Ke* cycle is broken due to an excess of one element. The "grandparent" element goes beyond the normal amount of control of the "grandchild" element so that it results in disease. This can be seen when one element is in excess and exerts too much restraint upon another element. For example, the Over-Acting Relationship would be occurring if Wood was so excessive that Metal cannot inhibit it. In this case Wood excessively inhibits Earth and causes a pathologic condition.

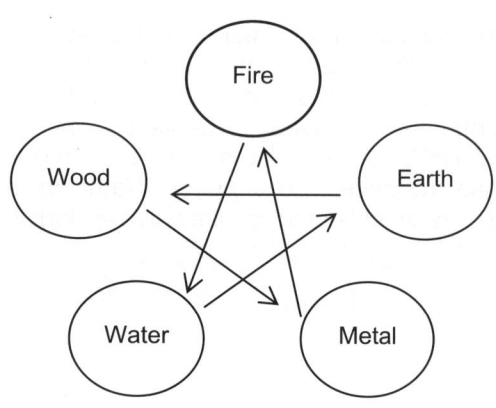

Inter-Insulting Relationship
Ru Cycle

This cycle occurs as a pathologic form of the Ke cycle when the balance of the normal Ke cycle is broken due to an insufficiency of one element. In this case, the Ke cycle is reversed. The "grandparent" element is weak, thus unable to exert a normal amount of control over the "grandchild" element. The flow of control is reversed and "grandchild" element restrains the "grandparent" element. For example, the Insulting Relationship can occur if Metal was weak or if there was an excess of Wood. In this case, the Wood will exert restraint upon Metal.

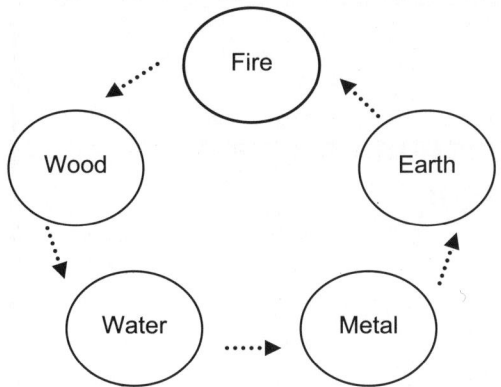

Son Element affects the Mother Element

This cycle occurs as a pathologic form of the *Sheng* cycle. In this case, the *Sheng* cycle is reversed. If the Child Element has a problem, it can transfer problems to the Mother Element. For example, if the Spleen is deficient, it may lead to a deficiency of the Heart.

One way of thinking about this is to imagine a sick child. The mother spends all her time and energy helping her sick child until she becomes ill herself.

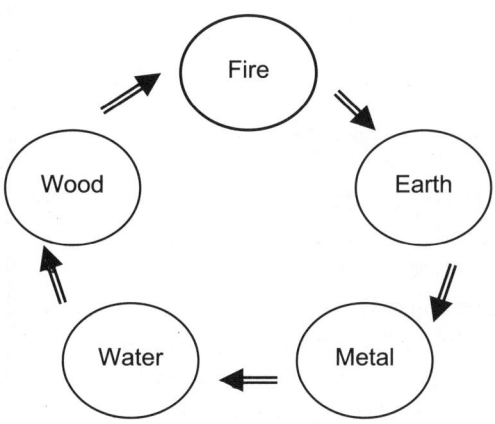

Mother Element affects the Son Element

This cycle occurs as a pathologic form of the *Sheng* cycle. In this case there is an imbalance in which the elements pass problems from Mother to Child. The mother element, which is ailing, is unable to maintain the proper balance within the cycle. Instead of supporting and nourishing the following element, the mother transmits problems to the child. For example a deficiency of Liver may eventually lead to a deficiency of the Heart, because the Liver is unable to properly nourish the Heart.

One could imagine an overworked, stressed parent who does not feel good. This parent comes home and does not want to interact with the child. This causes the child to become upset.

Example of Excessive Wood: **Example of Deficient Wood:**

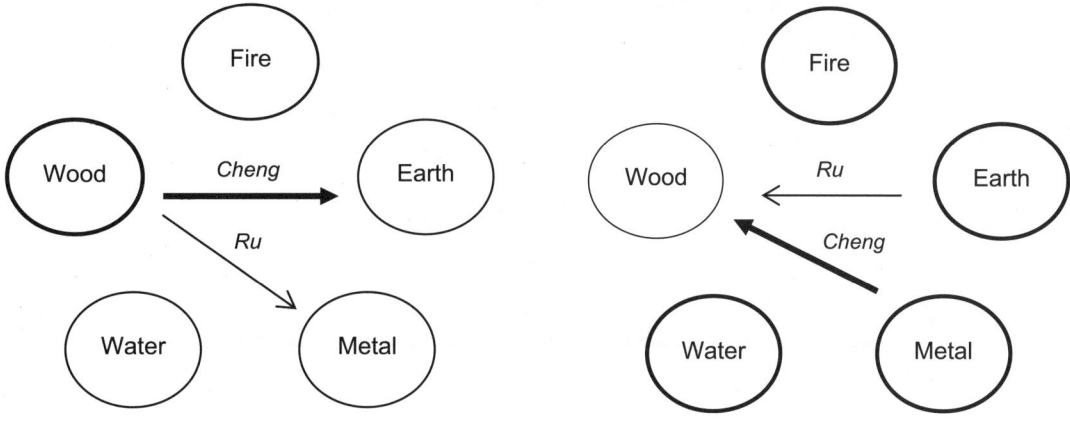

Identifying Small Animal Constitution Types in the Exam Room

Wood

- Confident
- Irritable, "Crabby"
- Active, Energetic, Athletic
- Aggressive, Angry
- Bites with little provocation
- Impatient

Fire

- Friendly
- Greets strangers warmly
- Noisy, Barking
- Excited, Hyper-excitable
- Difficult to keep still

Earth

- Friendly
- Enjoys sleeping or relaxing
- Eager to please
- Slow walker
- "Laid back"

Metal

- Clean hair coat
- Quiet
- Confident
- Disciplined
- Follows the owner's commands
- Organized, Knows what to do next or knows what to expect

Water

- Hiding behind owner or under the exam table
- Fear biter
- Not confident
- Watches what the veterinarian is doing
- Urine leakage
- Owner calls to cancel appointment because the cat is hiding under the bed.

Identifying Constitution Types
of Horses in the Barn

Wood

- Confident
- Irritable, "Crabby"
- Active, Energetic, Athletic
- Ears back
- Aggressive, Angry
- Kicks, Stomps, or Strikes
- Impatient
- Bites

Fire

- Friendly
- Noisy, Vociferous
- Loves to be touched or petted
- Excited, Hyper-excitable
- Difficult to keep still
- Very Sensitive

Earth

- Friendly
- Enjoys relaxing
- Easy going, mellow
- Eager to please
- Moves slow or walks

Metal

- Clean hair coat
- Quiet
- Organized
- Prepared for what happens next
- Confident
- Disciplined
- Follows the rules

Water

- Hides or runs away
- Kicks when afraid
- Not confident
- Watches the veterinarian
- Nervous when being examined
- May present rump and threaten to kick when examined

Case Examples

Case 2.1

Signalment: An eleven-year male, castrated Domestic Long Hair cat.

History and Physical Findings:

He is a very tolerant and friendly cat. He likes to dominate animals of equal strength, but he lets very young or very old animals dominate him. Although he likes to be petted, he hates to be groomed. He only wants attention on his own terms, when he wants it. He loves to be around people, but does not like to be the center of the party. He purrs both when happy and angry.

He prefers the support of furniture, shoes or folded rugs. He loves to sleep in the morning. He eats only when the owner eats or when the owner offers food, rarely eating when the owner is not home. When he was young, he was very fast and agile, catching birds and lizards; but, now he will not even catch a moth. He used to eat only what he caught; now he won't kill anything.

Recently he sleeps a lot and is sluggish. There is decreased muscle tone in both hind limbs. He used to breathe clearly, now his nose is congested chronically. Sometimes the nasal congestion is so bad that he has to use his mouth to breathe. His nasal discharge is clear and is worse on the right side. He coughs a lot recently, but it seems worse in the daytime.

His tongue is pale, and his pulse is deep and weak. Because of nasal discharge and congestion, he was given antibiotics and anti-histamines for the past month. The medications did not seem to help.

Case 2.1 Assessment:

This cat's tolerant, friendly attitude and his tendency to please others mark him as a typical Earth type cat. It is not uncommon for an Earth constitution cat to tend towards a deficient Spleen or Stomach. Deficient Earth might lead to deficient Metal (the Mother element affects the Child element). The chronic clear nasal discharge and congestion, the pale tongue, and the weak pulse indicate Lung Deficiency.

The treatment strategy is to tonify the Lung and Spleen. It is important to tonify the Spleen because the Spleen is the mother of the Lung. The acupuncture points LU-9 (the Earth point on the Lung Meridian) and BL-13 (the Lung association point) are recommended. Herbal formulas *Si Jun Zi Tang* (to tonify Spleen) and *Bai He Gu Jin Tang* (to tonify Lung) are recommended.

Case 2.2

Signalment: A thirteen year old Quarter Horse mare

History and Physical Findings:

She is always angry, irritable and "crabby". When the veterinarian examines her, she often has her ears pinned. The mare stomps her feet even tries to bite and kick the veterinarian.

Her tongue is red, purple and swollen. Her pulse is wiry and forceful. Her eyes are large, red, and watery.

Case 2.2 Assessment:

This is a typical Wood type mare. She has Liver Qi Stagnation and Liver Fire. The anger, irritability, aggressive behavior, purple tongue and wiry pulse are indications of Liver Qi Stagnation. A red and swollen tongue, red and swollen eyes, and a forceful pulse indicate Liver Fire. The treatment plan is to soothe the Liver Qi and clear Fire.

Treatment with the acupuncture points LIV-1, LIV-3, HT-9 and HT-8 are recommended. The herbal formula *Long Dan Xie Gan Tang* is also recommended to clear the Liver and to clear Fire.

Case 2.3

Signalment: An eight-year-old Paint gelding

History and Physical Findings:

He loves to run and to compete, but he has some anger problems. He is easily irritated and hyperactive. His tongue is purple. He is reactive on the entire Stomach Meridian of his neck, BL-20 (Spleen associate point), BL-21 (Stomach associate point), and *Dan Tian* (the stifle point). He is also very reactive at PC-1. His pulses are fast and wiry. His eyes are red. He had several episodes of laminitis. He also had history of colic and diarrhea. Recently his front feet seem to bother him.

Case 2.3 Assessment:

This gelding is a wood type of horse. He has liver Qi Stagnation (Liver Excess). The treatment strategy includes clearing the Liver Qi Stagnation and strengthening the Spleen.

The Wood (Liver) over-acts (Cheng) on the Earth (Spleen). This explains the sensitivity of the Stomach Meridian (the "husband" of the Spleen Meridian), of BL-20 (Spleen association point) and of BL-21 (Stomach association point). The stifle soreness is also considered a sign of a Stomach Meridian disorder.

The acupoints LIV-3, ST-45, GB-44, BL-20, BL-21, PC-9, and TH-1 are recommended. The herbal formula *Xiao Yao San* may also be beneficial.

The previous two cases have a core of similarity with slightly different clinical presentations. The root is the same: a Wood horse with Liver Qi Stagnation. The first case had secondary signs of Liver Fire, which were caused by the Liver Qi Stagnation because any long-term Stagnation may transform into Fire. The Liver Fire is a Yang factor which tends to flare upwards. Red and swollen eyes occur as a consequence because the eyes are the orifice of the Liver.

The second case also had Liver Qi Stagnation (Liver Excess). The Excessive Liver tends to affect the Stomach/Spleen (the Wood over-acts/*cheng* on the Earth), leading to sensitivity of the Stomach Meridian.

Since both cases have the same root (Liver Qi Stagnation), the primary treatment is the same: the acupoint LIV-3 and the herbal medication *Xiao Yao San*. However, since their secondary clinical presentation is different, the secondary treatment is different. For the first case, HT-8, HT-9 and the herbal formula *Long Dan Xie Gan Tang* are used to clear Liver Fire. For the second case, BL-20 and BL-21 are used to strengthen the Spleen and Stomach. PC-9 and TH-1 are used for the local foot soreness.

Case 2.4

Signalment: A thirteen year old, neutered, male cat

History and Physical Findings:

The cat had a history of fibrosarcoma. The tumor was surgically removed only to have it removed again when it reappeared many months later. Following the second surgery, the owner wanted to try holistic therapy.

The cat was bright and responsive. He was overweight and his coat was shiny. The cat was afraid of thunderstorms, loud noises, and strangers. However, the cat was very independent, stubborn and loud when he became hungry. He preferred to lie in the sun.

The cat's pulses were rapid and superficial. The upper and lower pulses were strong, and the middle pulses were slightly less strong. The tongue is pink with a normal coating. There was no pain on palpation of the alarm points. The mass was removed from the area around BL-20/21.

The treatment so far included diet modification and supplementation. He was given a natural diet that included fish, and he received omega-3 fatty acid supplements and antioxidants.

Case 2.4 Assessment:

This cat has a Water type personality. If the Water energy is deficient, a Water type of animal is prone to arthritis, intervertebral disc disease, and renal failure. If the water is excessive, the animal may develop problems due to counter-control (*Ru* Cycle) of the Earth, over-control (*Cheng* Cycle) of the Fire, or both. When the water is excessive, the result may be Spleen Qi Deficiency (gastrointestinal complaints or tumor) or Heart Deficiency (heart murmur or insomnia). The cat in this case is thirteen years old, but he is still bright and has a pink tongue, a strong pulse at the Kidney level, and a shiny coat. For these reasons, his condition is associated with a strong Water element.

Water over-controls Earth (Spleen) resulting in Spleen Qi Deficiency. The Spleen Qi Deficiency results in failure to produce enough Qi, including Wei-Qi. (Wei-Qi arises from Spleen Qi or food Qi.) When Wei Qi is insufficient, the T-cells fail to check the tissues for mutations and abnormal cells (Yin substances). Thus the body fails to move the Yin substances, and these substances accumulate eventually forming tumors or cancer.

The current therapy is intended as prevention. Thus, the focus of treatment should be on Spleen Qi Deficiency. Acupuncture points such as ST-36, SP-6, and BL-20/21 may be beneficial. Wei Qi Booster (Modified *Si Jun Zi Tang*), an herbal formula that assists Spleen Qi and Wei Qi, is also recommended.

Case 2.5

Signalment: A nine year old, spayed female mix breed dog

Primary Complaint: Urinary Incontinence

History and Physical Findings:

This dog has had urinary incontinence that is under control using Phenylpropanolamine. The owners would like to get her off the drug if possible. She is also on Thyroxine.

Her tongue is lavender and her pulses are weakest on the left. The pulses show weakness at Heart and Pericardium. She pants at night. She is a very excitable girl, wiggling and barking all the time. It is hard to keep needles in her. Her diet is a turkey and rice Purina food. She eats much and is over-weight. She prefers to lie on cool, hard surfaces.

Case 2.5 Assessment:

This dog has a Fire type constitution. The lavender indicates either cold or Yang Deficiency (Fire Deficiency). When the Heart Fire (emperor Fire) is deficient, it can lead to Ming-Men Fire (Minister Fire) weakness. Ming-Men Fire weakness is Kidney Yang Deficiency. The major complaint of urinary incontinence indicates Kidney Qi or Kidney Yang Deficiency. One of the major functions of the Kidney is to control urination.

The panting at night indicates Yin Deficiency. In this case it is a Heart Yin Deficiency. Since the dog is a Fire-type, the dog is prone to Heart Yin Deficiency by the nature of its constitution. (Fire consumes the body fluid easily and leads to Yin Deficiency).

Thus the TCVM diagnosis for this dog is both Yang Deficiency (Kidney) and Yin Deficiency (Heart). The recommended herbal formulas include *Suo Quan Wan* and *Jin Suo Gu Jin Wan* to tonify Kidney Qi and Kidney Yang. The acupuncture points including BL-28, BL-39, *Shen Shu* and CV-6 are recommended. After the Kidney Yang becomes stronger (normal urination), Yin tonification (HT-7, KID-3 and BL-23) can be used.

Case 2.6

Signalment: A five year old, neutered, male cat

History and Physical Findings:

As a kitten this cat had a portal shunt that was surgically repaired. For a while afterwards the cat did well, except for a couple of episodes of cystitis. Then the cat began acting strangely and was drooling intermittently.

On physical exam no dental problems were identified. There was no jaundice noted. The cat exhibited signs such as blindness, diminished hearing, seizures, poor appetite and occasional vomiting. The complete blood count and biochemical values were normal. An ultrasound of the liver was unremarkable, but the serum bile acids, both pre- and post-prandial, were grossly elevated. The cat was thought to have microvascular abnormalities resulting in diversion of portal blood flow from the normal detoxification path through the liver, but this was not confirmed by a liver biopsy. The tongue was pink to red and slightly dry. The pulses were very weak and difficult to palpate.

The cat's treatment included lactulose, metronidazole, and a low protein diet.

Case 2.6 Assessment:

This cat has a Liver Yin Deficiency pattern with Spleen Qi Deficiency. The red and dry tongue, blindness, seizure and elevated serum bile acids indicate Liver Yin Deficiency. Poor appetite, occasional vomiting and weak pulse indicate Spleen Qi Deficiency. Spleen Qi Deficiency can be secondarily caused by Liver Yang Rising due to Liver Yin Deficiency (the Wood over-acts the Earth).

The Liver Yin Deficiency may have resulted from Kidney Jing Deficiency. The cat had a severe developmental problem as a kitten, thus he was likely born with weak Kidney Jing. The Kidney (Water) is the mother of the Liver (Wood). If the mother is weak, she fails to nourish the child.

The treatment should focus primarily on the Liver and secondarily on the Spleen. After the Liver and Spleen problems are fixed, the treatment should include the Kidney. The acupoints BL-18, BL-20, KID-3 and SP-6 are recommended treatments. In addition, the herbal formulas *Yi Guan Jian* (to nourish Liver Yin) and *Xiang Sha Liu Jun Wan* (to tonify Spleen Qi) may be used. Afterwards, Epimedium Powder (*Sheng Jing San*) may be used to treat the Kidney.

Case 2.7

Signalment: A six year old, male, Arab-Trakehner cross-breed

History and Physical Findings:

This horse has previously been treated with acupuncture for allergies. He is allergic to molds and experiences intense pruritis. The horse will even self-mutilate his chest and ventral abdomen.

He seems to have a very "Yang" personality, as he is a bit hyperactive. The allergy problem tends to appear in the Spring.

Case 2.7 Assessment:

Where there is itching, there must be Wind. Both Wind and springtime are associated with the Wood element. In addition, a hyperactive, Yang personality may be consistent with a Wood type of animal.

The TCVM diagnosis is Wind Heat with Liver Yang Rising. Some suggested acupuncture points to help dispel the Wind and to sooth the Liver include GB-20, LIV-3, LIV-4, BL-10, LI-10, LI-11, and LI-4. *Xiao Yao San* is an herbal medication that can be used before spring to soothe Liver Qi and to prevent Liver Yang rising. When it is close to springtime, *Fang Feng Tang* can help to clear Wind Heat.

Case 2.8

Signalment: An eleven year old, Quarter Horse gelding

History and Physical Findings:

This horse has had chronic front foot soreness. He has not been completely sound for three years. Radiographs of his right front foot revealed multiple problems. There are some changes in the navicular bone of his right foot. It is also a slightly "clubbed" foot, and there is an angle problem in the pastern.

This horse was very fearful for a long time. He was difficult to catch and he would tremble when caught. He became calm and less fearful with the herbal medication, Shen Calmer (Modified *Tian Wang Bu Xin Dan*).

He was fat in the crest of the neck, and his eyes were red and draining. The gelding appeared to have Cushing's disease; however, he did not have colic, laminitis, or long hair. His tongue is red, dry and darker on the edges. His pulses are weaker on his left side.

Case 2.8 Assessment:

The TCVM diagnosis is Liver Heat with Kidney Yin Deficiency. The sore foot, the red eyes and the darker edges of the tongue indicate Liver Heat. Navicular bone changes, fear and a weak pulse on the left side indicate Kidney Yin Deficiency. Liver Heat can be caused by Yin Deficiency. Liver Heat can lead to Blood Stagnation and result in the sore foot.

The oral herbal medication, *Long Dan Xie Gan Tang*, may be beneficial in this case. If the foot is very painful (Blood Stagnation), Four Herbs Salve (*Si Sheng Gao*) may be added topically for two to three weeks. This herbal medication works very well for navicular disease and other severe sore foot problems.

Case 2.9

Signalment: A five year old, female, spayed Sheltie

History and Physical Findings:

She is scared and panics during thunderstorms or loud noises. She is very outgoing and sweet with strangers.

She has had a two-year history of reoccurring interdigital cysts. The red, firm, swollen, and painful areas are located on the left rear and right front paws. A change to hypoallergenic diet resolved the redness on the bottom of her paws, but the cysts continued. Examination by specialists, several surgical procedures, and medications did not resolve the problem.

Her diet is supplemented with Vitamins E and C and fatty acids. The dog has normal feces, normal thirst, normal urination, and no gastrointestinal complaints. She seeks cold floors to sleep on; however, she is not restless at night nor does she pant excessively. Her skin and hair coat are normal. She has a large scar on her left lumbar area from a bite wound three years ago. (The scar is lateral to the area of BL-24/25.) She has been healthy other than the interdigital cysts. The areas on the two paws where the cysts were removed are just slightly swollen, red, and cracked with a little clear, red, odorless discharge.

She was not sensitive at any alarm points. Her tongue was pink to red, a little dry, and had faint cracks. Pulses were normal to a little deep. The pulses may have been a little weak, especially in the Heart and Lung positions.

Case 2.9 Assessment:

Her personality is Fire. The problems with the paws may be considered part of the Wood element. The red and swollen cysts indicate Heat. Firm and painful cysts indicate Blood Stagnation.

Her TCVM pattern may be considered Liver Heat with Blood Stagnation. The recommended herbal medications are *Long Dan Xie Gan Tang* and Max Formula (Modified *Nei Xiao San*). The acupuncture points LIV-3, LIV-2, SP-10, LI-11, and LI-4 are recommended in this case to help sooth the Liver, nourish Blood, and eliminate Heat.

Case 2.10

Signalment: A ten year old, neutered, male Golden Retriever and Shepherd crossbreed

History and Physical Findings:

Twelve days previously, this dog was in a raccoon fight and he received bite wounds on his face. Eleven days after the fight, the owners noticed significant stiffness in the hind legs. He also developed orange, watery diarrhea.

He is very attached to the owner and becomes anxious and panics when she is not around. He tolerates other people and dogs well, but he only makes efforts to please his female owner (as opposed to her husband). He does not seem aggressive, but when there is something going on he wants to be part of it. For this reason, gets bitten first when chasing raccoons. Overall, he tends to be fairly high strung, but he will settle down especially if the owner gives him a massage.

He prefers soft surfaces such as a dog bed instead of hard ones such as a rug on the floor. The dog shows no preference for sun or shade. His thirst and urination are normal, but he will pant a lot. This dog always has a great appetite and would overeat if allowed. He is not an overly vocal dog, but he will always bark at any noise outside. This dog shares the house with another dog and a cat with which he has no difficulties. He loves to roll in rotten animals and to get dirty.

Lately, he has been very healthy with normal feces, urination, and hair coat and with no recent history of medical problems. However, three years ago, he fought with a raccoon and suffered bite wounds all over his lips. He subsequently developed coonhound paralysis ten days after the incident. During the illness, the dog had a weak to absent bark. Three days after the onset of clinical signs (stiffness), he suffered from flaccid paralysis. He seemed to make a complete recovery, although it was 75 days before he was able to stand up on his own. There appears to be a residual trembling of his hind legs since that time.

At the current presentation, the dog's vaccine status was noted to be current for Rabies and Distemper-Hepatitis-Leptospirosis-Parainfluenza-Parvovirus (DA$_2$LPP). The dog was panting and nervous. His tongue was pink/red without a coating. The pulse was normal to slow and very strong, almost bounding. He was weak in the hind end, and the neurological examination was consistent with lower motor neuron disease in the hind end. No problems were noted in the front end. The cranial nerve function appeared normal.

The next day, the dog was worse, but he could still get up and walk. His front legs were involved, and there was a dramatic bowing out at the elbows. There were lower motor neuron signs in the front end as well.

Case 2.10 Assessment:

He is not an Earth type because he does not seem to be laid back. Also, he is high-strung and is nervous/pants during the physical exam. Because he is not relaxed and laid-back, he is NOT typical of Earth.

He is not a Wood type because he is NOT the boss or the dominant dog. The Wood dog loves or tends to boss around the other dogs or cats. This dog, however, seems untroubled with other animals, and he leaves them alone.

He is NOT a Metal type because he is not clean and aloof.

He is NOT Water because he not afraid of other creatures; he is the first to fight with the raccoon. Being the first one to go to the action, such as fighting, is definitely NOT a Water trait.

Most likely, this is a Fire dog. A Fire dog tends to become excitable or anxious and will panic. For the fire dog, it is very important to be part of any event including barking, playing and even fighting.

The raccoon's saliva is considered a Toxin in TCVM. The toxin invades the body and then it consumes or damages the Qi or Yin. Consequently, a Qi or Yin Deficiency occurs. Weakness in the hind limbs and diarrhea indicate Qi Deficiency. Panting or nervousness in the exam room and a red tongue indicate Yin Deficiency.

The TCVM treatment strategies are to dispel the toxins, to tonify Qi, to strengthen the rear weakness, and to nourish Yin. Acupuncture points at the tip of the tail and the ears can be used to dispel toxins in acute cases. Additional useful acupuncture points include LI-4, ST-40, ST-36, *Bai Hui*, *Shen Shu*, KID-1, GB-34, GV-1, *Liu Feng*, KID-3, and SP-6. Electroacupuncture and aquapuncture may also be beneficial. The herbal formula *Bu Yang Huan Wu Tang* may be useful to tonify Qi and strengthen the rear weakness in this case.

Self Test

Question 2.1: Which is the correct order for the Sheng (promoting) Cycle?

    a. Wood → Fire → Metal → Water → Earth
    b. Wood → Metal → Water → Fire → Earth
    c. Wood → Fire → Earth → Metal → Water
    d. Wood → Earth → Water → Fire → Metal
    e. Wood → Fire → Water → Metal → Earth

Question 2.2: Which is the correct order for the Cheng (over-control) Cycle?

    a. Wood → Fire → Metal → Water → Earth
    b. Wood → Metal → Fire → Water → Earth
    c. Wood → Fire → Earth → Metal → Water
    d. Wood → Earth → Water → Fire → Metal
    e. Wood → Earth → Metal → Water → Fire

Question 2.3: The Season Spring belongs to which element?

    a. Wood
    b. Earth
    c. Fire
    d. Water
    e. Metal

Question 2.4: The Climate Damp belongs to which element?

    a. Wood
    b. Earth
    c. Fire
    d. Water
    e. Metal

Question 2.5: The color red belongs to which element?

    a. Wood
    b. Earth
    c. Fire
    d. Water
    e. Metal

Question 2.6: The fearful emotion belongs to which element?

    a. Wood

    b. Earth

    c. Fire

    d. Water

    e. Metal

Question 2.7: The direction West belongs to which element?

    a. Wood

    b. Earth

    c. Fire

    d. Water

    e. Metal

Question 2.8: The nose belongs to which element?

    a. Wood

    b. Earth

    c. Fire

    d. Water

    e. Metal

Question 2.9: The Fu organ Bladder belongs to which element?

    a. Wood

    b. Earth

    c. Fire

    d. Water

    e. Metal

Question 2.10: The bodily secretion saliva belongs to which element?

    a. Wood

    b. Earth

    c. Fire

    d. Water

    e. Metal

Question 2.11: A dog has a history of chronic ocular discharge and a hyperactive personality. According to the Five Element theory, which organ is most important?

    a. Spleen

    b. Lung

    c. Kidney

    d. Liver

    e. Heart

Question 2.12: According to the Five Elements, which organ should be tonified when the Lung is deficient?

    a. Heart

    b. Kidney

    c. Liver

    d. Spleen

    e. Bladder

Question 2.13: According to the Five Elements, which organ should be cleared (sedated) when the Heart is in excess?

    a. Liver

    b. Kidney

    c. Spleen

    d. Lung

    e. Bladder

Questions 2.14 and 2.15 are based on the following case.

Pete is a ten year old male Labrador Retriever who has a history of weakness and back pain for several years. Three weeks ago, Pete fell down several times. After prednisone therapy, the acute paresis seemed under control; however, he would no longer get up to urinate and would occasionally fall down. He was also very thirsty, but ice cubes seemed to help. A veterinary neurologist examined him and diagnosed chronic multifocal intervertebral disc disease (spondylosis deformans at C7-T1, T13-L1, L1-L3, and L7-S1). The owner does not want to pursue the surgical treatment approach.

Pete is a very friendly and excitable dog. He has been with the current owner since he was a puppy. He never acted aggressively towards humans or animals except for one instance when the owner returned home very late at night. According to the owner, he prefers cool or cold conditions. He wags his tail and is nice to everybody. During a TCVM examination, he fell down four times, rested for a short while, got up again, and walked across the slippery floor from the front room to the exam room (the whole distance is about 20 meters). Pete is overweight. He panted a lot while in the exam room, and he tried to avoid the acupuncture needling several times. The tongue is red and dry. The pulse is fast, thready and very deep/weak. The TCVM Diagnosis is Bony Bi syndrome due to Yin Deficiency.

Question 2.14: What is Pete's constitutional type?

    a. Wood
    b. Earth
    c. Fire
    d. Metal
    e. Water

Question 2.15: If Pete is an "Earth" dog, why does he show panting and restlessness during the examination?

    a. He has Excess Cold
    b. He is Deficient Cold
    c. He has Yang Deficiency
    d. He has Yang Excess
    e. He has Yin Deficiency

Question 2.16 and 2.17 are based on the following case.

Chief is a nine year old, male, castrated Japanese Chin dog with a history of chronic congestive heart failure and bronchitis. He was hospitalized due to lethargy, weakness and anorexia. Diagnostics revealed azotemia due to chronic renal failure (BUN: 88; Creatinine: 6.9). He was also diagnosed with mild pancreatitis and cervical disc disease.

Chief is a very confident and dominant dog. He does not fear anything, not big or small dogs, strangers, or thunderstorms. He loves to be in charge. He was very cooperative during the examination and acupuncture procedure. His nose was dry with a little crack line. His tongue is deep red and dry and his pulse is thready and thin. Chief prefers cool environments. His Shen is subdued. He eats well but is not thirsty. Chief also always holds his neck, back and hind limbs as if he feels pain or feels unhappy. He is reluctant to lower his head to eat or drink so the owner must lift the bowl to his mouth.

Question 2.16: What is Chief's constitutional type?

    a. Wood
    b. Fire
    c. Earth
    d. Metal
    e. Water

Question 2.17: What is the TCVM Diagnosis for him?

    a. Yang Excess
    b. Yin Deficiency
    c. Excess Cold
    d. Excess Heat
    e. Deficiency Cold

Question 2.18 is based on the following case.

Fireman is a 17 year old Quarter Horse-Thoroughbred cross gelding. He was diagnosed with navicular disease of the left front limb. Fireman is a friendly, sensitive and smart horse. He loves to be petted and touched but he becomes irritable and shows restlessness as soon as he realizes you will needle him. He is sensitive to acupuncture needling as well as the regular injections.

Fireman used to be the submissive to another horse (a 20 year old gelding who was the only other horse to share the pasture) until the old gelding died. The old gelding was always his boss. One year later, Fireman had a little pony to share the same pasture. He started to boss him around. He kicked and controlled the little pony. When the little pony left, a mare about his same age shared his pasture. He started to boss her around. The owner is very close with Fireman as she owned him since he was born. She often gives him treats. She rides him for pleasure about once or twice a week. He loves to run and play, but will let the mare go first if there is something unfamiliar ahead.

His left front lameness was grade 2 to 3. His tongue was purple and pulse was fast. The sensitive points on palpation using a needle cap include LI-18, LI-15, LI-16, BL-18 and 19, PC-1, BL-13 (worse at left side). The TCVM diagnosis is Qi and Blood Stagnation of the front foot (front foot lameness).

The horse was responding well after each treatment (3 to 5 weeks apart). He became completely sound after the 3rd acupuncture treatment. He had two episodes of mild left forefoot soreness six months and one year later, which resolved with acupuncture and herbal medicine.

Question 2.18: What is Fireman's personality?

 a. Wood
 b. Fire
 c. Earth
 d. Metal
 e. Water

CHAPTER THREE

QI, SHEN, JING, BLOOD AND BODY FLUID

Elements in the native (mineral) state are under domination of the material force. Elements in the body are under the control of the life force.

— James Monroe, *Physiologic Medication*

What is life? From one perspective, life may be defined as a self-contained information system with the ability to self-replicate or to perpetuate itself. Seven signs may indicate life: reproduction, growth, metabolism, respiration, excretion, sensation and locomotion.

According to Traditional Chinese Veterinary Medicine (TCVM), life exists only where there is Qi. DNA, merely a long, helical chain of linked molecules, forms the foundation of an organism's genetic code. It is the DNA that is passed from generation to generation, providing the information that regulates an organism's growth and development. Even a virus is nothing more than DNA chains surrounded by a little bit of protein. Yet, a virus is a life form, but the DNA itself is not. Why? The virus has Qi; the DNA does not. DNA is essential for an organism to function, but it is not what distinguishes between the animate and the inanimate. In this way, one may think that a living organism is more than the sum of its parts. The indefinable but recognizable quality that tells us something is alive is the Qi.

What maintains a normal life? In TCVM, life must be supported and controlled by the Five Treasures, Jing, Qi, Shen, Blood and Body Fluid. Those five treasures are the life forces and essential fundamental substances for the physiological activities of the Zang-Fu organs (the internal organs) and the whole body. The Zang-Fu organs need to be nourished and supported by Jing, Qi, Blood and Body Fluid. Qi, Blood and Body Fluid sprout from the Jing (Prenatal and Postnatal Jing) then disperse to the Zang-Fu organs and the whole body via the Meridians. The Shen rules the mind and the whole body. Health exists when the five treasures are abundant and properly moving and flourishing. Obstruction or insufficient quantities of the five treasures result in disease.

Qi

Qi gives life to the world. Where there is Qi, there must be life. Without Qi, life ceases to exist; it is Qi that gives our body life. *Zhuang Zi* states that "Qi gives birth to human beings; where Qi exists there is life, but the absence of Qi is death".

Qi exists in two states, the substantial Qi and the functional Qi. The substantial Qi is the foundation of the functional Qi, and it is comprised of the essential substances that maintain normal vital activities. Functional Qi refers to the physiological activity of each Zang-Fu organ.

CLASSIFICATIONS OF QI

There are eight major forms of Qi: Yuan Qi, Zong Qi, Gu Qi, Ying Qi, Wei Qi, Zang-Fu Qi, Jing Luo Qi, Zheng Qi. Each of these has different properties or functions.

Yuan Qi
(Primary Qi, Source Qi, Original Qi)

- Derived from the Kidney Essence or congenital Essence

- It is Essence in the form of Qi, rather than fluid.

- Requires supplementation and nourishment by the Food Essence (Gu Qi)

- Comprises the Primary Yin (Kidney Yin) and the Primary Yang (Kidney Yang)

- It is the original dynamic motive force of normal activities.

- Distributed to the whole body by the Sanjiao

- Impels the Zang-Fu organs to bring normal activities into play

- Maintains normal growth and development of the body

- Pathology: Yuan Qi Deficiency results in decreased disease resistance.

Yuan Qi is essential for proper function of the Zang-Fu organs. If the Yuan Qi is abundant, the Zang-Fu organs will function well and the animal will be ill less frequently. Deficiency of Yuan Qi results in decreased Zang-Fu function and increased pathological changes. Deficiency occurs due to Yuan Qi depletion during prolonged diseases or due to Deficiency of Congenital Kidney Essence (Jing).

Zong Qi

(Pectoral Qi, Gathering Qi, Ancestral Qi, Chest Qi)

- Formed by the combination of Gu Qi and Qing Qi (Cosmic Qi)

  Qing Qi is sometimes called universal clean air. It is the abundant, mostly invisible energy of the Universe made up of air, light, electromagnetic forces and various energetic particles in space and the atmosphere.

- Formed, gathered and stored in the chest

- Promotes the Lung's respiratory function (control of respiration)

- Promotes the Heart's circulatory function (governing Blood and vessels)

- Related to the voice, to respiration, and to the circulation of Qi and Blood

In the chest, the Food Qi formed by the Spleen/Stomach combines with the Qing Qi inhaled by the Lung to form the Zong Qi.

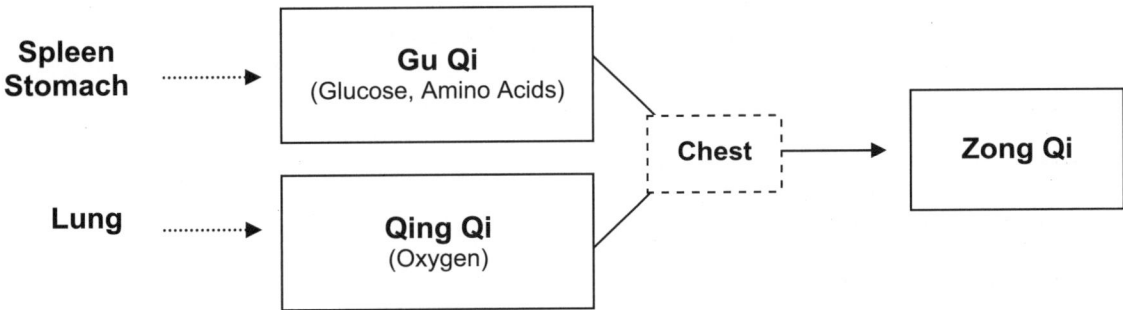

Figure 3.1: The Formation of Zong Qi

Gu Qi

(Food Qi or Food Essence)

- Formed from food by the Spleen

- The origin of the Ying Qi and the Wei Qi

- Replenishes the Yuan Qi and the Kidney Essence

Food enters the Stomach where it is rotted and decomposed. It is then transformed into Gu Qi (Food Essence) by the Spleen. The Gu Qi rises into the chest to the Lung. Here it combines with Qing Qi in the Lung to form Zong Qi.

Thus, Gu Qi is a substance produced by the Spleen's activity. This function of the Spleen occurs in an ascending direction. The Spleen should always send Gu Qi up to the Lung. In this way, the Spleen is a major source of Qi after birth, and it also controls the ascending movement of Qi. If the Spleen Qi descends, the food may not be properly transformed thus resulting in diarrhea.

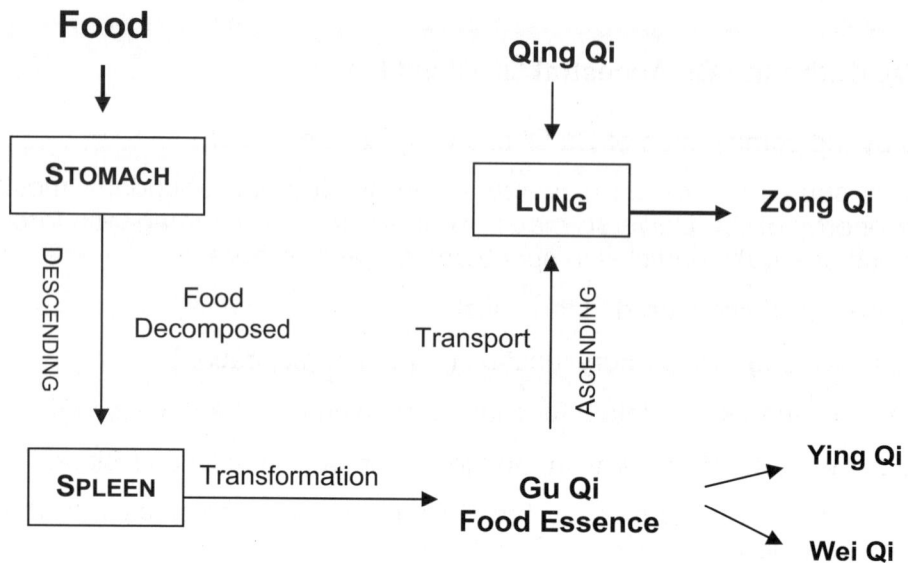

Figure 3.2: The path of Gu Qi

Ying Qi

(Nutrient Qi)

- Derived from Gu Qi

- Circulates in the blood vessels

- Produces Blood and nourishes the whole body

- Hemoglobin and other serum proteins are a part of Ying Qi

- Also called Nutrient Blood or Ying Blood due to its association with Blood and its flow within blood vessels

Wei Qi

(Defensive Qi)

- Derived from Gu Qi

- Circulates in superficial, extra-vascular parts of the body

- Protects the integument and musculature against the external attack of pathogens

- Controls the opening and closing of pores

- Regulates body temperature

- Moistens the skin and hair to warm up the Zang-Fu organs

- Also known as Defensive Yang or Wei Yang because it is part of the body's Yang Qi

Zang-Fu Qi

- Derived from Yuan Qi
- Zang-Fu organ's individual functions

This Qi represents the function of each of the internal organs:

- o Spleen Qi: The Spleen transports and transforms water and food.
- o Stomach Qi: The Stomach receives and decomposes food.
- o Heart Qi: The Heart controls the Blood and vessels.
- o Lung Qi: The Lung dominates Ascending-Descending movement.
- o Liver Qi: The Liver maintains the smooth flow of Qi.
- o Kidney Qi: The Kidney controls sexual function, governs water, and dominates bones.
- o Zhong Qi: The combination of both the Spleen Qi and Stomach Qi is known as Zhong Qi or Middle Qi. Its major function is to hold the internal organs in the proper position.

Jing-Luo Qi

(Meridian Qi)

- Derived from Yuan Qi
- The function of the Meridian itself
- Coordinates the activities of the Zang-Fu organs
- Provides communication between the Interior and the Exterior of the body
- Transmits the information from acupuncture point stimulation
- The "De-Qi" response is based on this type of Qi. The De-Qi response, otherwise known as the arrival of Qi, is the feeling or effect experienced as a result of the Meridian's transmission of the acupuncture stimulation.

Zheng Qi

(Antipathogenic Qi or Resistance Qi)

- A collective term for various kinds of functional activities in the body
- Body's total ability to resist disease
- Described in relation to Xie Qi (Pathogenic Qi or Pathogenic factors)

FUNCTIONS OF QI

Qi permeates and influences all parts of the body. There is not a place without Qi. If the movement of Qi ceases, the vital activities of the animal body will also cease. When there is abundant Qi, health is good, but Deficiency of Qi leads to disease. Qi has the following six functions: impelling, warming, defending, holding, activity, and nourishing.

Stimulating and Impelling Effect

- Yuan Qi is the original dynamic motive force of a body's vital activities
- Yuan Qi can impel the growth and development of the body
- Yuan Qi can impel the normal functions of the Zang-Fu organs and the Meridians
- Deficiency of Yuan Qi results in retarded growth and development

Warming Effect

In Traditional Chinese Veterinary Medicine, Qi is involved in temperature regulation. The Qi adjusts the body heat to maintain a normal body temperature. The Yang Qi or Yang is this special form of Qi that warms up the body.

- Heart Yang warms the entire cardiovascular system
- Spleen Yang warms the limbs and lips
- Kidney Yang warms the ear, back, and rear end
- Wei Qi (Wei Yang) warms the body surface
- Deficiency of the Yang Qi results in cold limbs or trunk

Defensive Effect

- Protects the body surface from invasion by the pathogenic factors
- Combats and eliminates pathogens when a disease occurs

Holding Effect

- Spleen Qi holds the Blood in the vessels
- Kidney Qi holds Essence and urine
- Wei Qi holds sweat
- Zhong Qi holds the Zang-Fu organs such as the uterus and rectum
- Deficiency of Zhong Qi may result in rectal or uterine prolapse

Qi Activity

(Activities of Vital Energy or *Qi Hua*)

Broadly defined as the mutual transformation among Essence, Qi, Blood, and Body Fluid

- Essence can be transformed into Qi or Blood by the Qi Activity
- Qi can be transformed into Essence
- Blood can be transformed into Body Fluid

Narrowly defined as the individual functions of the Zang-Fu organs.

- The Bladder stores urine then excretes it via the Bladder's Qi Activity

Nourishing Effect

- Ying Qi (Nutrient Qi) circulates in the Blood vessels and is a part of the Blood
- Ying Qi provides nourishment to the whole body

Table 3.1: Characteristics of the major Qi types

Name	Origin	Distribution	Functions	Zang-Fu
Zong Qi	Gu Qi + Qing Qi	Gathers in the chest and distributed in Lung and Heart	• Dominate Respiration • Promote circulation of Blood	HT LU
Zhong Qi	SP Qi + ST Qi	Distributed in the Middle-Jiao	• Generate Qi and Blood • Hold Zang-Fu organs • Dominate ascending/ descending movement of Qi	SP ST
Yuan Qi	Prenatal Jing	Stored in Kidney and distributed to whole body via San-Jiao	• Initiate Zang-Fu activities • Regulate growth, development, reproduction	KID
Ying Qi	Gu Qi	Distributed inside the vessels	• Generate Blood • Nourish the whole body	SP HT
Wei Qi	Gu Qi	Distributed outside of the vessels	• Protect the body surface • Resist any pathogens • Warm the Zang-Fu organs • Regulate excretion of sweat • Regulate body temperature	SP LU

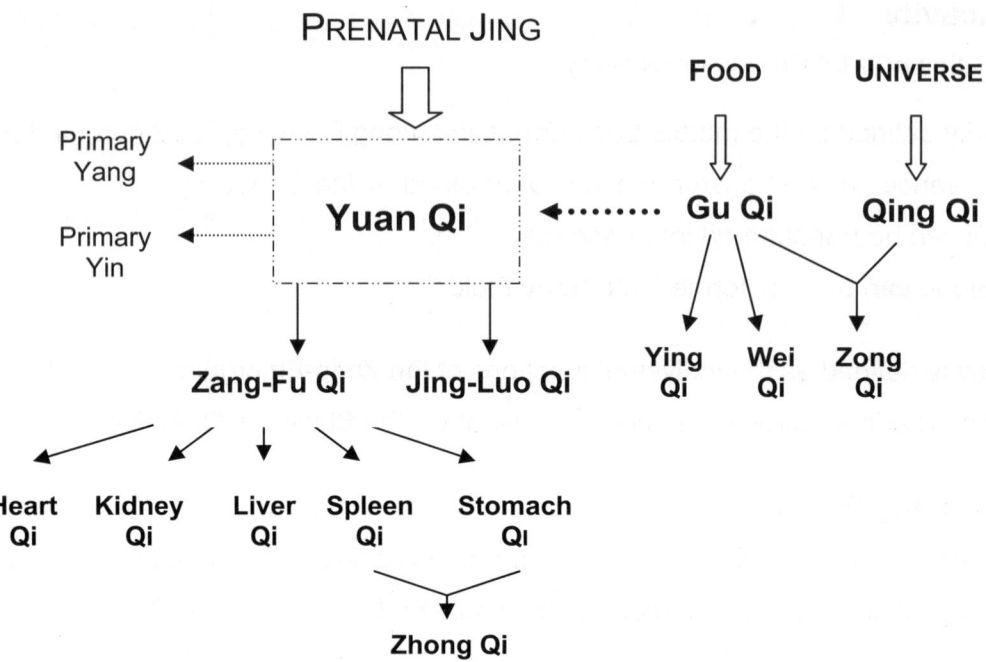

Figure 3.3: The origins of the major Qi types

QI PATHOLOGY

Qi plays a very important role in the body. Problems develop if there is an imbalance or a disruption of the normal Qi quantity or flow. Qi may exist in four pathologic states within the body: Deficiency, Stagnation, Rebellious, or Collapsed.

Qi Deficiency

If there is insufficient Qi to allow the organs to function properly, disease states can develop. Deficiency of Qi usually results in weakness.

Signs

- Fatigue
- Weakness in body and spirit (physical or mental exhaustion)
- Shortness of breath
- Weak pulse
- Pale tongue

Types

Heart Qi Deficiency:

- Palpitations
- Shortness of breath
- Spontaneous sweating (worse if moving)
- Irregularly or regularly intermittent pulse
- Easily frightened

Acupuncture points: HT-7, BL-15, CV-17, PC-6, LU-7
Herbal formula: *Yang Xin Tang* (Nourish Heart)

Lung Qi Deficiency:

- Weak, chronic cough or asthma (worse with movement)
- Appearance of an obvious groove (heaves line) along the rib arch in horses
- Constant recurrence of the common cold
- Spontaneous sweating
- Occurs in the course of chronic bronchitis or chronic pulmonary emphysema.

Acupuncture points: LU-9, BL-13, CV-17, ST-36, *Ding Chuan*
Herbal formula: *Bu Fei Tang* (Tonify Lung)

Spleen Qi Deficiency:

- Poor appetite
- Diarrhea
- Weight loss, difficulty in gaining weight or muscular atrophy
- Fatigue, weakness
- Hemorrhage, edema, or prolapse of anus
- Occurs in the course of poor absorption or chronic indigestion

Acupuncture points: ST-36, CV-6, CV-4, BL-20, GV-1
Herbal formula: *Si Jun Zi Tang* (Four Gentlemen)

Kidney Qi Deficiency:

- Arthritis (Bi syndrome)
- Weakness or pain in the lower back or rear limbs
- Urinary incontinence
- Deafness
- Infertility

Acupuncture points: BL-23, *Bai Hui*, CV-4, CV-6, KID-3
Herbal formula: *Jin Gui Shen Qi Wan*

Qi Stagnation

The Qi becomes blocked and does not flow properly. This leads to pain, stiffness and organ dysfunction. Any organ can experience Qi Stagnation; however, Stagnation of Liver Qi, Stomach Qi, and Large Intestine are most common.

Signs

- Local pain
- Stiffness

Examples

Liver Qi Stagnation:

- Hyperactivity
- Emotional stress
- Depression
- Anger
- Nervous
- Hypertension

Acupuncture points: LIV-3, LIV-4, GB-34, GB-39, TH-1
Herbal formula: *Xiao Yao San*

Stomach Qi Stagnation:

- Stomachache
- Vomiting
- Nausea

Acupuncture points: CV-12, BL-21, GB-34, ST-36, ST-25
Herbal formula: *Bao He Wan*

Large Intestine Stagnation:

- Impaction
- Constipation
- Gaseous colic

Acupuncture points: ST-37, ST-36, ST-25, BL-25
Herbal formula: *Da Cheng Qi Tang*

Rebellious Qi

The Qi is not moving in the proper directions.

Examples

Rebellious Stomach Qi:

- Hiccups
- Nausea
- Vomiting

   Acupuncture points: ST-36, GB-34, PC-6, CV-12
   Herbal formula: *Wei Chang He*

Rebellious Lung Qi:

- Cough
- Asthma

   Acupuncture points: BL-13, *Ding Chuan*, CV-22
   Herbal formula: *Su Zi Jiang Qi Tang*

Prolapsed Qi

This is the inability of the Zhong Qi (Middle Qi) to hold the organs in their normal place, resulting in prolapse of the rectum, uterus, or other organs.

Signs

- Prolapsed organs, such as the rectum or uterus
- Drooping of lips and drooling
- Chronic diarrhea

Treatment

Acupuncture points: GV-1, CV-1, GV-20
Herbal formula: *Bu Zhong Yi Qi Tang*

Shen

The translation of Shen may be the words Spirit or Mind. However, Spirit does not necessarily mean "spiritual" and its associated connotations. Shen refers to the outward appearance of the vital activities of the whole body. It rules the mind, mental activities, memory and sleep. It provides us with awareness and clear feeling. When Shen is healthy, it gives us inner peace. The animal with a healthy Shen will exhibit normal behaviors and will be alert and responsive to environmental stimuli. The Shen is housed in the Heart. It requires nourishment from the Heart Yin and Blood to remain healthy.

SHEN PATHOLOGY

Shen disturbances are often caused either by excessive Fire or by deficient Fire (Heart Yin/Blood Deficiency). General symptoms include restlessness, palpitations, anxiety, insomnia, forgetfulness, hyperactivity, frightening easily, and inability to focus attention.

Treatment

Acupuncture points: HT-7, PC-6 and *An Shen*
Herbal Formula: Shen Calmer (*Tian Wan Bu Xin Dan* modification)

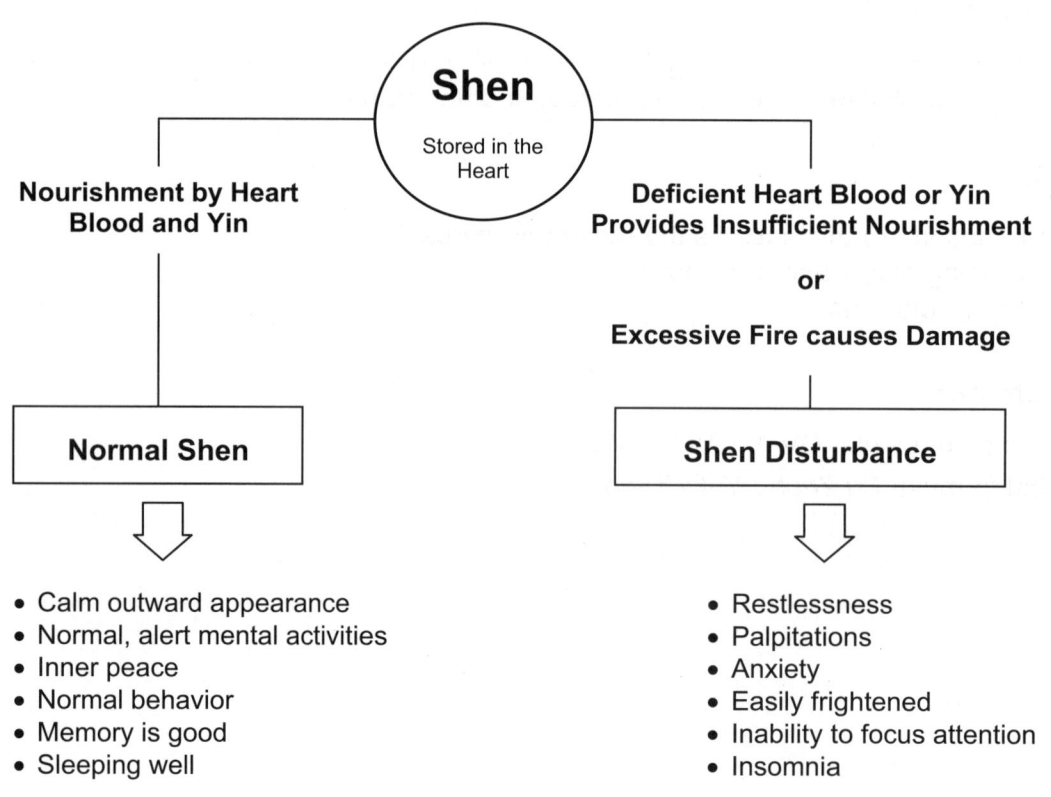

Jing

The translation of Jing is Essence. There are two types of Jing: Prenatal Jing and Postnatal Jing. Prenatal Jing, also called Kidney Jing, Congenital Jing or Natal Jing, is the seed of life. It is the basis for all growth, development, sexuality and reproduction. It manifests as sperm in males and as the ovum (the egg) and vaginal fluids in females. All the genetic materials (DNA, RNA, etc.) are stored in the Prenatal Jing.

Postnatal Jing is also called Acquired Jing or Zang-Fu Jing. Zang-Fu Jing is the Jing that each individual Zang organ possesses. This Jing is reflected in specific orifices of the head. The Jing of Liver opens to the eyes, keeping them clear and sparkling. The Jing of Kidney opens to the ears to stimulate acute hearing. The Jing of the Heart opens to the tongue to produce clarity of speech. The Jing of the Spleen opens to the lips and mouth, promoting the sense of taste and the production of saliva. The Jing of the Lung opens to the nose to promote an acute sense of smell.

Prenatal Jing is the foundation of life. An individual's lifetime supply of Congenital Jing is inherited from the parents and stored in the Kidney at birth. If there is a problem early in life, it is due to a Deficiency of the Prenatal Jing. Thus, Congenital Jing is never excessive and must be conserved. On the other hand, the Acquired Jing is extracted from Gu Qi (Food Qi) by the Spleen. When Acquired Jing is excessive, it may be saved or be transformed into Congenital Jing. Life, like a pilot light, constantly draws upon this Jing as a fuel throughout the years. Acquired Jing can provide supplemental energy for this life-flame. This often helps to decrease, but not completely eliminate, the draw upon the Congenital Jing. Jing is easily depleted, but it is very hard to replace. Thus, with age, the Jing gradually diminishes. The aging process itself is a sign of diminishing Jing, and natural death occurs with complete Jing depletion. Like a withering flower, Jing Deficiency gradually causes loss of vitality, dulling of the senses, lack of sexual desire, and inability to regenerate. The Jing is lost through over-work, excessive behavior patterns, too much sexual activity, lack of sleep, loss of fluids and chronic diseases.

Yuan Qi (Source Qi or Primary Qi) is the active form of Kidney Jing. The Yuan Qi is divided into Primary Yin and Primary Yang. Primary Yin refers to Kidney Yin while Primary Yang refers to the Ming-Men Fire (Fire of the life gate). It rules the uterus, vagina, penis, and reproductive ability; and it controls the seven-year (female) and eight-year (male) cycles of development and growth in human beings.

JING PATHOLOGY

Signs of Jing Deficiency

- Retarded or poor growth
- Developmental orthopedic diseases (DOD)
- Loss of vitality
- Infertility
- Early aging

Treatment principles

- Nourish Kidney Jing
- Tonify Spleen Qi

Treatment

Acupuncture points: KID-7, KID-3, KID-10, *Shen Shu*, SP-6
Herbal formula: *Sheng Jing San*

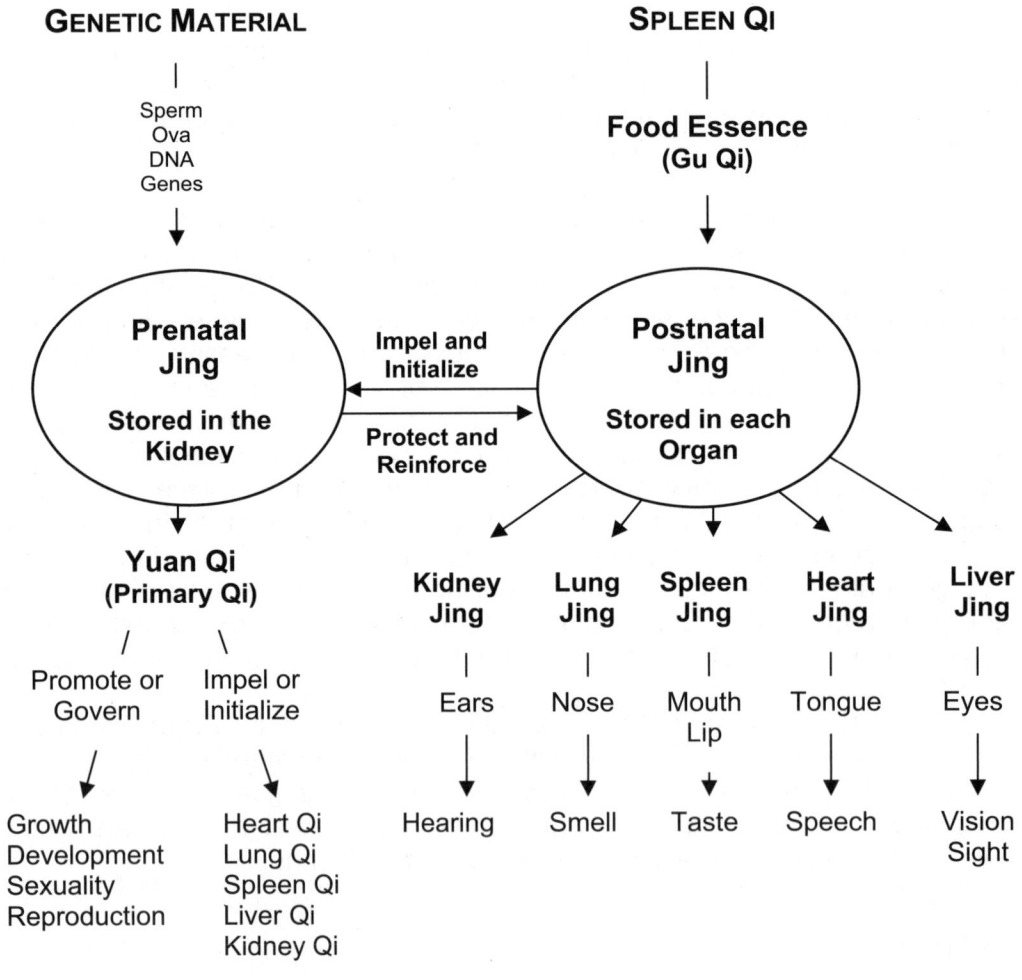

Figure 3.4: The pathways of Jing

Blood

It is a red liquid containing the Ying Qi and circulating in the vessels. The Heart Qi impels the Blood. It provides nourishment and moistens the body and Zang-Fu organs.

SOURCE AND FORMATION

There are four sources of Blood.

1. Food Qi

Blood is derived mostly from the Gu Qi produced by the Spleen. The Gu Qi ascends from the Spleen to the Lung and is distributed to the Heart. In the Heart, the Gu Qi is transformed into Blood.

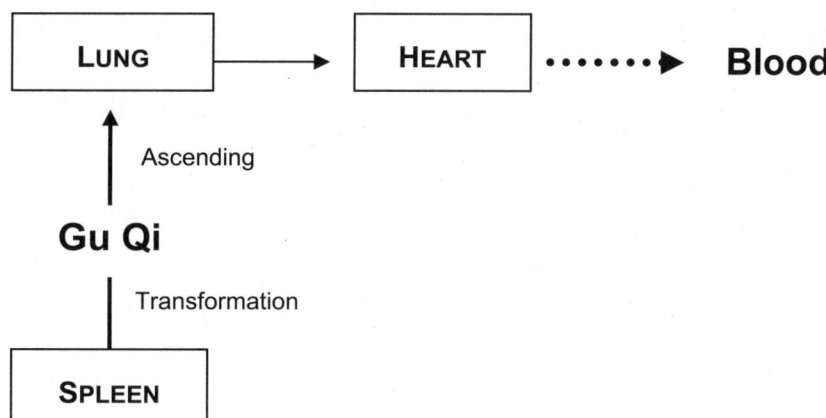

Figure 3.5: Transformation into Blood

2. Ying Qi

When Ying Qi flows into the vessels, it is transformed into Blood.

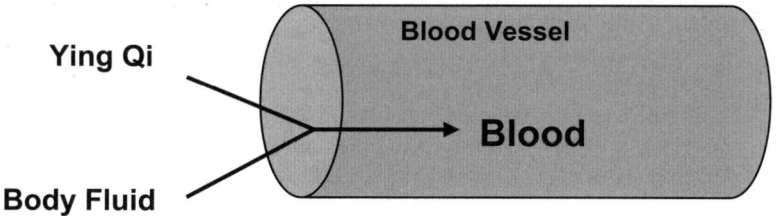

3. Jing - Essence

A relationship exists between Blood and Essence in which one transforms into the other.

- o If Blood is not consumed, it is transformed into Essence in the Kidney
- o If Essence does not leak out, it is transformed into Blood in the Liver

4. Body Fluid (*Jin Ye*)

Like Ying Qi, Body Fluid is transformed into blood when it flows into the vessels.

CIRCULATION OF BLOOD

Three organs are intimately related with the Blood: Heart, Spleen, and Liver. Each of these three controls Blood in a different way, and a disorder of any of these organs may negatively influence the Blood production and circulation. When these organs coordinate their actions, the continuous, smooth flow of Blood within the vessels is assured. The Heart acts as the pump, pushing the Blood along its path. The Spleen acts like the guard walls on the side of a road by preventing Blood leakage from the vessels. The Liver acts like a traffic police officer by keeping the Blood moving in a smooth, orderly fashion.

Organ	Relationship to Blood	Disorder Example
Heart	• Dominates the Blood and vessels • The impelling force of Blood circulation	Heart Qi Deficiency leads to Blood Stagnation.
Spleen	• Holds Blood • Prevents extravasation	Spleen Qi Deficiency leads to bloody feces.
Liver	• Promotes the smooth flow of Qi • Stores Blood • Readjusts Blood volume	Blood Stagnation

FUNCTIONS OF BLOOD

Nourishing and Moistening Effect

Blood circulates throughout the whole body. It passes through the Zang-Fu organs in the Interior as well as the muscles and tendons of the Exterior. This flow allows the Blood to nourish and moisten all the tissues of the body. This keeps the tissues functioning normally. For example, Blood in the Liver moistens the eyes and tendons maintaining normal vision and flexible tendons.

Carrying Effect

"Blood is the Mother of Qi, and Qi is the Commander or General of Blood"

The function of Blood is closely associated with Qi. The normal circulation of Blood requires propulsion by Qi. Blood carries Qi for distribution to the whole body. Thus a disorder with one will result in a disorder of the other.

Blood Deficiency	→	Failure to carry Qi	→	Qi Deficiency
Qi Stagnation	→	Failure to impel Blood	→	Blood Stagnation

BLOOD PATHOLOGY

Blood Deficiency:

- General weakness or deficiency
- Dizziness upon standing
- Pale complexion (lips and tongue)
- Cold extremities
- Dry hair coat or dandruff
- Poor growth of hooves (horse) or nails (dog or cat)
- Cracks in hooves or paw pads
- Subject to chills
- Thready pulse

Acupuncture points: BL-17, SP-10, ST-36, BL-20
Herbal formula: *Si Wu Tang* (Four Substances)

Blood Stagnation:

- Lumps
- Cysts
- Bruising
- Sharp stabbing pains

Acupuncture points: LIV-3, SP-10
Herbal formula: *Sheng Tong Zhu Yu Tang*

Blood Stagnation pain: (Substantial pain)	A stabbing, centrally located pain. Chronic, easily palpated or swollen, inflamed.
Qi Stagnation pain: (Non-substantial pain)	Dull aches that come and go. Not easily located upon palpation. No particular point of origin.

Blood Heat:

- Hives
- Rashes
- Dry skin
- Fast pulse
- Dry, red eye lids
- Red tongue
- Hemorrhage; A large amount of fresh, red blood without evidence of trauma

Acupuncture points: SP-10, LI-4, LI-11
Herbal formula: *Xi Jiao Di Huang Tang*

Bleeding:

There are three causes of bleeding: Qi Deficiency, Excess Heat, and Deficient Heat.

Qi Deficiency:

- Chronic hemorrhage, small amount with dark color
- General weakness
- Exercise intolerance
- Weak pulse
- Pale tongue

Acupuncture points: SP-10, BL-17, ST-36, CV-6
Herbal formula: *Gui Pi Tang*

Excess Heat

- Hemorrhage; A large amount of fresh, red blood without evidence of trauma
- Fever
- Hives or skin rashes
- Inflammation or infection

Acupuncture points: SP-10, LI-4, LI-11, GV-14
Herbal formula: *Xi Jiao Di Huang Tang*

Deficiency Heat:

- Hemorrhage; A small amount of fresh, dark blood
- Lower degree of fever
- Chronic inflammation or infection
- Red and dry tongue
- Thready and fast pulse

Acupuncture points: GV-14, KID-3, KID-6, HT-7
Herbal formula: *Xi Xian Cao* (Siegesbeckia Powder)

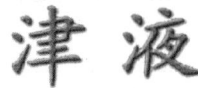

Body Fluid (*Jin Ye*)

Body Fluid is a collective term for all the normal fluids of the body:

Tears	Nasal discharge	Sweat
Urine	Saliva	Gastric juice
Joint fluid	Intestinal fluids	

FORMATION AND DISTRIBUTION

TCVM Water Metabolism

The formation, distribution, and excretion of Body Fluid is a complicated process. It involves the coordinated activities of the Spleen, Stomach, Lung, Kidney, Small Intestine, Bladder and Large Intestine. If there are problems with these organs, then the normal flow of fluid can be disrupted resulting in Body Fluid accumulation. Edema, diarrhea, or Phlegm can be products of a water metabolism disorder.

The Body Fluid originates from food and drink. The water an animal drinks is transformed and separated by the Spleen into a clear part and a turbid part. The clear part goes up to the Lung where the Lung separates this clear fluid once again into clear and turbid parts. The clear part is then distributed to the entire body. The turbid part is sent to the Kidney.

The Spleen and Stomach work as a team. The Spleen separates and transforms the food and drink then sends these products in an upward direction. The Spleen should only have an upward flow. The Stomach, however, has a downward flow. Thus it is the Stomach which sends the turbid part of the fluid down to the Small Intestine. The Small Intestine separates this turbid fluid into clear and turbid parts. The clear part goes to the Kidney, and the turbid part goes to the Large Intestine. The turbid part in the Large Intestine is excreted as feces.

The Kidney receives both the turbid part of the clear fluid from the Lung and the clear part of the turbid fluid from the Small Intestine. The Kidney separates this fluid into a pure and an impure part. The pure part is sent up to the Lung to be distributed to the body with the rest of the clear fluid. The impure part is sent to the Urinary Bladder for excretion as urine.

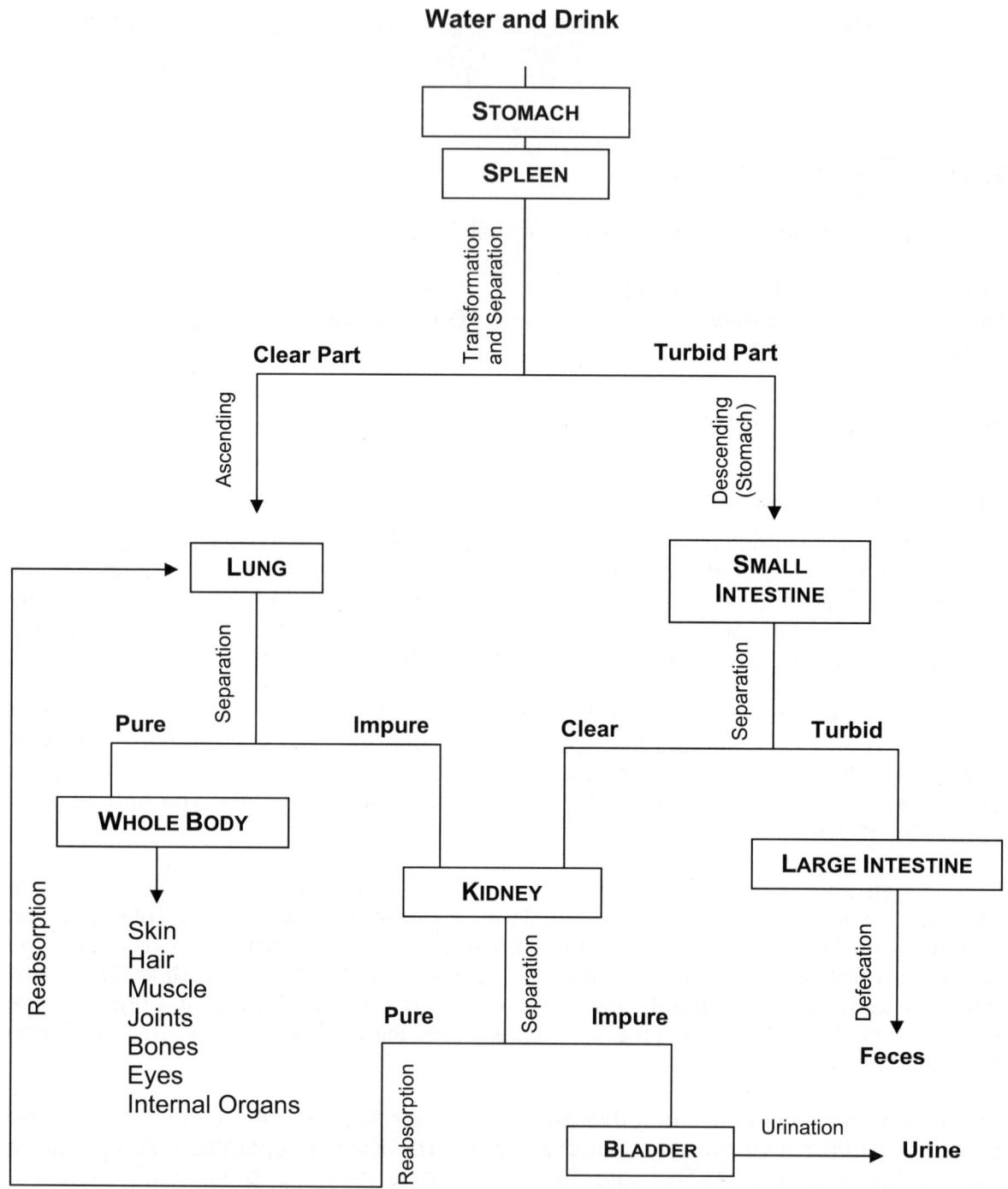

Figure 3.6: The pathway of water metabolism

FUNCTIONS OF BODY FLUID

Overall, the Body Fluid acts to moisten and nourish the body. There are two types of Body Fluid which have more specialized functions within this broad activity.

The clear and thin part of the Body Fluid is known as "Fluid" (Jin).

- o Distributed with the Wei Qi circulation to the surface, skin, and muscle
- o Warms and moistens the skin and muscles

The thick and heavy part is called "Liquid" (Ye).

- o Distributed by circulation within blood vessels to the Zang-Fu organs, Bone Marrow, Brain, joint cavities and orifices
- o Nourishes and strengthens these tissues or organs

Body Fluid, like Blood, originates from food and drink. Body Fluid and Blood are closely linked. When Body Fluid enters the vessels, it becomes a part of Blood. If there is a Body Fluid Deficiency, a Blood Deficiency will follow. Conversely, an excessive loss of Blood will result in a Deficiency of Body Fluid.

BODY FLUID PATHOLOGY

There are three major pathological conditions that involve Body Fluid. These are Internal Dryness, Edema, and Phlegm. These conditions arise due to a lack of sufficient Body Fluid, to an accumulation of too much Body Fluid, or to a modification in the Body Fluid quality which impedes its normal form and function. Pathological conditions involving Body Fluid occur when there is a disruption of the normal water metabolism system.

Internal Dryness

This occurs when there is insufficient Body Fluid to meet the needs of the tissues.

Signs

- Dryness of lips
- Dry skin
- Dry eyelids
- Joint stiffness
- Constipation

Treatment

Acupuncture point: KID-3, BL-23, KID-10
Herbal Formula: *Zeng Ye Tang*

Edema

This occurs as a consequence of Spleen Qi Deficiency or Kidney Qi Deficiency.

Sign

Water retention

Treatment

Acupuncture point: ST-36, CV-4, CV-6, BL-20, SP-9
Herbal Formula: *Shi Pi Yin*

Phlegm

Phlegm is a distorted form of Body Fluid which is often the cause of anything "strange" in the body. Phlegm develops due to Heat and Damp. Thus, there are two forms of Phlegm, Heat Phlegm and Damp Phlegm.

Heat Phlegm

Signs

- Fever and Upper airway infection
- Cough
- Red tongue
- Fast and forceful pulse

Treatment

Acupoints: LU-5, LU-9, PC-5, *Xiong Tang*
Herbal Formula: *Qing Qi Hua Tan Tang*

Damp Phlegm

Signs

- Wet Cough
- Pale tongue
- Slow and choppy pulse

Treatment

Acupoints: ST-36, ST-40, SP-6, SP-9
Herbal Formula: *Er Chen tang*

Case Examples

Case 3.1

Signalment: A two year old, female horse

Primary Complaint: Alopecia and dandruff

History and Exam:

This filly has a shiny, full coat, but she has areas of alopecia with crusts and dandruff. For a year she has been on a vitamin and mineral supplement which has helped the problem. The areas of alopecia this year are much smaller than those last year. The alopecia is mostly on her right rump.

Her tongue is pink and very wet. Her pulses are weaker on the right side, especially at the Kidney position. Overall she is a healthy horse.

Case 3.1 Assessment:

Chronic illness in early life indicates a Kidney Jing Deficiency. This horse may have a Kidney Jing Deficiency. Deficient Kidney Jing can cause Kidney Qi Deficiency and may lead to hair loss. This horse has a wet tongue and weak pulse on the right side. Both of these can indicate Kidney Qi Deficiency.

Treatment can include acupuncture at GV-3, KID-7, *Shen Shu* and BL-23. In addition, needles can be placed such that they surround the areas of alopecia. This is known as "Circle the Dragon". The herbal formula Epimedium Powder (*Sheng Jing San*) may be used for three to six months.

Case 3.2

Signalment: A twenty year old Morgan gelding

History and Exam:

This horse did a "split" several months previously. A rectal examination revealed a muscle tear, which was healing at a recheck exam a few weeks later. The horse has never totally recovered from this incident. He is stiff when he walks and when he gets up. Normally a gentle horse, he tries to kick with his good leg when someone tries to pick up his bad leg. The owners are unable to clean or trim that foot. His pulse is fast and strong. His tongue is purple.

Case 3.2 Assessment:

Muscle tears or secondary scar tissues due to injuries are considered Blood Stagnation. Blood Stagnation obstructs Qi flow, leading to Qi Stagnation. Thus the horse is painful to the touch. The TCVM diagnosis for this horse's condition is Blood Stagnation.

The acupuncture points *Shen Shu*, BL-54, *Lu Gu*, *Yan Chi*, BL-40, BL-67 and GB-44 may be used. Electroacupuncture at 20 Hz for 20 minutes may be performed once every one to three weeks. In addition, herbal medicines such as *Sheng Tong Zhu Yu Tang* may be beneficial.

Case 3.3

Signalment: A thirteen year old Quarter Horse mare

Initial History and Exam:

She became angry during an acupuncture treatment. After treatment she was fine for several months, but then she started to get a little "crabby". Upon examination, she pinned her ears, stomped her feet, and tried to bite and kick. Her eyes were red, swollen, and watery. Her tongue was red and dry. Her pulses were weak on the left side.

Initial Case 3.3 Assessment:

Red and swollen eyes, anger and an aggressive attitude indicate Liver Fire. The red, dry tongue and weak pulses indicate Yin Deficiency. The mare likely has a Liver Yin Deficiency which leads to Liver Yang rising. This causes Liver Fire, which disturbs the Shen. It is important to first treat the Excess (symptoms) then treat the underlying Deficiency. Initially, the treatment principle should be to clear the Liver Fire and to calm down the Shen. *Long Dan Xie Gan Tang* and Shen Calmer should be beneficial for this. After the symptoms of excess are cleared, *Yi Guan Jian* may be used to tonify Liver Yin.

Case 3.3 Reexamination:

Long Dan Xie Gan Tang and Shen Calmer were given to the horse for two months. She became about 60% better, but she is still aggressive to people. She swishes her tail and tries to bite and kick when touched. Her tongue is dark pink and her Liver pulse is deficient.

Case 3.3 Reexamination Assessment:

The dark pink tongue and weak Liver Pulse indicate a Liver Yin Deficiency. The aggressive attitude indicates Liver Qi Stagnation. *Yi Guan Jian* (to nourish Liver Yin) and *Xiao Yao San* (to soothe Liver Qi) should be used for two months.

Case 3.4

Signalment: An adult female dog

History and Exam:

The dog has eosinophilic myositis. She is unable to completely open her mouth, and she has temporal muscle atrophy. Her tongue is dark purple. Pulses are fast and forceful.

The only way to control this problem has been with prednisone. When she is taken off the prednisone, the myositis returns.

Case 3.4 Assessment:

Pain (inability to open her mouth) and a dark purple tongue indicate Blood Stagnation. Myositis and the fast, forceful pulse indicate Heat. Thus, the TCVM diagnosis is Blood Stagnation with Heat.

Topical application of *Bing Peng San* on the oral mucous membranes helps to move Blood and relieve pain. The herbal powder may be mixed with toothpaste to assist application. In addition, orally administered *Yu Nu Jian* (Jade Lady) can clear Heat. The acupoints LI-4 and ST-44 as well as local points may be used to move Qi and Blood and relieve pain.

Case 3.5

Signalment: A seven year old male Wire haired pointer

History and Exam:

This hunting dog presented with a sore right hind leg. He was hit by a car three months ago. According to the owner, the femur was fractured and the muscles were badly torn. The femur was set using a pin and wires. The dog is still non-weight bearing, and he holds his leg in a flexed position, letting his leg dangle below the tarsus. The muscles of his leg have atrophied severely. The dog permits massage and passive range of motion exercises. The owner reports that he lives outside, and he often cries in pain when it is cold.

Case 3.5 Assessment:

The TCVM diagnosis for this dog is Qi or Blood Stagnation. Acupuncture points such as BL-11 (influential for bone), BL-40, BL-54, and KID-3 (Kidney source point) and local points such as GB-29 and GB-30. *Du Huo Ji Sheng Tang* and *Sheng Tong Zhu Yu Tang* are beneficial herbal medications.

Case 3.6

Signalment: A ten month old English Pointer puppy

History and Exam:

This puppy suffers from acral mutilation syndrome (hereditary sensory neuropathy). This is a rare inherited condition; these dogs have a sensory neuropathy and decreased pain perception in their extremities. They lick and chew their paws and mutilate themselves, some actually chew their toes completely off. This puppy has just chewed ulcers on the legs because the owners have religiously kept the paws bandaged. This puppy is also very undersized or "stunted". There is no known conventional treatment for this condition.

Case 3.6 Assessment:

Licking and chewing can be considered as symptoms of Shen disturbance, usually caused by Heart Yin Deficiency. For the Shen disturbance, the herbal formula Shen Calmer (Modified *Tian Wan Bu Xin Dan*) may be beneficial. Topically, Golden Yellow Salve (*Ru Yi Jin Huang San*) can be used on skin lesions (ulcers). These may be used for one month. If there is no positive result, it may indicate that herbal medicines can not help the dog.

Case 3.7

Signalment: A seven year old, spayed, female dog

History and Exam:

This dog is overweight. Her most recent problem has been the growth of several lipomas.

Her eyes are red and have a mild mucoid discharge. Her gums are tacky to the touch, and her tongue is red. The pulses are mid-deep, strong and slightly fast. The dog likes warm, soft places and eats ravenously.

Case 3.7 Assessment:

The TCVM diagnosis for this dog is Phlegm Stagnation with Liver Yin Deficiency. Her red tongue and tacky gums indicate Yin Deficiency. The red eyes indicate involvement of the Liver. Lipomas are considered to be Phlegm. Acupuncture points including ST-40, ST-36, SP-6, LIV-3 and BL-18 are recommended. The herbal formulas *Er Chen Tang* and *Yi Guan Jian* may be beneficial.

Case 3.8

Signalment: A two year old, neutered, male, Labrador Retriever

History and Exam:

This dog was diagnosed with Type 1 cervical disk disease and underwent surgical fenestration. The pain returned after surgery and has been present ever since. The dog would only turn his neck 30 degrees in either direction. No neurological deficits were seen, and a repeat myelogram revealed a possible mild compression at C4-C5 which did not warrant further surgery. Also, he had a stiff hind end for several months. He was refusing to jump and suffered two short occasions of mild hind limb ataxia. Radiographs and a myelogram suggested some lumbosacral involvement. The dog improved significantly on oral non-steroidal anti-inflammatory drugs.

On physical exam, muscle wasting around shoulders, head and dorsal spinal region was noted. He had lost five kilograms body weight in the last six months. The dog had chronic bilateral otitis externa; mostly yeast, with a brown, sweet smelling, and thick discharge. He has a dry, flaky hair coat, a good appetite and little thirst. The diet is Purina HA formula. He also engages in coprophagia.

The tongue is pale pink with a moist white coating. The pulse is wiry and slippery. There is increased sensitivity at BL 20. The dog prefers soft surfaces, warm areas, and light touch. He has a sweet, friendly personality but is a bit worried.

Case 3.8 Assessment:

The Dog has an Earth constitution. The TCVM diagnosis is Cervical Qi Stagnation with Kidney Jing Deficiency. The local neck pain and disk disease indicate Cervical Qi Stagnation. The Kidney controls the bones and ears. Cervical and lumbosacral diseases, chronic bilateral otitis externa and medical problems at a young age indicate Kidney Jing Deficiency. Kidney Jing Deficiency tends to lead to Blood Deficiency, causing a dry and flaky hair coat. Kidney Jing Deficiency can also cause Deficiency of Ming Men Fire, leading to the secondary Spleen Qi Deficiency. The weight loss and muscle atrophy indicate Spleen Qi Deficiency. Coprophagia may be secondary to the Kidney Jing Deficiency.

The treatment strategies are to first treat the Cervical Qi Stagnation and then treat the underlying Kidney Jing Deficiency. For first two months, use dry needle acupuncture of the *Hua Tuo Jia Ji* points at C3-4, C4-5, and C5-6 as well as electroacupuncture bilaterally at BL-11, GV-20, GB-21, and SI-3. The herbal medication *Xiao Huo Lou Dan* and Cervical formula (*Ge Gen San*) may also be used.

When the cervical pain has resolved, tonify the Kidney Jing. The recommended treatments include the acupoints KID-3, KID-7, BL-23, ST-36, CV-4 and the herbal formula Epimedium Powder (*Sheng Jing San*).

Case 3.9

Signalment: A five year old intact male Golden Retriever

History and Exam:

This dog has a history of exercise intolerance. The Western physical exam revealed no problems. He is of normal size and weight and is well muscled. The owner reports that he seems to tire much more easily than the other dogs. The dog does well in field trials, but when he tires he will just lay down. Recently, after playing Frisbee and jumping up he became anxious and was unable to lie down. He cried when going down stairs.

As a young puppy he was quite ill. He had a severe food allergy to chicken. Before the food allergy was discovered, he was also obsessed with eating dirt. Currently he has occasional loose feces which are more grey in color than his normal stool. At night the dog moves from area to area looking for a cool area to sleep.

During the TCVM physical exam, the dog stared at the doorstopper on the wall. He would respond when called, but would return his attention to the doorstopper. His tongue was normal size, slightly paler than normal and dry. His pulses felt weaker on the right side. There was sensitivity over BL-23.

Case 3.9 Assessment:

The TCVM Pattern is Spleen Qi Deficiency, Qi Stagnation and Shen Disturbance. Exercise intolerance, the weak pulse on the right side and the pale tongue indicate Spleen Qi Deficiency. The crying when going down stairs and the inability to lie down after jumping indicate pain or Qi Stagnation. Eating dirt, staring at the doorstopper, cool-seeking behavior and dryness of the tongue indicate Shen Disturbance due to Heart Yin Deficiency.

The initial step in the treatment plan should be to focus on the Spleen Qi Deficiency and Qi Stagnation. For these, the herbal medicines *Si Jun Zi Tang* and Body Sore (*Sheng Tong Zhu Yu Tang*) are recommended. Acupuncture points including BL-20, ST-36, LIV-3 and *Shan Gen* should be used.

After this step, the dog should be more active and have more energy. If the dog still shows signs of Shen Disturbance, use Shen Calmer (*Tian Wang Bu Xin Dan*). Acupuncture points including HT-7, BL-15, BL-14 and *An Shen* may be used

Case 3.10

Signalment: A ten year old, castrated male Golden Retriever

History and Exam:

The dog has a large tumor in the Triceps muscle. The owner declined biopsy of the tumor, so the tumor type is unknown but it is considered malignant. The dog is very lame on affected leg. The owner reports that the dog is very lethargic and pants a lot. His blood work is within normal limits.

The dog is very friendly, excitable and sensitive. He wiggles his tail and talks all the time. The pulses are rapid, and surging, but are equal on both sides. The tongue is pale purple with a thin white coat. There is sensitivity at BL-20 and BL-21.

Case 3.10 Assessment:

The TCVM diagnosis is Blood Stasis with Qi Deficiency. The tumor, lameness and purple tongue indicate Blood Stasis. Long-term Blood Stasis may turn to Heat, leading to a rapid and surging pulse. The pale tongue, lethargy and sensitivity at BL 20-21 indicate Qi Deficiency.

The treatment should break up Blood Stasis and tonify Qi. It is, however, important to avoid acupoints that are too close to the tumor mass. The herbal formulas *Nei Xiao San* and *Si Jun Zi Tang* may be beneficial. Acupoints including GV-14, ST-36, LIV-3, LI-4 and BL-20 should also be used.

Self Test

Question 3.1: Spleen Qi is derived from which of the following?

      a. Kidney Essence or Yuan Qi
      b. Food Essence (Gu Qi)
      c. Blood
      d. Body Fluid
      e. Shen

Question 3.2: Defensive Qi (Wei Qi) is derived from which of the following?

      a. Kidney Essence or Yuan Qi
      b. the Food Essence (Gu Qi)
      c. Shen
      d. Blood
      e. Body Fluid

Question 3.3: The "De-Qi" (arrival of Qi) response during acupuncture treatment is related to which of the following?

      a. Wei Qi.
      b. Spleen Qi
      c. Jing-Luo Qi
      d. Zheng Qi
      e. Heart Qi

Question 3.4: Which of the following is a Source of Blood?

      a. Gu Qi
      b. Ying Qi (Nutrient Qi)
      c. Essence
      d. Body fluid
      e. All of the above (a, b, c and d)

Question 3.5: The Yuan Qi (Primary Qi) is derived from which of the following?

      a. Kidney Essence or congenital essence
      b. Gu Qi (Food Essence)
      c. Zong Qi
      d. Ying Qi
      e. Wei Qi

Question 3.6: Which of the following statements is NOT True?

    a. Qi is the Conveyor or Transporter of Blood while Blood is the Commander or General of Qi.

    b. Qi is the Commander or General of Blood while Blood is the Conveyor or Transporter of Qi.

    c. Blood Stagnation may cause Qi Stagnation.

    d. Qi Deficiency may cause Blood Deficiency.

    e. Qi Stagnation may cause Blood Stagnation.

Question 3.7: Which of the following statements is NOT true?

    a. Shen is housed in the Heart.

    b. Shen can be disturbed by Excess Cold.

    c. Shen can be disturbed by Deficient Heart Blood.

    d. Signs of Shen disturbance include abnormal behavior and anxiety.

    e. Shen refers to mental activities.

Question 3.8: Which of the following statements is NOT true?

    a. Where there is Qi, there must be life.

    b. Qi gives birth to human beings.

    c. The absence of Qi is death.

    d. Qi is always functional

    e. Qi can be substantial.

Question 3.9: Which of the following statements is True?

    a. Wei Qi circulates inside the blood vessels.

    b. Ying Qi circulates outside the blood vessels.

    c. Wei Qi warms the body surface.

    d. Ying Qi warms the whole body.

    e. Wei Qi holds blood in the vessels.

Question 3.10: Which of the following statements about Zong Qi is NOT true?

    a. Zong Qi is derived from Yuan Qi

    b. Zong Qi forms from the combination of Gu Qi and Qing Qi.

    c. Zong Qi is related to the voice.

    d. Zong Qi promotes the functions of the Heart and Lung.

    e. Zong Qi is formed in the Chest.

Question 3.11: Which statement about Zhong Qi (Middle Qi) is NOT true?

    a. Zhong Qi is the combination of Spleen Qi and Stomach Qi.
    b. Zhong Qi's major function is to hold the inner organs in the normal position.
    c. The signs of Zhong Qi Deficiency include prolapse of anus or uterus.
    d. Zhong Qi is formed in the Lower Jiao (Lower Burner)
    e. Zhong Qi (Middle Qi) is different from Zong Qi.

Question 3.12: Which of the following statements about Body Fluid is NOT true?

    a. Body Fluid is the collective term for all the normal fluids of the body
    b. Body Fluid acts to moisten and nourish the body.
    c. Edema and Phlegm are signs of Body Fluid disorder.
    d. A Disorder of Body Fluid is due to a water metabolism disorder.
    e. Dryness of the hair coat and nose may indicate accumulation (Excess) of Body Fluid

Question 3.13: Which of the following statements about water metabolism is NOT true?

    a. Water metabolism is associated with the Spleen, Lung and Kidney.
    b. The final waste product of Water metabolism is urine.
    c. Edema and diarrhea can be caused by a water metabolism disorder
    d. The Heart is directly associated with water metabolism.
    e. Small Intestine is related to water metabolism

CHAPTER FOUR

ZANG-FU PHYSIOLOGY

> The cure of many diseases is unknown to the physicians of Hellas, because they are ignorant of the whole, which ought to be studied also; for the part can never be well unless the whole is well. …This is the great error of our day in the treatment of the human body, that the physicians separate the soul from the body.
>
> – Plato, *Charmides*

Zang-Fu is the general term for the internal organs of the animal body. This includes the five Zang organs (sometimes described as the six Zang organs), the six Fu organs and the extraordinary Fu organs. The Liver, Heart, Spleen, Lung and Kidney are the five Zang organs. The Pericardium is occasionally considered the sixth Zang organ. The six Fu organs include the Gall Bladder, Stomach, Small Intestine, Large Intestine, Urinary Bladder and San Jiao (Triple Heaters). The brain, marrow, bones, vessels and uterus are known as the extraordinary Fu organs.

A Yin and Yang as well as an Exterior and Interior relationship exists between the Zang organs and the Fu organs. The Zang organs are the Interior or Yin organs, and the Fu organs are the Exterior or Yang organs. Zang and Fu organs may be thought of in pairs. The Zang organs are the "wives", and the Fu organs are their "husbands". Zang and Fu organs work together and support each other, but they are functionally and anatomically different from each other.

The Zang organs are solid; the Fu organs are hollow. The Zang organs mainly function to manufacture and store essential substances including Qi, Blood, and Body Fluid. The Fu organs primarily receive and digest food in addition to waste transport and excretion.

Despite the differences in form and function between the Zang and Fu organs, they are still connected to each other and to the entire body. The Meridians and collaterals form the structural and functional connections within the body. The Meridians join individual Zang and Fu organs into husband-wife pairs. The Zang-Fu organs are also joined to the five sense organs. In the end, every part of the body is combined into a whole.

This is the basis of the integrated concept. When applying these principles, the five Zang organs form the core of clinical investigation; however, all other relevant organs are also considered at the same time.

Table 4.1: Comparison of Zang, Fu and Extraordinary Fu organs

	Zang Organs	Fu Organs	Extraordinary Fu Organs
Metal	Lung (LU)	Large Intestine (LI)	
Earth	Spleen (SP)	Stomach (ST)	
Fire	Heart (HT) Pericardium (PC)	Small Intestine (SI) San Jiao (SJ, TH)	Vessels
Wood	Liver (LIV)	Gall Bladder (GB)	Gall Bladder Uterus
Water	Kidney (KID)	Urinary Bladder (BL)	Brain Marrow Bones
Structure	Solid	Hollow, Tube-like	Hollow
Function	Storage or Conservation	Transmission or Excretion	Storage or Conservation

The Zang Organs

THE HEART

The Heart is located in the thorax, and its Meridian connects with the Small Intestine. Described as the monarch of the Zang-Fu organs, it is the most important Zang-Fu organ. The Heart functions to dominate the Blood and vessels, to house the mind, to control sweat, and to open into the tongue.

Dominating the Blood and Vessels

The phrase "Dominating the Blood and Vessels" means that the Heart governs the circulation of Blood in the vessels. The Heart is the force that propels the flow of Blood. The vessels are the physical structures containing the circulating Blood.

The Heart's ability to maintain the Blood flow depends on the Heart Qi. Normally, the Heart Qi is vigorous, and the Blood circulates in the vessels supplying nutrients to all parts of the body.

Because there is a close relationship between the Heart, the Blood, and the vessels, changes in the amount of Heart Qi or Blood will influence the pulse and the tongue or mouth color. With vigorous Heart Qi and ample Blood, the pulse is regular and strong while the tongue or mouth is the color of a peach flower. Deficient Heart Qi and Blood result in weak, thready pulses and in a pale mouth color.

Housing the Shen

The Shen is the Spirit or Mind. It is the outward appearance of the body's vital activities. In Traditional Chinese Veterinary Medicine (TCVM), the Heart plays a role in mental activities, memory, and sleep. Thus, the Heart of TCVM has functions that are normally associated with the brain's mental activity in Western Medicine.

The functions, dominating the Blood and housing the mind, are interdependent. The Blood is the substance that becomes the foundation for mental activities. For instance, deficient Heart-Blood does not root the mind thus resulting in abnormal activities such as restlessness or anxiety. The Blood is like the rope and anchor of a sailboat. Without them, the boat is at the mercy of the winds and is unable to come to rest. Conversely, abnormalities of the Heart-mind will induce a Deficiency of the Heart Blood. The sailboat tosses about in a storm constantly pulling upon the anchor's rope. With time, the movement and tugging of the boat will cause the rope to weaken and fray.

Controlling the Sweat

Sweat comes from the Body Fluid, which is also an important component of Blood. Thus, Blood and sweat have a common origin. The Heart dominates the Blood; therefore, the Heart can also control perspiration.

The Heart Blood and the Body Fluid are mutually interchangeable. When the Blood is too thick, Body Fluid enters the blood vessels and thins down the Blood. A Deficiency of Heart Blood and Body Fluid will decrease sweat production. Conversely, too much sweating will cause a Body Fluid Deficiency followed by a Heart Blood Deficiency. Because the Heart Blood and the sweat share a close relationship, procedures that induce perspiration should not be used when there is Blood loss or hemorrhage. Similarly, procedures that may cause blood loss should not be used if there has been heavy perspiration. Therefore, diaphoretic medications are contraindicated in cases with blood loss, and hemoacupuncture is avoided in cases with excessive sweating.

Abnormal sweating often results from an imbalance of Heart functions. For example, a Deficiency of Heart Yang or Qi may result in spontaneous sweating. Meanwhile, a Deficiency of Heart Yin or Blood often causes night sweating.

- Excessive sweating ⇨ Deficiency of the Body Fluid ⇨ Deficiency of the Heart Blood

- Heart Yang/Qi Deficient ⇨ Failure to hold sweat ⇨ Spontaneous Sweating ⇨ Body Fluid Deficiency

- Heart Blood/Yin Deficient ⇨ Fails to control Heart Yang/Qi at night ⇨ Night sweating

Opening to the Tongue

The tongue may be considered a branch (or the opening orifice) of the Heart. It acts as a window giving a view of the Heart's condition. An interior portion of the Heart Meridian connects the tongue and the Heart. The Heart controls the color and appearance of the tongue, particularly the tip. In this way, the tongue reflects the physiological activities and pathological changes of the Heart. When the Heart performs normally, the tongue is moist, lustrous, freely moving, and bright red in color. If there is Deficient Heart Blood, the tongue will be pale. A dark red tongue reveals an accumulation of Heat in the Heart.

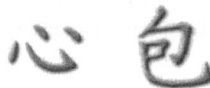

THE PERICARDIUM

The Pericardium, *Xin Bao Luo*, is a protective membrane surrounding the Heart. It is the sixth Zang organ, but it is often not recognized independently due to its close association with the Heart. The Pericardium connects with the Exterior San Jiao Meridian (Triple Heater Meridian).

Its main function is to protect the Heart. When the Xie Qi (pathogenic factors) attempt to invade the Heart, the Pericardium is the first to suffer attack and to battle the Xie Qi. In clinical practice, the Pericardium is regarded as an attachment of the Heart. The symptoms and treatment of pericardial diseases are same as those of the Heart.

THE LUNG

The Lung is located in the thorax. It connects upwards with the throat and opens into the nose. The Lung Meridian connects downwards with the Large Intestine. There is an Interior and Exterior relationship between these organs. The main physiological functions of the Lung are to govern Qi and respiration, to dominate ascending and descending, to regulate water passages, and to control the skin and hair coat.

Governing Qi and Respiration

Governing Qi and respiration is the most important function of the Lung. The Lung collects "Qing Qi" (Cosmic Qi containing oxygen) from the air through inhalation. The Qing Qi can then combine with Gu Qi (Food Qi) from the Spleen.

Qi is the energy that supports the vital activities of the body. "Governing Qi" means that the Lung controls both the Qi of respiration and the Qi of the whole body. The Lung performs a constant exchange and renewal of Qi through respiration. The Lung inhales the Cosmic Qi from natural air and exhales waste Qi from the Interior of the body. This includes the process of exchanging atmospheric oxygen for carbon dioxide from the body. By "getting rid of the stale and taking in the fresh", the Lung ensures an adequate supply of Qi for the whole body's physiological activities.

The Lung is an important organ because it provides Qi to the whole body. It influences the physiological activities of the whole body and participates in the formation of Zong Qi (Pectoral Qi). The Food Qi extracted from food by the Spleen combines with the Cosmic Qi from the Lung to form Zong Qi. Because the formation of Zong Qi occurs in the chest, the chest is called "the Upper Sea of Qi". After producing the Zong Qi, the Lung distributes the Qi all over the body. This provides nourishment for the body's tissues and helps to maintain the functions of these tissues. For example, Qi is essential for the Heart's ability to propel the circulation of Blood. Because the Lung governs Qi, the Lung also plays an important role in maintaining normal Blood circulation.

When the Lung functions normally, Qi passage is unobstructed, and respiration is normal. Lung Qi Stagnation results in respiration disorders such as cough or asthma. Lung Qi Deficiency results in weak respiration, a feeble voice, dyspnea, and weariness.

Dominating Ascending-Descending and Regulating Water Passage

When the Lung functions to "dominate ascending", it is distributing the Wei Qi (Defensive Qi) and Body Fluid to nourish the tissues of the whole body. Failure of the Lung Qi to ascend allows Stagnation thus resulting in coughing and obstructed respiration.

As a general rule, the upper Zang-Fu organs have the function of descending, and the lower Zang-Fu organs have the ascending function. The Lung is positioned as the highest Zang organ in the body. This position is known as the "lid" or "imperial carriage roof". By the nature of its position, the Lung's Qi must descend in order to promote the circulation of Qi and Body Fluid through the body. If this descending function of the Lung is abnormal, the result is cough and shortness of breath.

The Lung is also involved with regulating water movement by supervising Body Fluid circulation and excretion. As part of the ascending function of the Lung, the Lung distributes refined fluid from the Spleen to the skin, muscle, and other tissues. The distribution of Body Fluid to the Kidney and Bladder is part of the Lung's descending function. The Lung sends fluids to the Kidney, which vaporizes part of the fluids back up to the Lung and sends the rest down to the Bladder to become urine.

Controlling the Surface of the Whole Body, Skin and Hair

The body surface, also known as *Pi-mao* ("skin-hair"), includes the skin, the hair follicles, the hair coat and the sweat glands. It provides a protective screen, preventing invasion of the Xie Qi (pathogenic factors) into the body. The Lung and the skin-hair are related both physiologically and pathologically.

The sweat pores function to disperse Qi and sweat and to regulate respiration. This is part of the ascending function of the Lung. For this reason, the sweat pores are called the gate of Qi.

The Lung distributes Wei Qi and Body Fluid, which warms and nourishes the skin-hair. The connection between the Lung and the skin-hair joins them in pathological conditions as well. The skin-hair can reflect the symptoms of Lung problems, and a Xie Qi attack of the skin-hair may be transmitted to the Lung. For instance, a Lung Qi Deficiency will result in sweating, dry skin-hair, or hair loss. An exterior attack of Wind and Cold may cause nasal discharge and cough.

Opening into the Nose

The nose is a branch (or the opening orifice) of the Lung, acting as the pathway for respiration. The health of the nose depends on the function of the Lung. Normal Lung Qi maintains an acute sense of smell and unobstructed respiration. Stagnation of the Lung Qi due to Wind and Cold will cause nasal obstruction and nasal discharge. The accumulation of Heat in the Lung will lead to vibration of the ala nasi and shortness of breath. Because the nose is the offshoot of the Lung, it is also the pathway through which the Xie Qi (pathogenic factors) may invade the Lung. For instance, pathological Heat can pass through the nose and then invade the Lung.

The throat is a gateway of respiration and an organ of speech. It is connected with the Lung through the Meridians. Therefore, the Lung affects the function of the throat. For example, Lung problems will lead to abnormalities of the throat such as a hoarse voice or laryngeal paralysis.

THE SPLEEN

The Spleen is situated in the *Zhong-Jiao* (Middle-Burner). Its Meridian connects with the Stomach. The Stomach and Spleen exist with an Exterior-Interior relationship. The mouth is the offshoot of the Spleen. The Spleen's main physiological functions are to govern transformation and transportation, to control the Blood, to dominate the muscles and the limbs, and to open into the mouth and manifest upon the lips.

Governing Transportation and Transformation

Transportation implies transmission, and transformation implies digestion and absorption. The Spleen functions to transport and transform food and drink in order to extract the necessary substances for the body. This function replenishes energy in the body and nourishes the Zang-Fu organs, limbs, muscles, bone, and skin. Thus, the Spleen is known as the "root Essence of postnatal life" or "the mother of the five Zang organs".

There are two aspects to the transformation and transportation by the Spleen. The first is the method by which the Spleen metabolizes Food to create Food Essence. The second is the way that the Spleen acts upon the fluids of the body.

Transportation and transformation of Food Essence

The Spleen extracts nutrients (such as glucose and amino acids, called Gu Qi or Food Essence) from food and drink through digestion and absorption. The Spleen then transports the Food Essence to the Lung and Heart. The Food Qi is carried to the entire body by the Meridians in order to meet the requests of the tissues.

Therefore, the function of the Spleen in transporting and transforming Food Essences refers to the digestion, absorption, and transportation of nutrient substances. When the Spleen performs normally, the digestion will function well, and there will be a good appetite, normal absorption, and regular bowel movements. However, a Spleen Deficiency will impair this function resulting in a poor appetite, poor digestion, and diarrhea.

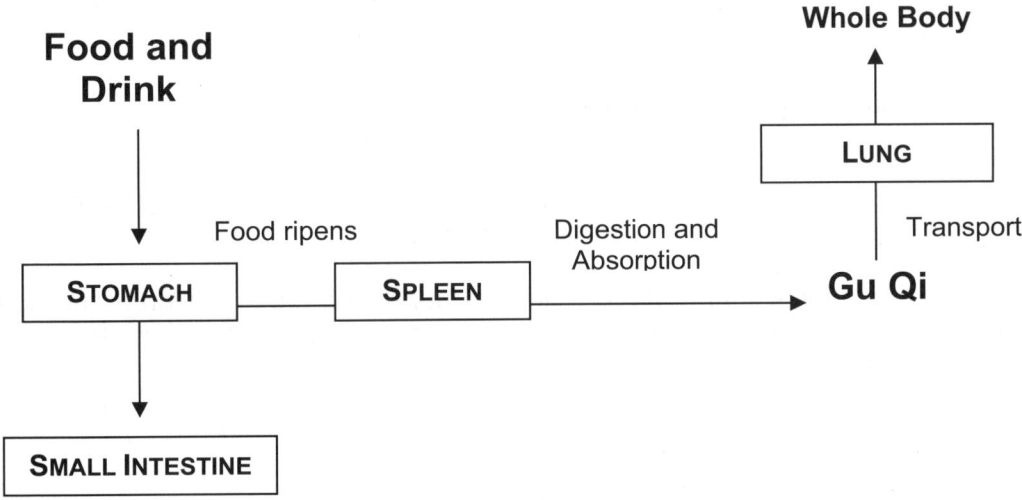

Figure 4.1: Food metabolism pathway

Transportation and transformation of water-dampness

The Spleen also controls the transformation, separation and transportation of water-dampness (such as the body fluids). This refers to water metabolism. The Spleen transports the water upward to the Lung for distribution to the skin and other parts of the body. The Spleen also helps discharge the fluid from the body after metabolism. The Spleen ensures that the various tissues of the body are both properly moistened and simultaneously free from water or Damp retention. Impairment of this function results in retention of water or Damp. Water or Damp that remains in the intestinal tract results in diarrhea. Damp in the abdominal cavity results in ascites. Edema results from Damp under the skin. Phlegm occurs with Damp retention in the respiratory tract.

The Spleen Qi is responsible for the ability to transport and transform both Food Essences and water-dampness. Normally, the Spleen Qi is always characterized by ascending movement in contrast to the descending movement of the Stomach Qi. This paired up-down motion between the Spleen and Stomach plays a key role in Qi flow. Disorder of this relationship can lead to a variety of illnesses. Prolonged diarrhea or rectal prolapse may occur if the Spleen Qi sinks. One treats sinking of the Spleen Qi by uplifting the Spleen Qi.

Controlling the Blood

The Spleen Qi keeps the Blood circulating within the vessels and prevents extravasation. If the Spleen Qi is healthy, Blood will circulate normally and stay within the vessels. A Spleen Qi Deficiency allows the Blood to spill out of the vessels resulting in various types of hemorrhage such as bloody feces, hematuria and petechiae.

Dominating the Muscles and the Limbs

The Spleen transports and transforms the Food Essences to nourish the whole body, especially the muscles and limbs. If this function is normal, the muscles and limbs remain well developed and strong. However, a Deficiency of Spleen Qi will lead to weakness, emaciation, or muscular atrophy.

Opening into Mouth and Manifesting the Lips

The mouth is an offshoot (the opening orifice) of the Spleen. The intake and chewing of food is closely related to the Spleen's function of transportation and transformation. Dysfunction of the Spleen results in a poor appetite.

The lips are the exterior aperture of the Spleen. They reflect the condition of the Spleen. When the Spleen functions normally, the lips are bright red like a peach flower. If the Spleen Qi is deficient, the lips are pale.

THE LIVER

The Liver is situated in the right flank. There is an Exterior and Interior relationship between the Gall Bladder and Liver. The main functions of the Liver are to store Blood, to maintain the smooth flow of Qi, and to control the tendons.

Storing Blood

The Liver stores Blood and regulates the volume of Blood in circulation. The volume of Blood circulating in various parts of the body changes according to the physical activity level. When an animal rests or lies down, a part of the Blood flows back to the Liver. When the animal is active, Blood in the Liver flows to the body to meet its physical needs. The Liver's ability to store Blood is closely related to the body's exercise tolerance levels. If there is sufficient Blood in the Liver, the body will not fatigue easily. When there is a Liver Blood Deficiency, the animal will quickly become tired.

Maintaining the Smooth Flow of Qi

Maintaining the smooth flow of Qi is the most important of all the Liver functions. In Traditional Chinese Veterinary Medicine, the flow of Qi is a general description of how the Zang-Fu organs are functioning. When the Qi flow is smooth (normal), the Zang-Fu organs function normally. If the flow of Qi is abnormal, there is disorder in the body.

Liver Qi is normally characterized as unrestrained and averse to depression. Disease results from Liver Qi Stagnation. There are three aspects to the Liver's function of maintaining smooth Qi flow. The Liver's ability to maintain the free flow of Qi is important for the digestive ability of the Spleen and Stomach, for the vital activities of the whole body, and for proper function of the Water metabolism pathways.

Ensuring the Spleen and Stomach digestive function

The Liver has an important influence on digestion. The Liver's control of Qi flow allows it to maintain smooth flow of the ascending and descending functions of the Spleen and Stomach respectively. It is also involved with bile secretion. When the Liver Qi flows smoothly, the Stomach can ripen and rot food, and the Spleen can extract and distribute the Food Qi. Stagnation of the Liver Qi causes disorder of the Qi flow. This may cause obstruction of food transport and transformation resulting in poor appetite, diarrhea, and abdominal fullness.

Maintaining normal vital activities of the whole body

Liver Qi, in addition to the Heart, is closely related to the body's vital activities. Only when the Liver maintains smooth Qi flow are the Qi and Blood harmonious and the vital activities normal. If the Liver Qi stagnates, mental depression may develop.

Ensuring the smooth flow of water-damp path

If there is Stagnation of Liver Qi, obstruction of the *San Jiao* (Triple Heater) or of the water metabolism pathways may occur. The end result is edema or ascites.

Controlling the Jin

Jin may be translated as fascia, sinews, ligaments and tendons. The Jin refers to the main tissues linking the joints and muscles, which are the means for movement of the limbs. The sinews' capacity to contract and relax depends on the nourishment and moisture from the Liver Blood. If Liver Blood is abundant, the sinews will be moistened and nourished thus ensuring both smooth movements of the joints and good muscle action. Deficient Liver Blood fails to moisten and nourish the tendons resulting in convulsion and weakness of the limbs.

Opening into the Eyes

The eyes are an offshoot (or the opening orifice) of the Liver. The Liver Meridian connects exteriorly with the eyes forming a link between them. If the Liver Blood is abundant, the eyes will be moistened normally. Deficiency of the Liver Yin and Blood may lead to dryness of the eyes. Excessive Heat of the Liver may cause redness, swelling, and pain of the eyes.

肾

THE KIDNEY

The Kidney is located on either side of the lumbar spine. Traditional Chinese Veterinary Medicine describes this area as "the home of the Kidney". The Kidney Meridian connects with the Bladder, and there is an Interior-Exterior relationship between the Kidney and Bladder. Its main functions are to store Essence, to govern water, to control the reception of Qi, to produce marrow to fill up the brain, to dominate bone, to open into the ears, and to control the two orifices.

Storing Essences

The Kidney Essence, the Kidney Yin or base Yin, forms the material base of the animal body. The Kidney Essence consists of two parts: Congenital Essence and Acquired Essence.

Congenital Essence is inherited from the parents. This is the base substance of an animal's vital activities. It nourishes the fetus before birth then controls development, growth, aging, and reproduction after birth. A Deficiency of Kidney Essence may cause infertility or retarded growth.

The Acquired Essence, also called the Essence of Zang-Fu, is the basic substance maintaining the vital activities. The Spleen extracts it from food during the transformation and transportation of Food Qi.

The Congenital and Acquired Essences rely on and promote each other. Acquired Essence replenishes the Congenital Essence. However, Acquired Essence is only produced with the assistance of the Congenital Essence.

One perspective may view the Congenital Essence as the total Life Force of an individual. Life continues as long as Congenital Essence remains; however, once the Congenital Essence has been depleted, life ceases. Starting with the first day of life, the Congenital Essence slowly decreases with each passing day.

Congenital Essence is like an oil lamp that remains lit from the day of birth. Each individual is born with a certain amount of oil that is his or her lifetime supply. The flame only exists as long as there is oil in the reservoir. The more brightly the flame burns, the more rapidly the fuel is diminished. Although there is no way to stop the use of this fuel, additional fuel sources can be used to support life. This is the Acquired Essence. The Acquired Essence allows the Congenital Essence flame to burn less brightly and to conserve the fuel. Acquired Essence is the alternative, renewable fuel that is gathered during life and supplements the base fuel. A healthy, balanced lifestyle with a good diet, exercise, and meditation promotes the production of Acquired Essence and reduces the depletion of the Congenital Essence.

Governing Water

According to the Five Element theory, the Kidney belongs to the Water element. It governs the transformation and transportation of body fluids. The Kidney Qi functions as a gate, regularly opening and closing to control the flow of Body Fluids. Failure of the Kidney Qi to open and close causes a disturbance of water metabolism and results in such problems as edema.

First, the Stomach receives the water that an animal drinks. The Spleen then transmits the water to the Lung. The Lung's descending function sends part of the fluid down to the Kidney. The Kidney Qi further divides the fluid into clear and turbid parts. The clear part is transmitted back up to the Lung while the turbid part flows down to the Bladder. The turbid part in the Bladder forms urine, which is then excreted.

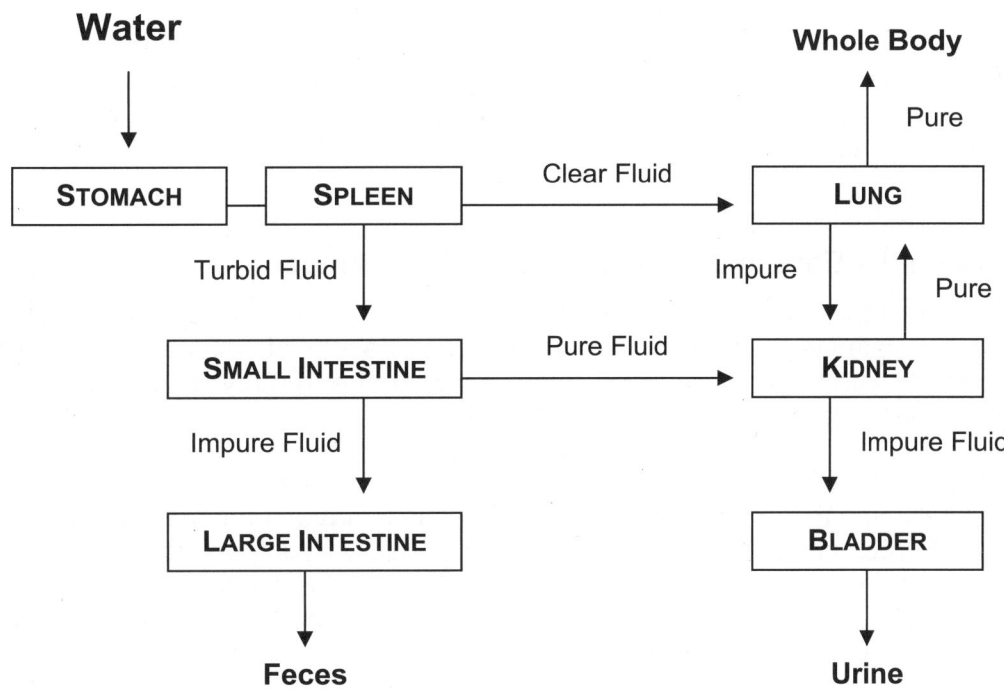

Figure 4.2: Water metabolism pathway

Controlling the Reception of Qi

Although the Lung controls the Qi and respiration, the Cosmic (Qing) Qi of the air inhaled by the Lung should go down to the Kidney. The Kidney responds by "holding down" or "grasping" this Qi. The Lung begins the process of inhalation, but the Kidney grasps the Cosmic Qi and pulls it down, thus assisting a deep intake of breath. If the Kidney fails to grasp Qi due to Kidney Qi Deficiency, the Lung's descending function will be affected, resulting in shortness of breath and asthma. This is a common cause of chronic heaves or asthma.

Dominating Bone, Producing Marrow and Filling up the Brain

The Essences, stored by the Kidney, can produce marrow. The marrow fills up the bone cavities and supports their growth and development. When Kidney Essences are abundant, the bone marrow has a rich source of production and the bones are well nourished and hard. However, with a Deficiency of Kidney Essence, the bone does not receive nourishment thus resulting in abnormal development or lumbar and hind limb weakness. Therefore, the acupuncture points (such as BL-23) or herbal medicines (such as Psoralea *Bu Gu Zhi*) that promote the Kidney also support the bones.

The marrow in Traditional Chinese Medicine refers to spinal marrow (spinal cord) and to bone marrow. The spinal marrow ascends to connect with the brain. When the Kidney Essences are abundant, the spinal marrow has a rich source of production, the brain is well nourished, and mental activities are normal.

Because teeth are considered the surplus of bone, both teeth and bones rely on nourishment by the Kidney Essences. When Kidney Essences are sufficient, the teeth are well nourished and strong. However, Deficiency of Kidney Essences may result in loose or missing teeth.

Opening into the Ears and Controlling the Two Orifices

The Kidney Essence also nourishes the ears; thus, they are physiologically and pathologically related to the Kidney. When the Kidney Essence is abundant, the ears are well nourished and hearing is acute. Deficiency of the Kidney Essence results in deafness or hearing loss.

The Kidney controls the function of the two orifices. These two orifices are the urethra/genitalia and the anus. The urethra and genitalia have the respective functions of urination and procreation. Therefore, the Kidney is also very important for reproduction in addition to urine excretion. Although urination is a Bladder function, the process requires Kidney Qi. A Deficiency of Kidney Qi results in frequent urination or lack of urination. The second orifice, the anus, has the function of discharging feces. The anus, although anatomically related to the Large Intestine, is functionally related to the Kidney. Deficiency of Kidney Qi results in constipation or diarrhea.

Table 4.2: Functions and locations of the Zang organs

Zang Organ	Element	Major Function	San Jiao Location
Heart	Fire	• House Shen (spirit and mind) • Govern Blood and vessels	Upper Jiao
Lung	Metal	• Govern Qi • Distribute Food Qi and Body Fluid	Upper Jiao
Spleen	Earth	• Transform and transport Food Qi and Body Fluid (water-dampness)	Middle Jiao
Liver	Wood	• Store Blood • Maintain free flow of Qi	Middle or Lower Jiao
Kidney	Water	• Store Essence (Jing) • Govern Water pathway • Govern bones	Lower Jiao

Table 4.3: Influences of the five Zang organs

Zang Organ	External Opening	Tissues Influenced	Major Five Treasure Associations
Heart	Tongue	Vessels Sweat	Shen Blood
Lung	Nose	Skin Hair coat Sweat glands	Qi Body Fluid
Spleen	Lips	Muscles Limbs	Qi Body Fluid Blood
Liver	Eyes	Tendons Ligaments Fascia	Qi Blood
Kidney	Ears	Bones Bone marrow Brain	Jing Body Fluid

Heart

The Heart is the King of the five Zang organs. It rules the entire body, and the entire body tries to protect the Heart. When the Heart is aversely affected, the problem is usually severe, difficult to treat, or requires a greater number of treatments. Shen disturbance is one of the major signs of Heart disease. This may show up as anxiety, restlessness or abnormal behaviors such as licking the toes, tail-chasing or barking at night.

Dominating the Blood and Vessels
- Heart Qi is the motive force propelling the Blood flow in the vessels

Housing Shen
- Shen is the outward appearance of the vital activities of the whole body
- Provides inner peace
- Maintains mental activities, memory, and sleep

Controlling the Sweat
- Excessive sweating ⇨ Body Fluid Deficiency ⇨ Heart Blood Deficiency
- Deficient Heart Yang/Qi ⇨ Spontaneous sweating ⇨ Body Fluid Deficiency
- Deficient Heart Blood/Yin ⇨ Uncontrolled night Heart Yang/Qi ⇨ Night sweating

Lung

The Lung, as the uppermost organ, is like a canopy. It protects and shelters all the other Zang-Fu organs. The Lung serves as the Prime Minister, helping the Heart rule the entire body. Despite this governing and protective role, the Lung is the most delicate organ in the body. It is vulnerable to attack by Wind, Heat, Cold, and Dryness. The worst enemy of the Lung is Pathogenic Dryness.

Governing Qi and Respiration
- Inhales Qing Qi (Cosmic Qi) from the natural air
- Exhales stale Qi (waste Qi) from the Interior of the body
- Includes the process of O_2 and CO_2 exchange
- Zong Qi (pectoral Qi) is formed from Qing Qi and Gu Qi and controls voice
- The chest, as the place of Zong Qi formation, is "the sea of Qi"

Dominating Ascending-Descending
Ascending:
- Distribution of Wei Qi to the surface
- Distribution of Body Fluid to the surface and other areas

Descending:
- Sends Qi down to the Kidney
- Sends Body Fluid down to the Kidney and Bladder

Regulating Water Passage
- Controls the circulation and excretion of Body Fluid
- Distributes Body Fluid to the body surface
- Sends Body Fluid down to the Kidney and Bladder

Controlling the Surface of the Whole Body, Skin, and Hair
- Forms a protective screen preventing Xie Qi invasion into the body

Spleen

The Spleen is the minister of the food department. It is the factory that generates Qi and Blood. Because Qi and Blood are essential for Zang-Fu organ function, the Spleen is known as "the mother of the five Zang organs". Also, excess Qi or Blood produced by the Spleen can be transformed into Kidney Essence. Thus, the Spleen is also called the "root of postnatal life". The Spleen prefers dryness and fragrance and dislikes dampness. Wet or Damp conditions antagonize the Spleen, but anything that is dry may help the Spleen.

Governing Transportation and Transformation (*Yun-hua*)
- Digestion and absorption of Food/Drink ⇨ Gu Qi ⇨ Nourish the entire body
- Food enters the Stomach and Spleen where it is rotted and digested. Waste products are sent down to the Small Intestine, and Gu Qi is sent up to the Lung for distribution to the whole body.

Normal:
- Spleen Qi always ascends
- Stomach Qi is always descending
- Spleen Qi Up with Stomach Qi down forms the key pivot of Qi Flow (Qi-Ji)
- Normal Qi-Ji maintained with ST-36 ⇨ Normal Zang-Fu functions

Abnormal:
- Spleen Qi descends ⇨ Diarrhea, Fatigue, Organ prolapse
- Stomach Qi ascends ⇨ Vomiting, Nausea, Belching
- Disordered Qi-Ji pivot ⇨ Many additional illnesses

Controlling the Blood
- Keeps the Blood circulating within the vessels, preventing extravasation

Dominating the Muscles and Four Limbs
- Spleen Qi Deficiency leads to weakness of the limbs, emaciation, muscular atrophy

Liver

The Liver is the General or commander of the body. It is unrestrained and freely moving, abhorring stress. Any stress, whether from emotion or drugs, will lead to Liver Qi stagnation. Liver Qi is never deficient, but there can be a Liver Blood or a Liver Yin Deficiency. If a disorder does occur, the Liver Qi is always either excessive or stagnant.

Storing Blood
Regulates the Blood volume in circulation
- Blood storage in the Liver while at rest provides a reservoir of Blood
- Blood leaves the Liver while active to meet the body's physical needs

Determines the body's threshold for fatigue
- Sufficient Liver Blood ⇨ Does not tire easily ⇨ Good athlete
- Deficient Liver Blood ⇨ Tires easily ⇨ Poor athlete

Regulates Menstruation and Estrous cycling

Maintaining Smooth and Free Flow of Qi
- Smooth Qi flow is a basic requirement for the Zang-Fu organs, especially the Spleen and Stomach
- Permits Bile secretion
- Balances emotions and maintains a good mood

Controlling the Sinews
- Influences the ligaments, tendons, paws, nails, and hooves

Kidney

The Kidney is the Minister of the Water pathway. The Kidney is the root of prenatal life. With age, the Kidney essence gradually diminishes. Kidney essence should be always conserved. If there is a disorder, the Kidney is almost always deficient.

Storing Jing (Essences)

Congenital Jing:
- Inherited from the parents
- Congenital foundation of life (Genetic materials: DNA, genes)
- Nourishes the fetus before birth
- Regulates development, growth, aging, and reproduction after birth
- Deficiency of Kidney Jing ⇨ Infertility and retarded growth
- Controls the 7-year (female) and 8-year (male) cycles of development and growth

Acquired Jing:
- Also called Essence of Zang-Fu
- Basic substance for maintenance of the vital activities
- Extracted from Food Qi by Spleen

Governing Water Metabolism
- Acts as the gate of water

Controlling the Reception of Qi
- Holds or pulls Qi down from Lung
- It is in charge of inhalation

Dominating Bone, Producing Marrow, and Filling up the Brain
- Influences bones and the central nervous system

Relationships among the Five Zang Organs

HEART AND LUNG

Qi and Blood

The Heart rules the Blood. The Lungs govern Qi. Qi moves blood, and Blood carries Qi. Thus, the Qi from the Lung is required to move the Blood of the Heart.

Qi Stagnation may cause Blood Stagnation, and Blood Stagnation may cause Qi Stagnation. Qi Deficiency leads to Blood Stagnation or Deficiency. Blood Deficiency leads to Qi Deficiency.

Zong Qi

Zong Qi influences both Lung and Heart. Zong Qi dominates respiration and promotes blood circulation. Some texts consider Zong Qi a combination of Lung Qi and Heart Qi.

A weak voice indicates weakness of the Zong Qi. Lung Qi weakness may lead to Heart Qi Stagnation which may cause Heart Blood Stagnation with signs such as palpitations, chest pain, and a purple tongue. Deficient Heart Qi or Yang may lead to a disorder of Lung functions resulting in cough and asthma.

Five Element Theory

According to Ke cycle, Fire (Heart) controls Metal (Lung). Excessive Heart Fire dries up Lung Yin causing a dry cough, a dry nose, and thirst.

HEART AND SPLEEN

Blood

The Heart rules the Blood. The Spleen generates and holds the Blood.

Deficient Spleen Qi can lead to a Heart Blood Deficiency. Overwork or too much worry leads to a Spleen Qi Deficiency (poor appetite, fullness in abdomen, loose stool, and fatigue) which then may cause a Heart Blood Deficiency (palpitations, insomnia, poor memory, anxiety, restlessness, dizziness, and pale tongue or complexion).

Five Element Theory

According to the Five Elements, Fire creates the Earth. The Spleen requires two types of Fire: Emperor's Fire and Minister's Fire. The Emperor's Fire refers to the Heart Yang; the Minister's Fire refers to Kidney Yang or Ming-men Fire (life-gate Fire). If the Heart is deficient then Spleen Qi may become deficient.

HEART AND LIVER

Blood

The Heart rules the Blood. The Liver stores Blood and regulates its volume.

Blood Deficiency may be either Heart Blood Deficiency or Liver Blood Deficiency. Liver Blood Deficiency may cause Heart Blood Deficiency, and Heart Blood Deficiency may cause Liver Blood Deficiency. Patients with both Heart and Liver Blood Deficiency are commonly seen in practice. This condition is called a whole Blood Deficiency. The clinical signs include a pale complexion or tongue, palpitations, poor memory, insomnia, dizziness, numbness of limbs, and pale, scant menses.

Shen

The Heart houses the Shen, and the Liver dominates the free flow of Qi and emotions. Stress, whether emotional, environmental or medication-related, often causes Liver Qi Stagnation. Liver Qi Stagnation easily transforms into Fire, which disturbs the Heart Shen (mother-child cycle) and results in insomnia, restlessness, hyperactivity, anxiousness, red eyes, and a short temper.

HEART AND KIDNEY

The Connection of the Heart Fire and the Kidney Water

According to the Five Elements, the Heart belongs to Fire and the Kidney belongs to Water. If there is no cooling system, the Heart Fire easily becomes excessive and transforms into pathogenic Heat. On the other hand, the Kidney Water easily becomes pathogenic Cold if there is no warming system. Water and Fire have a Yin-Yang relationship, each supporting and controlling the other.

In normal physiological conditions, the Heart Fire and the Kidney water assist each other across their bonds. The Heart Fire should go down to warm the Kidney, while the Kidney water rises up to cool the Heart. This physiological process is called "*Xin Shen Xiang Jiao*" which means "Connection between Heart and Kidney". If the Heart and Kidney do not connect with each other, it is called *Xin Shen Bu Jiao*.

Disconnection of the Heart and Kidney

Xin Shen Bu Jiao, the disconnection between the Heart and Kidney, is a common clinical problem. As a result of this disconnection, there is too much Heat in the Heart (the upper jiao) and/or there is too much Cold in the Kidney (the lower jiao). The symptoms of this condition include hyperactivity, restlessness, insomnia, ulcers on the tongue, impotence, tinnitus, dizziness, and weak, cold hind limbs and back.

The TCVM treatment strategy for this problem is to tonify (warm) the Kidney and to clear (cool) the Heart Fire. The acupuncture points KID-3 and HT-7 may be selected. *Jiao Tai Wan*, an herbal formula consisting of Coptis *Huang Lian* and Cinnamon *Rou Gui*, is designed for this problem. Coptis clears Heart Fire, and Cinnamon warms Kidney Yang.

Water Freezes the Heart

Shui Qi Ling Xin, water over-controlling or freezing the Heart, is another common problem. When Kidney Yang is weak, it fails to control water resulting in water retention. It further causes the Heart to become frozen, and both Heart and Kidney develop Yang Deficiency. The clinical signs include edema, heart failure, palpitations, purple tongue, cool extremities and poor circulation. The treatment principle is to warm the Kidney Yang and to clear the water. Moxibustion on acupoints such as *Bai Hui*, GV-4, CV-4 and CV-6 may be useful. *Zhen Wu Tang*, an herbal formula, is designed for this purpose.

LUNG AND SPLEEN

Qi and the Five Elements

The Spleen generates Gu Qi. The Lung distributes Qi throughout the whole body.

When Spleen Qi is weak, the production of Lung Qi is impaired. This is known as Earth not nourishing Metal. Its clinical signs include lethargy, fatigue, weakness of the limbs, weak voice, weak panting, shortness of breath, exercise intolerance, loose stool, and poor appetite. Strengthening the Earth to generate Metal is the treatment.

Body Fluid metabolism

Both Spleen and Lung have important effects on Body Fluid movement throughout the body. When Spleen Qi is weak, fluids may stagnate and develop into phlegm. Phlegm is commonly stored in the Lung where it impairs Lung functions and causes coughing or asthma.

LUNG AND LIVER

Qi Ji, the flow of Qi

The Liver sustains the free, smooth flow of Qi. Normally, the Liver Qi moves upward, which helps the Lung to exhale (ascending function). The Lung's descending function (inhalation) prevents the Liver Qi from aggressively or excessively rising. If the Liver Qi rises too much (Liver Yang Rising), it will transform into Fire and will result in red eyes, tears, dry eyes, and dizziness.

Liver Fire Insulting Lung

The Liver Qi stagnates and transforms into Fire. The Liver Fire flares up to damage the Lung Yin (Fire melts the Metal) and results in a dry cough, hemoptysis, asthma, red eyes (red face), hyperactivity, and anger.

Lung Over-Controls the Liver

With sustained Lung Heat, the Lung over-controls (Cheng cycle) the Liver. This results in Stagnation of Liver Qi. The clinical symptoms include cough, hypochondriac pain, painful breathing, and depression.

LUNG AND KIDNEY

Water transportation

The Lung regulates water movement. The Lung's descending function sends fluids down to the Kidney. The Ming-men Fire (Kidney Yang) evaporates some of the fluids. This mist from the Kidney floats back up to the Lung where it provides moisture to the Lung.

When Lung Qi is weak, the Lung's ability to send fluids down to the Kidney and Bladder is impaired, leading to Kidney Qi Deficiency. The clinical signs of patients with this disharmony typically include urinary incontinence, edema, water retention, cough or asthma, and hind limb weakness.

When Kidney Yin is deficient, there is an overall reduction of fluids in the lower jiao. Subsequently, the Kidney is unable to send enough fluids up to the Lung. The Lung is inadequately moistened and a Lung Yin Deficiency develops. Clinically, this appears as a dry throat in the evening and night, a dry, hacking cough, night panting or sweating, and warm paws.

Qi

The Lung governs Qi, and the Kidney holds down (grasps) Qi. When Lung Qi and Kidney Qi both are deficient, the patient exhibits shortness of breath, asthma, exercise intolerance, general fatigue, difficult inhalation and weakness of the hind limbs and back.

LIVER AND SPLEEN

Qi flow

The direction of flow for both Liver and Spleen Qi is upward. The major role of the Liver is ensuring the smooth flow of Qi throughout the entire body. It assists the upward flow of Spleen Qi. Liver Qi is also responsible for the flow of bile. This sets up the digestive process in preparation for the Spleen's transformation, separation and transportation of ingested food and water.

Liver Over-controlling the Spleen

When Liver Qi stagnates due to emotional, environmental, or pharmaceutical stress, the ability of Spleen Qi to flow upwards becomes disrupted. The resulting clinical signs include abdominal distention, hypochondriacal fullness or pain, loose stool and poor appetite.

Spleen Insulting the Liver

When Spleen Qi is weak, it permits food accumulation and retention in the middle jiao. This accumulated food easily transforms into Damp-Heat which is capable of restricting Liver Qi flow. In this way, the Spleen counter-controls the Liver (Ru cycle). The clinical signs include abdominal distention, hypochondriac pain, irritability, vomiting, poor appetite, and a yellow tongue.

LIVER AND KIDNEY

Essence and Blood

Blood is stored in the Liver, just as Jing is stored in the Kidney. Liver Blood nourishes Kidney essence and helps to renew its supply. Kidney Jing produces bone marrow, which in turn is responsible for producing Liver Blood. Thus, it is said that there is "the same origin of both Liver and Kidney" or that there is "the same origin of Jing and Blood".

Kidney Jing Deficiency can lead to Liver Blood Deficiency. The clinical symptoms are dizziness, blurred vision, tinnitus, infertility and lower back pain.

Five Element Theory

By virtue of the Sheng-cycle between Water and Wood, a Kidney Yin Deficiency can cause a Liver Yin Deficiency. Deficient Liver Yin fails to constrain the Liver Yang, resulting in Liver Yang Rising. Clinical signs of this condition include irritability, headaches, dizziness, tinnitus, and blurred vision. Nourishment of Water (nourishing Kidney Yin) is the key to treating this disorder.

SPLEEN AND KIDNEY

Sources of Jing

The Kidney is the root of Prenatal Jing. The Spleen is the root of postnatal Jing. Prenatal Jing is continually depleted by the day to day Qi requirements of the body. The Postnatal Jing, created by the Spleen Qi from food (Gu Qi), can replenish the Prenatal Jing.

When Spleen Qi is weak, inadequate Qi is produced to maintain the body stores of Kidney Jing. Patients with both Spleen Qi Deficiency and Kidney Qi Deficiency will show anorexia, dizziness, low back pain, and tinnitus.

When Spleen Qi is deficient, the Spleen fails to transform and transport body fluids. This results in the accumulation of dampness, which can damage the Kidney's ability to govern water.

Ming-men Fire (Life Gate Fire)

The Prenatal Qi is an active form of Prenatal Jing. It consists of Prenatal (Kidney) Yin and Yang. Kidney Yang (Prenatal Yang) provides the Fire needed for the digestive and transformation processes controlled by the Spleen.

When Kidney Yang is deficient, the Ming-men Fire cannot warm the Spleen. Without warmth from the Ming-men Fire, the Spleen is unable to transport and transform food. This results in watery or cold diarrhea and chilliness. This disharmony is known as Fire failing to nourish Earth. In addition, Deficient Kidney Yang cannot provide the Fire that Spleen needs in order to transform the body fluids. This results in the accumulation of dampness, which leads to diarrhea, cold and edema.

In summary, the Kidney is the most important organ of prenatal origin while the Spleen is the most important of postnatal origin. The Kidney Yin is the source of the global body fluid (whole body Yin). The Kidney Yin nourishes the Liver Yin, Heart Yin, Spleen Yin, and Lung Yin. A Deficiency of Kidney Yin easily leads to a Deficiency of Liver, Heart, Spleen or Lung Yin. The Kidney Yang (Ming-men Fire) is the Minister Fire that supports the Heart Fire (Heart Yang) or Emperor Fire. The Kidney Yang is also a major source of Spleen Yang. Weakness of Kidney Yang may cause a Spleen Yang Deficiency. On the other hand, a chronic Spleen Yang Deficiency may cause a Kidney Yang Deficiency because more Kidney Yang is consumed when Spleen Yang is weak.

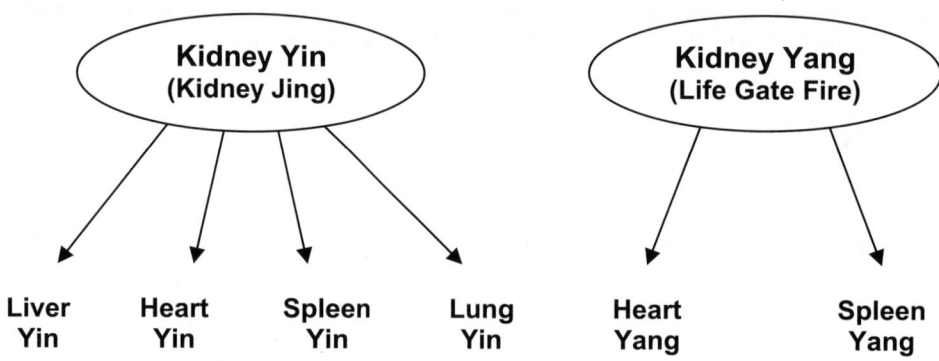

Figure 4.3: The source of Zang organ Yin and Yang

The Spleen is the center of the five Zang organs. The Spleen Qi generates Food Qi and Blood, which nourish the internal organs and whole body. Thus, the Spleen is called "the root of postnatal life", or "the Mother of Five Zang Organs".

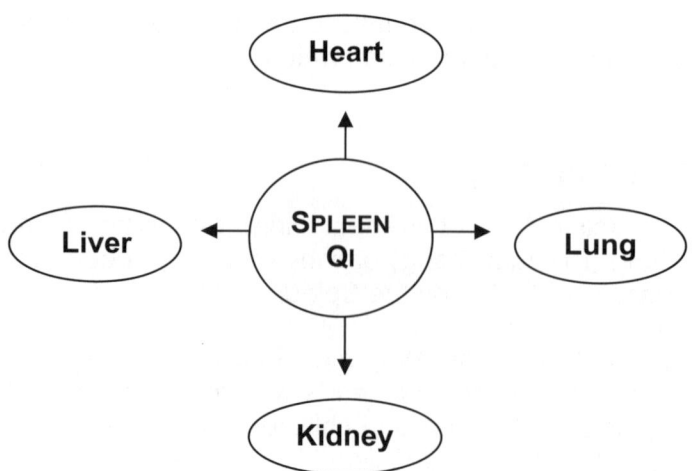

The Fu Organs

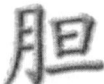

THE GALL BLADDER

The Gall Bladder is attached to the Liver, and it has an external-internal relationship with the Liver. Although the horse does not have a Gall Bladder sac, it does have a bile duct.

Similar to the transportation function of the other Fu organs, the Gall Bladder functions to store and excrete bile and to assist digestion. The Gall Bladder occupies a special place among the six Fu organs because it is the only one that does not deal with food, drink, and their waste products. For this reason it is classified as a member of both the six Fu organs and the extraordinary Fu organs.

When the Gall Bladder functions normally, its Qi descends and it excretes bile into the intestines to aid digestion. When its Qi is stagnant, the bile may go the wrong way, resulting in jaundice. Even though Liver Qi is never deficient, the Gall Bladder Qi can be deficient. The major clinical sign of a Gall Bladder Qi Deficiency is the inability to make a decision or judgment.

THE STOMACH

The Stomach is located in the front part of abdomen. It connects cranially with the esophagus and caudally with the small intestines. It functions mainly to receive food and to rot or decompose food. Food enters the Stomach where it is rotted and ripened. The essential substances are then transported and transformed by the Spleen to supply the whole body. After transformation in the Stomach, the food is passed down to the small intestines for further separation and absorption.

The Stomach prepares the ground for the Spleen to separate and extract the refined Essence from food. The Stomach and Spleen, acting in conjunction, are the organs mainly responsible for digestion and absorption, and they are the origin of Qi and Blood. Therefore, Stomach and Spleen are called "the acquired foundation".

The Stomach Qi is responsible for the functions of receiving and digesting food. The Stomach Qi has a downward movement. Normally, the Stomach sends transformed food downward to the Small Intestine. Thus, digestion is normal if Stomach Qi descends, but disturbance of that downward movement results in decreased appetite, indigestion, or vomiting (dog or cat).

小 肠

THE SMALL INTESTINE

The Small Intestine connects cranially with the Stomach and caudally with the Large Intestine. Its main functions are to receive food and drink from the Stomach and Spleen, to further digest food, to absorb essential substances, and to separate the ingesta into "clean" or "turbid" parts.

The Small Intestine separates the clean part, which includes essential substances and water, from the turbid part. The Spleen and Lung transmit the clean part to the whole body. The Small Intestine transmits the turbid parts to their respective organs. The residue of food goes to the Large Intestine, and the residue of water goes to the Kidney and Bladder. Because the Small Intestine is involved with separations of the food and water-fluid (drink), dysfunction of the Small Intestine may adversely influence digestion as well as interfere with the processes of defecation and urination.

大 肠

THE LARGE INTESTINE

The Large Intestine connects cranially with the Small Intestine and caudally with the anus. Its main functions are to receive the waste materials from the Small Intestine, to reabsorb some of the fluids, and to form the remainder into feces for excretion. If the Large Intestine fails to reabsorb fluid, loose feces or diarrhea may occur. If there is extreme Heat, which consumes the fluid of the Large Intestine, constipation may occur.

膀 胱

THE BLADDER

The Bladder is situated in the back part of abdomen. It functions to store and to excrete the urine. The turbid part of Body Fluid, from the Small Intestine or the Lung, goes to the Kidney to form urine. The urine descends to the Bladder, where it will be discharged via the Kidney Yang activity. A Kidney Yang Deficiency may cause frequent urination or urinary incontinence. The accumulation of Heat-Damp in the Bladder may lead to difficult or painful urination or to bloody urination.

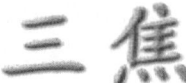

THE SANJIAO

The Sanjiao, also known as the Triple Heater, Triple Burner or Triple Warmer, is located separately from the Zang-Fu organs in the body.

The San-jiao's exact nature and form have been disputed for centuries. Generally, there are four meanings of San-jiao: 1) It is a Channel pathway on the body surface (commonly called the Triple Heater Meridian, TH); Its Channel connects with the Pericardium. 2) It is considered one of the six Fu organs, and it shares an external-internal relationship with the Pericardium. 3) It is divided into three parts: the Upper Jiao, the Middle Jiao, and the Lower Jiao (Burner, Heater). 4) It is the general pathway for distribution of Yuan Qi (Source Qi) and Body Fluid.

The Upper Jiao is located from the head to the diaphragm. It is like mist or fog. It mainly functions to govern respiration and the blood vessels and to distribute the nutrients from food and water to the body. The Upper Jiao contains the Heart and Lung.

The Middle Jiao is located from the diaphragm to the navel. It is concerned with maceration. It functions to rot, digest and absorb food; thus, it is associated with the digestive and absorptive functions of the Spleen and Stomach.

The Lower Jiao is located from the navel to the feet. It acts as a drainage system. Mainly it functions to separate the clear fluid from the turbid and to excrete unwanted water and food residues from the body. It is closely related to the Kidney, Bladder, Small and Large Intestines.

Therefore, food reception, digestion, absorption, distribution and excretion are performed through Qi Activity that is closely related to the Sanjiao. The Sanjiao governs the Qi Activity, and it acts like the passageway for transport of nutrients, water, and excreta.

The Extraordinary Fu Organs

In addition to the regular five Zang and six Fu organs, there are also six Extraordinary Fu organs: the Brain, Marrow, Bones, Vessels, Gall Bladder and Uterus. These have the hollow shape of Fu organs, but they function similar to Zang organs because they store essential substances. Their differences from both Zang and Fu organs warrant their label as Extraordinary Fu organs. Each of these Extraordinary Fu organs stores the Kidney Essences, marrow, Blood, or bile. Functionally they are directly or indirectly related to the Kidney.

THE BRAIN

The Brain is located in the skull, and it connects with the spinal marrow. It is also called the "Sea of the Marrow" or the "House of the Mind and Spirit ". It controls memory, spirit, consciousness, and thought.

Because the Kidney Essence and the Heart Blood replenish the Brain, it is functionally related to the Kidney and Heart. Therefore, many diseases of the brain are associated with the Kidney and the Heart.

THE MARROW

The marrow includes the brain, the spinal cord, and the bone marrow. The Kidney Essences are the origin of marrow. Its main functions are to fill up and to nourish the brain and the bone.

THE BONE

Anatomically, the Bone is the same as in Western veterinary medicine. According to Traditional Chinese Veterinary Medicine, the Kidney controls the bone. Its main functions are to store the marrow and to form the skeleton of the body.

THE VESSELS

The Vessels are also called the "House of Blood". The Qi and Blood circulate in the Vessels. The Vessels are indirectly related to the Kidney because the Kidney Essences are another origin of the Blood.

THE GALL BLADDER

The Gall Bladder is a special organ. Since it is hollow, it is one of the regular Fu organs. However, it stores bile and functions like one of the Zang organs. Therefore, it is also considered one of the six extraordinary Fu organs.

THE UTERUS

The Uterus controls estrus and pregnancy and nourishes the fetus. It is closely related to the Kidney, the Chong Mai (Penetrating Vessel), and the Ren Mai (Conception Vessel).

Case Examples

Case 4.1

Signalment: A ten year old, male, castrated Domestic Shorthair Cat

History and Exam:

The presenting complaint was weight loss and decreased appetite. The cat may also have been vomiting. He lived in a multi-cat household so the owner was unable to describe an individual cat's habits in detail. This cat was normally very shy and was often hard to find.

Upon examination, a moderate heart murmur was auscultated. This murmur had been present for many years. A mass was palpated in the abdomen. The tongue was slightly pale and possibly thin. The pulse was deep and weak.

The bloodwork revealed hypoalbuminemia and leukocytosis (with neutrophilia). Ultrasound revealed hypertrophic cardiomyopathy, a bowel mass, and enlarged lymph nodes. The Western differential diagnoses included lymphosarcoma and inflammatory bowel disease.

Case 4.1 Assessment:

Weight loss, decreased appetite, pale tongue, and weak, deep pulses indicate a Spleen Qi Deficiency. Vomiting indicates rebellious Stomach Qi (or Stomach Qi Stagnation). The abdominal mass, bowel mass, lymph node enlargement and hypertrophic cardiomyopathy indicate Phlegm (which can be secondary to the Spleen Qi Deficiency). The heart murmur can be caused by Phlegm in the Heart Channel. Shy behavior and hiding indicate a Water-type personality. A strong Water constitution can pathologically over-control the Spleen (Earth) especially when the Earth energy is weak.

Thus, the TCVM diagnosis is Spleen Qi Deficiency with Stomach Qi Stagnation and Phlegm. The acupuncture points ST-36, CV-12 and BL-20 and herbal formula Four Gentlemen (*Si Jun Zi Tang*) may be used to tonify the Spleen Qi and to build up muscle. In addition, ST-40, GB-34 and the herbal formula *Wei Chang He* may be used to resolve the Stomach Qi Stagnation and Phlegm. When the clinical signs are under control, *Nei Xiao San* can be used to address the mass in the gastrointestinal tract.

Case 4.2

Signalment: A twelve year old, spayed female Great Dane

History and Exam:

In September of 1999, the dog presented with a history of weight loss (loss of 30 lb), poor appetite and lethargy (exercise intolerance) for several months. She also had been losing hair for the past two months. No vomiting, changes in thirst, itching, lameness, or diarrhea had been observed.

On physical exam, the dog appears depressed and skinny. She is a laid-back, friendly dog. She barks when someone visits the house, and she will vocalize in a different tone if barking at another dog. She has never bitten any people or other dogs.

Upon examination, her Shen was low. Her tongue was pale, and her pulse was deep and weak. Palpation revealed sensitivity at BL-20, BL-21 and BL-23.

Case 4.2 Assessment:

She was a typical Earth dog. The weight loss, emaciation, poor appetite, lethargy, pale tongue and weak pulse indicated a Spleen Qi Deficiency. Hair loss can be a sign of Spleen Qi Deficiency because the deficient Spleen Qi fails to generate enough Blood to nourish the hair follicles, thus it fails to hold onto the hair coat. Thus, the TCVM Diagnosis was Spleen Qi Deficiency. The herbal medicine *Si Jun Zi Tang* and electroacupuncture at BL-21, BL-20, ST-36, LI-10 and *Shan Gen* were the recommended treatments.

Re-examination of Case 4.2:

Within four to five weeks after two subsequent acupuncture treatments and daily herbal medication, the dog showed great improvement. She had gained body weight (20 lb), had more energy, and had re-growth of her hair. She was doing great until March 2001.

She had a decrease in appetite for three days. Her feces consisted of watery, brown diarrhea (especially in the morning). She had vomited a small amount of yellow, mucoid fluid several days previously. She has also been slightly more lethargic in the morning and has been weak in the hind end. Her tongue was pale and purple, and her pulse was weak on the right side. She was sensitive to palpation at BL-23.

Case 4.2 Reassessment:

She is an Earth dog with a history of Spleen Qi Deficiency. Watery diarrhea indicates a Spleen Qi Deficiency. Early morning diarrhea, weakness in the hind end, a purple tongue, and sensitivity at BL-23 indicate a Kidney Yang Deficiency. Therefore, her TCVM Diagnosis at this time was Spleen Qi and Kidney Yang Deficiency. For this condition, the herbal formula Four Immortals (*Si Shen Wan*) was recommended. Treatment also included electroacupuncture at GV-4, *Bai Hui*, BL-20, BL-21, BL-23, ST-36, and GB-34 as well as aquapuncture at BL-21, BL-20, GV-1, and *Bai Hui*.

Re-examination of Case 4.2:

By her May 2001 follow-up visit she continued to gain weight, maintain a good appetite and have normal stool since her last treatments. However, she had experienced several episodes of collapse in the last two months. At these times her pulse is irregular and she seems unaware her surroundings, but she does not lose consciousness. In addition, she becomes a little incontinent during these episodes.

On physical exam, her skin was scaly and smelled. Her stool was of normal consistency, but she was sometimes unable to wait to defecate outdoors. She loves to lean on somebody or to have support for her rear limbs when she stands. She was lethargic, had weakness of her hind limbs and had severe gingivitis. There was muscle atrophy bilaterally of her rear legs. Her Shen was good. Her tongue was pale purple, and her pulse was weak and slow and worse on the right side. She was sensitive to palpation of BL-14, BL-20 and BL-23.

Case 4.2 Reassessment:

The falling down, unawareness of her surroundings and irregular pulses during the episodes of collapse indicate a Heart Qi/Yang Deficiency. The rear end weakness, muscle atrophy, lethargy, pale purple tongue, and slow, weak right pulse still indicate a Spleen Qi and Kidney Qi Deficiency. The scaly, smelly skin and gingivitis indicate a Yin Deficiency. Her current TCVM diagnosis is Heart and Kidney Yang Deficiency and a Spleen Qi Deficiency with Yin Deficiency. The recommended treatment should include *Bu Yang Huan Wu Tang*. In addition, dry needle acupuncture at GB-20, KID-3, BL-20, GV-4, *Bai Hui*, LIV-3, and ST-36 may be combined with aquapuncture (0.5 cc of vitamin B_{12}) at CV-17, CV-4, CV-6 and ST-36. Further neurologic workup is recommended if the problems with falling down do not resolve.

Case 4.3

Signalment: An eight year old, castrated male Rottweiler

History and Exam:

Historically, the dog had an acute onset of lameness of his left rear limb at three years of age. A torn left anterior cruciate ligament and mild degenerative changes of left stifle were later diagnosed. The torn ACL was addressed with surgery and regular Adequan® injections.

Recently, the dog developed dyspnea which was due to chylothorax. Thoracocentesis was performed weekly, and three to five liters of fluids were removed from the chest cavity. The dog was diagnosed with torsed left cranial and middle lung lobes. A left cranial and middle lung lobectomy was performed. He was doing well after surgery, but several months later he was found recumbent and suffering from increased dyspnea. His chest was drained and he was prescribed Rutin, a compound that may help resolve the pleural effusion.

The dog has lived with the owner since six weeks of age. He is a tolerant, laid-back, friendly dog who sleeps a lot. He interacts well with other animals. His appetite is fine, but he is not overly motivated by food. Since the problem with the cruciate ligament, he has been unable to raise his leg to urinate. Previous acupuncture treatments (about five times) seemed to help relieve the soreness of his rear limbs.

Upon examination, the dog was bright and alert, but he panted a lot in the exam room. He was ataxic when he walked. His skin was a little dry. His pulses were weak and deep (worse on the right side). His tongue was dark red. His nose was wet. No sensitive back *shu* and front *mu* acupoints were located.

Case 4.3 Assessment:

This dog has an Earth-type personality.

Hydrothorax indicates deficient Spleen Qi which fails to transport and transform water and body fluids. The wet nose and dyspnea indicate a Lung Qi Deficiency. A dark red tongue and dry skin indicate Yin Deficiency.

This TCVM diagnosis is Spleen and Lung Qi Deficiency with Yin Deficiency. The formula *Shi Zao Tang* is recommended for treatment. In addition, dry needle acupuncture at CV-17, LU-9, LU-7, SP-9, CV-4 and CV-6, as well as daily moxibustion at CV-17 may also be beneficial.

Case 4.4

Signalment: An eleven year old female, spayed Rottweiler

History and Exam:

This dog first presented to a referral hospital in July 1997. She was then diagnosed with bilateral carpal degenerative joint disease (DJD) and a right cranial cruciate ligament tear. She was seen again in August 2000 for an evaluation of dermal lumps. By March 2001, she had grown more lumps and was diagnosed with a benign dermal melanoma. The owner is an acupuncture student and has been pursuing acupuncture for the dog's DJD, cruciate ligament problems and dermal lumps for past three years. Clinically, the DJD and cruciate ligament problems have completely resolved.

During May 2001, the dog presented with the major complaints of separation anxiety, thunderstorm phobia and urinary incontinence. She has been non-painful and has had no new cutaneous growths. She walks and runs normally. The owner reported some episodes of urinary incontinence particularly related to excitement or fear.

She prefers to stay in cooler places. Her tongue is dark and her pulse is weak and thready on the left side. The skin and Shen appear good. She is a timid and shy dog who hides under the table and tries to run away during examination and needling.

Case 4.4 Assessment:

She is a typical Water dog. Her TCVM diagnosis includes Shen Disturbance due to Yin Deficiency, urinary incontinence due to Kidney Qi Deficiency, and Phlegm. Separation anxiety and thunderstorm fear indicate Shen Disturbance. Yin Deficiency is diagnosed because of the dark tongue; the weak, thready, left-sided pulse; and cool-seeking behavior. Urinary incontinence is often related to Kidney Qi Deficiency. Benign dermal melanomas or lipomas are considered to be Phlegm.

The Shen Disturbance seems to be the most urgent problem right now because it is the major concern and the thunderstorm season is coming. The urinary incontinence will also be addressed at this time. After the Shen becomes stable and normal, the next step is to focus on treating the phlegm.

The acupuncture treatment consists of dry needling KID-10 which is a Kidney Yin tonic point (He-sea point for the Kidney) as well as electroacupuncture at the following points. Stimulation of *Bai Hui* and *Shen Shu* helps tonify the Kidney Qi and resolve urinary leakage. The acupoints BL-23, KI-3, and KI-7 nourish Kidney Yin. The lower He-sea point for TH, BL-39 can help regulate the water pathway and resolve urinary leakage.

The herbal formulas *Suo Quan Wan* (to strengthen Kidney Qi and to resolve urinary incontinence) and Shen calmer (to nourish Yin and to calm down the Shen) may also be beneficial. In an addition, she should be fed cooling, Yin foods such as fish, sweet potatoes, carrots, watermelon and bananas. She should avoid hot, Yang foods including chicken, turkey, mutton, deer meat, garlic, ginger, or onion.

Case 4.5

Signalment: A three year old Female Spayed Poodle

History and Exam:

This poodle suffers from chronic recurrent bouts of inflammatory bowel disease (IBD), which occurs as vomiting and diarrhea that is sometimes bloody. She has been in and out of many veterinary clinics since she was born.

She suffers terribly from separation anxiety and has been on a homeopathic remedy, which does not seem to help. She always responds to Metronidazole and Metoclopramide. At her most recent visit, she had been vomiting and has had foul-smelling diarrhea with fresh red blood for two days.

The poodle was a shy and timid dog. Her tongue appeared dry, and the tip of tongue looked red. The pulse was very rapid and easily palpated. She was very thin.

Case 4.5 Assessment:

In TCVM, inflammatory bowel disease (bloody diarrhea with a foul odor) is considered an Intestinal Damp-Heat. Vomiting may be considered Stomach Qi Stagnation or rebellious Qi. Separation anxiety is often caused by Heart Yin Deficiency. Redness of the tip of tongue and a rapid pulse are also signs of a Heart Yin Deficiency. Thus, her TCVM diagnosis includes Intestinal Damp-Heat and Heart Yin Deficiency with Stomach Qi Stagnation.

Treatment should include the acupoints ST-36, GB-34, BL-20, BL-23, GV-1, LI-10, and LI-11. In addition, the herbal formula *Wei Chang He* may be used to regulate Stomach Qi for three months. *Da Xiang Lian San* may be used to clear Damp-Heat of the intestinal tract for one to three weeks only when the IBD occurs. This herbal medication should be discontinued as soon as the clinical signs resolve. To assist with the separation anxiety and nourish Heart Yin, Shen Calmer can be used starting one month prior to separation.

Case 4.6

Signalment: A five year old, female Old English Sheepdog

Primary Complaint: Urinary Incontinence

History and Exam:

The dog's urinary incontinence has become progressively worse over the past two years. Her current medication is diethylstilbestrol (DES), but the incontinence is not responding well.

Her tongue is pale and wet without a coating. She is very weak in the hind limbs and often has trouble getting up. She has sensitivity at BL-23. Her pulses are deep and weak. She is very friendly, but she growls and barks when the acupuncture begins; she seems frightened. She prefers soft rugs to hard, cold, wood floors. She is worse at night and when she just wakes up (she has accidents in the house).

Case 4.6 Assessment:

Because she is scared and sensitive when performing acupuncture but is very friendly, she may be a Fire-type personality. Dogs with Fire constitutions tend to have Yin Deficiency. Her preference for cold floors and the worsening of the problem at night indicate Yin Deficiency. The urinary incontinence itself is a Kidney Qi Deficiency. The pale and wet tongue, the deep and weak pulse and the rear weakness also indicate Kidney Qi Deficiency. Therefore, her TCVM diagnosis is Kidney Qi with Yin Deficiency.

Dry needle and aquapuncture may be performed once every one to two weeks at points such as BL-23, BL-39, KID-3, *An Shen*, and HT-7. The herbal formula *Suo Quan Wan* helps to tonify Kidney Qi and Rehmannia Six helps to nourish Kidney Yin.

Case 4.7

Signalment: A ten year old male cat

History and Exam:

This cat presented with severe dehydration, weakness, and inability to stand. According to the owner he had been normal one week previously.

Blood work revealed leukocytosis, elevated creatinine, elevated BUN, and elevated liver enzymes. He was cold and weak. His treatment included fluids, antibiotics, and acupuncture. He was painful and resisted palpation along his back from T10 to the lumbosacral area. He gained some strength later in the day. He was alert, and he stood and allowed people to stroke his back. However, his appetite was poor and he had been vomiting.

The next day his tongue appeared shrunken, dry, and pale. His pulse was slow, weak and deep. His ear tips were cool, and temperature over the cervical and thoracic area felt warm. The skin over T10 to the lumbosacral area was noticeably colder. He was much stronger and alert and active, but not eating on his own. He did keep down some canned food which was force-fed.

He was diagnosed with acute pyelonephritis.

Case 4.7 Assessment:

Inability to stand, weakness, poor appetite and pale tongue indicate Spleen Qi Deficiency. Deep, slow, weak pulses, cool ears, a cold, sore back indicate a Kidney Yang Deficiency. Dehydration and a dry tongue indicate Yin Deficiency. This cat's TCVM diagnosis is Kidney Yang and Spleen Qi Deficiency with Yin Deficiency.

The treatment could include dry needle acupuncture at KID-3, KID-7, *Shen Shu*, ST-44, and GB-34. A dilute B_{12} solution (1 cc of B_{12} with 3 cc of saline) may be injected (0.3 cc per point) at BL-23, *Bai Hui*, CV-4, CV-6, and ST-36 for extra stimulation of these points. The Chinese herbal formulas *Xiang Sha Liu Jun Zi Wan* and *Rou Gui Wan* are also recommended to tonify Spleen Qi and Kidney Yang.

Case 4.8

Signalment: A nine year old Tennessee Walking Horse mare

Presenting Complaint: Chronic Diarrhea

History and Exam:

This horse had a diarrhea that was difficult to manage. The volume of diarrhea has decreased over time; however, she still continued to produce very loose feces. Her appetite was poor. She had severe ventral edema and cold extremities. Her pulse was deep, rapid, and weak. Her tongue was red with a yellow coating. She also had a small rectal prolapse and is eight months pregnant.

She had received two acupuncture treatments, but no changes were noted in her condition.

Case 4.8 Assessment:

The diarrhea, cold extremities, poor appetite, ventral edema, and rectal prolapse indicate that this mare has a Spleen Qi and Yang Deficiency.

The acupuncture points GV-1, *Bai Hui*, GV-3 and BL-21 are recommended. Dilute vitamin B$_{12}$ may be used for aquapuncture at *Qi Hai Shu*. In addition, moxibustion at *Bai Hui* and CV-6 may be performed for five to ten minutes daily for about a week. The herbal formula *Bu Zhong Yi Qi Tang* may be used for two to three weeks.

Case 4.9

Signalment: A fifteen-year-old Appaloosa mare

Presenting Complaint: Recurrent uveitis

History and Exam:

Past treatments for her uveitis have included acupuncture and the Chinese herbal formula *Jue Ming San* (Haliotis Powder). She does not eat the herbal formula well, so she only ingests about one dose a day. She continues to have episodes of conjunctivitis and corneal opacities.

Her pulses are weak on the left side. Her tongue is pale pink with darker edges.

Case 4.9 Assessment:

Corneal opacities, weak pulses on the left side, a red tongue and dark edges of the tongue indicate a Liver Yin Deficiency. Acute episodes of conjunctivitis indicate Liver Heat. Thus, this mare's TCVM diagnosis is Liver Yin Deficiency with Heat

The herbal formula *Yi Guan Jian* nourishes the Liver Yin. In addition, "Picrorrhiza Eye Drop" (*Hu Huang Lian*) may be used topically three to five times daily. The acupuncture points GB-37, GB-34, BL-18, KID-3, BL-1, GB-1 and ST-1 are also recommended.

Case 4.10

Signalment: A fourteen year old female cat

History and Exam:

This cat had an acute onset of hyphema. She was hypertensive with a diastolic blood pressure of 240.

On physical exam she was quiet, well hydrated and of normal body condition. Her pulse rate was over 200 beats per minute. It felt fast and thin. She also had a grade 2/5 heart murmur. Her tongue was red with a mild clear coating. She is blind in both eyes from the detached retinas. The owners feel that she drinks a lot of water. She prefers cool places and has a good appetite most of the time.

Her owners describe her independent, laid back, and very protective of the dogs in the house. Her treatment has included a natural diet and Lotensin® to get the blood pressure down into a safe range.

Case 4.10 Assessment:

Acute onset of hyphema and hypertension indicate Liver Yang Rising. A fast, thin pulse, a red tongue and cool-seeking behavior indicate Yin Deficiency. Thus, this cat's TCVM diagnosis is Yin Deficiency with Liver Yang Rising.

The herbal formula *Yi Guan Jian* may be beneficial to nourish the Liver Yin and anchor the Liver Yang. Acupuncture points including GB-34, LIV-3, LIV-2, GB-37, KID-3 and BL-18 are recommended.

Case 4.11

Signalment: An eight year old female spayed cat

History and Exam:

About 1½ years ago she presented with cough and dyspnea. A specialist felt that she had a rare, unusual lung cancer. Her radiographs revealed multiple areas of consolidation and an interstitial pattern.

Currently she is maintained on 20 mg prednisone and 37.5 mg of Furosemide per day. Periodically, antibiotics are used for acute crises which are thought to be secondary bacterial infections. She is still somewhat tachypneic with these medications, but without them she has great difficulty breathing. She is showing worsening signs of Cushing's disease including enlargement of her fat pads, thin skin, oily coat with small flakes, and hair loss on her ears, behind her elbow and on her abdomen and flanks.

She has a picky appetite. Radiographs showed a possible huge hairball. Generally, she's timid and anxious. She sleeps well. Initially her tongue was red with a dry white coat, and she was reactive over the BL-20 and BL-23 points.

Following two acupuncture sessions and dietary supplements including antioxidants, her tongue is deep pink with a thin white coat. Her pulse is rapid and thready. Her back *shu* points are reactive over BL-13 (the Lung association point). Her front *mu* points are normal.

Case 4.11 Assessment:

Chronic cough indicates a Lung Qi/Yin Deficiency. Very chronic dyspnea indicates Lung and Kidney Qi Deficiency. A picky appetite and a huge hairball indicate food stasis. The thin skin, oily hair coat with small flakes, red tongue and rapid, thready pulses indicate Heat due to a Yin Deficiency. The enlargement of fat pads can indicate Qi Deficiency. Thus, this cat's TCVM diagnosis is Lung and Kidney Qi/Yin Deficiency with Food Stasis.

The herbal formulas *Ren Shen Ge Jie San* and *Wei Chang He* may be beneficial. Acupoints including LU-9, LU-7, *Ding Chuan*, CV-22, CV-17, KID-7, KID-3 and BL-13 are recommended.

Self Test

Question 4.1: The Heart houses which of the following?

    a. Shen
    b. Qi
    c. Jing
    d. Body Fluid
    e. Blood

Question 4.2: Which organ controls the sinews (ligaments/tendons) and paws/hooves?

    a. Spleen
    b. Lung
    c. Liver
    d. Kidney
    e. Heart

Question 4.3: Which organ dominates blood vessels?

    a. Spleen
    b. Lung
    c. Liver
    d. Kidney
    e. Heart

Question 4.4: Which group of organs is most closely associated with Blood?

    a. Kidney, Liver, Lung
    b. Spleen, Liver, Heart
    c. Spleen, Lung, Heart
    d. Kidney, Lung, Spleen
    e. Lung, Liver, Heart

Question 4.5: Which Zang organ dominates the Muscles?

    a. Spleen
    b. Lung
    c. Liver
    d. Kidney
    e. Heart

Question 4.6: When we hear "the root of prenatal life", we connect it with the function of which of the following Zang organs?

    a. Spleen
    b. Lung
    c. Liver
    d. Kidney
    e. Heart

Question 4.7: The phrase "the Mother of Five Zang Organs" refers to which of the following organs?

    a. Spleen
    b. Lung
    c. Liver
    d. Kidney
    e. Heart

Question 4.8: Which of the following statements is NOT true?

    a. The Fu (Yang) organs are hollow while the Zang (Yin) organs are solid.
    b. The Fu organs are relatively Exterior while the Zang organs are relatively Interior.
    c. The major function of Fu organs is to excrete while that of the Zang organs is to store.
    d. The Gall Bladder is one of Six Fu organs as well as one of Extraordinary Fu organs.
    e. The Bone is not one of the Six Extraordinary Fu Organs.

Question 4.9: If a 10-year old Thoroughbred mare has a history of chronic heaves and cough, which organ should you closely examine according to the Five Elements?

    a. Spleen
    b. Lung
    c. Kidney
    d. Liver
    e. Heart

Question 4.10: According to the five element theory, which is the organ to examine if the dog has a history of chronic eye discharge and hyperactive personality?

    a. Spleen
    b. Lung
    c. Kidney
    d. Liver
    e. Heart

Question 4.11: Which of the following is NOT a clinical sign of Spleen Qi Deficiency?

    a. Weight loss or muscle atrophy
    b. Poor appetite
    c. Loose stool or diarrhea
    d. Exercise intolerance (weakness of limbs or fatigue)
    e. Urinary incontinence

Question 4.12: Which of the following statements is TRUE?

    a. Kidney stores blood.
    b. Spleen stores Jing (Essence).
    c. Liver is responsible for the body's tolerance of fatigue
    d. Lung is responsible for producing marrow
    e. Heart is responsible for water metabolism

CHAPTER FIVE

THE MERIDIANS

Anatomy is to physiology as geography to history; it
describes the theatre of events.

– Jean Fernel, *On the Natural Part of Medicine*

Having learned of the interconnectedness of so many aspects within living, healthy
organisms, questions arise about what makes this possible and what is the underlying
structure of this integrated whole. By what mechanism are the *Sheng* and *Ke* cycles able
to balance the Five Elements of the body? How is the connection between the "wife" and
"husband" Zang-Fu organs formed? How are the five treasures (Qi, Blood, Shen, Jing
and Body Fluid) able to support the Zang-Fu physiological activities? It is the special
system called "Jing Luo" that provides the connections or pathways essential for the
body's co-operative functions.

The Jing Luo system is the pathway through which Qi and Blood circulate. It regulates
the physiological activities of the Zang-Fu organs. It extends over the Exterior of the
body, but it pertains to the Zang-Fu organs located on the Interior. It connects and
correlates all the tissues and organs, forming a network which links the tissues and
organs into an organic whole. Chapter 33 of *Ling Shu (Miraculous Pivot)* states that
"Twelve Regular Channels are connected with the Zang-fu organs internally and with the
joints, limbs, and body surfaces externally".

The classical traditional Chinese veterinary medical text *Yuan Heng Liao Ma Ji* (*Yuan-
Heng's Therapeutic Treatise of Horses*, 1608) considers the Jing Luo to be so important
that "it determines life and death of an animal, treats all the diseases, and regulates both
the Deficiency and Excess Patterns". Therefore, this text recommends that veterinarians
gain a thorough understanding of this system. Despite the tremendous amount of
scientific research dedicated to studying the anatomy of Jing Lou system, no one in the
past 40 years has been able to exactly describe the Jing Luo system.

There are two major components in the Jing Luo system: *Jing Mai* and *Luo Mai*. *Jing* can
be translated as Meridian, Channel, or major trunk. *Mai* means vessels. *Luo* is a
collateral or branch. Thus, *Jing Mai* translates as major trunk vessel, and it is also known
as the Channel. *Luo Mai* refers to the collateral or branch vessels. These Channels are
the body's equivalent of telephone lines, airways, rivers, highways, and city roads, which
provide a means of communication and transport. The *Jing Mai* is like a major telephone
carrier, a main telephone line, a major highway, a state/city/county road, an international
airport, or a large river. The Luo Mai is like a telephone extension, a small street, a small
connection airline, or a small river.

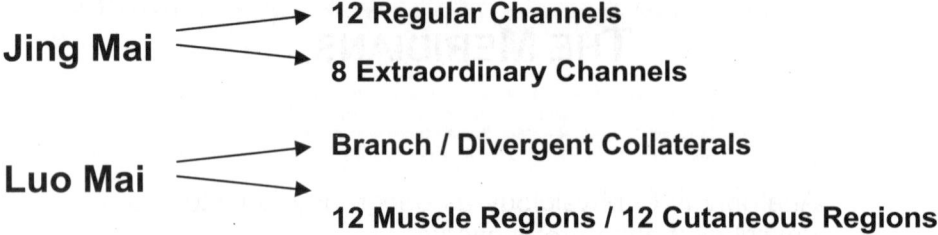

Nomenclature of the Twelve Regular Channels

There are twelve Zang-Fu organs; six are Zang (Yin) organs and six are Fu (Yang) organs. Each organ has a Channel of its own. The nomenclature of the Twelve Regular Channels is based on three factors: 1) the location on a thoracic or pelvic limb; 2) the association with either one of three Yin (Tai Yin, Shao Yin, Jue Yin) or the three Yang (Yang Ming, Tai Yang, Shao Yang); 3) the relationship with one of the Zang-Fu organs.

Each thoracic and pelvic limb is supplied by three Yin and three Yang Channels. Because the Twelve Regular Channels are bilaterally symmetrical, there are twenty-four Channels in the body.

Table 5.1: The Twelve Regular Channels

Channel Location	Zang Fu Organ	Abbreviation
Tai Yin of the thoracic limb	Lung	LU
Tai Yin of the pelvic limb	Spleen	SP
Shao Yin of the thoracic limb	Heart	HT
Shao Yin of the pelvic limb	Kidney	KID
Jue Yin of the thoracic limb	Pericardium	PC
Jue Yin of the pelvic limb	Liver	LIV
Yang Ming of the thoracic limb	Large Intestine	LI
Yang Ming of the pelvic limb	Stomach	ST
Tai Yang of the thoracic limb	Small Intestine	SI
Tai Yang of the pelvic limb	Urinary Bladder	UB
Shao Yang of the thoracic limb	Sanjiao	SJ / TH / TB / TW
Shao Yang of the pelvic limb	Gall Bladder	GB

*TH = Triple Heater; TB = triple Burner; TW =Triple Warmer

The Channels that relate to Yin organs are Yin Channels, and the Channels that relate to Yang organs are Yang Channels. The Yin and Yang Channels are each divided into three types. Yin consists of Tai Yin, Shao Yin, and Jue Yin. Yang consists of Yang Ming, Tai Yang, and Shao Yang. The energy levels dissipate with the flow from one Yin or

Yang level to the next level. Yangming (brightest Yang) and Taiyin (greatest Yin) are each in the highest, strongest level. Taiyang (greatest Yang) and Shaoyin (smallest Yin) are in the next level, which is not as strong as the first. Shaoyang (smallest Yang) and Jueyin (diminishing Yin) are part of the third level, which is the weakest of the three. The greatest Yin can never be as great as the brightest Yang, but the weakest Yang can never be as small as the lowest Yin.

Table 5.2: The Levels of the Twelve Regular Channels

	Limbs	Three Yang	Fu Organs	Zang Organs	Three Yin	Limbs
1st Level	Thoracic	Yangming	LI	LU	Taiyin	Thoracic
	Pelvic		ST	SP		Pelvic
2nd Level	Thoracic	Taiyang	SI	HT	Shaoyin	Thoracic
	Pelvic		BL	KID		Pelvic
3rd Level	Thoracic	Shaoyang	TH	PC	Jueyin	Thoracic
	Pelvic		GB	LIV		Pelvic

The General Pathways of the Twelve Regular Channels

The Zang organs belong to Yin, and the Fu organs belong to Yang. The medial aspect of the limb is Yin, while the lateral aspect is Yang. Thus, the six Channels for the Zang organs are Yin Channels, which are distributed on the medial aspect of the limbs. Likewise, the six Channels for the Fu organs are Yang Channels, which are distributed on the lateral aspect of the limbs. The Yin Channels, which belong to the Zang organs, are also able to communicate with the Fu organs. Similarly, the Yang Channels, which belong to the Fu organs, are able to communicate with the Zang Organs. In this way, an Exterior-Interior or a husband-wife relationship develops between the Yin and Yang Channels and their Zang-Fu organs.

The three Yin Channels of the thoracic limb start from the chest, circulate along the medial aspect of the thoracic limb, and terminate at the end of the front feet. The three Yang Channels of thoracic limb start from the end of front feet and circulate along the lateral aspect of the thoracic limb to end at the head. The three Yang Channels of the pelvic limb start at the head, circulate along the back (except the Stomach Channel which runs along the ventral abdomen) and the lateral aspect of the pelvic limb, and terminate at the end of the hind feet. The three Yin Channels of pelvic limb start from the end of the hind feet, circulate along the medial aspect of the pelvic limb, and travel along the abdomen to end at the chest (Table 5.3).

All three Yang Channels of the thoracic limb end on the head, and all three Yang Channels of the pelvic limb begin there. Thus, the head is known as the "Gathering

House of all the Yang". In a similar fashion, all three Yin Channels of the thoracic limb start from the chest and all three Yin Channels of the pelvic limb end there. Thus, the chest is called the "Gathering House of all the Yin".

On the thoracic limb, three Yin Channels run along the medial side and three Yang Channels run along the lateral side. The Lung Channel of Taiyin supplies the cranial and medial border of the limb. The middle of the medial forelimb is home to the Pericardium Channel of Jueyin. The Heart Channel of Shaoyin resides along the caudomedial border of the limb. On the lateral forelimb, the Large Intestine Channel of Yangming supplies the cranial edge. The Sanjiao Channel of Shaoyang runs along the middle of the lateral side. The Small Intestine Channel of Taiyang lies along the caudolateral part of the limb (Table 5.4).

On the pelvic limb, three Yin Channels run along the medial side and three Yang Channels travel along the lateral side. The Stomach Channel of Yangming supplies the cranial border of the lateral aspect of the pelvic limb. The Gall Bladder Channel of Shaoyang resides in the center of the lateral hind leg. The caudolateral part of the hind limb is home to the Bladder Channel of Taiyang. Moving to the medial side of the leg, one finds the Spleen Channel of Taiyin along the cranial border of the pelvic Limb. The Liver Channel resides along the middle of the medial side. The Kidney Channel of Shaoyin is located along the caudolateral part of the pelvic limb (Table 5.4).

Table 5.3: The general pathways of the Twelve Regular Channels on the body

Channel	Origin	Pathway	Terminus
The three Yin Channels of the Thoracic Limb	Chest	Medial aspect of the thoracic limb	End of front feet
The three Yang Channels of the Thoracic Limb	End of front feet	Lateral aspect of the thoracic limb	Head
The three Yin Channels of the Pelvic Limb	End of hind feet	Medial aspect of the pelvic limb and the ventral abdomen	Chest
The three Yang Channels of the Pelvic Limb	Head	Lateral aspect of the pelvic limb and the back	End of hind feet

Table 5.4: The general pathways of the Twelve Regular Channels on the limbs

Location on Limb	Cranial	Middle	Caudal
The medial aspect of the thoracic limb	LU	PC	HT
The lateral aspect of the thoracic limb	LI	TH	SI
The lateral aspect of the pelvic limb	ST	GB	BL
The medial aspect of the pelvic limb	SP	LIV	KID

Table 5.5: The Circadian Flow of the Twelve Regular Channels

	Circadian Clock	Yin Channels	Yang Channels	Circadian Clock	
Tai Yin	3 am to 5 am	LU	LI	5 am to 7 am	Yang Ming
	9 am to 11 am	SP	ST	7 am to 9 am	
Shao Yin	11 am to 1 pm	HT	SI	1 pm to 3 pm	Tai Yang
	5 pm to 7 pm	KID	BL	3 pm to 5 pm	
Jue Yin	7 pm to 9 pm	PC	TH	9 pm to 11 pm	Shao Yang
	1 am to 3 am	LIV	GB	11 pm to 1 am	

The Twelve Regular Channels join with one another in a fixed order (Table 5.5, Figure 5.1 and Figure 5.2). Along this course, there is an endless, cyclical flow of Qi and Blood within the Channels. The flow always passes from one Channel to the next in a specific order throughout the day; however, the Qi dominates within certain Meridians at designated times. This is the TCVM Circadian rhythm, which provides the body with its own internal clock. Disorders of this rhythm can be used to assist with Pattern identification and TCVM diagnosis.

The cycle begins at 3:00 am with the Lung Channel at the chest. The energy dominates in each Meridian for two hours before passing on to the next Channel. Thus the flow passes to the Large Intestine Channel at 5:00 am and remains there until 7:00 am. Next, the Qi moves to the Stomach Channel from 7:00 to 9:00 am. The Spleen Channel follows from 9:00 am to 11:00 am. In such a manner, the Qi moves from thoracic Yin to thoracic Yang to pelvic Yang to pelvic Yin. It makes a complete circuit around the body while passing from wife to husband and husband to wife. Once back at the chest, it is the Heart Channel's turn from 11:00 am to 1:00 pm. The husband of the Heart, the Small Intestine Channel, then carries the energy from 1:00 pm to 3:00 pm. On the head, the Qi passes to the yang channel of the same energy level, the Urinary Bladder Channel. From 3:00 pm to 5:00 pm, the Bladder holds the Qi flow until it passes through Kidney, the wife of the Bladder, from 5:00 pm to 7:00 pm. Now back at the chest, the Qi flows down the Pericardium Channel of the thoracic limbs from 7:00 pm to 9:00 pm. Her husband, the Triple Heater Channel, next carries the Qi from 9:00 pm to 11:00 pm. At the head, the Gall Bladder Channel takes the flow to the hind limb from 11:00 pm to 1:00 am. From 1:00 am to 3:00 am, the Liver Channel brings the flow back to the chest for the cycle to begin again with the Lung Channel at 3:00 am.

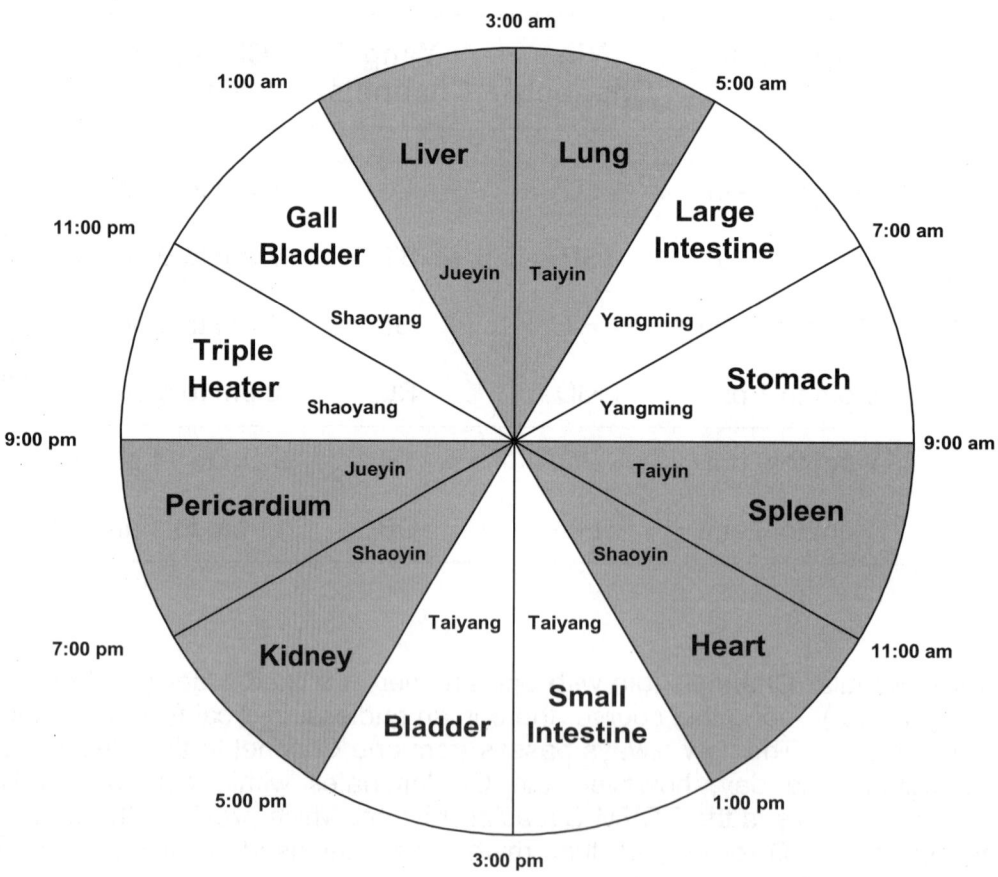

Figure 5.1: TCVM Circadian Clock of the Twelve Regular Channels

The following figure, Figure 5.2, is a concise illustration of the relationships between Yin-Yang, Zang-Fu, Thoracic-Pelvic, the Levels, and the individual organs. Each concentric circle represents one level with the outermost demonstrating the first level. After traveling around the circle in a counter-clockwise direction, it flows into the next level. Along the way it passes through each quadrant with its own associated organ. When reaching the end of the center circle, it skips back to the first level where it starts again.

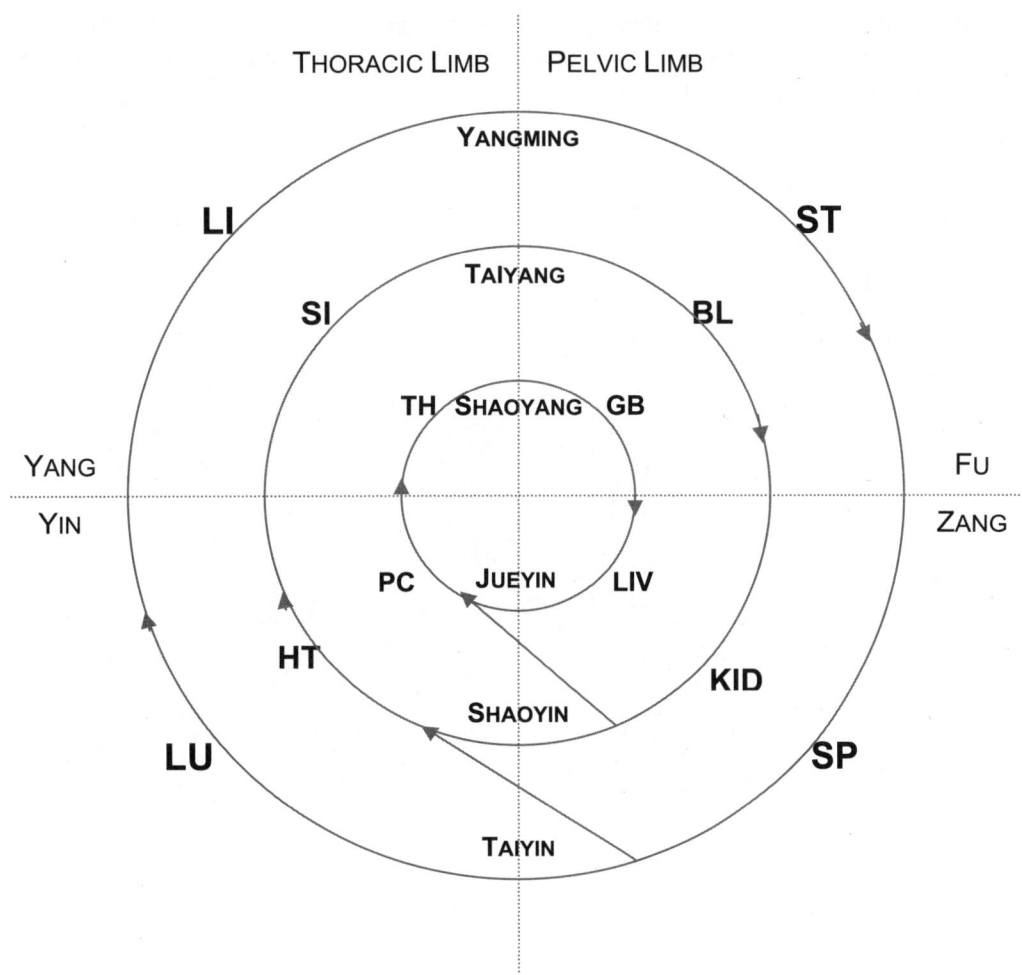

Figure 5.2: A summary of the Levels and Organ associations

The Meridians exist internally and externally as they connect all parts of the body together. The following images will trace these pathways on the human, dog/cat, and horse. The Meridians, especially including the internal branches, are well described in humans. Omissions in the animal Meridian descriptions may be extrapolated from the human model; however, differences in anatomy may require some modifications of the pathway in various species.

The Unit of Measurement of the Body

Acupuncture points may be located at certain distances from a body landmark or another point. Because of the differences in size between one individual and the next, we can not use absolute measurements such as inches or centimeters. In acupuncture practice, it is common to the unit "*cun*" to measure the body. The cun is a relative or proportional measurement unit which is used to locate the *Jing-luo* and acupuncture points. For example, there are always 12 cun between the wrist and elbow of every human being, so the distance between the wrist and the elbow is the same whether the person is 7 feet tall or only reaches 4 feet.

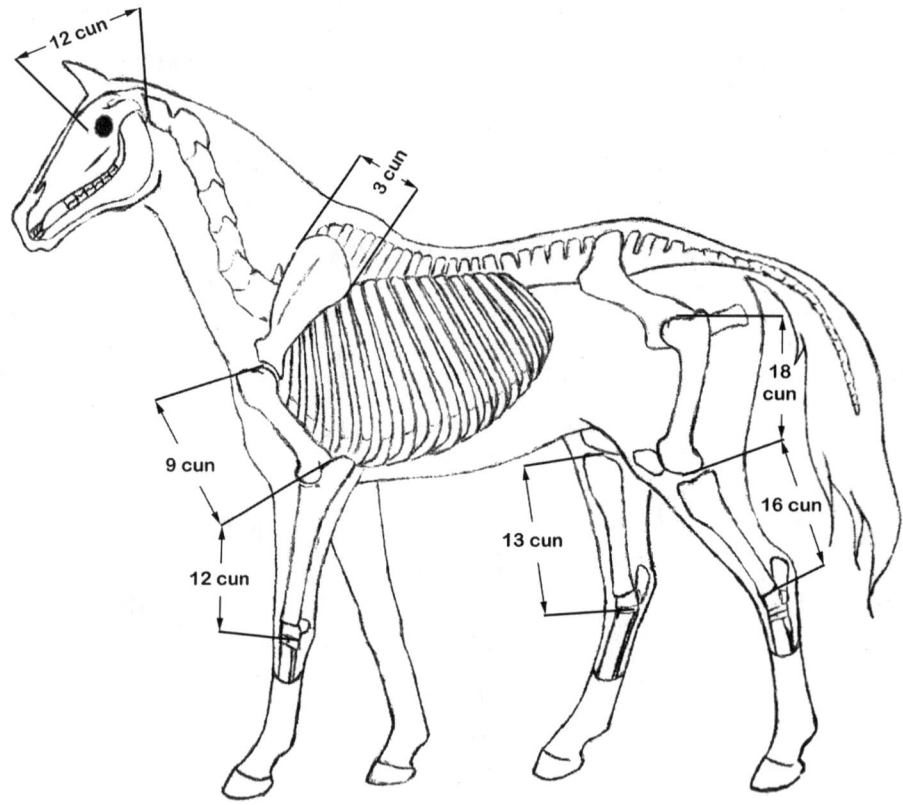

Figure 5.3: Cun measurements for the horse

As shown in Figure 5.3, the distance from the point of the hip (the greater trochanter) to the center of the stifle is 18 cun. On the lateral leg, it is 16 cun from the center of the stifle to the center of the hock, but it is 13 cun on the medial leg. The scapula is 3 cun wide from cranial to caudal edge at its widest part. The distance from the point of the shoulder (the greater tubercle) to the elbow is 9 cun. The leg is 12 cun from the center of the elbow to the center of the carpus. On the head, the distance along the midline from the back of the skull to just cranial to the eyes is 12 cun.

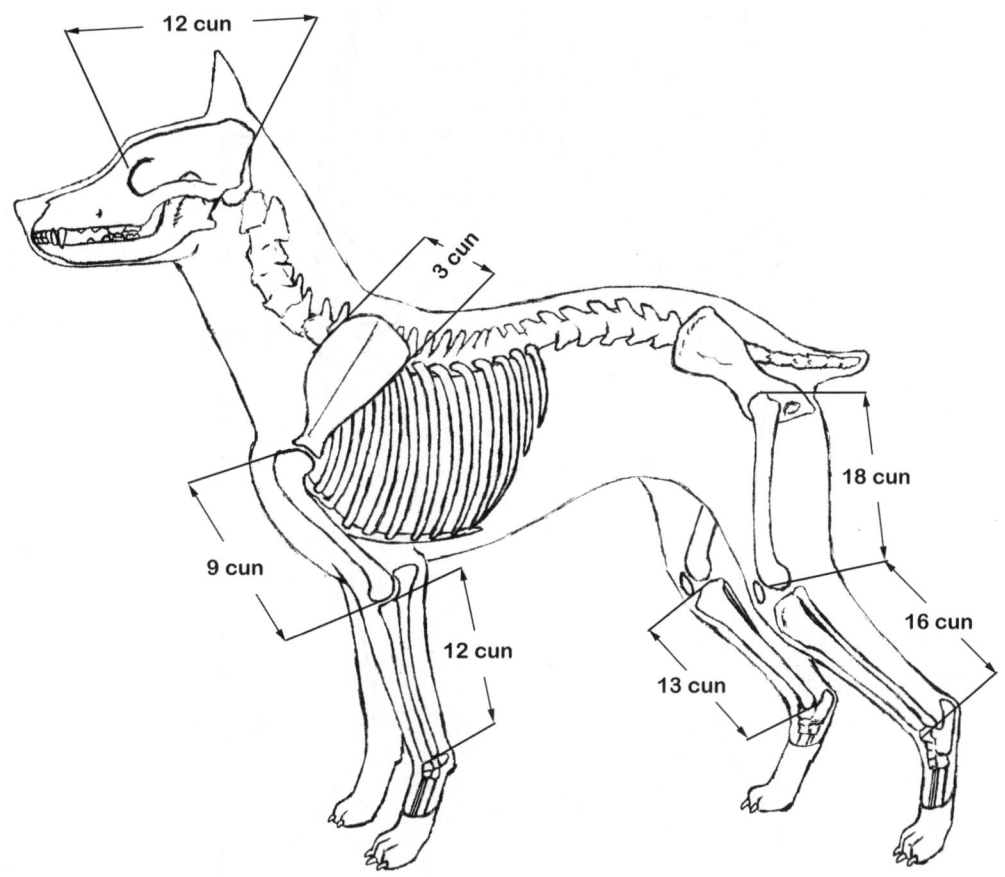

Figure 5.4: Cun measurements for the dog

As shown in Figure 5.4, the distance from the greater trochanter to the center of the stifle is 18 cun. On the lateral side, it is 16 cun from the center of the stifle to the lateral malleolus, but on the medial side it is 13 cun from the medial epicondyle of the tibia to the medial malleolus. The scapula is 3 cun wide from cranial to caudal edge. The distance from the greater tubercle to the elbow is 9 cun. The front leg is 12 cun from the center of the elbow to the area just proximal to the carpus. On the head, the distance from the back of the skull to just cranial to the eyes is 12 cun along the midline.

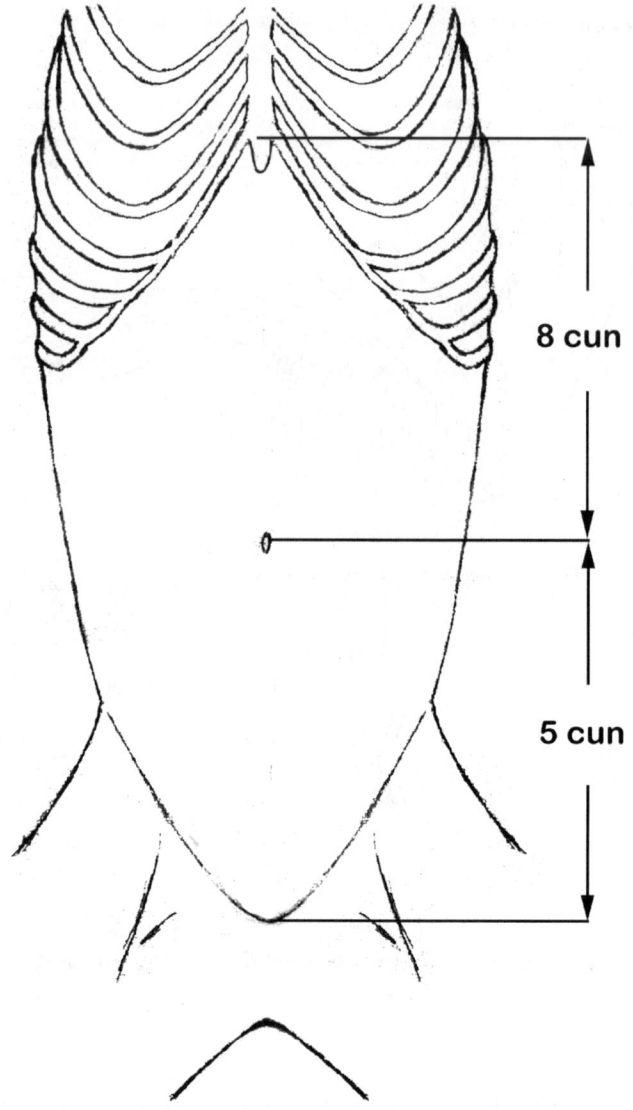

8 cun

5 cun

Figure 5.5: Cun measurement of the ventral abdomen

As demonstrated in Figure 5.5, the distance from the pubis to the umbilicus is 5 cun. The distance from the umbilicus to the xiphoid process (just cranial to the xiphoid cartilage) is 8 cun. CV-12 is located halfway between the xiphoid process and the umbilicus. CV-14 is halfway between CV-12 and the xiphoid process. If the space between the pubis and the umbilicus is divided into five equal parts, the first and last points relate to CV-2 and CV-8 respectively. CV-2 is just cranial to the pubis and CV-8 is the center of the umbilicus. CV-3, CV-4, CV-5, and CV-7 are located sequentially on each of the equidistant subdivisions. CV-6 is located halfway between CV-5 and CV-7.

LUNG CHANNEL

Human

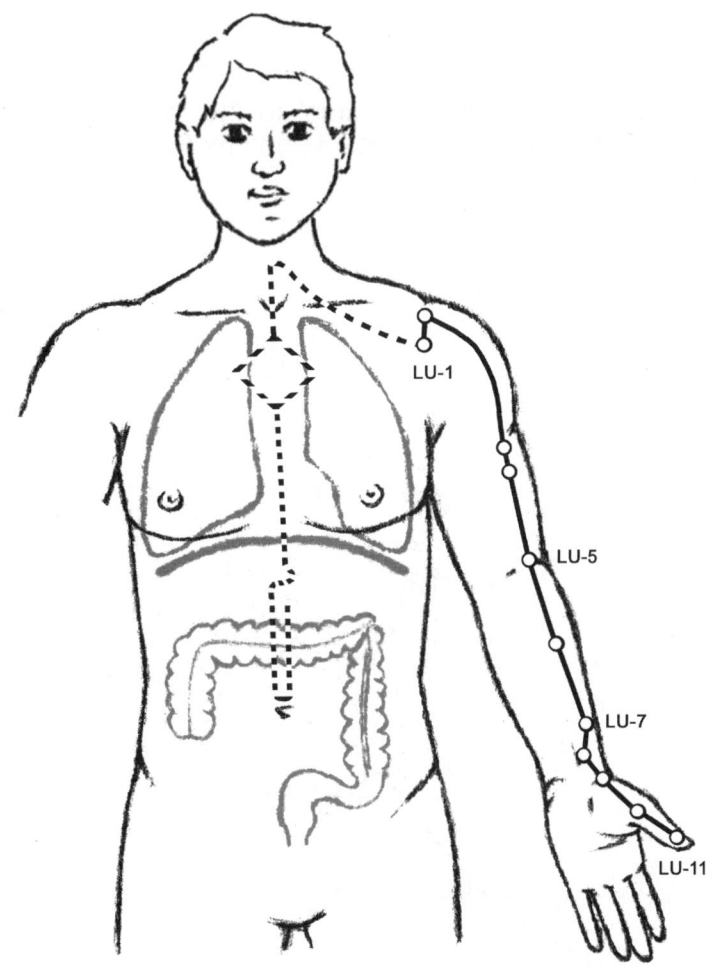

Internal Branch

The Lung Channel (LU) originates from the Middle Jiao (Stomach), and it runs downward to connect with the Large Intestine. Turning back, it travels along the lower gate of the stomach (pylorus) and the upper gate of the stomach (*ostium cardiacum*). It passes upward through the diaphragm to enter its pertaining Organ, the Lungs. From there, it ascends to the throat, and finally emerges on the body surface at the first Lung Meridian point *Zhong-fu* (LU-1). LU-1 is located on the median edge of the brachiocephalicus muscle, medial to the lesser tubercle of the humerus in the first intercostal space.

Lateral Branch

This branch travels along the surface of the body. From LU-1, the LU channel descends along the medial aspect of the upper arm to reach the cubital fossa of forelimb (LU-5). It then goes along the anterior portion of the radial side in the medial aspect of the forearm to enter *Cunkou* (the radial artery at the carpus for pulse diagnosis). It passes above the radial artery of the carpus to LU-9 (medial aspect of the carpus, immediately distal to the radial styloid process). It finally emerges at the LU-11 (the medial coronary border of the first phalanx of the arm).

Extra Branch

From LU-7 (medial aspect of the arm, proximal to the radial styloid process), it runs directly to the radial side of the tip of the second phalanx (LI-1) to connect with the Large Intestine Channel (LI).

Small Animal

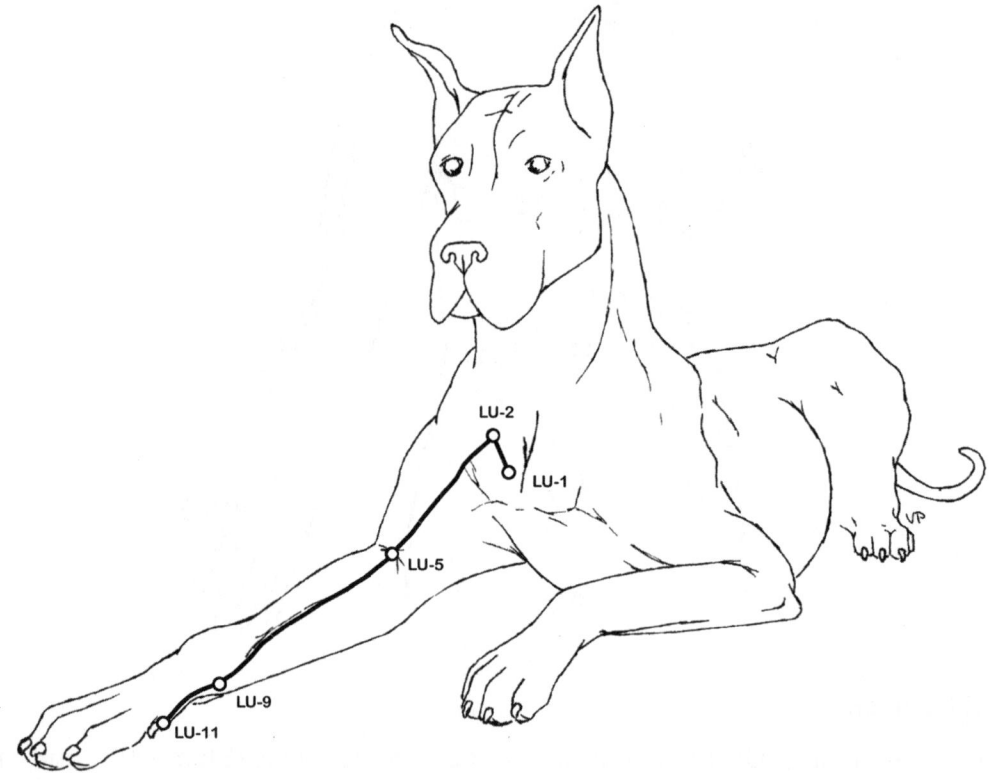

The Lung Channel begins on the chest at the first intercostal space. From there it travels along the craniomedial aspect of the foreleg to reach the elbow crease. The channel passes just lateral to the biceps tendon and runs distally toward the carpus. At the carpal crease, the channel flows parallel to the radial artery on the radial side. From here the Lung Channel travels to the first digit where it ends at the medial nail bed. A small extra branch runs from LU-7 distally to connect with the Large Intestine Channel on the first digit.

Horse

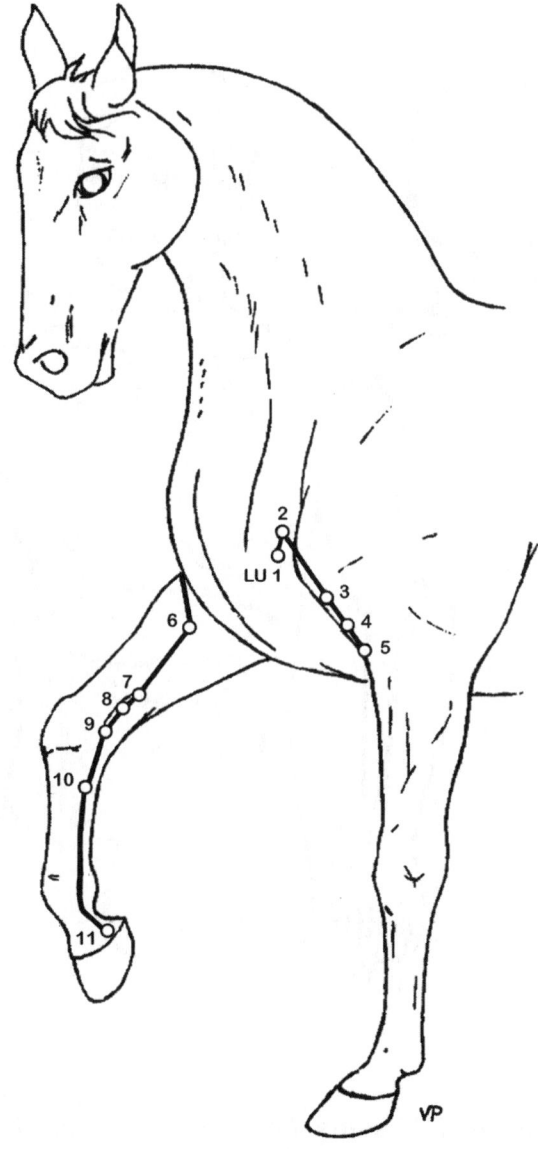

The Lung Channel originates from the Middle Jiao (Stomach). It runs downward to connect with the Large Intestine organ. Turning back, it goes along the Stomach, passes upward through the diaphragm to enter its pertaining organ (the lungs). From there, it ascends to the throat, descends the jugular grooves to the *Shuang-fu-mai* (carotid artery, a location for equine pulse diagnosis), and emerges at LU-1 (*Zhong-fu*). LU-1 is located in the first intercostal space medial to the humerus, over the muscularis pectoralis descendens, directly medial to the cephalic vein.

From LU-1, the Lung channel descends to reach the medial side of cubital crease and cranial edge of the elbow region (LU-5, *Chi Ze*). It then goes along the medial aspect of the forearm and craniomedial edge of the radius to an area just proximal to the carpus. It then passes caudal to the carpus and metacarpus. It terminates at a point just proximal to the coronary band and cranial to the medial collateral cartilage (LU-11, *Shao Shang*).

LARGE INTESTINE CHANNEL

Human

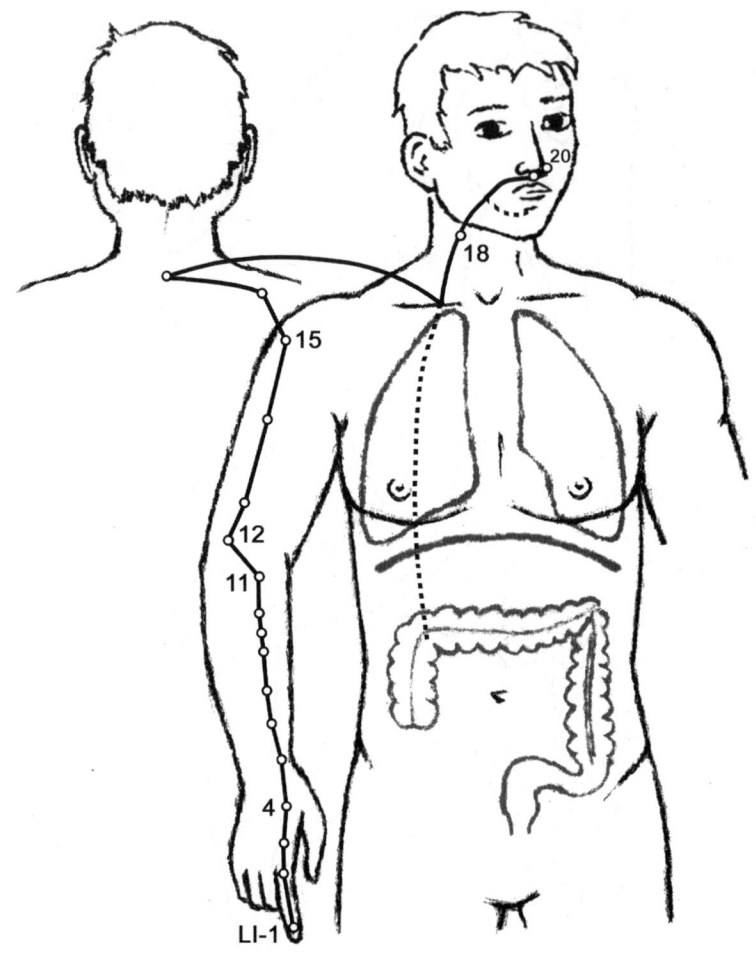

Major Surface Branch

The Large Intestine Channel (LI) starts from the tip of the index finger (LI-1), runs upward along the radial side of the index finger. It passes through the space between the first and second metacarpal bones (LI-4). From there, it goes upward along the anterior border of lateral aspect of the forearm and upper arm to the highest point of the shoulder (LI-15). It then goes to the seventh cervical vertebra (GV-14, the confluence of six Yang Channels) to connect with the Governing Vessel Channel (GV). From there, it descends to the supraclavicular fossa to connect with its Extra Surface Branch and its Internal Branch.

Extra Surface Branch

It begins at the supraclavicular fossa and runs upward to the neck. It passes through the cheek, and enters internally the gums of lower teeth. Exteriorly, it curves around the upper lip and crosses through the philtrum (GV-26) to enter the opposite side of nose (LI-20) and connect with the Stomach Channel.

Internal Branch

Beginning at the supraclavicular fossa, it enters the body interior to connect with the Lung. It then passes through the diaphragm and enters the pertaining Organ, Large Intestine.

Small Animals

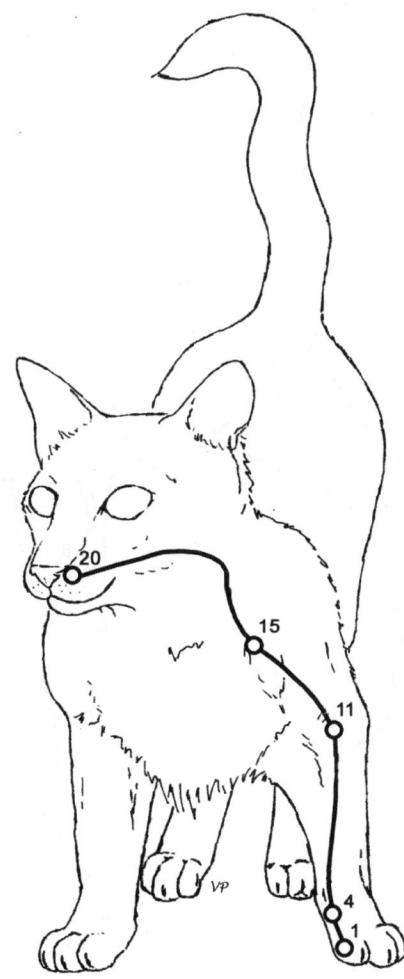

The Large Intestine Meridian begins on the distal foreleg at the medial nail bed of the second digit. The Meridian travels proximally along the radial side of the second digit and between the first and second metatarsal bones. It continues along a cranial and lateral path up the foreleg to the lateral side of the elbow. It continues to flow cranially past the shoulder and turns up the neck toward the head. The Meridian ends on the face lateral to the nostril (LI 20).

Horses

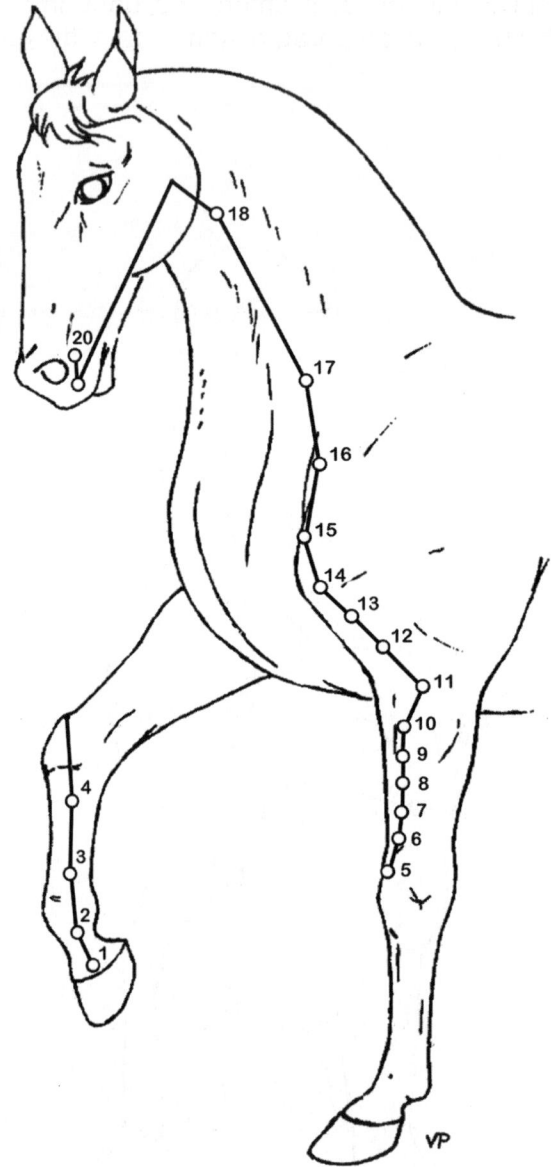

The Large Intestine Meridian begins on the distal foreleg at a point proximal to the craniomedial aspect of the coronary band. The Meridian travels proximally up the medial pastern and metacarpus and along the cranial aspect of the carpus. At the carpus, it moves laterally and continues proximally along the craniolateral foreleg up to the ventral neck. It continues along the larynx and mandible and ends at a point lateral to the ventral border of the nares.

STOMACH CHANNEL

Human

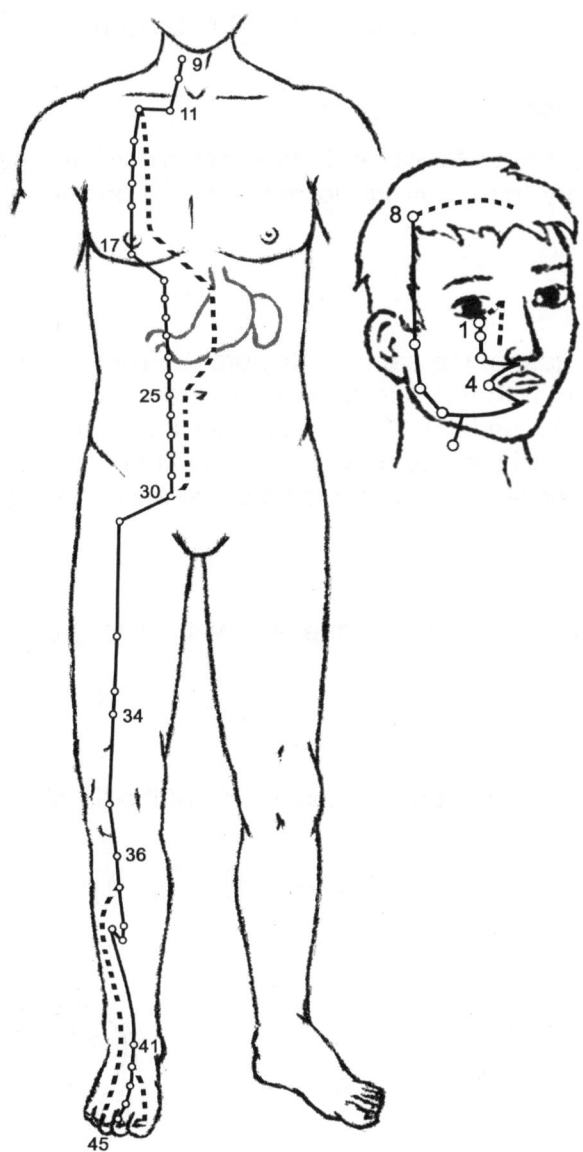

Lateral Branch

The Stomach Channel (ST) begins internally at LI-20 (the lateral side of ala nasi) where the Large Intestine Channel terminates. It ascends to the bridge of the nose to meet the inner corner of the eye (BL-1). It then emerges under the eyes to ST-1 and descends along the lateral side of the nose and enters the upper gums. It curves around the lips and descends to meet CV-24, the mentolabial groove. From there, it turns upward and runs along the lower jaw to ST-5 (the lower portion of the cheek). Along the angle of the mandible, it ascends in front of the ear and follows the anterior hairline to reach the forehead (GV-24).

Facial Branch

It starts at ST-5. From there, it runs downward to ST-9 and along the throat. It enters the supraclavicular fossa. It then descends to pass through the diaphragm, and enters the stomach, its pertaining organ, and connects with the Spleen.

Supraclavicular Branch

It starts from supraclavicular fossa and runs downward to the nipple. And then it descends and passes by the umbilicus to enter ST-30 on the lateral side of the lower abdomen.

Stomach Branch

It starts from the lower gate of the stomach (pylorus). From there, it descends inside the abdomen and then joins with the Supraclavicular Branch at ST-30. From there, it runs downward through ST-31 and ST-32 to reach the knee. It then continues downward along the anterior border of the lateral aspect of the tibia. It passes through the dorsum of the foot and ends at the lateral side of the tip of the second toe (ST-45).

Tibial Branch

Starting at ST-36 three cun below the knee, it travels distally and enters the lateral side of the middle toe.

Foot Branch

It starts at ST-42 and terminates on the medial side of the tip of the big toe and connects with the Spleen Channel.

Small Animals

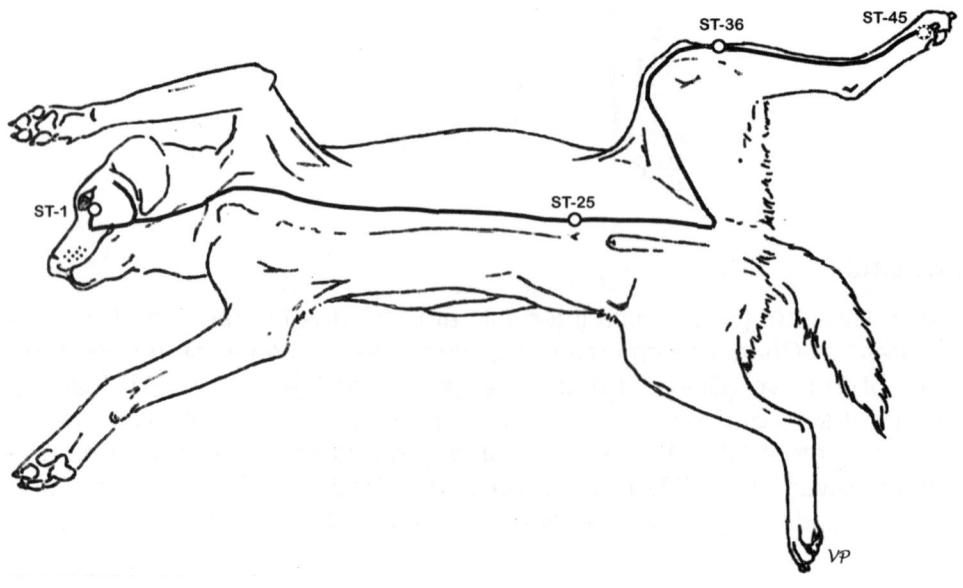

The Stomach Meridian begins on the head directly below the pupil within the orbit. It descends lateral to the nose, curves around the edge of the lips, and it curves upward along the angle of the jaw in front of the ear. It then travels downward and caudally along the ventral surface of the neck, chest, and abdomen. The Meridian travels along the cranial-lateral surface of the thigh to the lateral side of the stifle. From there it travels distally along the craniolateral leg and passes between the second and third metatarsals to end at the lateral nail bed of the second digit.

Horses

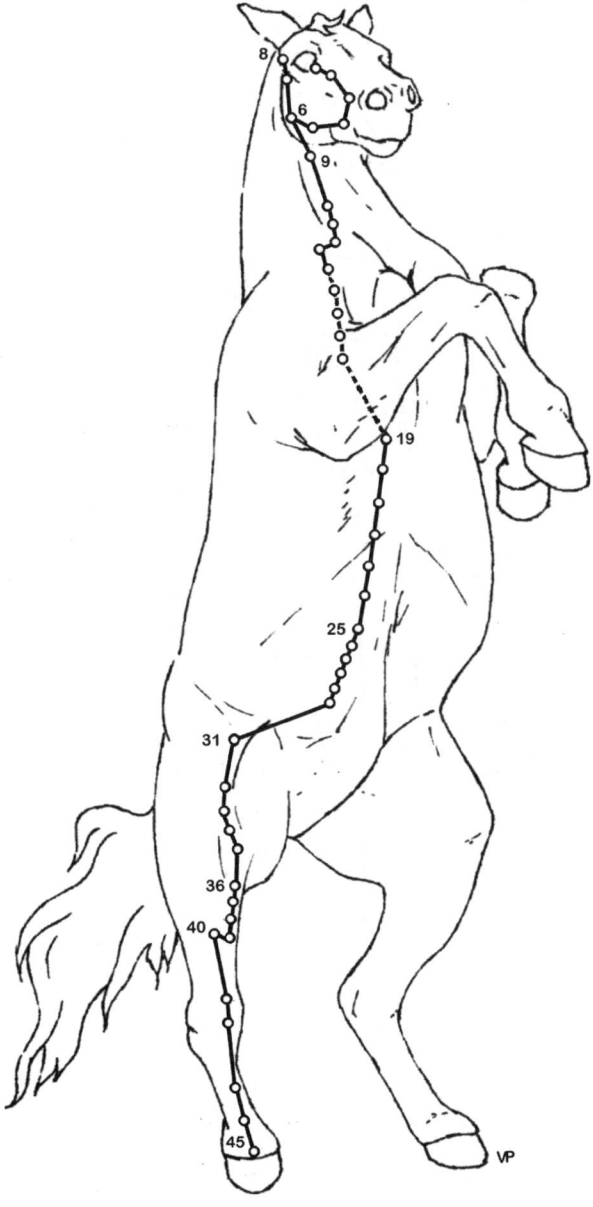

The Stomach Meridian begins on the head just ventral to the eye at the midpoint. It descends to curve around the edge of the lips, and then it turns along the angle of the jaw in front of the ear to the temporomandibular joint. Subsequently coursing along the ventral aspect of the neck and chest, it runs parallel to the ventral midline at a distance of about 1.5 cun. After meeting the groin, it runs towards the ventral aspect of the tuber coxae, and it travels along the cranial-lateral surface of the hind leg. It ends on the craniolateral aspect of the coronary band.

SPLEEN CHANNEL

Human

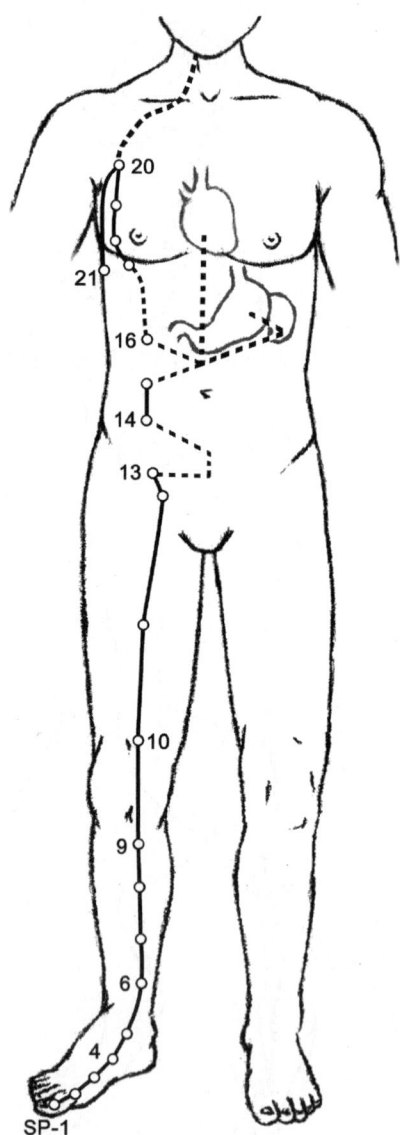

Lateral Branch

The Spleen Channel (SP) starts at the tip of the medial aspect of the big toe, and it runs along the medial aspect of the foot. Turning in front of the medial malleolus, it ascends along the medial and posterior aspect of the leg. Traveling along the posterior aspect of the tibia, it crosses in front of the Liver Channel at a level eight cun dorsal to the medial malleolus. It continues its ascent along the anterior medial aspect of the knee and thigh, and it enters the inguinal area and the lower abdomen. From there, it runs perpendicular and four cun lateral to the abdominal midline. It travels straight up to the last ribs, and then turns laterally to a distance six cun lateral to the abdominal midline. It ascends perpendicularly to the abdominal midline to reach the second intercostals space.

Internal Branch

Starting at the abdomen, the branch enters the abdominal cavity, meets the Spleen, its pertaining organ, and connects with the Stomach. It passes through the diaphragm and reaches the esophagus. It then runs upward alongside the esophagus and larynx, and then reaches the root of the tongue and spread over the lower surface of the tongue.

Extra Internal Branch

It starts at the stomach, and then goes upward through the diaphragm. It flows into the Heart to link with the Heart Channel.

Small Animals

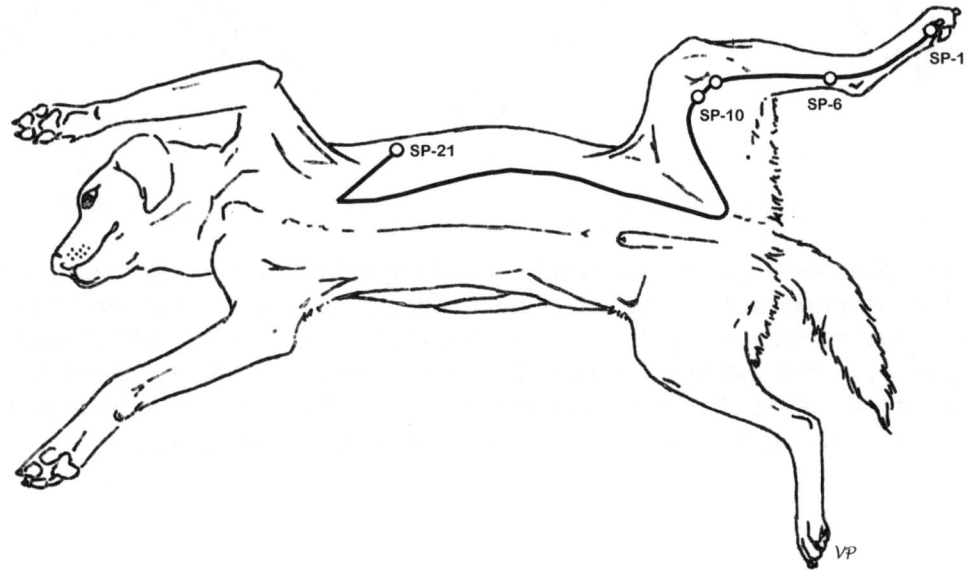

The Spleen Channel begins on the hind foot at the medial nail bed of the most medial toe (the first or second phalanx). It travels proximally along the medial aspect of the most medial toe up to the hock. The Channel continues towards the groin following a path along the caudomedial border of the tibia and past the medial aspect of the stifle. On the medial thigh, the Channel flows along the cranial aspect of the leg and then runs along the ventrolateral body wall to end on the chest.

Horses

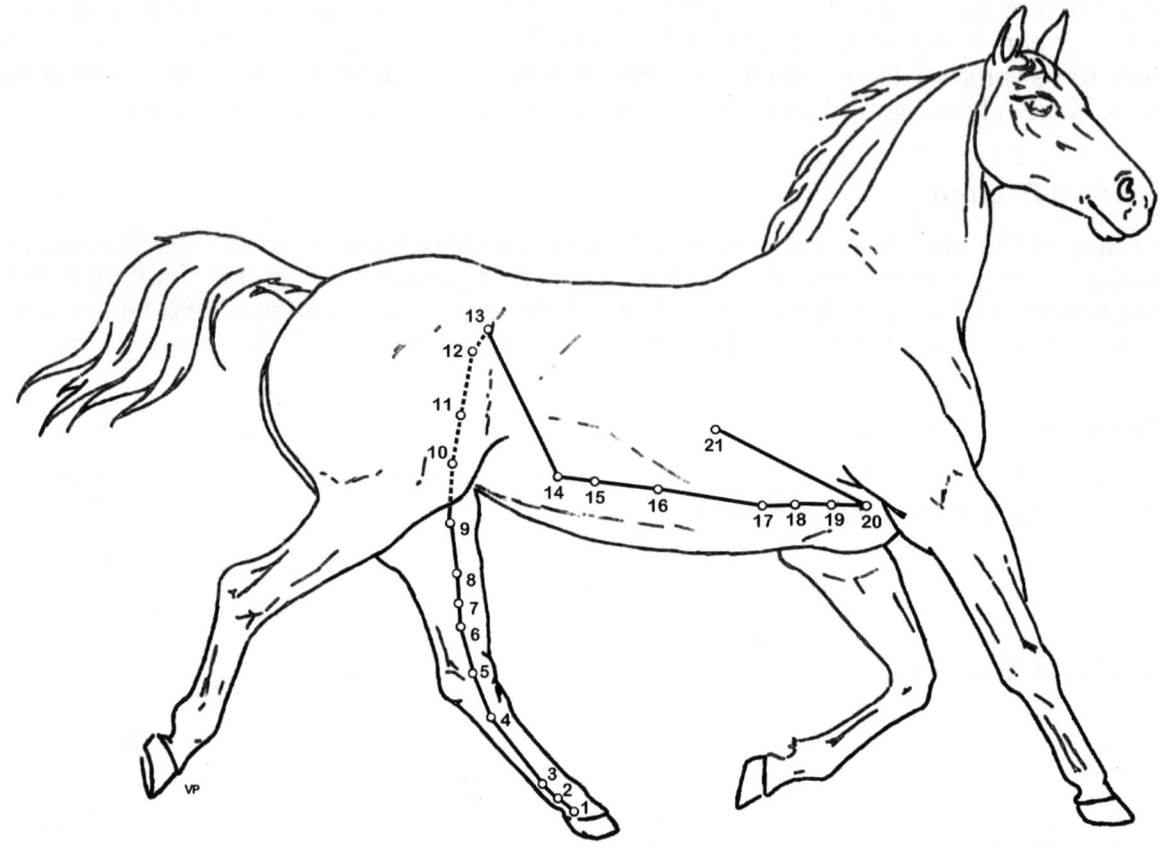

The Spleen Channel begins on the caudomedial aspect of the coronary band of the hind limb. It travels proximally along the medial aspect of the pastern and metatarsus. Traveling more cranially along the middle of the tibia, it crosses the medial aspect of the stifle and ascends to a location cranial to the tuber coxae. As it moves cranially, it curves along the ventral chest to the fourth intercostals space. It then turns caudally and ends at a point in the fourteenth intercostals space at the level of the shoulder joint.

HEART CHANNEL

Human

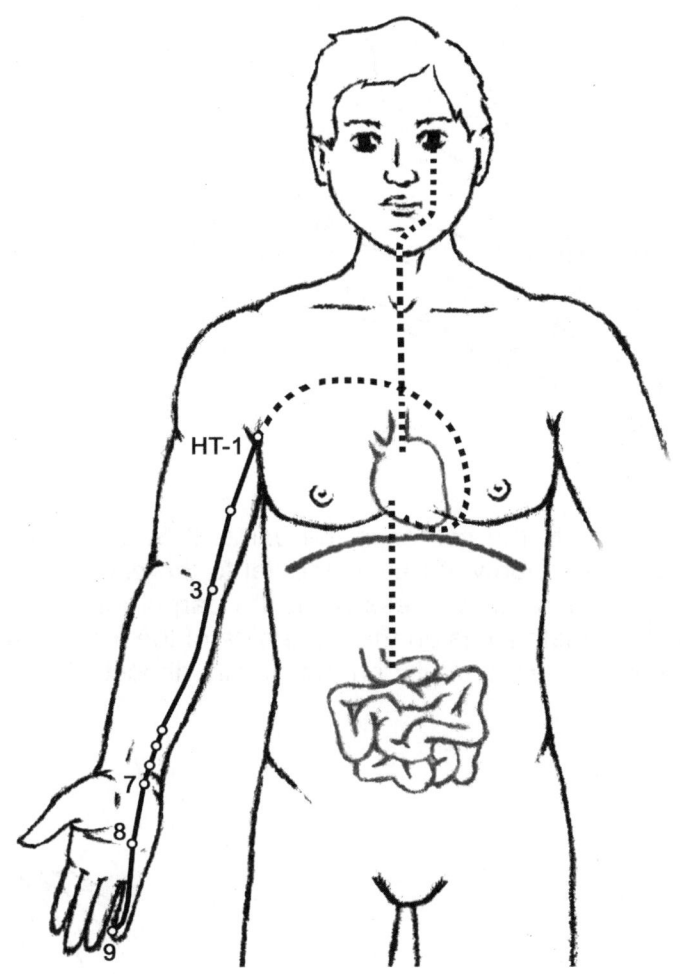

Internal Branch

It originates from the Heart. It emerges and spreads over the "Heart system". From there, it is divided into three portions: It descends and passes through the diaphragm to connect with the small intestine. It ascends and runs alongside the esophagus to connect with the eyes. It goes upward to the Lung, and then runs downward to emerge at the center of axilla (HT-1).

Lateral Branch

It starts at the axilla and runs downward. It travels along the posterior and medial border of the upper arm to enter the cubital fossa. Continuing along the posterior border of the medial forearm, it reaches the pisiform region of the palm. From there, it follows the medial aspect of the little finger, enters the tip of medial aspect of the little finger, and connects with the Small Intestine Channel.

Small Animals

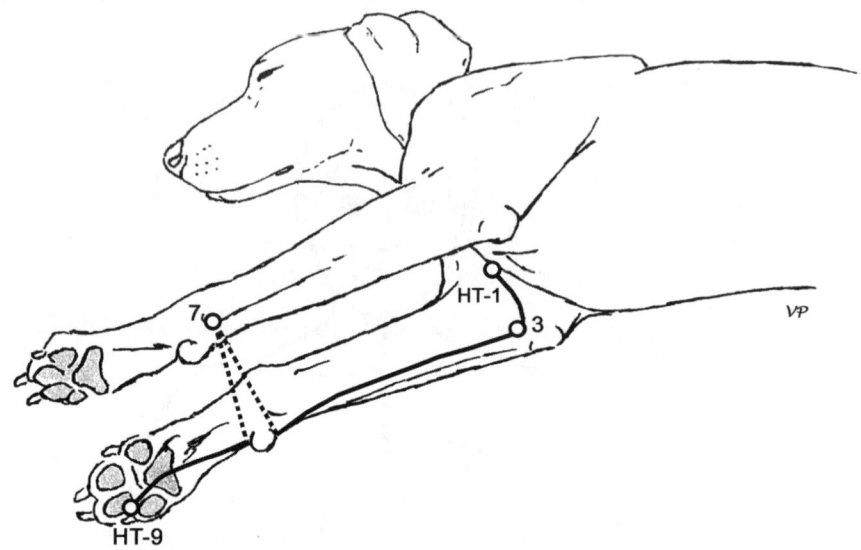

The Heart Channel begins in the center of the axilla. It flows distally along the medial aspect of the foreleg. At the elbow, it travels medial to the cubital crease and continues distally to intersect with the large depression at the carpal joint adjacent to the carpal pad. From there, the Channel travels on the underside of the foot between the fourth and fifth metacarpals. It comes back dorsally on the medial aspect of the fifth digit to end at the nail bed.

Horses

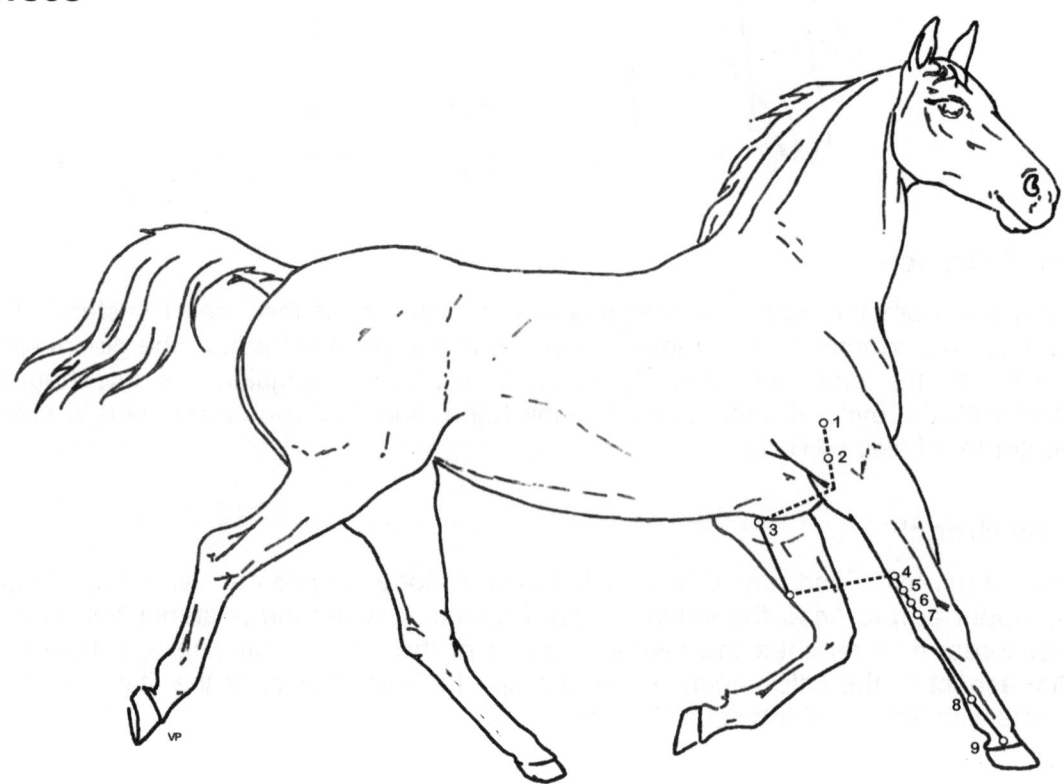

The Heart Meridian begins at the Heart. It emerges on the body surface at a point caudomedial to the shoulder joint. Traveling distally down the foreleg, it follows the caudomedial side of the ulna to the caudal aspect of the carpus. At the carpus it crosses laterally and continues distally. It ends on the craniolateral aspect of the coronary band.

SMALL INTESTINE CHANNEL

Human

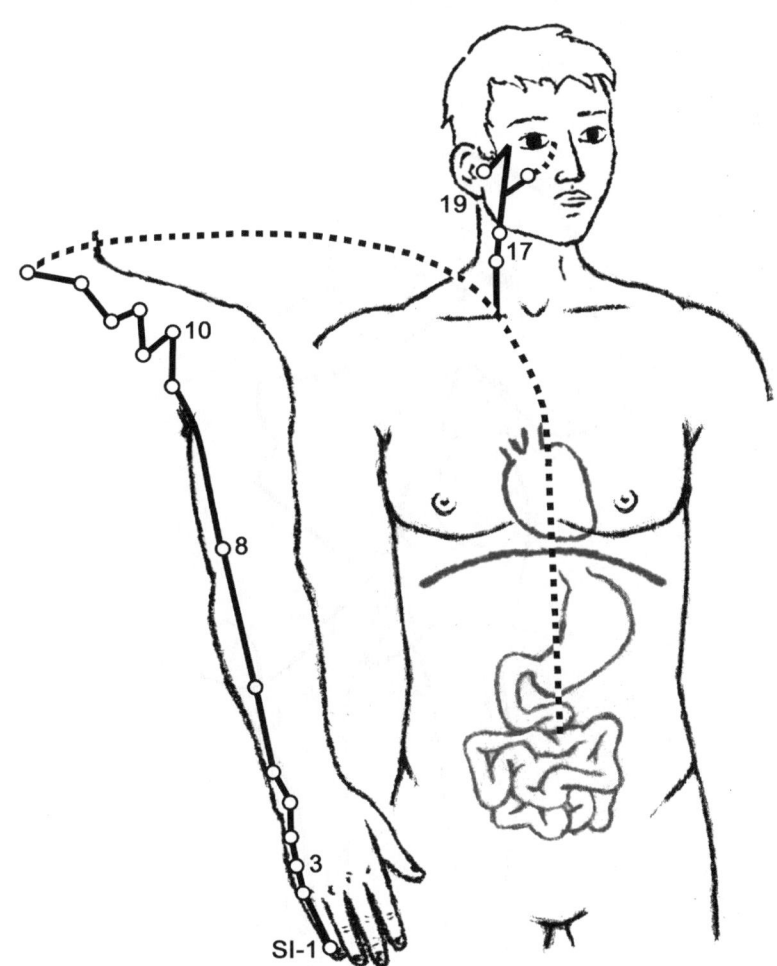

Lateral Branch

The Small Intestine Channel (SI) begins at the ulnar (medial) side of the tip of the little finger (SI-1) and runs along the ulnar side of the palm to the wrist. It then passes upward along the posterior border of the lateral forearm and runs between the olecranon of the ulna the medial epicondyle of the humerus. It then goes upward along the posterior border of the lateral upper arm, circles behind the shoulder, and reaches the cervical and thoracic conjunction (GV-14) where it connects with the GV Channel. From there, it turns to the supraclavicular fossa, ascends along the side of the neck to the cheek and lateral canthus of the eye, and reaches the ear (SI-19).

Extra Lateral Branch

This branch starts from the cheek. It then ascends to the medial canthus (BL-1) to connect with the Bladder Channel (BL).

Internal Branch

It starts at the supraclavicular fossa and enters internally to the heart. Then it descends along the esophagus, passes through the diaphragm and the stomach. Finally, it reaches the Small Intestine, its pertaining organ.

Small Animals

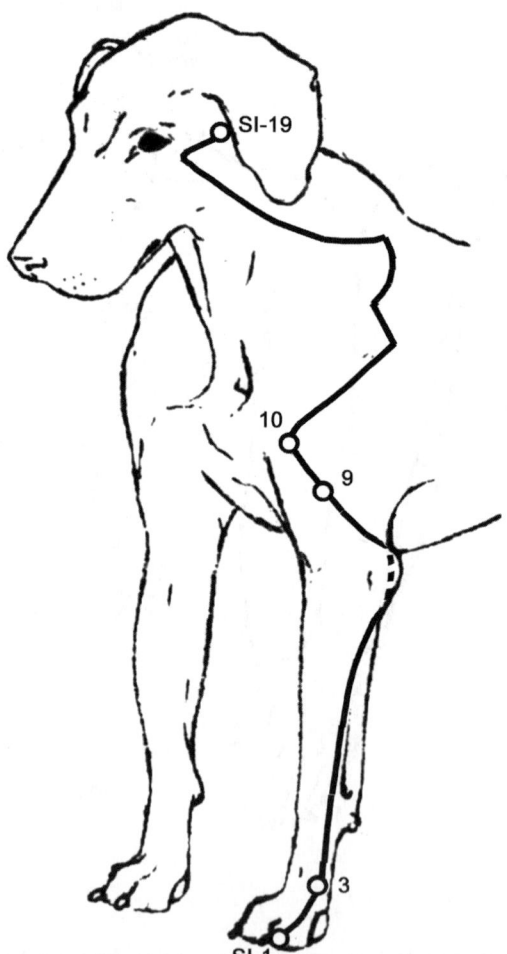

The Small Intestine Channel begins on the fifth digit of the foreleg. From the lateral nail bed, the Channel flows proximally along the lateral and caudal border of the leg. The Channel runs medial to the point of the elbow, but then returns to the lateral side beyond the elbow. Continuing up past the shoulder and along the neck, the Channel comes to an end rostral to the tragus of the ear.

Horses

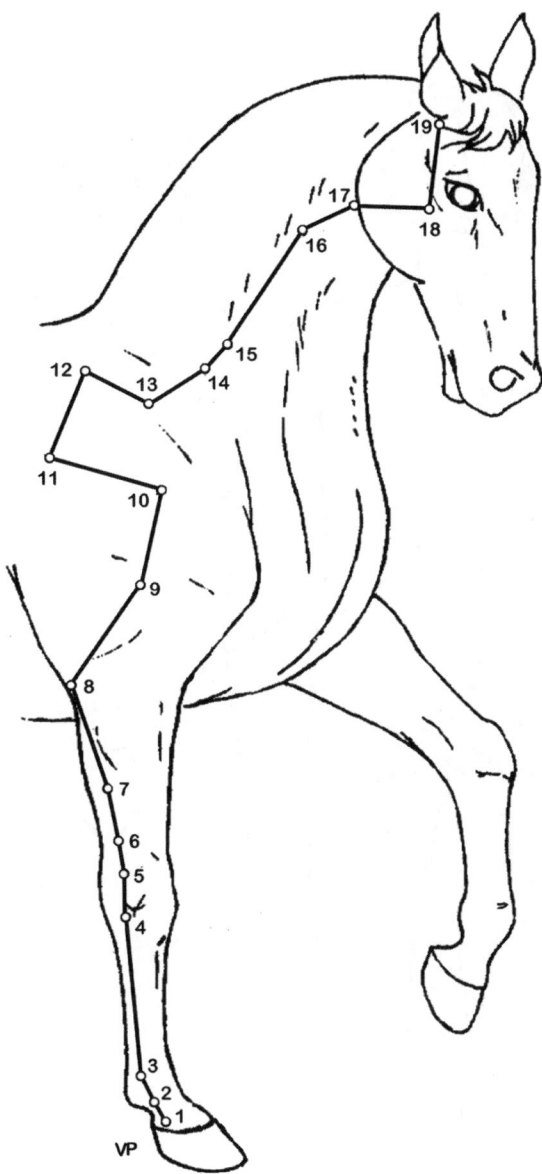

The Small Intestine Channel begins on the caudolateral aspect of the coronary band. It travels proximally along the craniolateral aspect of the forelimb. After passing over the triceps muscle and scapula, it moves cranially up the neck dorsal to the cervical vertebrae. It ends on the lateral side of the ear base.

URINARY BLADDER CHANNEL
Human

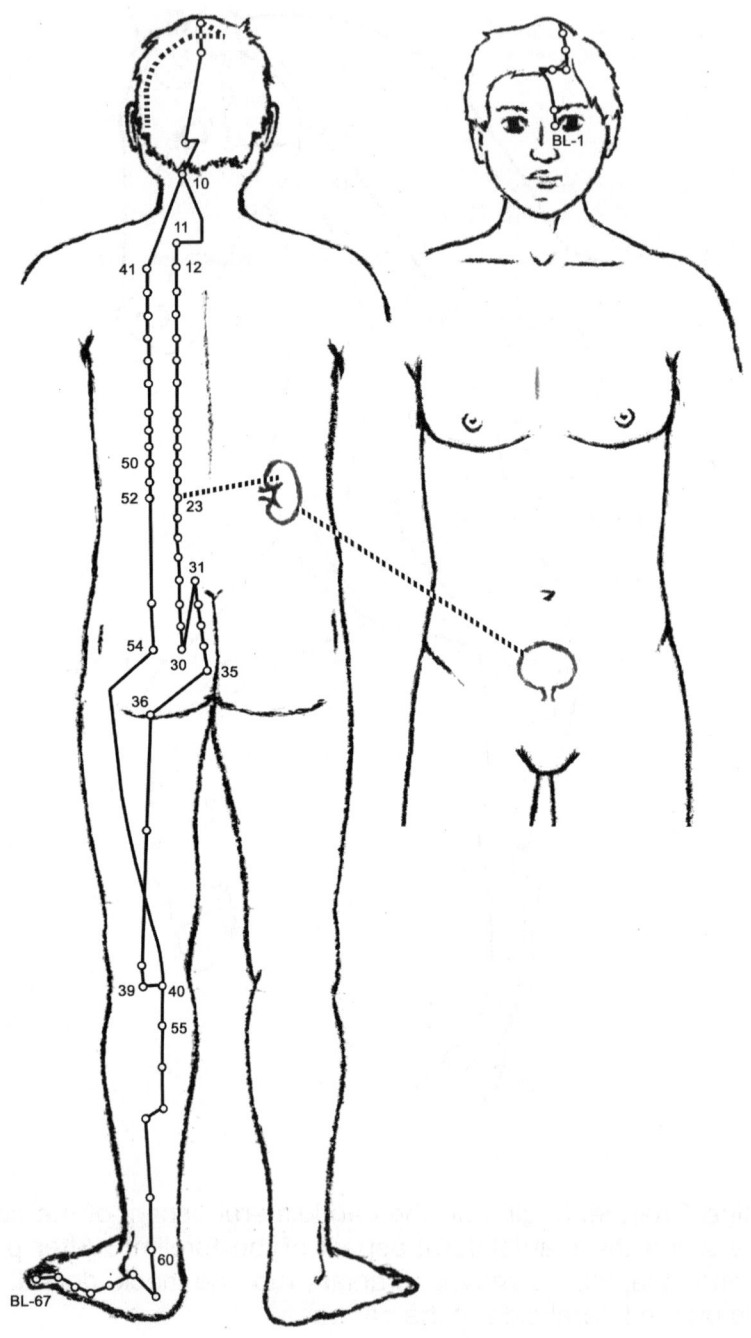

Lateral Branch

The Urinary Bladder Channel starts at the medial canthus (BL-1) and ascends across the forehead to cross at the vertex of head (GV-20). From GV-20, it bifurcates and runs alongside the dorsal midline to reach the occipital areas. From the occiput, it enters the skull (cranial cavity) to connect the brain. It then emerges at BL-10 and bifurcates into the inner branch and outer branch.

Inner Branch: From BL-10, it descends alongside the medial aspect of the scapula region and runs parallel to the vertebral column at a distance 1.5 cun lateral to the dorsal midline. It runs downward through the gluteal region and ends in the popliteal fossa (BL-40) to merge with the outer branch.

Outer Branch: It starts from BL-10. It then runs straight down the back at a distance three cun lateral to the dorsal midline. It passes through the gluteal region and crosses with GB-30. It then descends along the posterior border of the lateral thigh to enter the popliteal fossa (BL-40) and merge with the inner branch.

The merged branch then descends, passing through the gastrocnemius muscle to enter the posterior aspect of the external malleolus. It then runs along the lateral side of the fifth metatarsal bone to reach the lateral tip of the little toe (BL-67) and to connect with the Kidney Channel.

Internal Branch

It starts at the middle lumbar area (BL-23) and enters the body cavity where it reaches the kidneys. It then joins the bladder, its pertaining organ.

Extra Internal Branch

It starts at the occipital area, and enters the skull (cranial cavity) to connect with the brain.

Small Animals

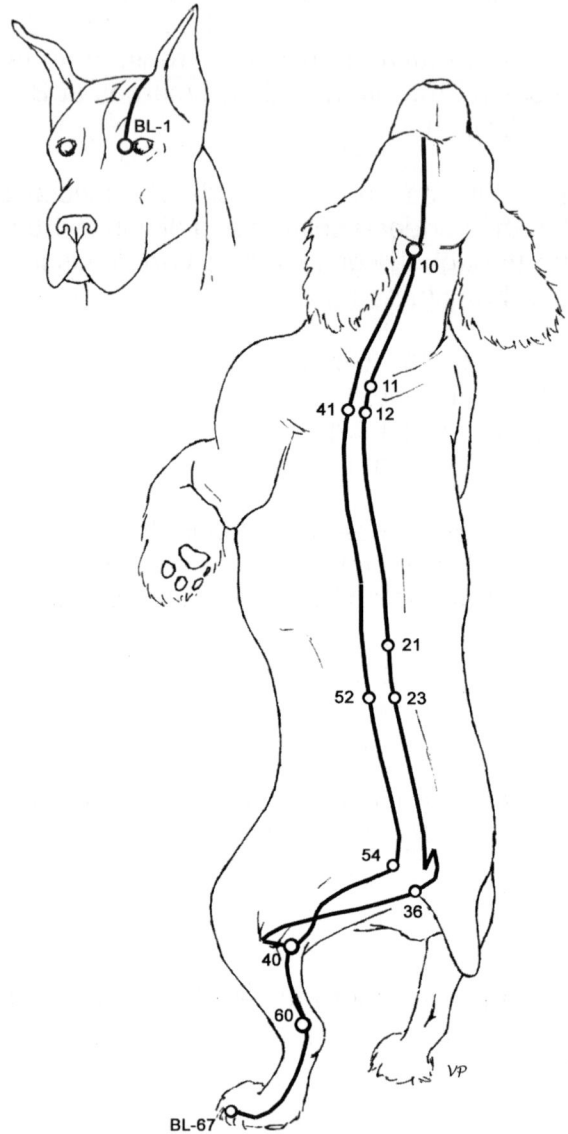

The Urinary Bladder Channel begins on the head. The Channel runs caudally from the medial canthus of the eye. The channel splits into two beyond the head and travels as two parallel channels caudally along the entire back. At the rump, the Channels continue to run distally along the caudal part of the hind leg. At the level of the stifle, the two Channels join again. The Channel continues along the caudal and lateral aspect of the distal leg until it ends on the lateral nail bed of the fifth digit.

Horses

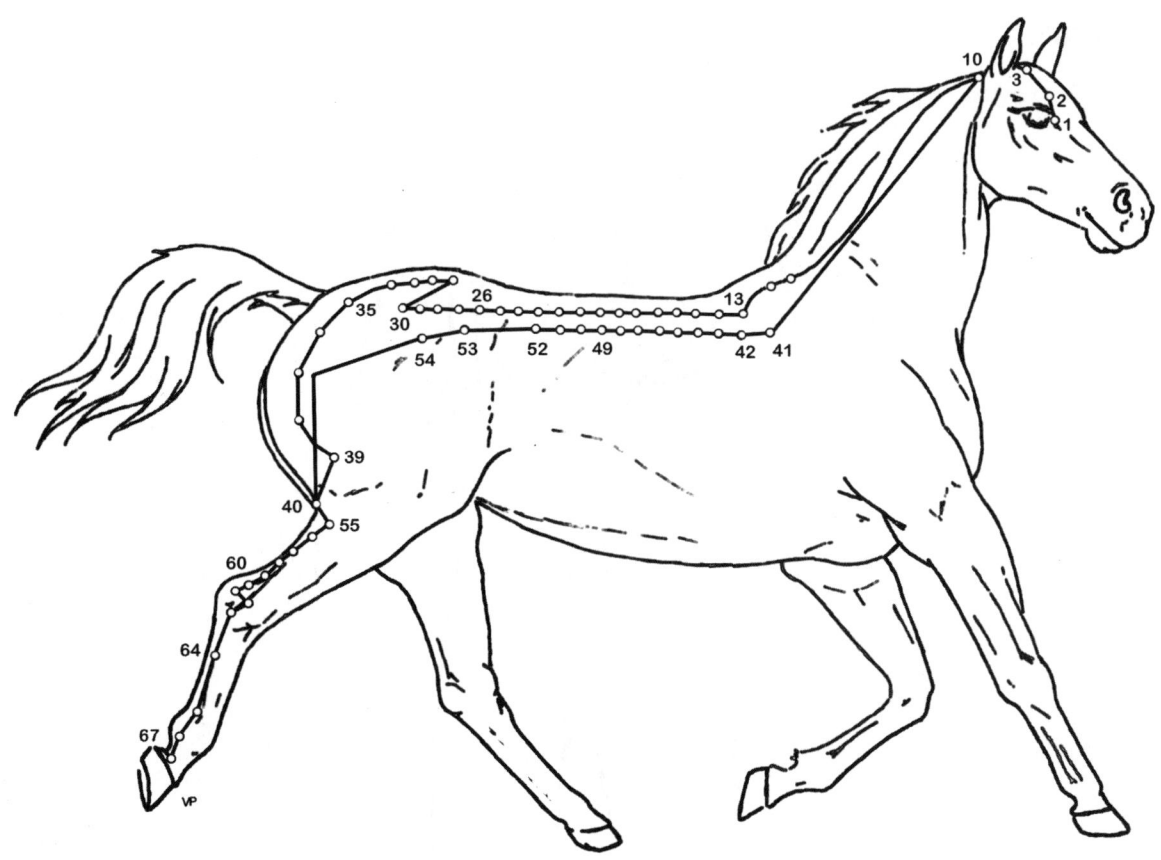

The Bladder Channel starts at the medial canthus of the eye. It continues caudally over the head parallel to the dorsal midline and medial to the ear. Running past the wings of the atlas, it travels down the dorsal portion of the neck to reach a point caudal to the scapula where it splits into two branches. The inner branch runs parallel to the spine at a distance three cun lateral to the dorsal midline and the outer branch runs similarly six cun lateral to the midline. At the popliteal fossa, the two branches join. The Meridian continues distally along the caudolateral aspect of the hind leg. It ends on the caudolateral aspect of the coronary band.

KIDNEY CHANNEL
Human

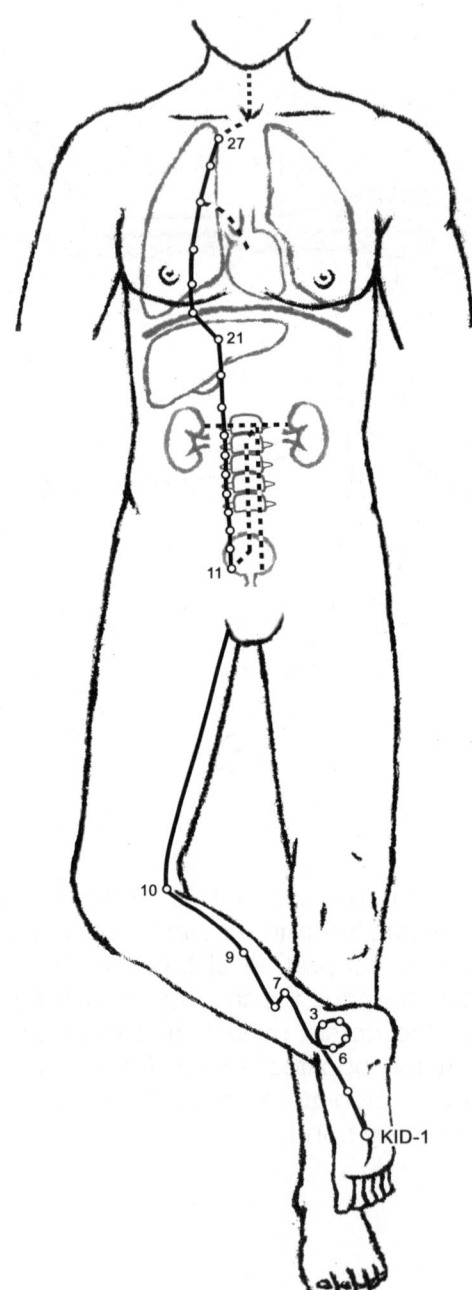

Lateral Branch

The Kidney Channel (KID) starts at the inferior aspect of the small toe, and runs obliquely towards the sole (KID-1). From KID-1, it emerges along the arch of the foot and runs upward between the heel and the inner ankle (the medial malleolus). It then runs medially along the posterior border of the leg towards the vertebral column (GV-1). It then connects to the Inner Branch which meets the kidney and bladder.

Extra Lateral Branch

It starts with the Internal Branch at the pubic bone, and then runs upward parallel to and 0.5 cun lateral to the ventral midline. At KID-21 (0.5 cun lateral to the ventral midline and 6 cun dorsal to the umbilicus), it runs obliquely laterally to KID-22 (two cun lateral to the ventral midline at the fifth intercostal space). From KID-22, it runs straight upward to end at KID-27 (lower border of the clavicle, two cun lateral to the ventral midline).

Internal Branch

From GV-1, the Kidney Meridian enters the body where it reaches the kidneys and connects the bladder. Then, it moves upward, passing through the liver and diaphragm to enter the lungs. Continuing along the throat, it terminates at the root of the tongue.

Extra Internal Branch

It starts at the lungs and passes through the heart. Entering the chest, it connects with the Pericardium Channel.

Small Animals

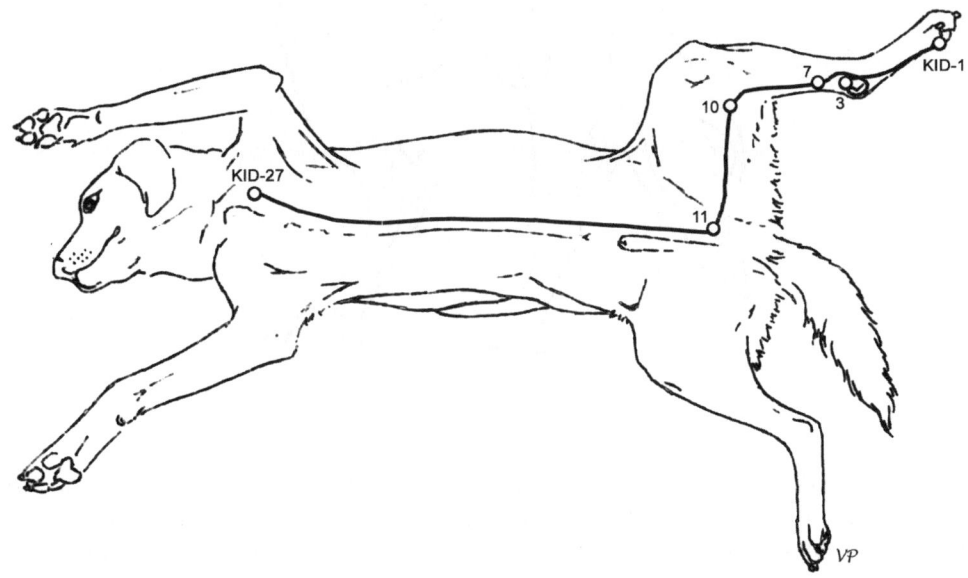

The Kidney Channel begins below the center of the metacarpal pad. The Channel travels up to the medial aspect of the tarsus where it circles around the medial malleolus before continuing proximally along the caudomedial leg. It then runs along the ventral aspect of the abdomen to end at the chest.

Horses

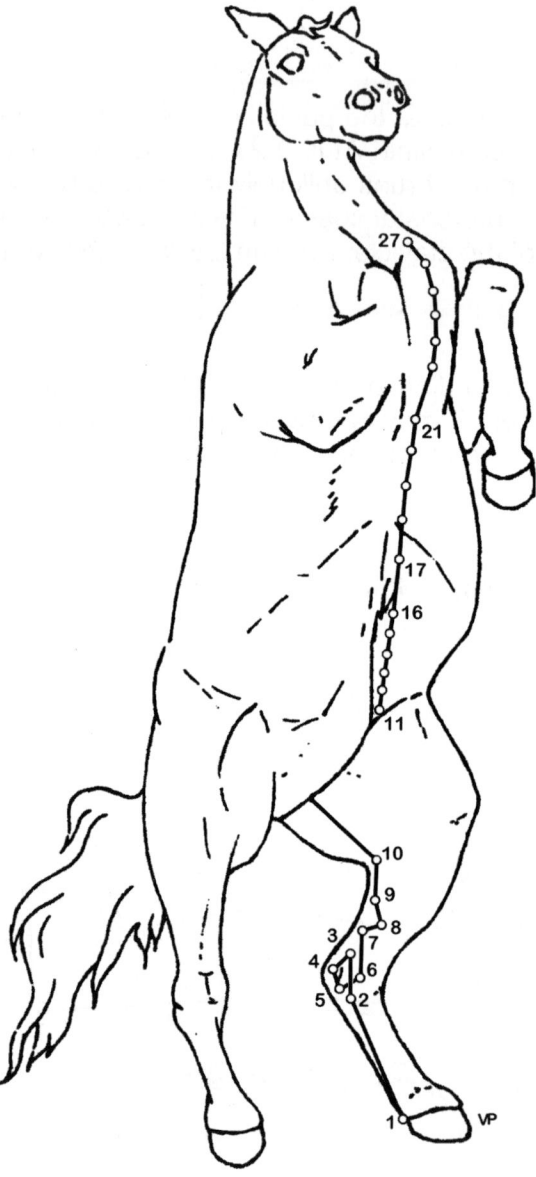

The Kidney Channel begins on the hind limb at a point between the bulbs of the heel. It courses proximally up the caudomedial aspect of the hind leg. At the abdomen, it runs cranially one cun parallel to the ventral midline. It ends between the sternum and the first rib.

PERICARDIUM CHANNEL

Human

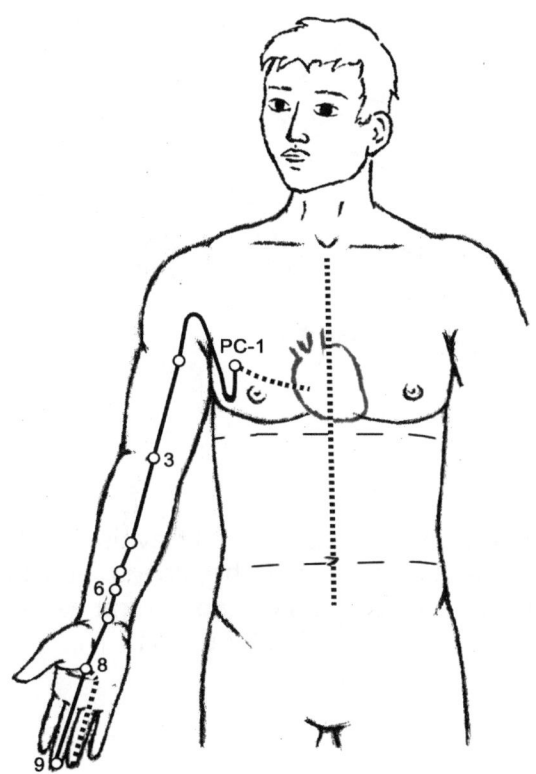

Internal Branch

The Pericardium (PC) Channel originates from the chest and enters its pertaining organ, the Pericardium. It then descends through the diaphragm to link the Upper, Middle, and Lower Jiao. A branch arising from the chest runs inside the chest and emerges at the point PC-1 (3 cun ventral to the center of axilla).

Lateral Branch

It originates from PC-1, and ascends to the center of axilla. From there, it runs down the medial aspect of the upper arm to the elbow crease. It descends further down the forearm and the palm to pass through PC-8 (on the transverse crease of the second and third metacarpal bones). The Channel ends at the tip of the middle finger. A short branch splits off at PC-8 and runs along the fourth digit to connect with the San Jiao Channel at the tip of the ring finger.

Small Animals

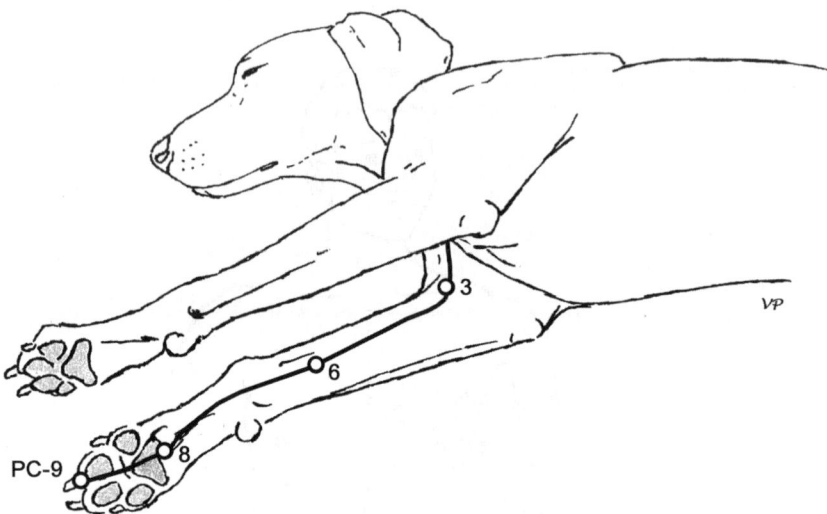

The Pericardium Channel begins on the chest and travels distally on the medial forelimb. At the elbow, it flows past the medial side of the biceps muscle tendon. Distally, it runs between the second and third metacarpals on the ventral aspect of the foot. At the end, it moves dorsally to end at the nail bed of the third digit.

Horses

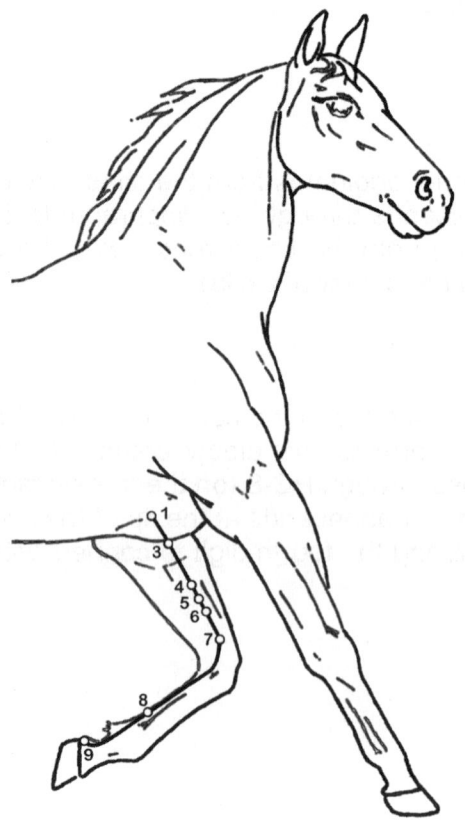

The Pericardium Channel begins in the pericardium. It emerges on the surface between the fifth rib and the medial aspect of the elbow. Moving distally along the medial foreleg, it courses along the caudomedial aspect of the leg between the Lung Channel and the chestnut. It continues past the accessory carpal bone and down the metacarpal bone to end at a point between the bulbs of the heel.

TRIPLE HEATER CHANNEL

Human

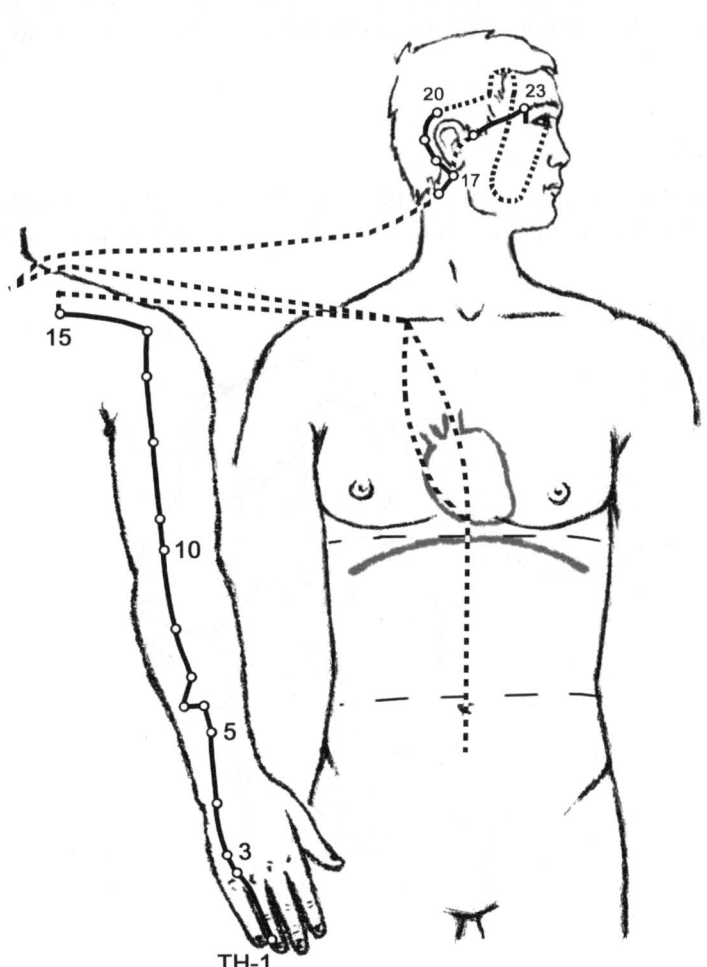

Lateral Branch

Triple Heater (TH) Channel originates at the lateral tip of the ring finger (TH-1). Then it runs upward between the fourth and fifth metacarpal bones over the back of the hand to meet the wrist. It ascends further along the lateral aspect of the forearm between the radius and ulna. It passes through the olecranon and along the lateral aspect of the upper arm. Next, it then reaches the posterior shoulder region and then runs forward to enter the supraclavicular fossa and to connect with its Internal Branch.

Internal Branch

From the supraclavicular fossa, it enters the chest and connects with the Pericardium Channel. It descends through the diaphragm, and then proceeds downward to connect the Upper Jiao, Middle Jiao and Lower Jiao. Extra internal branch splits off at the chest, emerges from the supraclavicular fossa to connect its Extra Lateral Branch.

Extra Lateral Branch

It starts at the supraclavicular fossa. It runs upward the neck and reaches the posterior border of the ear (TH-17). It ascends further and enters the anterior hairline at the level of the ear apex (TH-20). Then it turns downward to the cheek and terminates in the infraorbital region.

Auricular Branch

It arises from the retroauricular region and enters the ear. Then it emerges in front of the ear, and reaches the lateral canthus (GB-1) to link with Gallbladder Channel.

Small Animals

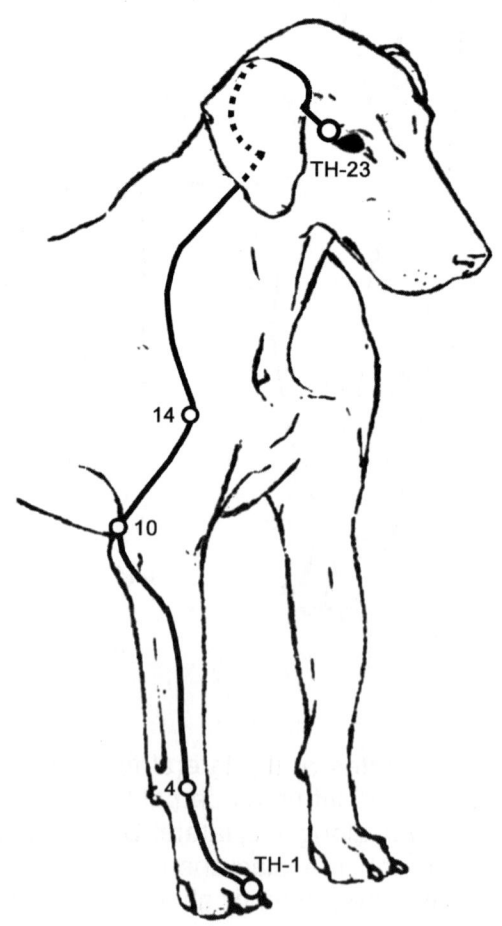

The Triple Heater Channel begins on the distal forelimb. From the lateral fourth digit nail bed, the Channel moves proximally on the dorsal aspect of the paw between the fourth and fifth metacarpals. Traveling on the lateral aspect of the forelimb, the Channel continues past the caudal edge of the shoulder up to the ventral ear. At the ear, the Meridian flows up and around the backside of the ear to arrive at the top of the ear. It swings down in front of the ear and then moves rostrally to end lateral to the eyebrow.

Horses

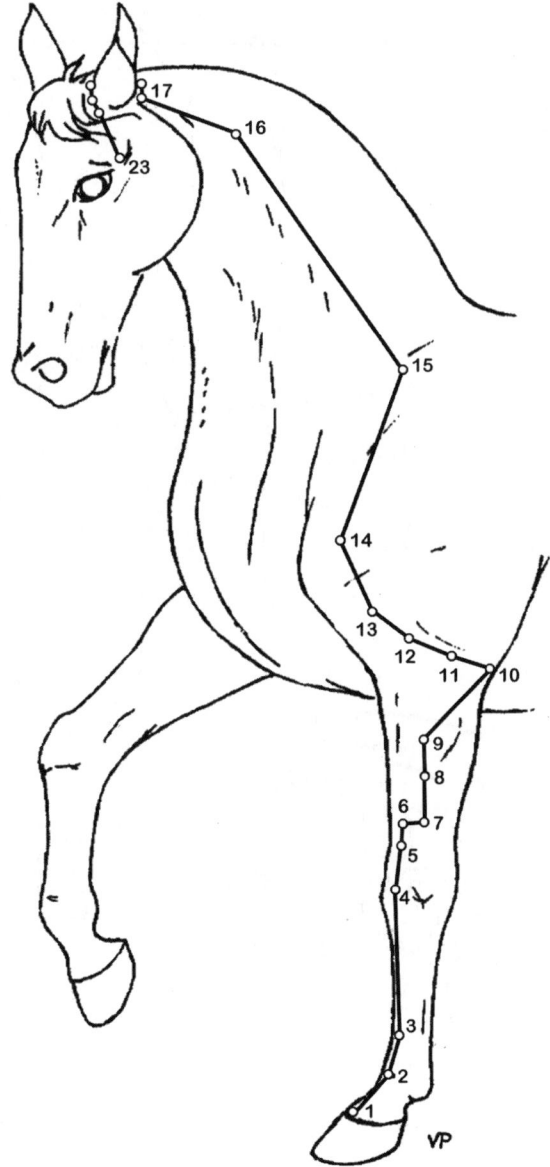

The Triple Heater Channel begins on the forelimb at the cranial aspect of the coronary band. It runs proximally up the craniolateral aspect of the pastern and metacarpus to the lateral carpus. From the middle of the radius, it travels past the elbow and shoulder to run past the cranial border of the scapula. It moves along the lateral neck and around the back of the ear. It comes to an end dorsal to the lateral canthus of the eye.

GALL BLADDER CHANNEL
Human

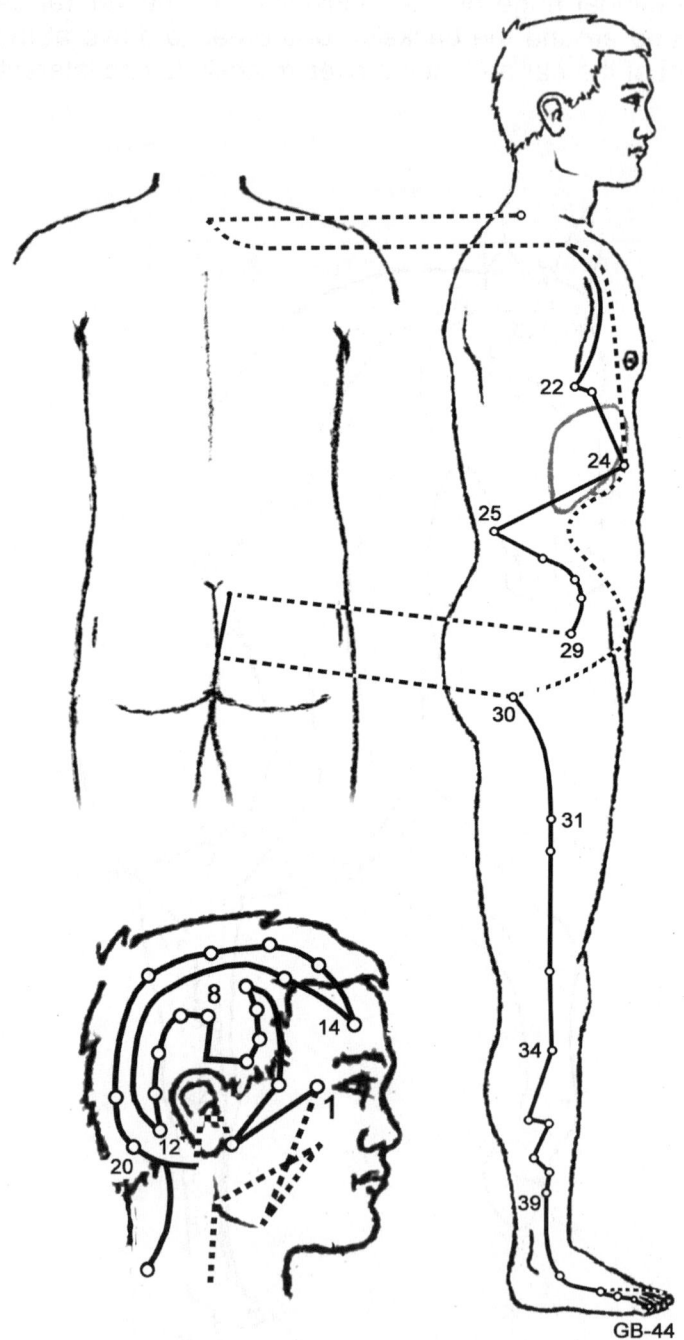

GB-44

Main Lateral Branch

The Gallbladder (GB) Channel originates at the lateral canthus (GB-1). It ascends to the corner of the forehead (GB-4) and then runs downward and curves to the retroauricular region (GB-12). It then winds back and ascends to the point GB-14 (1 cun dorsal to the eyebrow). From there, it winds back and descends to GB-20 and runs further down along the neck to the shoulder. It then goes forward to the supraclavicular fossa and circles downward to the axilla. Continuing downward along the lateral aspect of the chest and abdomen, it reaches the hip (GB-30). From there, it descends along the lateral aspect of the thigh to the lateral side of the knee. It runs down the side of the lower leg and past the front of the outer ankle. Crossing the dorsum of the foot, it terminates at the lateral tip of the fourth toe (GB-44).

Auricular Branch

It starts from the retroauricular and enters the ears. It then emerges at front of the ears and reaches the lateral canthus.

Eye Branch

It starts from the lateral canthus, runs downward to ST-5 and meets the TH Channel in the infraorbital region. Then it passes through ST-6, descends the neck and enters the supraclavicular fossa where it merges with the Main Lateral Branch.

Foot Branch

It starts from the dorsum of foot (GB-41), runs between the first and second metatarsal bones, and terminates at the distal portion of the big toe (LIV-1), where it links with the Liver (LIV) Channel.

Internal Branch

It starts at the supraclavicular fossa, and enters the chest. It passes through the diaphragm to connect the Liver and enter its pertaining organ, the Gallbladder. Then, it runs inside the hypochondriac region and comes out from the lateral side of the lower abdomen near the femoral artery at the inguinal region. From there, it circles superficially along the margin of the pubic hair and goes transversely into the hip region (GB-30) to merge with the Main Lateral Branch.

Small Animals

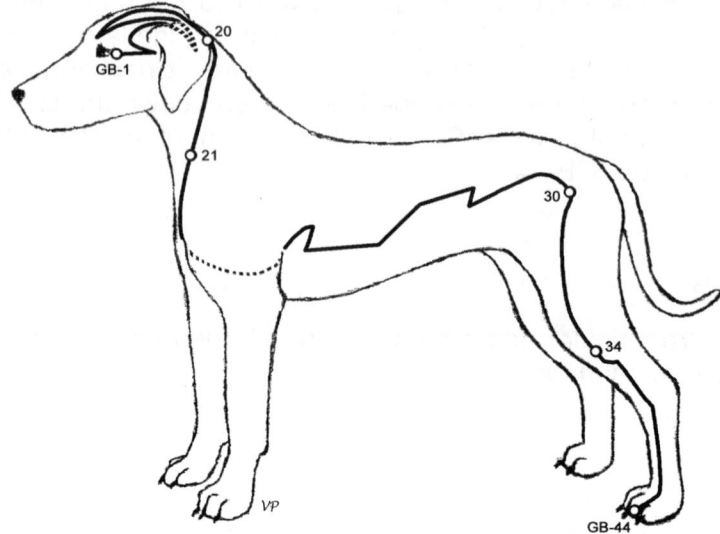

The Gall Bladder begins on the head near the lateral canthus of the eye. On the head, it makes several back and forth movements before it finally runs caudally over the top of the head. It travels down the neck and across the lateral aspect of body. The Channel continues distally along the center of the lateral aspect of the hind leg. It ends on the lateral aspect of the fourth toe nail bed.

Horses

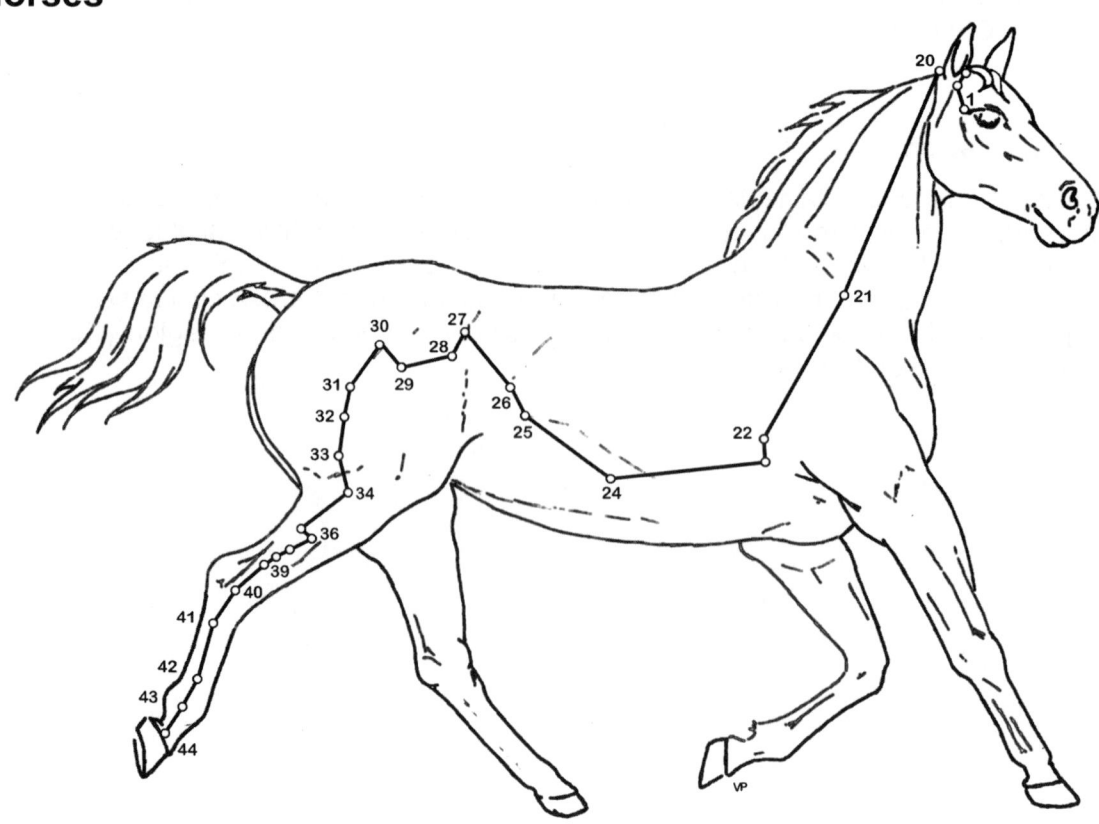

The Gall Bladder begins on the head near the lateral canthus of the eye. It runs to the medial side of the ear to the occipital condyle. It continues along the dorsal edge of the neck and across the chest to the fifteenth intercostals space. Moving past the caudal aspect of the eighteenth rib, it curves around the hip and travels distally along the lateral hind leg. It comes to rest at the craniolateral aspect of the coronary band.

LIVER CHANNEL

Human

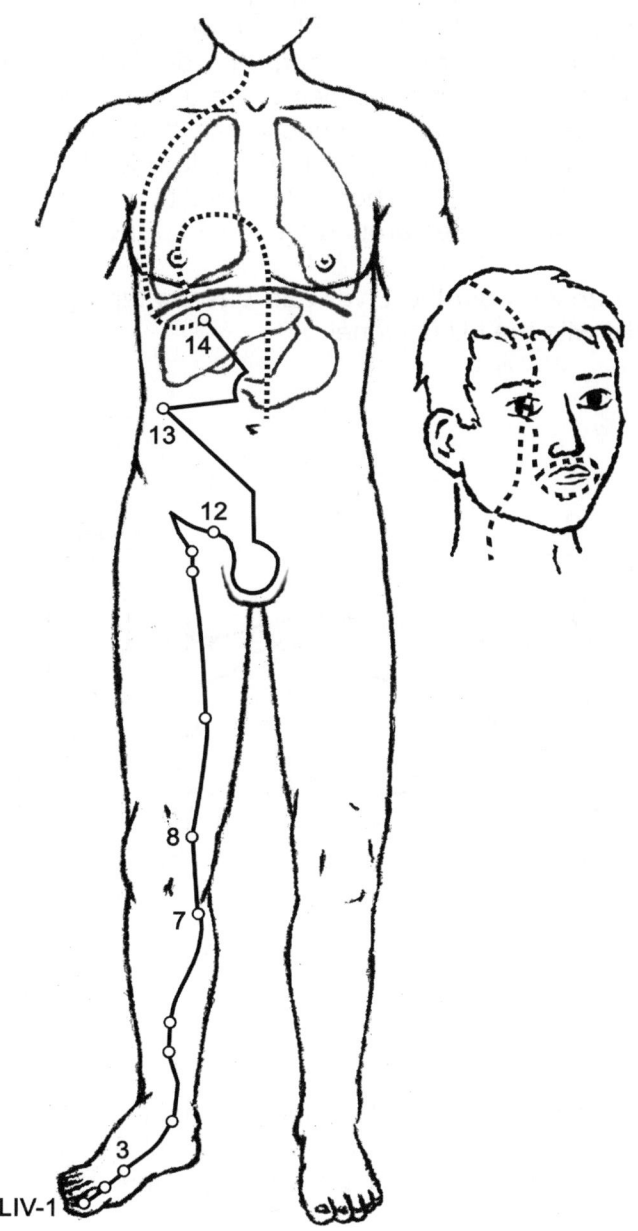

Lateral Branch

The Liver (LIV) Channel starts from the dorsal hairy region of the big toe (LIV-1), transverses the top of the foot, and ascends in front of the inner ankle and along the medial aspect of the lower leg and knee. It runs further upward along the medial aspect of the thigh to the hairy pubic region, where it encircles the external genitalia. From there, it goes up to the lower abdomen and reaches the free end of the eleventh rib (LIV-13). It continues upward to the hypochondriac region.

Internal Branch

It starts from the lower abdomen and enters the abdominal cavity. From there, it curves along the Stomach to enter the Liver, its pertaining organ, and connects with Gallbladder. It runs upward and passes through the diaphragm and spreads out in the costal and hypochondriac region. It continues upward along the posterior aspect of the throat, reaches the nasopharynx, and connects with the "eye system" (including optic nerve). It runs further upward and emerges from the forehead and meets the Governing Vessel (GV) Channel at the vertex. A short branch splits off from the "eye system", runs downward into the cheek and curves around the inner surface of the lips.

Another short branch arises from the Liver and passes through the diaphragm. It runs into the Lung and links with the LU Channel.

Small Animals

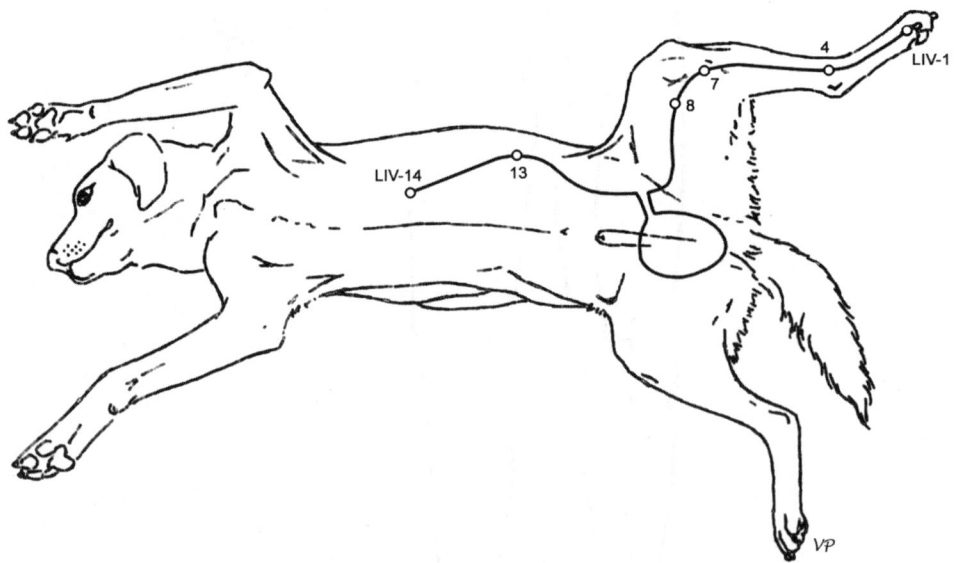

The Liver Channel begins on the distal hind leg. It runs along the most medial aspect of the hind foot, but is located dorsal to the Spleen Channel. The Meridian continues along the medial aspect of the hind leg. It comes to an end on the chest.

Horses

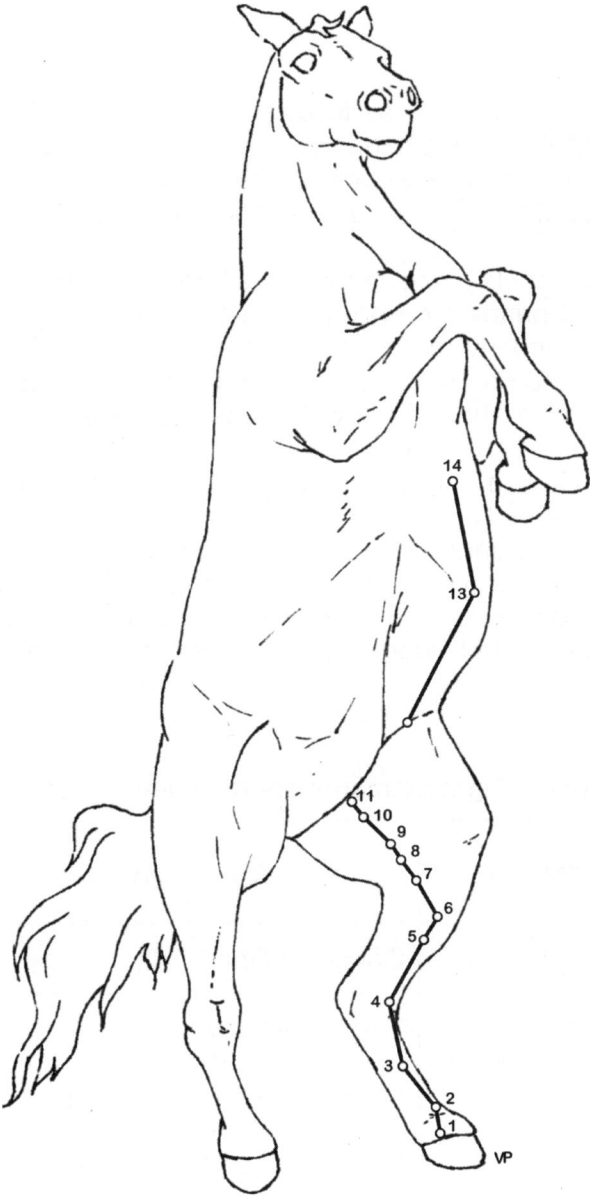

The Liver Channel begins on the distal hind leg at the craniomedial aspect of the coronary band. It runs proximally along the craniomedial aspect of the pastern and metatarsus. From the cranial aspect of the tarsus, it continues past the caudal aspect of the medial condyle of the femur to the inguinal area. Moving cranially, it runs past the tip of the eighteenth rib and ends in the fourteenth intercostal space at the level of the elbow.

The Eight Extraordinary Channels

Qi Jing Ba Mai

The translation of *Qi Jing Ba Mai* is as follows: Qi means special or extraordinary. Jing means Meridian, and Mai means Channels. Ba is the number eight. Thus the phrase Qi Jing Ba Mai refers to the Eight Extraordinary Channels (8-EC). These eight channels are named Du, Ren, Chong, Dai, Yang-Qiao, Yin-Qiao, Yang-Wei, and Yin-Wei.

The Extraordinary Channels have several differences from the Twelve Regular Channels. First, these Channels do not pertain to either Zang or Fu organs. Second, they are not exteriorly-interiorly related each other as are the Regular Channels. Third, most of these Channels do not have their own acupoints. Du and Ren do have their own acupoints, but the rest share their points with a few of the Regular Meridians.

As assistants to the Regular Channels, the Extraordinary Channels acquire similar functions to those of nearby Regular Channels. This occurs because the Extraordinary Channels coordinate and balance the Qi and Blood within the Regular Channels they link. These Extraordinary Channels form a conduit that connects, coordinates, and facilitates communication among the Twelve Regular Meridians. In addition, the Extraordinary Channels control, store, and regulate the Qi and Blood of the Twelve Regular Meridians.

Table 5.6: Distribution of the Eight Extraordinary Channels

Channel Name		Location	Meridian Connections
Du	Governing Vessel	Dorsal Midline	Ren (CV), ST
Ren	Conception Vessel	Ventral Midline	Du (GV), ST
Chong	Penetrating	Parallel to Kidney Meridian	KID
Dai	Girdle	Encircling Lumbar Region	GB
Yang-Qiao	Yang Motility	Lateral Hind Limb Extremities, Shoulder and Head	SI, BL, LI, ST, GB
Yin-Qiao	Yin Motility	Medial Hind Limb Extremities, Eye	KID, SI
Yang-Wei	Yang Linking	Lateral Stifle, Shoulder	Du, SI, BL,TH, GB, ST
Yin-Wei	Yin Linking	Medial Hind Limb, Neck	Ren, GB, SP, LIV

Du Channel

Human

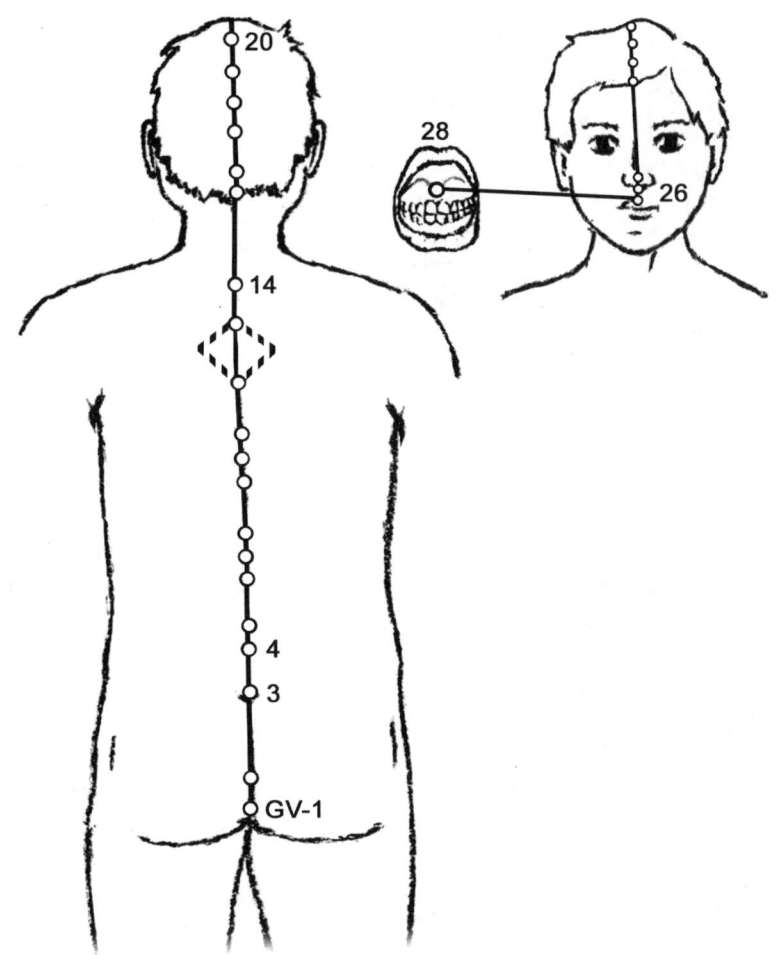

This Meridian is known as the Governing Vessel or the Du Channel. The Governing Vessel (GV) Channel originates from the lower abdomen (from the uterus and ovaries in women or the prostate and testes in men). It emerges from the perineum and passes through the tips of the coccyx. From there, it runs upward along the middle of the spinal column and reaches the head to penetrate the brain. Continuing up to the vertex of the head, it then descends across the forehead and nose and terminates inside the upper gum (GV-28). An internal branch splits off at the spinal column of the lower back and enters the pelvic cavity to reach the Kidney.

Animal

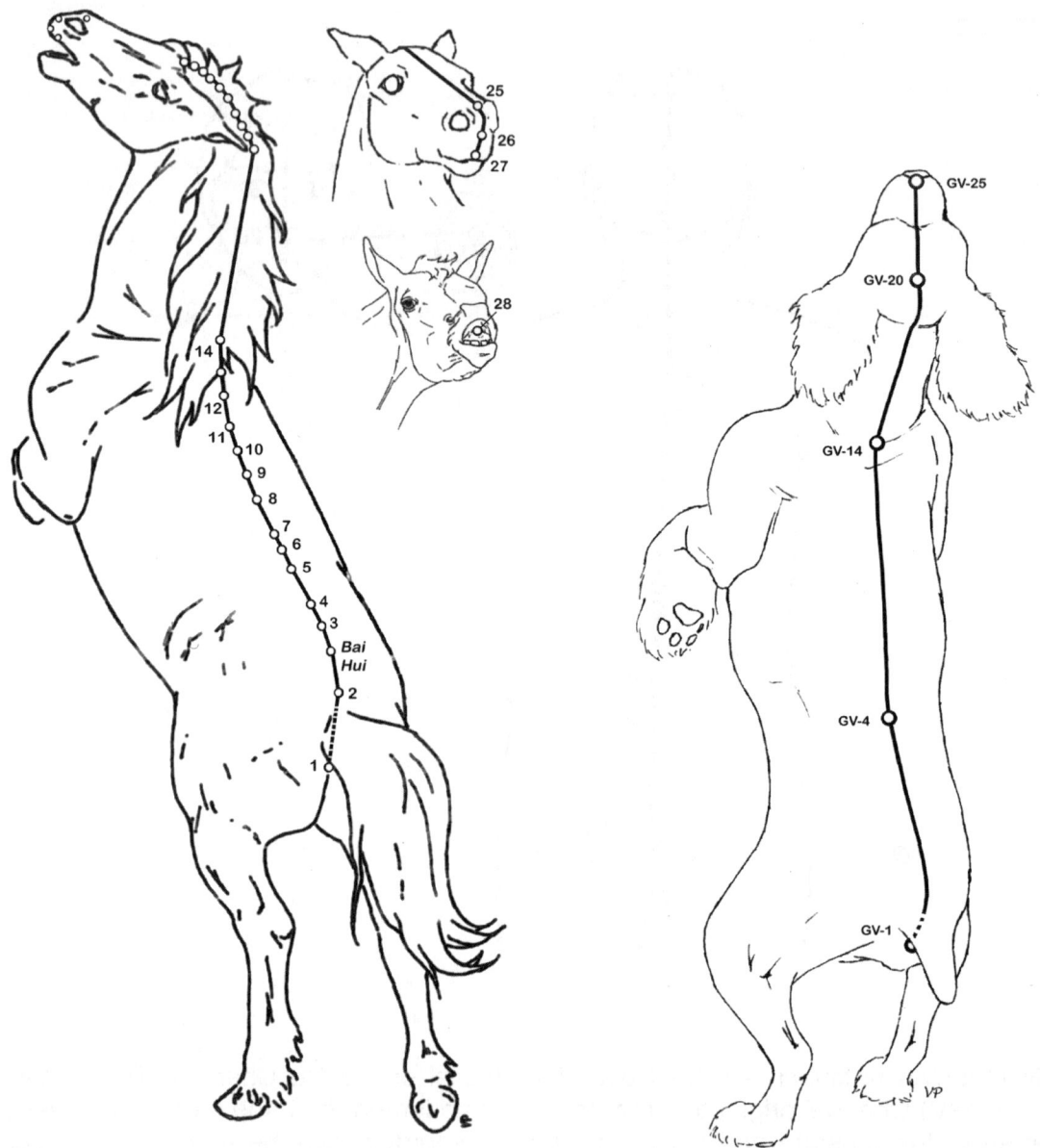

The Du Channel originates from the uterus. It travels within the lower abdomen to emerge at the perineum. The first point on the Channel is GV-1, which is located on the midline between the anus and the underside of the tail base. A branch extends to the tip of the tail to the point GV-1b (*Wei Jian*). The main branch of the Channel continues cranially along the dorsal midline. Along the way it passes through *Bai Hui*, GV-3 (*Yao Yang Guan*), GV-4 (*Ming Men*), and *Tian Ping* to reach GV-20 at the top of the head. At this point, the Channel descends down the midline of the face through GV-26 at the nasal philtrum to end inside the upper gum at GV-28 (*Nei Chun Yin*).

As it courses along the dorsal midline, the Du Channel connects with all six Yang Meridians (Small Intestine, Large Intestine, Stomach, Bladder, Triple Heater, Gall Bladder), the spinal cord, and the brain. It is known as "the sea of Yang Meridians".

These connections allow the Du Channel to govern the Qi of all the Yang Meridians. The Du Channel may be used for treating problems involving the spinal cord, disc disease, Heat Patterns, mental disorders, and Yang Deficiency Patterns.

REN CHANNEL

Human

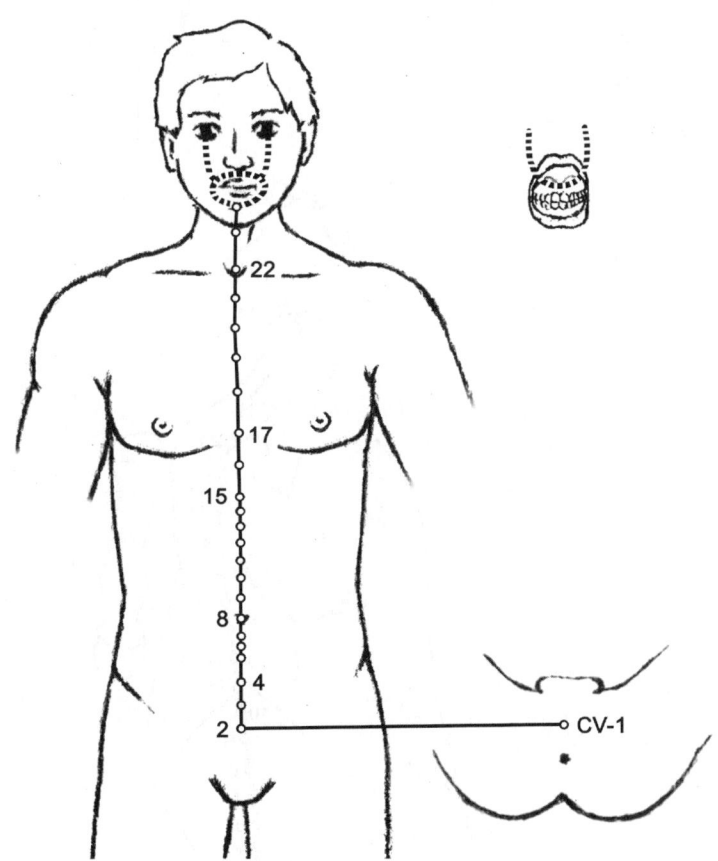

This Meridian is known as the Conception Vessel or Ren Channel. The Conception Vessel (CV) Channel originates from the lower abdomen (from the uterus and ovaries in women or the prostate and testes in men). It emerges from the perineum (between the anus and external genitalia) and passes through the pubic region. From there, it runs upward along the midline of the abdomen, chest, and throat to the lower jaw. Here, it penetrates internally to encircle the lips, to pass through the cheek and to enter the infraorbital region. An internal branch arises from the uterus (female) or prostate (male), transverses backward to cross the GV Channel and terminates at the lower back.

Animals

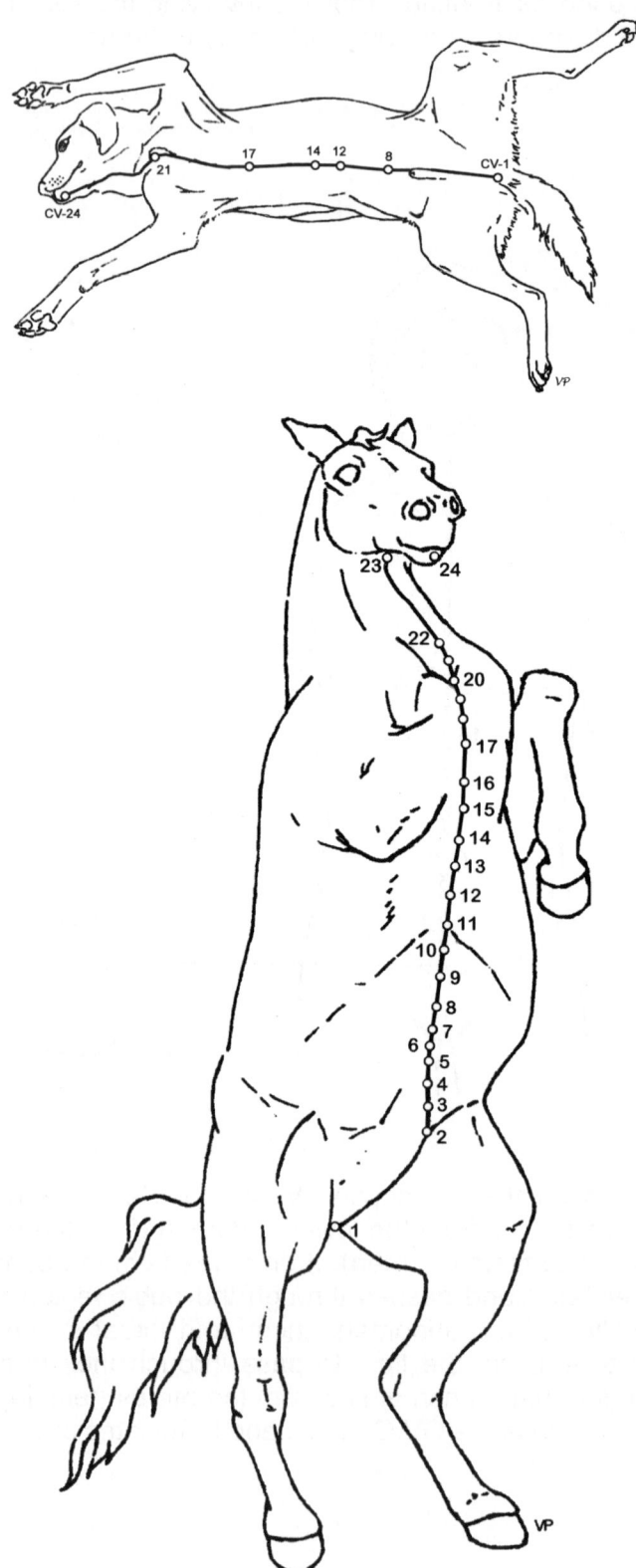

The Ren Channel originates from the uterus. From inside the pelvic cavity, the Channel emerges at the perineum between the anus and the external genitalia (CV-1). It then runs cranially along the ventral midline of the abdomen, chest, throat, and mandible to end at CV-24.

Along its path, the Ren Channel connects with all the Yin Channels (Spleen, Lung, Kidney, Liver, and Heart). Also known as "the sea of the Yin Meridians", this Channel receives and regulates the Qi of the Yin Meridians. The Ren Channel nourishes the uterus and regulates pregnancy. It is useful for treatment of reproductive complaints, Yin Deficiency, and sore throats.

CHONG CHANNEL

Human

The Chong Channel arises from the lower abdomen (from the uterus and ovaries in women or the prostate and testes in men). It emerges from the perineum and passes through the point ST-30 (*Qi Chong*). From there, it merges with the Kidney Channel, goes upward to the throat, and curves around the lips.

Animals

The Chong Channel originates from the uterus. From the uterus, the Channel travels along the ventral abdomen and chest parallel to the Kidney Meridian. It continues from the chest up to the infraorbital region.

This Channel connects with the Du and Ren Channels as well as the Twelve Regular Meridians. It is also known as "the sea of the twelve Meridians" or as "the sea of Blood". The Chong Channel functions as a reservoir for the Qi and Blood of the Twelve Regular Meridians. It may be useful for treatment of infertility, estrous disorders, postpartum disorders, incontinence, and difficult urination or defecation.

DAI CHANNEL

Human

The Dai Channel originates below the hypochondriac region and runs obliquely downward through GB-26 (*Dai Mai*), GB-27, and GB-28. At the level of the umbilicus and the point GV-3, it travels around the waist like a belt.

Animals

The Dai Channel originates at the flank. It obliquely through GB-26, GB-27, and GB-28 and circles the abdomen to meet at *Bai Hui*. The pathway of the Dai Channel is like a belt or girdle. This Channel may be used for hind limb weakness or Yang Deficiency.

YANG-QIAO CHANNEL

Human

The Yang-Qiao Channel originates from the lateral side of the heel (BL-62). It runs upward along the external ankle and the posterior border of the fibula. It then goes onwards along the lateral side of the thigh and posterior side of the hypochondrium to the posterior axillary fold. From there, it passes through the shoulder, the neck and the corner of the mouth. Entering the medial canthus of the eye (BL-1), it connects with the Yin-Qiao Channel. Then it runs upward along the Bladder Channel over the head to meet GB-20.

Animals

The Yang-Qiao Channel begins at BL-62 and travels proximally through BL-61 to run along the posterior border of the fibula. It continues along the lateral side of the thigh and moves cranially toward the shoulder. The Channel runs rostrally to the medial canthus of the eye and then travels caudally to end at GB-20.

Together, the Yang-Qiao and Yin-Qiao Channels control the hind limb motion. They dominate the movement of Yang and the inactivity of Yin. Individually, the Yang-Qiao Channel may be beneficial for ataxia, unbalanced movement, Wobblers disease, Equine Protozoal Myeloencephalitis (EPM), insomnia, and eye problems

YIN-QIAO CHANNEL

Human

The Yin-Qiao Channel originates from the posterior aspect of the navicular bones (KID-6). It then moves proximally along the upper portion of the inner ankle and the posterior border of the medial thigh to reach the external genitalia. From there, it continues upward along the abdomen and chest to the supraclavicular fossa. Passing through ST-9 and the zygoma, it reaches the medial canthus (BL-1) to connect with the Bladder Channel and the Yang-Qiao Channel.

Animals

The Yin-Qiao Channel begins at Kid-6 and travels proximally along the caudomedial border of the thigh. It continues cranially to the chest and head.

As stated earlier, the Yin-Qiao Channel may collaborate with the Yang-Qiao Channel to control the hind limb motion and to dominate Yang movement and Yin inactivity. The Yin-Qiao Channel itself may be used for hypersomnia or difficult urination.

YANG-WEI CHANNEL

Human

The Yang-Wei Channel starts at the point GB-63 (the lower border of the external ankle). It runs upward along the GB Channel and passes through the hip region. Continuing upward along the hypochondriac and costal regions, the axilla, the shoulder and the neck, it reaches the forehead. It runs upward to the top of head and descends the neck to connect with the GV Channel at GV-16 and GV-15.

Animals

The Yang-Wei Channel starts at BL-63 from where it moves proximally and merges with Gall Bladder Meridian. The Channel flows along the Gall Bladder Meridian to the hip and then moves cranially to the shoulder and forehead. It then ends on the back of the neck.

The Yang-Wei Channel is connected with all the Yang Meridians. It dominates the Exterior of the whole body. Together with the Yin-Wei Channel, the Yang-Wei Channel maintains the coordination and equilibrium between the Yin and Yang Meridians. The Yang-Wei Channel may be beneficial for back pain, influenza, and Cold Patterns.

YIN-WEI CHANNEL

Human

The Yin-Wei Channel arises from the point KID-9 on the medial aspect of the leg. It runs upward along the medial aspect of the thigh to the abdomen. Here it communicates with the Spleen Channel. From there, it continues upward and crosses with LIV-14. Then it runs up the chest to communicate with the Ren Channel at CV-22 and CV-23.

Animals

The Yin-Wei Channel begins at KID-9 and travels proximally along the medial aspect of the thigh. Moving cranially along the abdomen, it connects with the Spleen Meridian. On the chest, the Yin-Wei Channel connects with CV-22 and ends on CV-23.

The Yin-Wei Channel is connected with all the Yin Meridians, and it dominates the Interior of the whole body. This Channel, along with the Yang-Wei Channel, also helps to balance the Yin and Yang Meridians. The Yin-Wei Channel may be beneficial for treatment of depression or chest pain.

Fourteen Regular Channels

The Twelve Regular Channels together with the Du Channel and the Ren Channel constitute the Fourteen Channels. The Twelve Regular Channels are distributed symmetrically on the left and right sides of the body. The Ren and Du Channels, however, are unpaired. The Ren Channel runs along the ventral midline, and the Du Channel courses along the dorsal midline.

Within the Twelve Regular Channels, Qi and Blood circulate along each Meridian in a specific order over the course of a twenty-four hour period. There is also cyclical Qi flow within the Fourteen Regular Channels, which takes the Du and Ren channels into account. The Lung Channel, which is the beginning of the Twelve-Regular-Channel cycle, sends a branch to the Ren Channel. Thus the Qi flows from the Lung Channel to the Ren Channel, and then it runs cranially along the Ren Channel. At the mouth, the Qi flows into the Du Channels and runs caudally along the back. Upon reaching the perineum, the Qi enters the Ren Channel again and flows back to the Lung Channel. Thus, the cyclical flow of Qi and Blood in the Fourteen Channels includes the circulation through the Du and Ren Channels along with the flow within the Twelve Channel cycle.

During Qi Gong meditation, one places the tip of the tongue against the palate behind the upper incisors. This connects the Du and Ren Channels. The Qi flow between these two Channels becomes the focus of meditation. It is possible to imagine this pathway as a shortcut which allows the Qi to circle the body while bypassing the Twelve Regular Channels. Unlike the Twelve Regular Channels, the flow between Du and Ren does not dominate at a certain time of day. Rather, the Qi constantly cycles between the two Channels throughout the day.

The Qi is always flowing through the Fourteen Regular Channels. Within the Twelve Regular Channels, it has a predictable direction of flow from one Channel to the next. However, even when one Channel dominates during its two hour period, the Qi continues to flow along the remaining Meridians as well. The Qi flow of the Twelve Channels is like cargo boats on a river with multiple ports along its length. As a boat travels down the river, it may spend a short while in each of the ports in sequence. When numerous boats come to a specific port at a specific time, that port is very important during that time. Although this location may be a center of commerce for the moment, it does not prevent other ships from continuing along the river.

On the other hand, the flow within the Du and Ren channels is like a freeway encircling a city. The Qi flows smoothly around in a large loop around the body. The traffic may travel in either direction (i.e. It may take Du to Ren or Ren to Du) all times of the day and night.

Functions of the Jing Luo

The Jing Luo system is closely connected with all the tissues and organs of the body, and it plays an important role in animal physiology, in pathology, and in treatment with acupuncture or herbal medicine.

THE PHYSIOLOGICAL ASPECTS

1. Transporting Qi and Blood and Nourishing the Body

All the body's tissues require nourishment by Qi and Blood in order to maintain their normal physiological activities. The Meridians are passages that transport the Qi and Blood. Therefore, failure of the Meridians to transport Qi and Blood prevents Qi and Blood from reaching the Zang-Fu organs and results in organ malfunction.

2. Coordinating Zang-Fu Organs and Connecting the Whole Body

The Meridians connect with all the tissues and organs of the body. The connection through the Meridians keeps the Interior and Exterior, the front and hind, and the left and right parts of the body in close association. This communication allows the Zang-Fu organs to coordinate their activities and to maintain equilibrium between the organ systems.

3. Preventing Invasion of the Body Surface and Resisting Pathogens

The Meridians, with the help of the Defensive Qi, shield the body surface and resist the attack of pathogens (Xie Qi). The Meridian system has many small branches that distribute Qi and Blood to strengthen the muscles, tendons, and skin. This fortifies the body's natural barriers to infection or pathogen invasion. In addition, the Defensive Qi flows outside of the Meridian pathways to make sure this remains an impermeable defense.

THE PATHOLOGICAL ASPECTS

The Meridians also play a role in disease conditions. They may transmit pathogenic factors, or they may reflect the disease states of internal systems.

1. Transmitting the Pathogenic Factors

If pathogenic factors invade the body, the Meridian system initially participates in combating these pathogens on the surface before they reach deeper tissues. However, when the Zheng Qi is weak and Yin and Yang become unbalanced, the pathogenic factors overcome the resistance of the Meridians. The pathogens may then use the Meridian pathways to migrate into the Interior from the Exterior. For instance, an unresolved Exterior Wind-Cold Pattern will allow the pathogenic Wind-Cold to follow the Lung Channel to the Lung, resulting in cough and asthma.

2. Reflecting Symptoms of Diseases

In pathological conditions, the Meridian system may reflect signs of internal problems onto the surface of the body. Because there are small branches of the Meridians that connect the Zang-Fu organs with their external organs or body areas, disease in the Zang-Fu organs will result in changes of these external organs. A clinician may then examine these external structures for evidence of internal disease. For instance, extreme Heat or Fire of the Heart may lead to ulceration on the tongue because the

Meridians connect the Heart with the tongue. Similarly, extreme Heat of the Liver may cause congestion and swelling or the eyes. Deficient Kidney Yang may result in lumbar weakness.

THE THERAPEUTIC ASPECTS

1. Transmitting the Effect of Herbal Medications

Chinese herbs may have specific actions on certain Zang-Fu organs or Channels. This quality is known as the Channel-tropism of the drugs. For example, Coptis root (*Huang Lian*) functions to eliminate Heart Fire, and Scutellaria root (*Huang Qin*) can eliminate Lung Fire.

2. Transmitting the Acupuncture Stimulation

The Meridian system is important in the treatment of diseases. This system transmits the signal from acupoint stimulation by acupuncture or moxibustion. The stimulus from an acupuncture point travels along the Meridian to the relevant Zang-Fu organs along that Meridian. As a consequence, the Zang-Fu organs regain their balance and the normal flow of Qi and Blood is restored. When treating a Stomach Heat Pattern, hemoacupuncture at the point Yu-Tang sends the stimulation along the Stomach Channel to the Stomach. The point Dai-Mai may be stimulated for treatment of diarrhea because this point is located on the Spleen Channel.

The De-Qi (the arrival of Qi) response is a phenomenon in acupuncture which is the feeling or effect experienced as a result of the Meridian's transmission of the acupuncture stimulation. The De-Qi response manifests in different ways for each individual. It may feel like heaviness, tingling, soreness, or pressure. A human patient can tell the acupuncturist when he or she feels the sensation. In veterinary acupuncture, observation of muscle twitching, flinching, or attempts to bite may indicate De-Qi with stimulation of the needles.

The therapeutic results are closely related to De-Qi response. Without a De-Qi response, there will be less benefit from the acupuncture treatment. Inducing the De-Qi response regulates the Qi flow, which is vital to effective acupuncture treatments. No acupuncture treatment can be successful without this ability of the Meridians to transmit the acupuncture stimuli.

Self Test

Question 5.1: How many Regular Channels are in the body?

    a. 4

    b. 8

    c. 12

    d. 13

    e. 16

Question 5.2: How many Extraordinary Channels are in the body?

    a. 4

    b. 8

    c. 12

    d. 14

    e. 16

Question 5.3: Where do the Large Intestine Channel and Lung Channel connect?

    a. on the head

    b. on the abdomen/chest

    c. on the front feet

    d. on the rear feet

    e. on the tail

Question 5.4: Where do the Liver and Gall Bladder Channels connect?

    a. on the head

    b. on the abdomen/chest

    c. on the front feet

    d. on the rear feet

    e. on the tail

Question 5.5: Where do the Bladder and Stomach Channels connect?

    a. on the head

    b. on the abdomen/chest

    c. on the front feet

    d. on the rear feet

    e. on the tail

Question 5.6: According to the TCM circadian clock, when does the Bladder dominate?

    a. 3 am to 5 am

    b. 5 am to 7 am

    c. 3 pm to 5 pm

    d. 5 pm to 7 pm

    e. 7 pm to 9 pm

Question 5.7: According to the TCM circadian clock, when does Pericardium dominate?

    a. 3 am to 5 am

    b. 5 am to 7 am

    c. 3 pm to 5 pm

    d. 5 pm to 7 pm

    e. 7 pm to 9 pm

Question 5.8: The thoracic limb Shaoyin is which of the following?

    a. Spleen Meridian

    b. Kidney Meridian

    c. Heart Meridian

    d. Lung Meridian

    e. Pericardium Meridian

Question 5.9: The pelvic limb Taiyang is which of the following?

    a. Gall Bladder Meridian

    b. Small Intestine Meridian

    c. Large Intestine Meridian

    d. Stomach Meridian

    e. Bladder Meridian

Question 5.10: Based on the human Triple Heater Channel, how many points are on the channel? In other words, what is the number of the last point on the TH Channel?

    a. 67

    b. 44

    c. 23

    d. 19

    e. 9

Question 5.11: Based on the human Conception Vessel Channel, how many points are on the channel? In other words, which is the last point on the CV Channel?

    a. 28
    b. 24
    c. 23
    d. 21
    e. 20

Question 5.12: Which of the following points is closest to the eye?

    a. ST-45
    b. BL-1
    c. SI-1
    d. GB-23
    e. SP-1

Question 5.13: How many cun are there between the carpus and elbow?

    a. 12
    b. 9
    c. 8
    d. 5
    e. 4

Question 5.14: All of the following are true of the TCM Meridians EXCEPT:

    a. The Meridians are the pathways through which Body Fluid and Jing circulate
    b. There are 12 Major/Regular Channels
    c. The Meridians are the networking system in which all the Zang-Fu organs are connected
    d. The Meridians reflect symptoms of diseases and transmit the pathogenic factors
    e. The Meridians protect the body surface and resist attach of pathogens

CHAPTER SIX

ETIOLOGY AND PATHOLOGY

> Patients should have rest, food, fresh air, and exercise – The quadrangle of health.
> – William Osler

In Traditional Chinese Veterinary Medicine (TCVM), etiology is the study of the causes of disease. Pathology is the study of the bodily processes involved in disease as well as the understanding of the physical changes and developments induced by disease.

In the normal physiological state, the body exists in equilibrium with the external environment on one hand and the Zang-Fu organs on the other. This equilibrium is in a constant state of flux; the body regularly readjusts itself to maintain its normal functions in the face of the various external and internal forces. If certain forces overwhelm the capacity of the body to adjust, the body is unable to maintain the delicate balance and disease results. There are numerous forces, which are capable of impairing this equilibrium and causing disease; these are called Pathogens. They can be divided into exogenous factors, internal factors, secondary factors and others.

Different pathogens produce different symptoms within the body. Thus, it is by analyzing the clinical manifestations of a disease that a practitioner of Traditional Chinese Veterinary Medicine is able to identify the cause of a disease. This is known as "seeking the cause of a disease by identifying patterns". In addition, the treatment principle depends upon the cause of the disease. This is otherwise known as "treatment according to the cause". It is the TCVM practitioner's role to recognize a patient's symptoms as a result of a certain pathogen and then to administer a specific treatment regimen to resist the previously diagnosed pathogen. For example, if a sick horse exhibits alternate leg lameness, a TCVM practitioner identifies these as signs characteristic of pathogenic Wind and Damp and applies a treatment that eliminates Wind and Damp.

Because the TCVM diagnosis relies heavily on gathering information about the clinical signs and then determining how they fit with known pathogens, both Western and traditional Chinese medical diagnostic principles can be used in combination for disease diagnosis. Conventional Western diagnostic tests and physical exam complement the traditional Chinese history and physical exam. A Western diagnosis of disease can be beneficial as a component of the TCVM diagnosis, and a TCVM diagnosis can further clarify a Western diagnosis. For example, radiographs are an invaluable tool to visualize the joints of the body and may provide a Western diagnosis of degenerative joint disease or arthritis. However, Chinese medicine can further define which type of arthritis it is based upon the patient's collective clinical signs.

CLINICAL SKETCH: A fourteen year old Labrador Retriever has had stiffness of his limbs for three years. After a full physical exam and radiographs, the Western diagnosis is osteoarthritis of the hip and stifle. Upon further questioning, the owner relates that the condition is worse after a change from warm to cold weather or after exposure to a cold environment. From a TCVM perspective, this is now classified as a Cold type of osteoarthritis (Bi Syndrome). The TCVM treatment principle is to clear Cold and Wind-Damp. Thus the treatment in this case includes moxibustion at GV-3 and Bai Hui and administration of the herbal formula Ba Ji San.

Exogenous Etiologic Factors

The exogenous factors, which include the Six Excessive Qi and the Noxious Epidemic Qi, invade the body through the skin, mouth, or nose. They are also called the Xie Qi.

THE SIX EXCESSIVE QI

Wind, cold, summer-heat, damp, dryness and fire (heat) are the six climatic changes found in nature. Under normal conditions, they do not produce pathological changes in the body and are thus known as the "six types of Qi" in the natural environment. These six types of Qi will cause disease only when the climatic changes are sudden or extreme and the body's resistance to them fails. It is when these six types of Qi are able to cause disease that they become known as the Six Excessive Qi. Therefore, The Six Excessive Qi are merely abnormal forms of the six natural climates that become the six pathogenic factors when they enter the body. These include Wind, Cold, Summer Heat, Dryness, Damp and Fire (Heat).

Diseases due to the Six Excessive Qi are closely related to the nature of an individual's environment and the weather, especially seasonal changes. For example, a Heat Pattern mostly occurs in the summer, a Cold Pattern in the winter and a Damp Pattern in late summer. However, things are not always that simple. The Six Excessive Qi may also cause disease in much more complex ways. Under certain circumstances, one type of Excessive Qi can even transform into another. It is possible for a Cold Pattern to occur in the summer. Also, an Extreme Heat Pattern can change into Wind, or an Extreme Wind Pattern may transform into Dryness.

The Six Excessive Qi usually invade the body from the Exterior via the skin, mouth, or nose. However, when there is a disorder of the Zang-Fu organs, similar pathological changes may occur without external invasion of the Xie Qi. In contrast to the Six Excessive Qi, these pathogens are known as Internal Wind, Internal Cold, Internal Damp, Internal Dryness, and Internal Fire (Heat).

Each of the Six Excessive Qi may affect the body singly or in combination. For instance, Summer Heat alone causes Sunstroke, but the common cold is due to a combination of Wind and Cold.

EXAMPLE 6.1: The heat during a Florida summer can sometimes be quite intense. Summer Heat leads to anhidrosis (non-sweating) in horses during this time. Since the pathogen is Summer-Heat, the treatment principle is to clear Summer-Heat. The acupoint Tai Yang and the herbal formula Xiang Ru San are used for treatment.

EXAMPLE 6.2: It can be very dry in Colorado during the fall, resulting in pathogenic Dryness. Dryness combined with Wind leads to Lung Wind-Dryness. This condition is often evidenced by nosebleeds. The treatment principle, therefore, is to clear the Wind and the Dryness. Sang Ren Tang Plus and the acupoint LU-7 are part of the treatment.

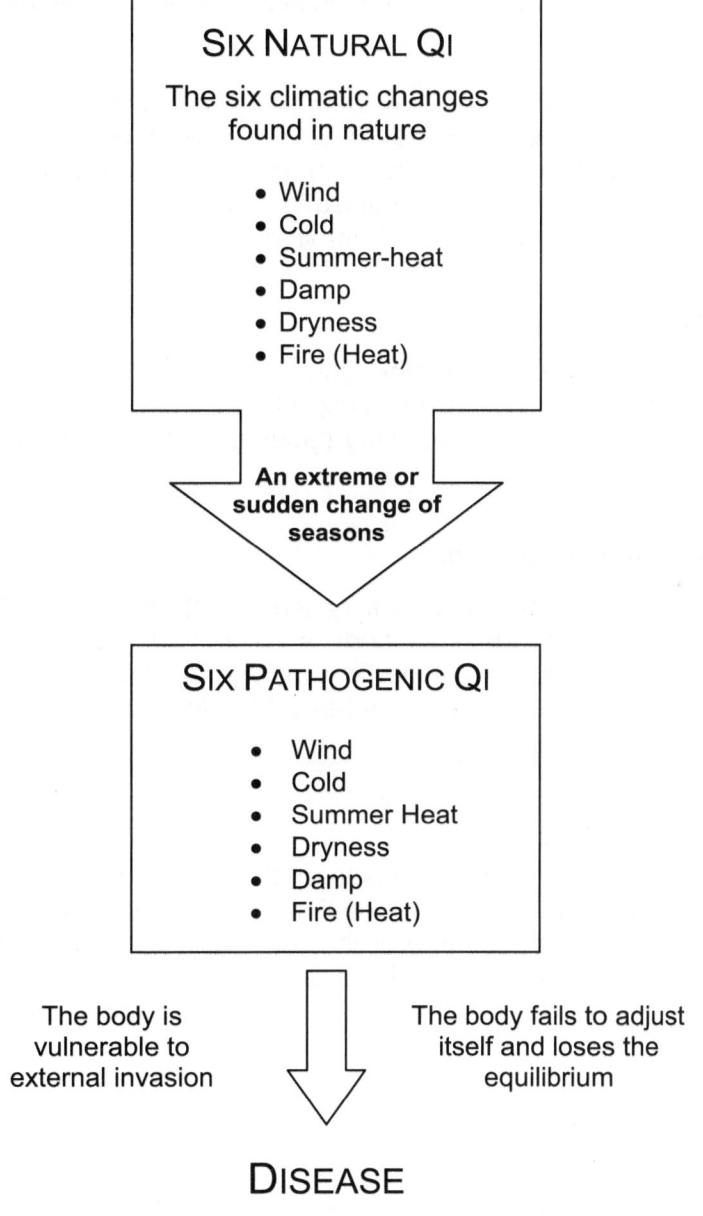

Figure 6.1: The Six Exogenous Qi and Disease

Wind

Wind is the predominant Qi of spring, but it may occur in any of the other seasons. Many exogenous diseases are concerned with Wind; thus, Wind is considered the primary cause of disease. Wind, often joined by another one of the Excessive Qi, invades the body from the external environment. This type of Wind is known as Exogenous Wind. In contrast, Internal Wind is closely related to dysfunction of the Heart, Liver or Kidney. It is especially common with disorders of Liver function; therefore, the Internal Wind is also called the Liver Wind.

There are several characteristics unique to Wind. Wind is often the primary pathogen upon which all the others depend in order to gain access to the body. Wind also tends to affect the upward and outward most parts of the body. Rapid changes and fluctuations in a condition are common in Wind induced diseases. Wind is the sudden storm that strikes the woods leaving the trees swaying and trembling.

The Primary Pathogen

Wind is the number one pathogenic factor. Cold, Heat, Damp and Dryness all depend on Wind in order to invade the body. Wind transports the other Xie Qi into and around the body. Thus it is not uncommon to see Wind causing a Wind-Heat Pattern, a Wind-Cold Pattern or a Wind-Damp Pattern.

Upward and Outward Dispersion

Wind is a Yang pathogenic factor, and it typically distributes itself in an upward and outward fashion. It easily invades the body surface and the upper part of the body including the head and face. This superficial attack results in abnormal opening and closing of the pores. Common clinical manifestations include nasal obstruction, itching, sweating, and aversion to Wind.

Rapid Movement and Changes

Wind rapidly changes and moves. A disease due to Wind has no fixed place; the affected area of the body is variable. In addition, the clinical signs have an acute onset and subsequent changes in the course of the disease occur very quickly. For instance, shifting-leg lameness or pain often characterizes rheumatism due to Wind-Damp. Similarly, hives due to Wind are swellings that may arise suddenly in a variety of places on the body.

Vibration or Oscillation

Wind is characterized by constant trembling. The diseases due to Wind exhibit convulsions of the limbs and rigidity of the neck. In TCVM, tetanus, with its distinctive muscle spasms, is related to Wind. Similarly, diseases such as epilepsy, which produce spastic, uncontrolled movements, are also related to Wind (Internal Wind). The trembling appearance of a scratching patient marks pruritus as a Wind condition.

Common Wind Patterns

1. Wind-Cold Pattern
2. Wind-Heat Pattern
3. Wind-Damp Pattern (or Wind-Cold-Damp Pattern)
4. Wind-Dryness Pattern
5. Internal Wind Pattern due to Extreme Heat
6. Internal Wind Pattern due to a Liver Yin Deficiency
7. Internal Wind Pattern due to a Liver Blood Deficiency

Cold

Cold is the predominant Qi of winter although it may also occur in other seasons. Prolonged exposure to a cold environment, especially after sweating, can lead to invasion of Cold. Wading in cold water during winter or becoming soaked in a rainstorm also promote Cold invasion.

There are several important characteristics of Cold. As a Yin Xie Qi, it can disrupt the Yin-Yang balance and subsequently affect the temperature regulation and metabolism within the body. Cold also promotes Stagnation which causes painful conditions. In addition, it causes closure or contraction of body structures, which impairs their function. Cold is the frozen wasteland where all life is buried deep within itself to escape the glacial environment. It is the ice-filled river that impedes aquatic travel.

Yin Pathogenic Factor and Impairment of Yang Qi

Cold is a Yin pathogenic factor, which easily impairs the Yang Qi of the body. This damages the warming ability of the Yang Qi. If the Cold invades the Exterior, it may injure the Defensive Yang (Defensive Qi), which is one of the body's outer defenses. This causes an Exterior Cold Pattern identified by signs such as aversion to cold and cold extremities. If the Cold directly attacks the Spleen and Stomach, it impairs the Spleen Yang. This Cold Pattern causes cold limbs and trunk as well as watery feces with undigested food.

Stagnation and Pain

Cold causes Stagnation. The Cold freezes the fluids and tissues making the flow and movement sluggish or even promoting an obstruction. Cold invasion easily results in Blood and Qi Stagnation, which causes pain. In Traditional Chinese Veterinary Medicine, there is pain only if there is Stagnation present. For instance, when a horse drinks cold water (pathogenic Cold) and develops enterospasm, the primary clinical sign is pain or colic.

Contraction

Cold makes the tissues contract, just as a cold environment makes a person want to curl up in a warm place. Cold invasion of the body surface causes contraction (closing) of the pores and obstruction of the Defensive Qi, which produces signs such as fever, aversion to cold, and absent perspiration. Cold invasion of the tendons and Meridians causes contraction of these structures resulting in cold limbs and restricted limb movement.

Common Cold Patterns

1. Wind-Cold Pattern
2. Cold Pattern of the Spleen and Stomach
3. Internal Cold Pattern, usually due to a Deficiency of the Kidney and Spleen Yang

Summer Heat

Summer Heat is the predominant Qi in the summer and it only occurs during that season. Excessively high temperatures induce the diseases due to Summer Heat. Overexposure to the blazing sun or remaining in a scorching hot environment for too long will produce patterns characteristic of Summer Heat.

There are several characteristics of Summer Heat. Summer Heat is associated with extreme heat conditions, and it is often combined with Damp when invading the body. In addition, the Summer Heat tends to move upward and affect the highest levels of the body.

Extreme Heat

Summer Heat is characterized by extreme Heat. This Yang pathogenic factor had gained in intensity when transformed from Fire. High fever, thirst, and profuse sweating are some clinical signs of Summer Heat diseases.

Upward Dispersion

Summer Heat, like warm air, tends to move upward. This tends to distribute the effects of Summer Heat at the surface and highest parts of the body. The pores open, and there is profuse sweating. This consumes Body Fluid and Qi. A patient suffering from a Summer Heat condition has a dry mouth, a great thirst and desire to drink, weakness, and shortness of breath. In severe cases, Summer Heat may disturb the mind resulting in shaking, ataxia or even coma.

Combination with Damp

As summer is often accompanied by high humidity, Summer Heat frequently combines with Damp when invading the body. So, not only does the patient suffer from the effects of the extreme Heat, but also the patient endures conditions associated with the Damp. Thus, in addition to fever, the clinical signs include loose feces, poor appetite and general lassitude.

Common Summer Heat Patterns

1. Sunstroke or Heatstroke
2. Summer Heat with Damp Pattern
3. Anhidrosis (inability to sweat) in horses

Damp

Damp is the predominant Qi of late summer. Throughout China, the period between summer and autumn is a hot and rainy season with abundant dampness. Living in damp conditions, frequent exposure to water, and prolonged periods of rain promote diseases due to Damp.

Damp has several important characteristics. Damp is viscous, bringing to mind a stagnant swamp or some primordial ooze. It is wet and heavy; it clings to the body and hinders Yang activity. It slowly erodes strength, like walking along the water-soaked sand at the seashore, which sucks down every footstep.

Obstruction of Qi Flow and Impairment of the Spleen Yang

Damp, a Yin pathogenic factor, impairs Yang and obstructs the Qi Flow (*Qi Ji*). Because the Spleen prefers dryness, Damp easily affects the Spleen Yang Qi. Damp in the Spleen impairs its food transformation and transportation functions. The result is edema, diarrhea, poor appetite, and a painful, bloated abdomen, slippery pulse.

Heaviness and Turbidity

Damp is heavy and turbid. The clinical manifestations of Damp-related diseases include difficult movement with heaviness, stiff or weak movement, turbid bodily discharges (e.g. turbid urine), mucoid or bloody feces, suppurative lesions, and weeping eczema.

Viscosity and Stagnation with Long Disease Course

Damp also is viscous and tends to stagnate. Additional Damp-related clinical signs may include tenesmus due to viscous feces, obstructed urination, and prolonged courses of disease or difficulty resolving a disease.

Common Damp Patterns

1. Wind-Damp Pattern
2. Damp-Toxin Pattern
3. Damp-Heat Pattern
4. Cold-Damp Pattern
5. Spleen Yang Deficiency Pattern (Internal Damp Pattern)
6. Kidney Yang Deficiency Pattern (Internal Damp Pattern)

Dryness

Dryness is the predominant Qi of autumn. Dryness Patterns often occur in autumn because this season is usually very dry. However, it may occur during other seasons if an area's climate is dry all year such as that of Arizona.

Dryness is the arid desert environment. The land itself, so thirsty for rain, draws the fluids right from the body. The sweat quickly evaporates making a traveler feel like a raisin in the sun. The parched throat and lungs burn in the waterless air.

Consumption of Body Fluid

Dryness consumes Body Fluid. Dryness Patterns typically have Body Fluid Deficiency signs such as a dry mouth and nose, dry feces or constipation, reduced urination, dry skin and dull hair. In addition, a Body Fluid Deficiency due to Dryness can lead to a secondary Blood Deficiency.

Impairment of the Lung

Since the Lung is a delicate organ with the functions of ascending, descending and moistening, Dryness easily impairs the Lung function. This results in a dry cough without phlegm.

Common Dryness Patterns

1. Cool Dryness
2. Warm Dryness
3. Deficiency of Yin and Blood (Internal Dryness Pattern)
4. Intestinal Dryness (Internal Dryness Pattern)
5. Lung Dryness (Internal Dryness Pattern)

Fire (Heat)

Fire and Heat have the same properties, but they vary in degree. In Traditional Chinese Veterinary Medicine, Fire is considered to be extreme Heat, while Heat is mild Fire. Fire and Heat often occur in summer, but they may be seen in other seasons.

The characteristics of Fire or Heat within the body can mirror those of Fire in nature. Fire moves upward, not unlike the flames that provide the warm, buoyant air of the hot air balloon. Also, Fire burns, whether in the body or outside. The Heat evaporates fluids and damages tissues just as sunburn makes the skin red, hot, dry and painful.

Scorching Heat and Upward Direction

Fire, as a Yang pathogenic factor, is characterized by a scorching heat and an upward direction. Its clinical manifestations include high fever, thirst, restlessness, a deep red tongue with a yellow coating, and full pulse.

Burning of Blood Vessels and Extravasation of Blood

Fire easily burns and damages the blood vessels. It allows the blood to circulate outside the vessels, which results in various forms of hemorrhage. Bloody urine, bloody feces, epistaxis, and skin hemorrhage are some signs seen with Fire or Heat conditions.

Consumption of Body Fluid

As a Yang pathogenic factor, Fire easily consumes the Body Fluid. The clinical manifestations of Heat conditions include increased thirst, dry mouth and tongue, reduced urination, dry feces or constipation, and high fever.

Common Heat Patterns

1. Wind-Heat
2. Damp-Heat
3. Dryness-Heat
4. Heat-Toxins

THE NOXIOUS EPIDEMIC QI

Like the Six Excessive Qi, the Noxious Epidemic Qi are also exogenous factors of disease. Their characteristics are similar to those of Fire; however, they are severely toxic and infectious. The Noxious Epidemic Qi can result in the sudden onset of severe diseases such as plague, anthrax, cattle plague, and hog cholera.

Some diseases due to Noxious Epidemic Qi are seasonal and some are non-seasonal. Influenza and Swine Encephalitis type B are both seasonal diseases. Influenza occurs mostly at the end of autumn, while swine encephalitis typically occurs in the summer (the major mosquito season).

Table 6.1: The Major Effects of Pathogens in the Body

Pathogen	Major Effects on the Body
Wind	• Penetrates to all parts of the body surface leading to skin problems • A Master Pathogen that brings other pathogens into the body • Induces convulsions and seizures
Heat or Fire	• Consumes Body Fluid • Causes hemorrhage and Blood Stagnation • Disturbs Shen
Damp	• Obstructs Spleen Qi creating gastrointestinal disorders • A heavy, downward moving pathogen causing heaviness and stiffness • Clings to the body making healing difficult
Summer Heat	• Extreme Heat overheats the body • Disturbs Shen • Combines with Damp thus adding Damp-associated problems
Dryness	• Dries up Lung Yin • Consumes Body Fluids • Causes Blood Deficiency
Cold	• Freezes and blocks Qi flow leading to Qi Stagnation and pain • Injures Yang causing Spleen or Kidney Yang deficiencies • Obstructs Wei Qi to cause fever without sweating

---

General Principles of Xie Qi Identification

- Where there is itching, there is Wind
- Where there is redness, there is Heat
- Where there is exudate or discharge, there is Damp
- Where there is pain, there must be blockage of Qi flow
- Where there is dandruff, there is a Blood Deficiency

Internal Etiologic Factors

The Internal causes of disease include emotional factors, dietary programs, and daily activities (exercise, training, or breeding management).

EMOTIONAL FACTORS

Experiencing each of the emotions can be healthy. It is only when the emotional state lasts too long or is too intense that it leads to disease. Emotional imbalance can impair Qi Flow (Qi-Ji) and can affect the five Zang organs.

There are seven emotions: *Kong* (Fear), *Jing* (Fright), *Xi* (Joy), *Nu* (Anger), *Si* (Worry), *Bei* (Grief), and *You* (Melancholy). Each of these emotions is associated with a Zang organ. Fear relates to the Kidney. Joy and Fright belong to the Heart. Anger relates to the Liver. Worry describes the Spleen. Grief and Melancholy relate to the Lung. (Grief is sadness that is visible externally such as crying, but melancholy is sadness which remains inside.) Both the Lung and Heart each have two emotions because they are in the upper jiao; they are closest to the brain and are in the highest positions (King and Prime Minister).

Anger

According to *Plain Questions (Su Wen)*, intense or prolonged anger causes Qi rebellion. The Qi is forced upward and the Liver Yang and Blood rise to affect the upper body and head. Clinically this is apparent as a red face and eyes, headache, restlessness, or coma.

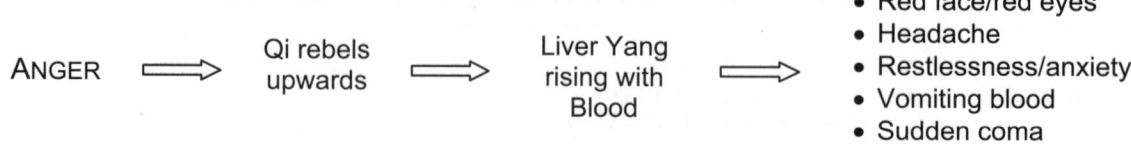

Joy

According to *Plain Questions (Su Wen)*, joy slows the Qi flow. In normal situations, joy or happiness allows the Qi to flow slowly and smoothly thus leading to longevity. Too much joy, however, can dissipate the Heart Qi. The Shen is then able to escape from its house (the Heart) which results in mental disorders and inability to focus.

| ABNORMAL JOY | ⇒ | Heart Qi Dissipates | ⇒ | Shen moves outside of the house (Heart) | ⇒ | • Difficulty focusing
• Easily distracted
• Mental disorder |

Worry

According to *Plain Questions (Su Wen)*, *Si* (Worry) may lead to Qi Stagnation. Constant thought or worry obstructs the Qi flow, which leads to Spleen and Stomach Qi Stagnation. This appears clinically as a poor appetite and fullness of the abdomen.

| THINKING DELIBERATING WORRYING

Careful Consideration | ⇒ | Obstruction of Qi flow | ⇒ | Qi Stagnation of SP/ST | ⇒ | • Poor appetite
• Abdominal fullness |

Grief and Melancholy

According to *Plain Questions (Su Wen)*, excessive sadness (including grief or melancholy) can lead to Qi dissipation. The sadness impairs the Zheng Qi and Lung Qi leading to Deficiency of both. The result is fatigue, depression, a hoarse voice and shortness of breath.

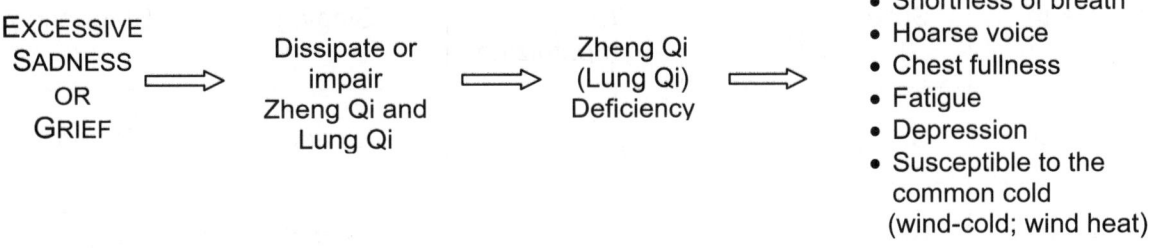

| EXCESSIVE SADNESS OR GRIEF | ⇒ | Dissipate or impair Zheng Qi and Lung Qi | ⇒ | Zheng Qi (Lung Qi) Deficiency | ⇒ | • Shortness of breath
• Hoarse voice
• Chest fullness
• Fatigue
• Depression
• Susceptible to the common cold (wind-cold; wind heat) |

Fear

According to *Plain Questions (Su Wen)*, fear leads to Qi leakage. Fear allows the Qi to flow downwards and leak. When this happens, the Kidney Qi is not firm, thus resulting in incontinence, hind limb weakness, and abortion. The Chinese word *kong* refers to Fear which is associated with the Kidney. An animal that experiences Fear will become scared and run away.

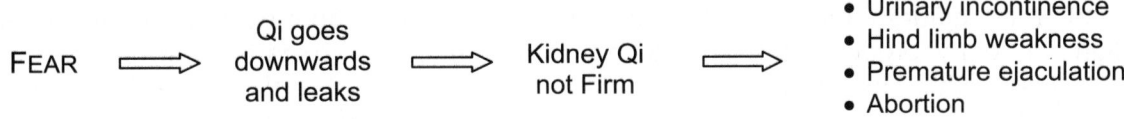

| FEAR | ⇒ | Qi goes downwards and leaks | ⇒ | Kidney Qi not Firm | ⇒ | • Urinary incontinence
• Hind limb weakness
• Premature ejaculation
• Abortion |

Fright

Fright (*Jing*) differs from Fear (*Kong*). The Chinese word Jin refers to fright that is associated with the Heart. An animal which becomes frightened will be scared but will not know how to deal with it. The animal may panic but will still remain in place; its Shen is out of control.

According to *Plain Questions* (*Su Wen*), fright can lead to Qi disorders. If an animal remains scared, the Qi flow becomes disordered which affects the Heart. Thus the patient suffers from panic, palpitations, insomnia or mental disorder.

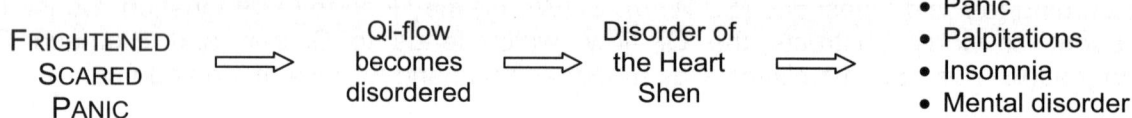

FRIGHTENED SCARED PANIC ⟹ Qi-flow becomes disordered ⟹ Disorder of the Heart Shen ⟹
- Panic
- Palpitations
- Insomnia
- Mental disorder

Table 6.2: The Organs, Emotions, Expressions, and Qi Disorders of the Five Elements

Five Elements	Zang Organ	Five Emotions		Expression	Qi-flow Impairment
Wood	Liver	*nu*	Anger	Shouting	Rebellious
Fire	Heart	*xi* *jing*	Joy Fright	Laughing	Distraction
Earth	Spleen	*si*	Thinking Worrying Sympathizing	Singing	Stagnation
Metal	Lung	*bei* *lu*	Grief Melancholy	Crying	Dissipation
Water	Kidney	*kong*	Fear	Groaning	Leakage Disorder

DIETARY FACTORS OR FEEDING PROGRAM

The foods that an animal eats are very important for maintaining health. Diets should be balanced to maintain optimum wellbeing. Disease results if the food is unhealthy or if the diet is unbalanced.

Foods have different properties that must be taken into account when preparing a diet. High fat, dairy products are considered Damp foods. High carbohydrate foods are associated with Heat/Fire, and dry foods are associated with Dryness. A TCVM practitioner designs a feeding program by combining this information with knowledge of an individual's constitutional type, environmental living conditions, and disease states. If these are not considered, a disease may develop or worsen. For example, providing dairy products to a patient with a Damp condition or an Earth constitution may make a problem worse.

The quantity and the quality of the food also are very important. Food is converted into Gu Qi which is a major Qi source for the body. Thus the food directly impacts upon the Qi of the whole body. Malnutrition can easily lead to disease.

Undernutrition or Poor Diet Quality

This sort of malnutrition results from an inadequate intake of good food and water due to poor feeding practices. Either an insufficient quantity of food or a poor quality of food prevents the animal from acquiring the required nutrients for maintaining normal body function. This lack of sufficient food and water for long periods is also known as an Over-Hungry condition. In such a state, there is a failure in Qi and Blood construction. The clinical signs include weight loss, slow growth of young animals, and weariness.

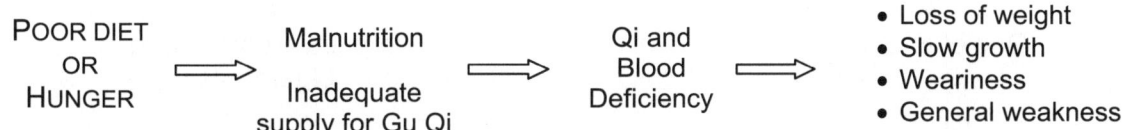

Overnutrition or Overfeeding

The quantity of food intake should be appropriate for the requirements of the body. This type of malnutrition occurs when food quantities above the appropriate amounts are ingested. Overfeeding, especially in individuals that have suffered thirst and starvation (stray animals), will impair the Spleen and Stomach function. A lot of food or water in an unprepared Stomach may thus result in sour regurgitation, abdominal distention, and loss of appetite. Regular overfeeding can result in obesity, which also promotes other disease conditions. An old TCM maxim states "eat until you are not hungry; do not eat when you are full".

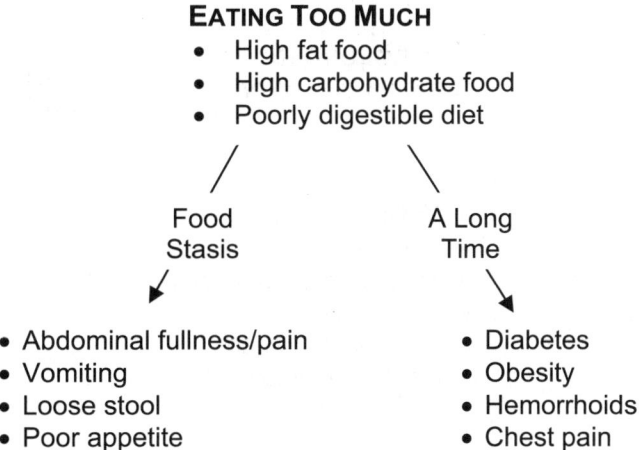

DAILY ACTIVITY

The daily activities of an individual include various types of work, exercise, and performance events. To remain healthy, a balance must be achieved between activity and rest. If there is imbalance, there is disease.

Physical Work

Overwork, prolonged or hard work, will consume the Body Fluid and Qi. In the long run, overwork will cause lassitude and weakness. It also places strain on muscles and ligaments and may damage these tissues.

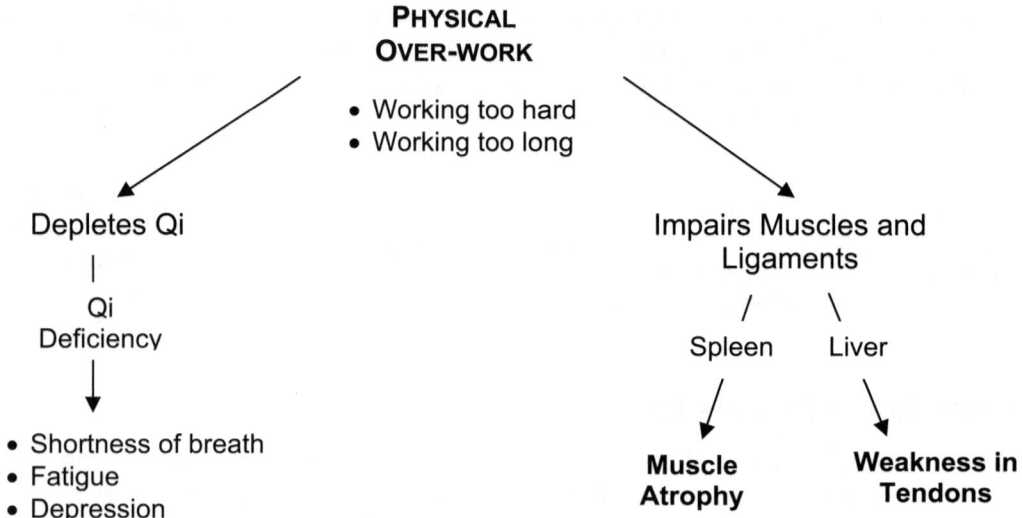

Sexual Activities

Animals that are heavily involved in breeding programs may overwork their bodies and deplete their Kidney Jing. They may show such signs as hind limb weakness, impotence, and premature ejaculation.

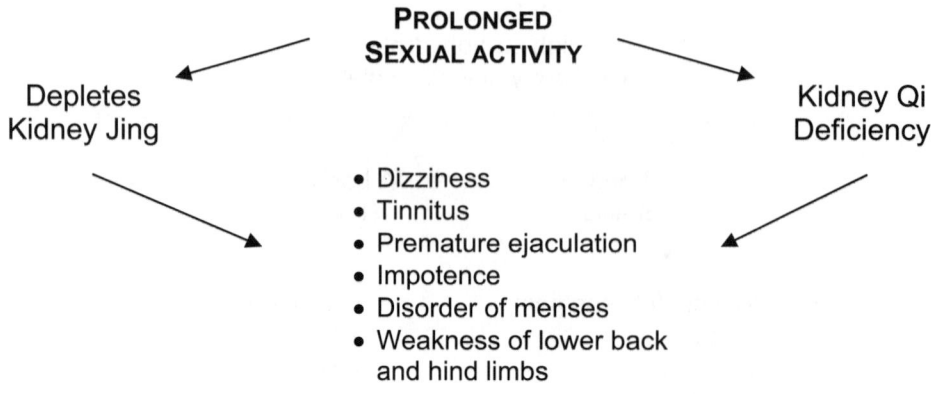

Mental Work

Long periods of mental activity or situations requiring intense concentration or alertness can wear down the body. Most anyone who has studied for a final examination can understand that it can be almost as exhausting as running a marathon. Prolonged mental activities may result in such problems as insomnia, poor appetite, and poor memory.

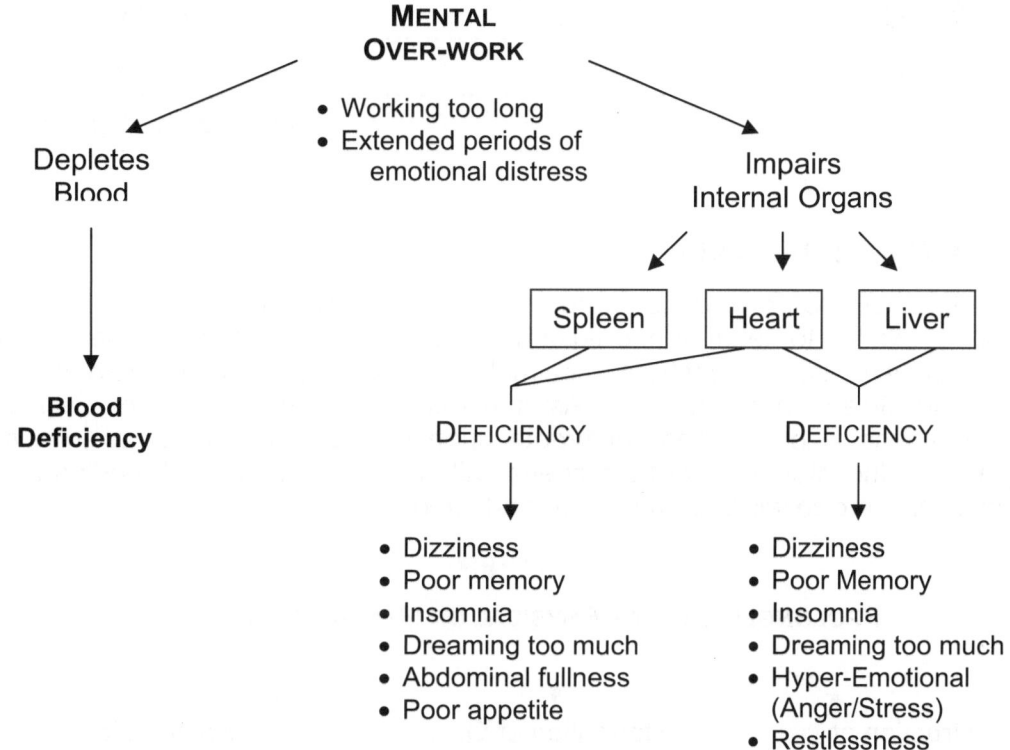

Special Activities

There are five additional activities that can also cause disease if an individual engages in these activities for prolonged periods of time. These activities are excessive observation/reading, sitting, lying, standing, or walking. Typically a healthy individual will engage in each of these throughout the day in a balanced fashion.

If one spends too much time engaging in demanding visual activities such as reading or carefully watching television, it may deplete the Liver Blood. A Deficiency of Liver Blood will fail to provide the eyes with adequate nourishment thus resulting in dry eyes or poor vision. Too much time spent lying down impairs the Qi and leads to Qi Deficiency. Extended periods of sitting, standing, and walking respectively impair the muscles, bones, and tendons.

Table 6.3: The Effects of Excessive Activities

Excessive Activity	Disease Condition	Affected Tissue
Reading or Watching	Liver Blood Deficiency	Vision, Dry Eye
Reclining or Lying down	Qi Deficiency	Qi
Sitting		Muscles
Standing		Bones
Walking		Tendons and Ligaments

Insufficient Work or Inactivity

Just as it is important to not work too hard, it is also important to not work too little. The body requires balance to keep Qi and fluids flowing properly. Extended periods of time without physical exercise can obstruct the circulation of Qi and Blood and can affect the function of the Spleen and Stomach. As a result, the individual suffers decreased appetite, weakness, and shortness of breath upon exertion. If this occurs in a male breeding animal, the vital activity of the sperm will decrease. A female breeding animal lacking physical exercise will become obese and infertile.

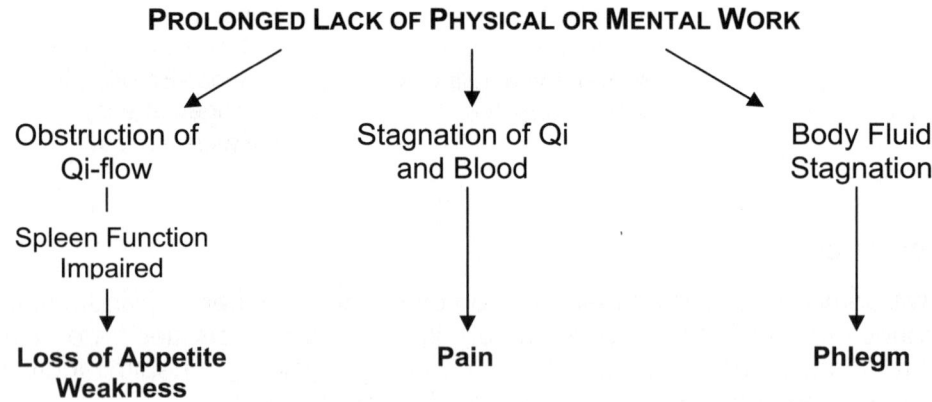

Secondary Etiologic Factors

The secondary pathologic factors that cause disease include phlegm, stagnant blood, stones and food stasis. Those secondary pathogens are caused by the primary factors which may include the Six Exogenous Xie Qi (e.g. Heat), the Internal Etiologic Factors (e.g. emotional stress) or trauma.

PHLEGM AND RETAINED LIQUID

Phlegm and Retained Liquid are the pathological products of Zang-Fu organ dysfunction. They are considered to be the accumulation of Body Fluid due to Lung, Spleen and Kidney dysfunction, which may have originally been caused by exogenous Heat or Cold. Figure 6.2 and Figure 6.3 illustrate the normal and abnormal water metabolism processes.

Phlegm is a turbid, thick and Damp material. Diseases due to phlegm include a variety of syndromes depending upon the body region affected. Retention of phlegm in the Lung, for instance, may lead to cough and asthma. Obstructed phlegm in the Meridians may give rise to subcutaneous nodules or suppurative inflammation of deep tissues. Phlegm afflicting the Heart may cause Shen disturbance, loss of consciousness or coma.

Retained Liquid is clear and dilute fluid. Retained Liquid is caused by a Yang Deficiency of the Spleen and Kidney. Retained Liquid in or under the skin may cause edema. Retained Liquid in the thoracic may cause hydrothorax. Retained liquid in the abdomen may cause ascites. Retained liquid in the gastrointestinal tract may cause diarrhea.

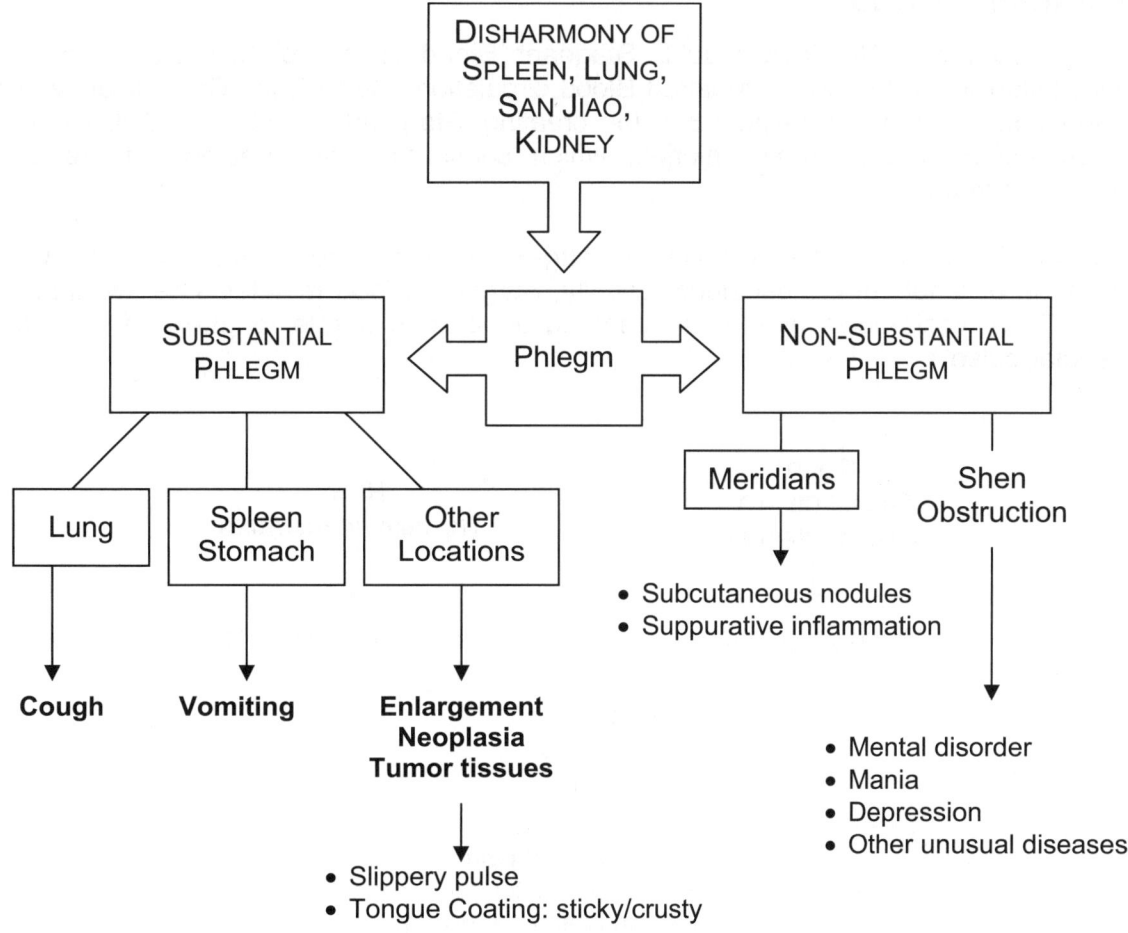

Figure 6.2: Water-Damp metabolism (the distribution of body fluids)

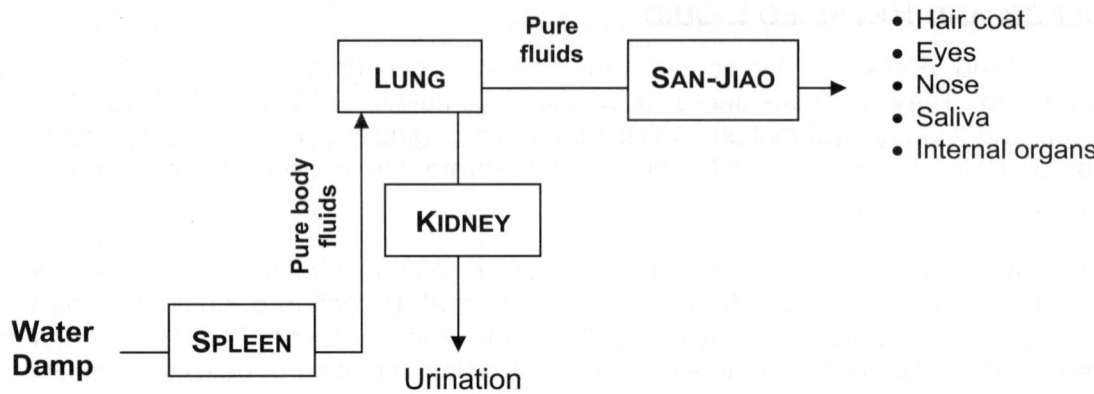

Figure 6.3: The Pathway of Water Damp Transformation

STAGNANT BLOOD

Like phlegm and Retained Liquid, Stagnant Blood is the pathological product of dysfunction within the body. Impaired Blood circulation due to Cold, Qi Deficiency or Qi Stagnation is primarily responsible for creating Stagnant Blood. In addition, blood accumulation from traumatic injuries, which cause internal bleeding, can result in Stagnant Blood.

Stagnant Blood afflicts the associated Zang-Fu organs, tissues and Meridians, which results in a variety of clinical signs. Locally, Stagnant Blood manifests as swelling and pain. On a whole-body level, it is observed as a deep purple tongue and a choppy, irregular pulse.

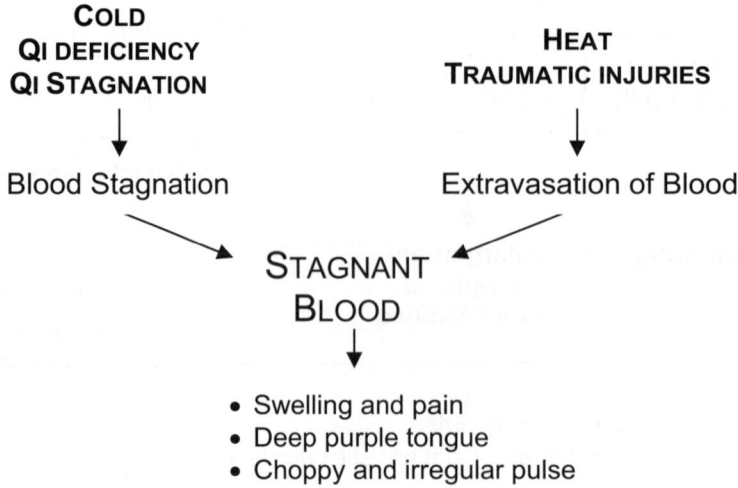

LITHIASIS

The formation of calculi in the body is also due to imbalance or Xie Qi. If there is an insult to the Liver due to stress or accumulation of Damp-Heat, then Gall Bladder stones may develop. Similarly, if Damp-Heat causes an imbalance within the Lower Jiao then Kidney or Bladder stones may form.

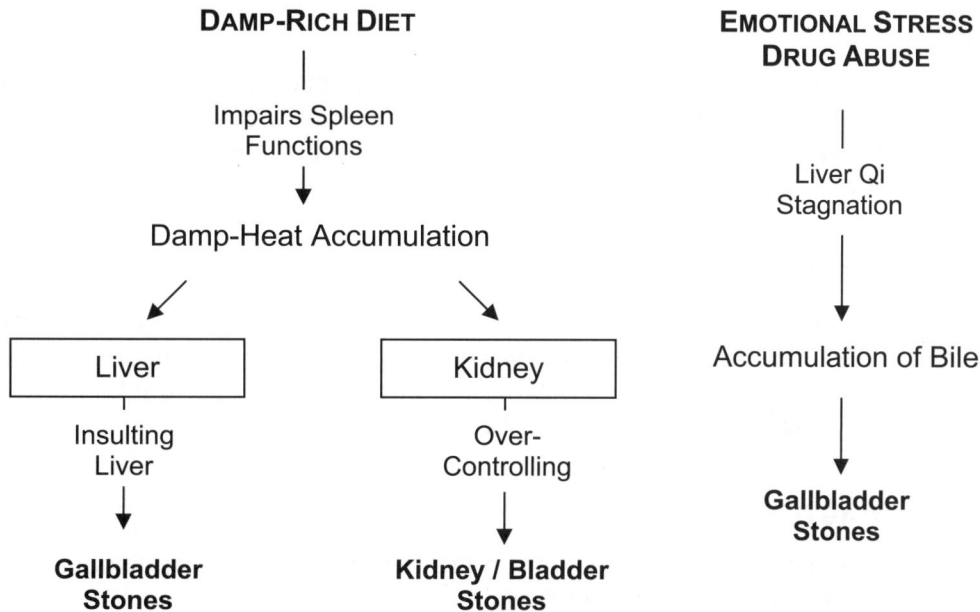

FOOD STASIS

Food Stasis occurs when an animal is over-fed, is fed a poor quality diet, or has a Spleen Qi Deficiency. Food Stasis will be discussed in Chapter 8.

Other Etiologic Factors

In addition to all the etiologic factors discussed previously, there are also other causes of disease. These include traumatic injury, parasites, poisoning, iatrogenic factors, and congenital factors.

TRAUMATIC INJURY

Damage to the body, especially due to external physical forces, is considered traumatic injury. This includes gunshot wounds, incisions, contusions, sprains, scalds, and burns. Wounds due to the bite of a poisonous snake, a rabid dog or other animals are also considered traumatic injury. The problems associated with a traumatic injury may include muscular swelling and pain, Blood Stagnation, bleeding, tendon injury, fracture of bones, and joint dislocation.

PARASITES

A parasite, as an organism that lives upon or within another organism, gains personal advantage at the expense of its host organism. Parasites feed upon or migrate through their host and may lead to damage or death of the host animal. They may include internal organisms such as intestinal worms or external organisms such as biting flies.

POISONING

Poison is a substance that may cause structural or functional damage to a body. A poison may enter the body in a variety of ways including inhalation, ingestion, and absorption. Some examples of poisons include toxic plants, toxic gasses, adulterated foods, and dangerous chemicals.

IATROGENIC FACTORS

When disease results from the activity of a medical practitioner, it is considered an iatrogenic cause. For example, a dog may develop signs of hyperadrenocorticism due to the administration of corticosteroids. Similarly, an iatrogenic allergic reaction may result due to an injected substance such as a vaccine.

CONGENITAL FACTORS

There are a variety of diseases that exist from the time of birth. These diseases may be inherited or due to an environmental insult while in the womb.

Table 6.4: Pathology of Exogenous Diseases

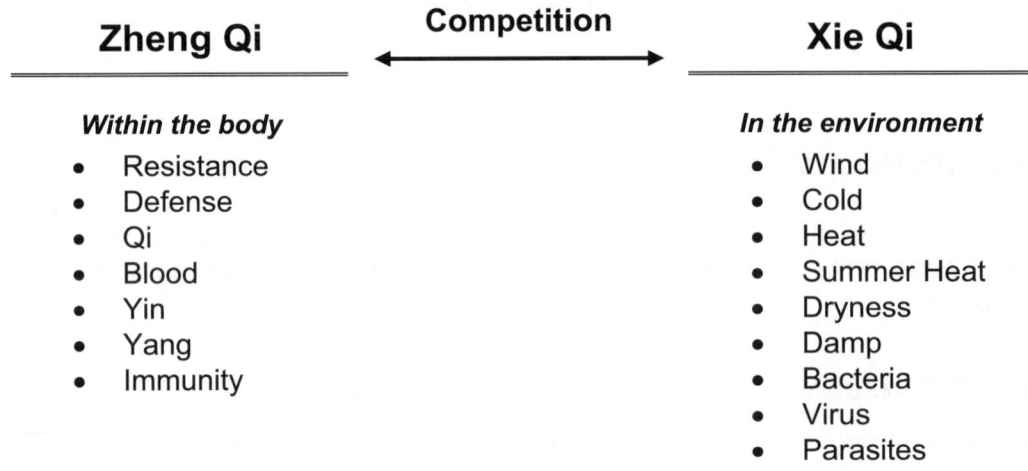

Zheng Qi	Competition	Xie Qi
Within the body		**In the environment**
• Resistance		• Wind
• Defense		• Cold
• Qi		• Heat
• Blood		• Summer Heat
• Yin		• Dryness
• Yang		• Damp
• Immunity		• Bacteria
		• Virus
		• Parasites

Pathology

Pathology, in TCVM, is the study of the bodily processes involved in disease occurrence, development and transformation. Despite the possible complications and variations among diseases, they generally may be categorized into three pathological processes: the conflict between the Zheng Qi and the Xie Qi, the disharmony of Yin and Yang, and the development of abnormal Ascending and Descending Qi Flow.

Zheng Qi is the whole body's power to kill and/or resist any Xie Qi. The Xie Qi, the Pathogenic Qi, refers to all the various causative factors of disease. Yin refers to the essential substance of the body; Yang relates to the functional activities of the body. Qi Flow, *Qi Ji*, normally circulates through the whole body with Ascending, Descending, Inward and Outward Movements.

The Zheng Qi, the Anti-pathogenic Qi, includes the body's functional activity and the ability to resist diseases. There are three aspects of the Zheng Qi which relate to the body's defensive ability, adaptability, and ability to maintain homeostasis:

1. Zheng Qi is involved in the body's ability to resist pathogens. This function also includes Wei Qi.
2. Zheng Qi assists the body in maintaining the Yin and Yang balance. This includes Ying Qi, Wei Qi, Blood, Body Fluid, Yin and Yang.
3. Zheng Qi is important in the body's ability to survive. This includes Shen, Yuan Qi and Jing.

Three TCVM Pathological Processes

- Conflict between the Zheng Qi and the Xie Qi
- Disharmony between Yin and Yang
- Disorder of Qi Flow

CONFLICT BETWEEN THE ZHENG QI AND THE XIE QI

The conflict between the Zheng Qi and the Xie Qi refers to the struggle between the body's resistance and the pathogenic factors. The outcome of this battle determines the occurrence, progression and transformation of the disease. There are five possible scenarios in this combat. 1) Zheng Qi is relatively weak and Xie Qi invades. 2) Zheng Qi is sufficient and the Xie Qi is strong. 3) Zheng Qi is deficient and Xie Qi is strong. 4) Zheng Qi is deficient and Xie Qi disappears. 5) Zheng Qi recovers and Xie Qi disappears.

1. The Relative Weakness of the Zheng Qi and Strength of the Xie Qi

When the Zheng Qi in the Interior of the body is strong, the Xie Qi can not invade the body despite the fact that it continually surrounds the body. Whenever the Xie Qi tries to attack or invade the body, the Zheng Qi immediately arrives to combat the Xie Qi. If the Zheng Qi is stronger than the Xie Qi, the Zheng Qi will defeat or eliminate the Xie Qi thus preventing disease. However, if the Xie Qi is much stronger than the Zheng Qi, the Xie Qi will invade the body and cause disease.

2. Sufficiency of the Zheng Qi and Strength of the Xie Qi

This state is common in the early stages of a disease. Although the Zheng Qi is sufficient, the Xie Qi is strong. They fight each other violently, but neither one can defeat the other. Clinically this is visible as an Excess Pattern or a Heat Pattern. For example, Heat invades the body and accumulates in the interior resulting in Heat Pattern.

3. Deficiency of the Zheng Qi and Strength of the Xie Qi

This is a consequence of a long battle between the Zheng Qi and the Xie Qi. If the Zheng Qi can not defeat the Xie Qi or if the treatment is incorrect, the Zheng Qi is consumed. This results in a Zheng Qi Deficiency with an Excess of the Xie Qi. For instance, when a Heat Pattern lasts a long time, it will consume the Body Fluid and Blood. This causes a Deficiency of Yin and Blood that results in constipation.

4. Deficiency of the Zheng Qi and Disappearance of the Xie Qi

This may be the immediate consequence of treatment. The treatment effectively eliminates the Xie Qi, but the body has not recovered from the effects that pathogen leaves behind. It is also possible that the Zheng Qi finally prevails over the Xie Qi. Even though the Zheng Qi is deficient after the long battle, the Xie Qi disappears. Clinically this manifests as a Deficiency Pattern. For instance, if a Heat Pattern is treated with herbs that eliminate Heat, the Heat disappears, but the Body Fluid has already been consumed resulting in a Yin Deficiency Pattern.

5. Recovery of the Zheng Qi and Disappearance of the Xie Qi

This is the final stage or recovery stage in the course of a disease. After treatment, the Zheng Qi recovers, the Xie Qi disappears, and the disease is cured.

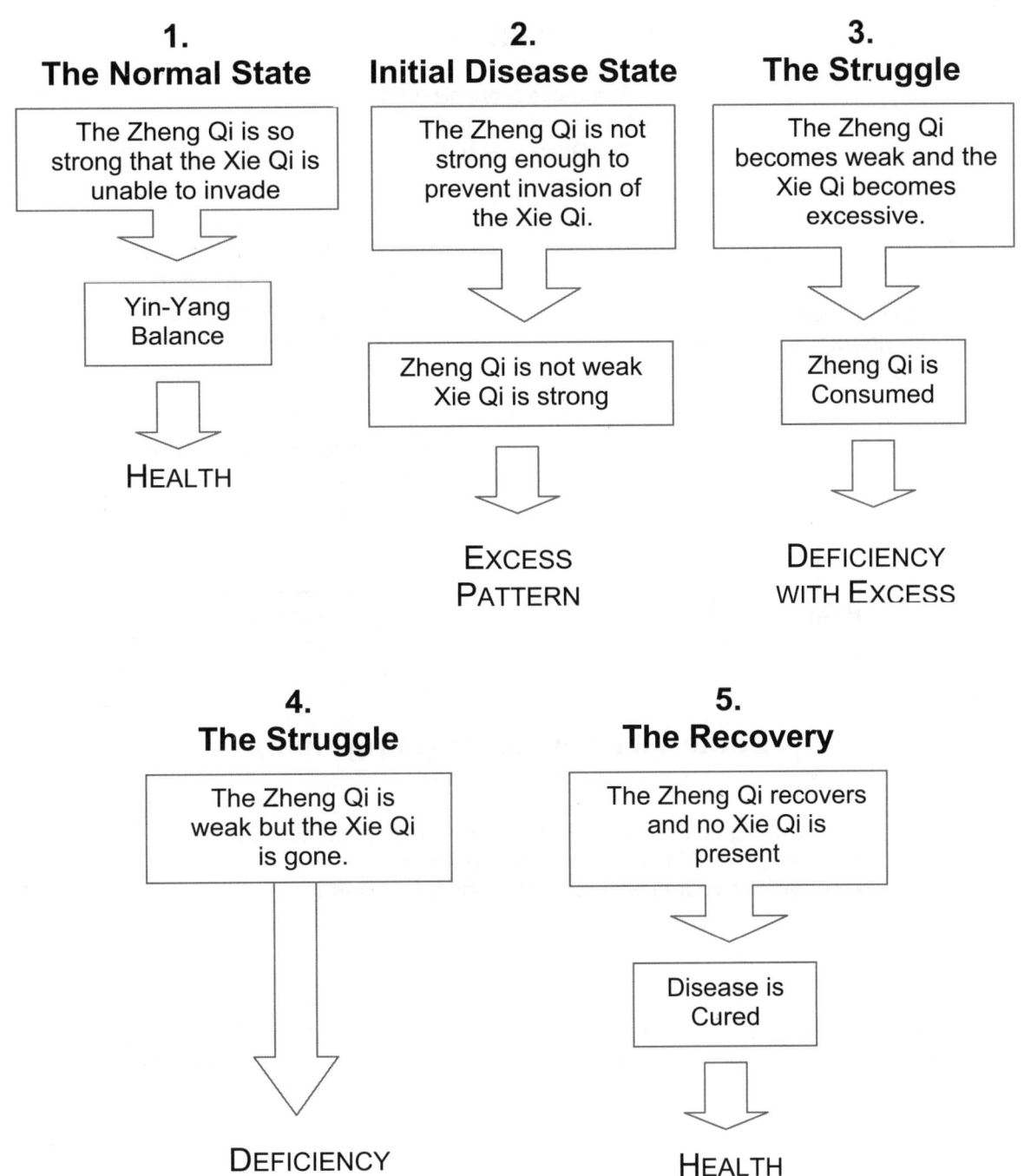

Figure 6.4: The interaction of Zheng Qi and Xie Qi

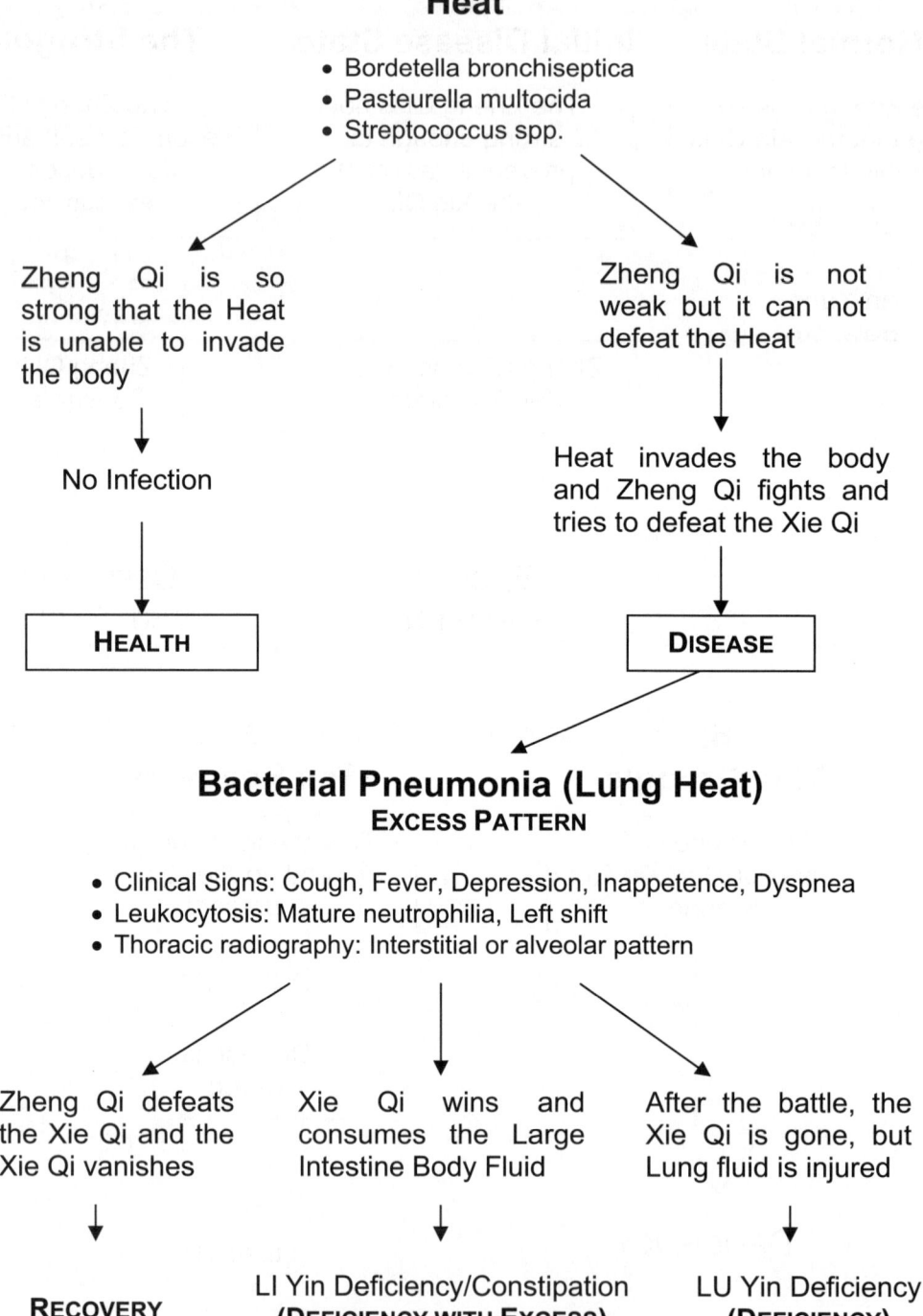

Heat

- Bordetella bronchiseptica
- Pasteurella multocida
- Streptococcus spp.

Zheng Qi is so strong that the Heat is unable to invade the body

No Infection

HEALTH

Zheng Qi is not weak but it can not defeat the Heat

Heat invades the body and Zheng Qi fights and tries to defeat the Xie Qi

DISEASE

Bacterial Pneumonia (Lung Heat)
EXCESS PATTERN

- Clinical Signs: Cough, Fever, Depression, Inappetence, Dyspnea
- Leukocytosis: Mature neutrophilia, Left shift
- Thoracic radiography: Interstitial or alveolar pattern

Zheng Qi defeats the Xie Qi and the Xie Qi vanishes

RECOVERY

Xie Qi wins and consumes the Large Intestine Body Fluid

LI Yin Deficiency/Constipation
(**DEFICIENCY WITH EXCESS**)

After the battle, the Xie Qi is gone, but Lung fluid is injured

LU Yin Deficiency
(**DEFICIENCY**)

Figure 6.5: The possible outcomes of the Zheng Qi and Xie Qi struggle

THE IMMUNE SYSTEM AND ZHENG QI

The body's immune system is involved in the three following physiological activities: defense, homeostasis, and immunosurveillance. The immune system has an important role in maintaining balance within the body. When it functions well, it benefits the body, but malfunction of the immune system can lead to disease.

The immune system defends the body through both adaptive and non-adaptive immunity. The non-adaptive immunity is often general in nature, and it includes complement, phagocytes, interferons and Natural Killer cells. These will react to many foreign substances, invading agents or abnormal cells. The adaptive immunity is more specific. It involves the B cells which have specific receptors for foreign antigens. For instance, B cells may produce protective antibodies against bacterial antigens encountered during a previous infection or vaccination.

When these two defense systems work together properly, the immune system helps to remove foreign antigens from the system. This helps to prevent or to fight against infection, thus keeping the body healthy. However, if the body reacts excessively to innocuous antigens, then allergies may result. On the other hand, a deficient response of the immune system to an antigen may result in recurrent infections.

The immune system also is involved in maintaining homeostasis. It performs this duty by recognizing normal cells and removing old or damaged cells. If the immune system views the body's own cells as foreign antigens, autoimmune diseases develop. The body attacks its own normal cells instead of just the abnormal cells.

This is similar to the immunosurveillance function of the immune system. Once again the immune system patrols the body for abnormal cells. Poor function of the immune system can thus result in cancer. In this case, the body fails to remove abnormal, mutated cells before they begin to multiply out of control.

The Zheng Qi relates to the immune system overall. The various aspects of the immune system are further related to different types of Qi; Yuan Qi, Food Qi, Ying Qi, and Wei Qi each support a certain part of the system. Therefore, in order for Zheng Qi to be strong and promote a strong immune system, the Qi of each of the component parts must also be strong.

The process begins in the Bone Marrow. Here, the pluripotent stem cells are part of the Kidney Essence. If Yuan Qi is normal, the bone marrow will contain adequate numbers of healthy stem cells to supply the body with the blood cells it will need. The Food Qi then takes part in the transformation of the stem cells into the lymphoid, myeloid and erythroid series cells within the bone marrow. For example, iron, copper, and vitamin B are needed to form normal red blood cells. When these cells further develop into their mature forms such as neutrophils, lymphocytes, and erythrocytes, they enter the bloodstream and become a part of the Ying Qi.

Some of these cells such as lymphocytes, neutrophils, and macrophages may leave the bloodstream and enter the tissues. At this time they become part of the Wei Qi or extravascular body defense. In some situations, such as lymphocytes entering lymph tissues, these cells may enter the blood vessels to become part of the Ying Qi again.

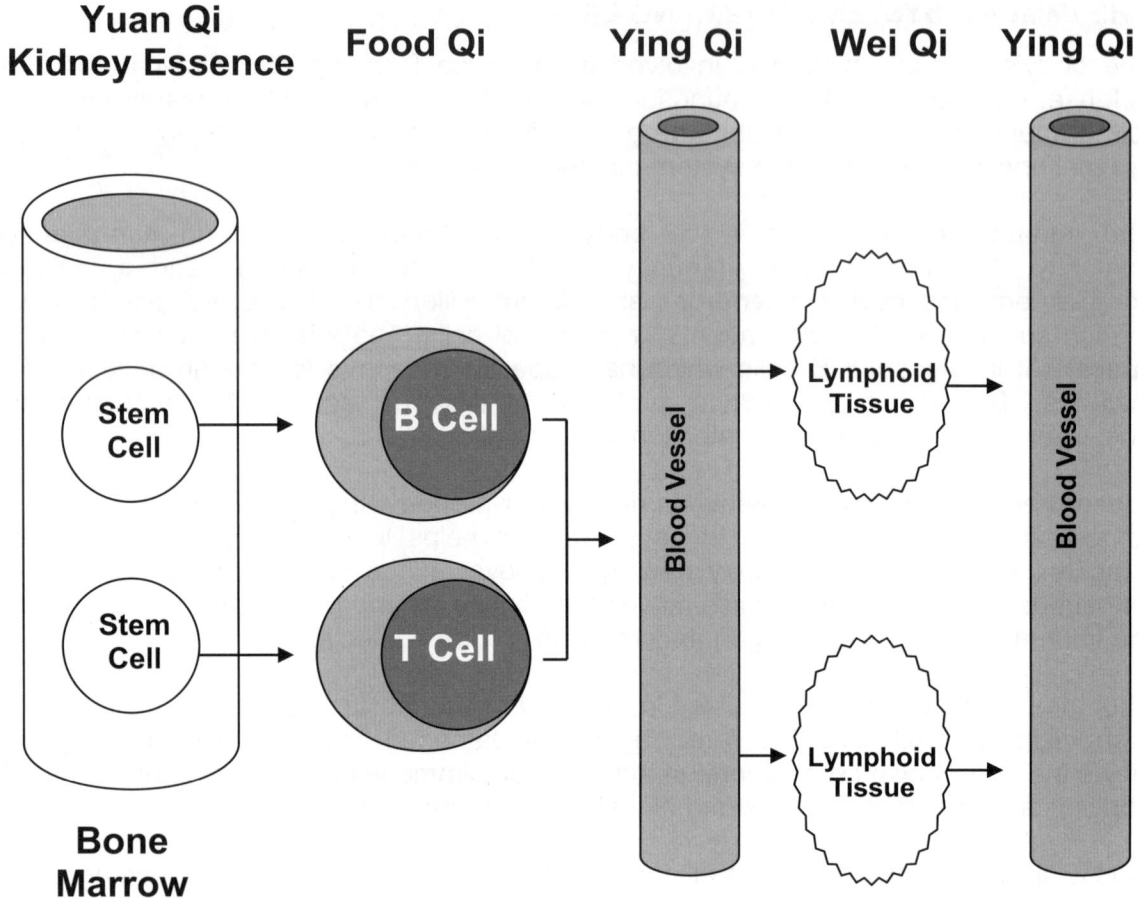

Figure 6.6: General view of Zheng Qi in relation to the immune system structures

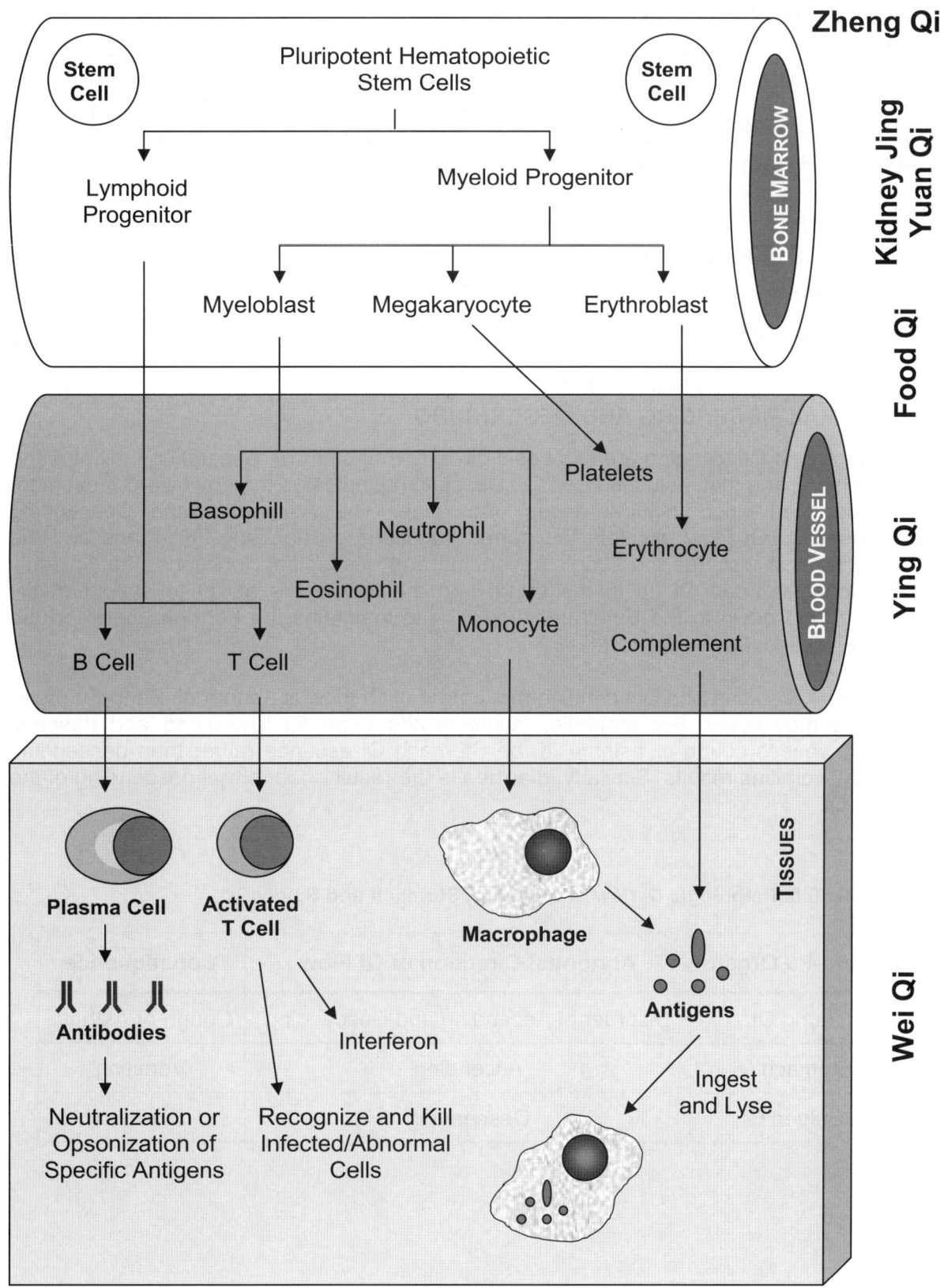

Figure 6.7: Interactions of the physical bodily structures associated with Zheng Qi

DISHARMONY OF YIN AND YANG

When the Xie Qi invades the body, it produces pathological changes that cause disharmony of Yin and Yang, producing either Excess or Deficiency of Yin or Yang. Disease occurs only if the body is invaded by pathogenic factors that cause derangement of Yin and Yang in the Interior. As discussed previously in Chapter 1, there are four basic forms of disharmony between Yin and Yang:

1. Yang Excess or Excess Heat

2. Yin Excess or Excess Cold

3. Yang Deficiency or Deficient Cold

4. Yin Deficiency or Deficient Heat

ABNORMAL ASCENDING AND DESCENDING

Ascending and Descending are two basic directions of Qi Flow. Ascending indicates the rising, clear Yang that includes Food Qi. Descending indicates the downward movement of turbid Yin, which includes feces and urine. The Ascending and Descending movements of Qi Flow maintain the normal functions of the Zang-Fu organs and the Meridians. This includes the Lung's ascending and descending functions, the Spleen's ability to send Food Qi up to the Lung, and the Stomach's ability to send partially digested food down to the Small Intestine. It also maintains the harmony between the Heart (Fire) and Kidney (Water).

When the Ascending and Descending movement of Qi Flow is abnormal, Zang-Fu organ disorders may result. For example, failure of the Lung Qi to ascend and descend normally causes cough or asthma. If the Stomach Qi ascends rather than descending normally, vomiting results. Similarly, diarrhea is the result of abnormal descending of the Spleen Qi.

Table 6.5: Pathologic Qi flow of the Lung, Stomach and Spleen

Zang-Fu Organ	Abnormal Direction of Qi Flow	Consequence
Lung Qi	Disorder of Ascending and Descending	Cough or Asthma
Stomach Qi	Ascending	Vomiting
Spleen Qi	Descending	Diarrhea

Summary of TCVM Principles of Disease Etiology

Health
- A state of equilibrium between the body and the external environment
- A state of equilibrium among the Zang-Fu organs of the body
- This equilibrium is not static, but is a state of constant self-adjustment

Disease:
- This equilibrium is impaired by a certain factor and the body is unable to adjust to restore this equilibrium.

"Identifying the cause of a disease by analyzing the signs"

Different causes of a disease
↓
Different symptoms or signs

Analyzing the clinical manifestations
↓
Discover the cause of disease

Exogenous Causes of Disease:
- *Six Excessive Qi:* Wind, Cold, Summer Heat, Damp, Fire/Heat, Dryness
- *Noxious Epidemic Qi:* Severely toxic/infectious; acute (plague, anthrax, hog cholera)

- The Six Excessive Qi and the Noxious Epidemic Qi (both known as the Pathogenic or Xie Qi) enter the body via the skin, mouth, or nose and cause disease.

- One Pathogenic Qi can transform into another:
- Extreme Heat can change into Wind
- Extreme Wind can change into Dryness

Internal Causes of Disease:
- Emotional Imbalance: Anger, Joy, Fright, Worry, Grief, Melancholy, Fear
- Poor Diet or Feeding Program: Undernutrition, Overfeeding
- Daily Activity: Physical, Mental, Sexual activities and Inactivity

Secondary Causes of Disease:
- Phlegm, Stagnant Blood, Stones, Food Stasis

Other Causes of Disease:
- Traumatic injury, Parasites, Poisoning, Congenital factors, Iatrogenic factors

Wind Summary

1. Master Pathogen
- The number one pathogenic factor causing disease.
- Cold, Heat, Damp and Dryness all depend on Wind to invade the body.

2. Upward and Outward Dispersion
- A Yang pathogenic factor: Very light
- Invades the upper parts (head/face) and superficial parts of the body
- Abnormal opening and closing of the pores
- Nasal obstruction, itching, sweating, and aversion to Wind

3. Rapid Mobility
- No fixed affected place (the affected place is changeable)
- Urticaria (wheals); Papules/swellings moving from place to place very fast

4. Rapid Changes
- A sudden onset of headache, which then quickly develops into nasal discharge

5. Vacillating and Wavering
- Epilepsy; Convulsion/wavering of the body/limbs; Internal Wind

Cold Summary

1. Yin Pathogenic Factor and Impairment of Yang Qi
- A Yin pathogenic factor
- Impairs warming function of the body's Yang Qi
- Cold in the Exterior impairs Wei Qi
- Exterior Cold Patterns result in aversion to cold and cold ears and nose
- Cold in the Spleen/Stomach impairs SP/ST Yang and results in cold limbs, watery stool, colic

2. Blockage/Stagnation and Pain
- Cold causes obstruction and Stagnation of Qi and Blood, which causes pain.
- Cold water ingested causes Qi Stagnation of the Stomach and Intestines which results in colic.

3. Contraction
- Cold invades the body surface causing contraction (closing) of the pores and obstruction of Wei Qi.
- Signs include fever without sweating and aversion to cold

Summer Heat Summary

1. Extreme Heat
- A Yang pathogenic factor which is transformed from Fire
- Clinical signs: high fever, thirst, profuse sweating.

2. Upward Dispersion
- Causes the pores to open resulting in profuse sweating
- Impairs Body Fluid and Qi
- Clinical signs: thirst, desire to drink, dry mouth, weakness, shortness of breath

3. Mostly Combined with Damp
- High humidity in the summer time; Summer Heat (+ Damp)
- Clinical signs: loose stool, poor appetite, general lassitude, non-sweating horses

Damp Summary

1. Impairment of the Spleen Yang
- A Yin pathogenic factor which impairs Yang
- Obstruction of the Qi Flow or *Qi Ji*
- Because Spleen favors dryness and dislikes dampness, it easily impairs the Qi Flow of the Spleen
- Impairs Spleen's ability to transport/transform food/drink
- Clinical Signs: edema, diarrhea, poor appetite, abdominal fullness and pain

2. Heaviness and Going Downwards
- Damp is heavy and sinks
- Clinical signs: difficulty walking, walking with heaviness and stiffness, weakness

3. Turbidity
- Clinical signs: turbid bodily discharges
- Turbid urine, mucoid or bloody feces, suppurating lesions, weeping eczema

4. A Long Course of a Disease
- Damp is viscous and sticky
- Clinical signs: Difficult defecation or urination; Prolonged, difficult to cure diseases

Dryness Summary

1. Consumption of Body Fluid
- Dryness consumes the body fluid which causes a Deficiency of Body Fluid
- Clinical signs: dry mouth or nose, dry feces or constipation, reduced urination, dry skin, withered hair

2. Impairment of the Lung
- The Lung is a delicate organ that cannot withstand dryness
- Impairment of the Lung's function of ascending and descending
- Clinical sign: dry cough without phlegm

3. Damages Blood
- Dryness dries up Body Fluid and causes Blood Deficiency

Heat Summary

1. Scorching Heat and Upward Direction
- A Yang pathogenic factor
- Clinical signs: high fever, thirst, restlessness, deep red tongue with yellow coating

2. Impairing Blood Vessels and Extravasation of Blood
- Damage to blood vessels
- Impels blood to circulate outside the vessels
- Clinical signs: hemorrhage: bloody urination, bloody feces, epistaxis, skin hemorrhage

3. Consumption of Body Fluid
- As a Yang pathogenic factor, it easily consumes the Body Fluid
- Clinical Signs: thirst, dry mouth and tongue, reduced urination, dry feces or constipation, high fever

4. Disturbing Shen
- Fire goes upwards and impairs the Heart Yin
- Heart fails to house Shen resulting in Shen disturbance

5. Extreme Heat Transformed into Wind
- Fire impairs the Liver Yin
- The Liver fails to nourish ligaments and tendons resulting in Internal Wind (convulsions)

Case Examples

Case 6.1

Signalment: An adult female spayed Greyhound

Primary Complaint: Persistent vaginitis

History and Exam:

After three weeks of antibiotics based on the culture of a vaginal swab, some of the symptoms have improved. Reexamination revealed a yellow discharge and a purple, inflamed vaginal vault.

Her tongue is not very red; it is more lavender or pink with a scant coating. The dog does have Middle Jiao Heat, vomits yellow bile, eats grass and has lost a little weight. Bismuth subsalicylate (Pepto Bismol®) does help.

Case 6.1 Assessment:

Vaginitis and vomiting bile indicate a TCVM diagnosis of Liver Damp-Heat. The external genitalia are associated with the Liver, and bile is associated with the Gall Bladder, which is the husband of the Liver.

The herbal formula *Long Dan Xie Gan Tang* may be beneficial. Acupoints including *Wei Jian*, GB-34, LIV-2 and LIV-13 may be used.

Case 6.2

Signalment: An adult Thoroughbred mare

Primary Complaint: Chronic laminitis

History and Exam:

The laminitis began in January, and it has persisted for several months. The condition is very severe. Her front hooves smell very bad. She has not been able to stand up very well. She is recumbent and has splints on all four limbs. She is not very receptive to touch due to the bedsores all over her skin.

Overall, the horse appears painful. She is very painful on her front limbs and her shoulders are very reactive. Her back is sore. Her hips and pelvic limbs are so painful due to the compensation for the front feet that she appears as though she may sit down.

Case 6.2 Assessment:

Laminitis can sometimes be a big challenge. It is crucial to control the pain and inflammation. Pain signifies Stagnation. Inflammation and a bad smell point to Heat and Toxin. Thus, from a TCVM perspective, this means that one must apply treatments that will clear the Heat, detoxify, and remove Stagnation.

Some suggested acupoints include *Bai Hui*, SI-9, BL-18, BL-19, BL-60 and PC-1. In addition, electroacupuncture can help release beta-endorphin to block pain. Electroacupuncture can be performed at the following points: 1) *Shen Shu*, bilateral and 2) *Bai Hui* with either left or right SI-9

Hemoacupuncture may be performed at TH-1 and ST-45 using a 20- or 21- gauge needle. Allow up to 100 cc of blood to flow from each hoof. This is the fastest way to clear Heat, to detoxify and to remove Stagnation. If 100 cc is too much for those observing the procedure, try to bleed as much as possible because any amount of stale blood that comes out of the hoof will help the laminitis. Do not repeat the acupuncture at the same points within 10 days. If it is necessary to bleed again, it is possible to use the rest of the ting-points such as LI-1, SI-1, GB-44, and LIV-1.

After the acute conditions are under control, local points such as PC-9, KID-1 and systematic points including BL-11, BL-18, and BL-19 will be beneficial. In addition, local massage will help to move the blood. Four Herbs Salve (*Si Sheng Gao*) may be used as a topical pain reliever.

Case 6.3

Signalment: Herd Health of Pregnant mares

Primary Complaint: Abortion storms

History and Exam:

Many mares began have abortions occurring between 60 and 75 days of pregnancy. At first the abortion rate was significant, but the rate slowed with time. Mares sent for breeding developed pleuritis and their foals began showing signs of severe uveitis, which in some cases results in blindness.

Case 6.3 Assessment:

From a TCVM perspective, these mares have too much "Liver Heat Toxin", which invades the fetus and eventually causes abortion. Thus, cooling the Blood is the key for both treatment and prevention.

For the mare and foal, *Yi Guan Jian* may be a good formula to cool the blood, to clear the Liver, and to nourish Liver Yin.

Case 6.4

Signalment: A Quarter Horse Colt

History and Exam:

The primary concern is lameness that has become progressively worse. The secondary concern is a hard swelling on the left front leg between the pastern and fetlock.

The colt was born with his tongue sticking out of his mouth. He was doing well until about two months ago when he ate moldy hay and almost died. He was treated with IV LRS, Banamine®, a triple antibiotic, Bactrim® and Acetazolamide. Within two weeks his left front pastern to fetlock became severely swollen. No fracture was seen on radiographs.

About a week later, the muscles on the left side of his neck (the same side as the catheter) were in a large knot. His tongue was pale and dry. His pulses were deep and weak (worse on the left). He was very sensitive at LIV-14, but the sensitivity has diminished with time. He is growing, has a great appetite, and is getting much stronger. The swelling has gone down, but the lameness has gotten worse.

Treatments have included Bach Flowers, Milk Thistle, Homeopathics (Apis, Silica, and Hypericum), and acupuncture. He has received weekly acupuncture treatments that help for three to four days, and then he gets worse again.

Case 6.4 Assessment:

The TCVM diagnosis can be considered Blood Stasis (Blood Stagnation).

Acupuncture can be beneficial. Perform hemoacupuncture at SI-3 on the palmar vein using 21-gague needle to bleed. Let up to 100 cc of blood flow. Only perform this once every two weeks. Do not reuse the same bleeding points during the two-week time period. Hemoacupuncture is a fast and effective way to get rid of blood stasis because "fresh blood can not be generated until the stale blood is resolved". Use dry-needle acupuncture at TH-1, SI-1, LU-11, LI-1, once every one to three weeks. Also use aquapuncture at TH-15, BL-13, SI-9, BL-18, once every one to three weeks

The herbal recommendation includes topical *Huo Xue Hua Yu Gao* (Relief Salve). Local massage before application of the topical medication may assist movement of blood.

Case 6.5: Topic Discussion

Topic: Inflammatory Bowel Disease (IBD)

Question: How does one differentiate the TCVM classification of Inflammatory Bowel Disease as opposed to other regular diarrhea types?

Discussion:

Inflammatory Bowel Disease is not a TCVM diagnosis; TCVM considers it a diarrhea disease. Basically, it is viewed as a "Heat" or "Fire" pathogen in the early stage because it is inflammatory.

There may be four basic types of IBD Patterns.

Heat Toxin Pattern:	• Very acute • Bright, red blood • Fever
Damp Heat Pattern:	• Acute • Blood and/or mucus • Unpleasant odor • This is most common form of IBD in dogs.
Yin Deficiency Pattern:	• Chronic • Diarrhea not severe • Dehydration • Prolonged Heat damages Yin/Body Fluid causing Yin Deficiency
Qi Deficiency:	• Very late stage • No Heat signs (red tongue, foul odor of diarrhea) are observed. • "Yin fails to support Qi or Qi follows Yin to become deficient"

If a dog with IBD responds to an antibiotic, the disease may be one of the first two types (especially first one). Antibiotic is cold, and it can clear Heat or Heat Toxin.

Self Test

Question 6.1: The Six Exogenous Pathogens are

    a. Wind, Cold, Air, Summer Heat, Fire, Damp
    b. Wind, Cold, Damp, Summer Heat, Fire, Dryness
    c. Wind, Cold, Heat, Fire, Damp, Dryness
    d. Wind, Cold, Heat, Fire, Air, Dryness
    e. Wind, Cold, Summer Heat, Fire, Air, Dryness

Question 6.2: What is the worst enemy of the Spleen?

    a. Wind
    b. Cold
    c. Damp
    d. Dryness
    e. Fire

Question 6.3: The most significant clinical sign of a disease caused by Wind is

    a. Fever
    b. Anorexia
    c. Diarrhea
    d. Thirst
    e. Seizure

Question 6.4: Which of the following statements about Wind is NOT true?

    a. Wind is the Master pathogen.
    b. Wind usually brings in or combines with other pathogens when invading the body.
    c. Where there is itching, there must be Wind.
    d. Where there is cough, there must be Wind.
    e. The disease caused by Wind usually has a short course.

Question 6.5: Which of the following is NOT a clinical sign of a disease caused by Heat/Fire?

    a. Fever
    b. Anxiety
    c. Hemorrhage
    d. Thirsty
    e. Urinary incontinence

Question 6.6: Which of the following statements is NOT true about Heat/Fire?

    a. Extreme Heat/Fire may transform into Wind

    b. Heat/Fire may consume Body Fluid

    c. Heat/Fire may lead to Damp

    d. Where there is redness, there must be Heat/Fire

    e. Often, inflammation or infections can be considered as Heat/Fire.

Question 6.7: Which of the following statements is TRUE about Damp?

    a. Damp often occurs in the Springtime.

    b. Damp often leads to fever.

    c. The disease caused by Damp often has a long course.

    d. Extreme Damp can transform into Cold.

    e. Damp often obstructs Lung Qi

Question 6.8: Which of the following clinical signs is caused by Cold?

    a. Pain

    b. Redness

    c. Swelling

    d. Fever

    e. Seizure

Question 6.9: Which of the following statements is True about Cold?

    a. Spleen Yang and/or Kidney Yang Deficiency often cause internal Cold.

    b. Where there is excretion/discharge, there must be Cold.

    c. Cold often leads to Yin Deficiency

    d. Extreme Cold can transform Wind

    e. Cold often opens the pores of skin and causes sweat.

Question 6.10: Which of the following statements is NOT true about Summer Heat?

    a. Summer Heat often leads to high fever.

    b. Summer Heat often leads to diarrhea.

    c. Summer Heat is often combined with Damp.

    d. Summer Heat can cause non-sweating (anhidrosis) in horses.

    e. Summer Heat often occurs in late Summer.

Question 6.11: Which of the following statements is NOT true about Dryness?

    a. Dryness often leads to Yin Deficiency.

    b. Where there is dandruff, there must be Dryness.

    c. Dryness often leads to Blood Deficiency.

    d. Dryness is always combined with Heat/Fire.

    e. Dryness often leads to Deficiency of Body Fluid

Question 6.12: Which of the following statements is NOT true about Zheng Qi?

    a. Zheng Qi is the whole body's ability to resist any pathogens.

    b. Zheng Qi protects the body from being invaded by virus and bacteria.

    c. Zheng Qi includes Wei Qi, Ying Qi, and Yuan Qi.

    d. Zheng Qi Deficiency often leads to immune deficiency.

    e. Zheng Qi is Yin.

Question 6.13: Which of the following statements is True?

    a. Ascending Stomach Qi (or rebellious Stomach Qi) leads to vomiting.

    b. Ascending Spleen Qi leads to vomiting.

    c. Ascending Spleen Qi leads to diarrhea.

    d. Ascending Stomach Qi leads to diarrhea.

    e. Descending Stomach Qi leads to diarrhea.

Question 6.14: Which of the following statements is NOT true?

    a. Yin Excess is Cold.

    b. Yang Excess is Heat.

    c. Yang Deficiency leads to Cold.

    d. Yin Deficiency leads to Cold.

    e. Yin Deficiency leads to Heat.

CHAPTER SEVEN

DIAGNOSTIC METHODS

We must turn to nature itself, to the observations of
the body in health and disease to learn the truth.

–Hippocrates

In any medical system, effective treatment of disease hinges upon accurate, complete diagnoses. This places *Bian Zheng*, the diagnostic system of Traditional Chinese Veterinary Medicine (TCVM), as the most important part of medical practice. *Bian*, which is differentiation and identification, and *Zheng*, which is a type or pattern of illness, together indicate that the TCVM diagnostic system relies upon pattern differentiation. Therefore, a correct TCVM diagnosis and a subsequent effective treatment depend upon the practitioner's ability to analyze a patient's symptoms and to identify the *Zheng* (pattern of illness).

The *Zheng* is a major difference between TCVM and conventional Western medical disease diagnosis. Western medicine identifies a disease and its cause by analyzing the individual symptoms. However, TCVM takes all symptoms into consideration in order to identify a special *Zheng* in addition to naming the disease. For example, consider the cases of bloody diarrhea in two horses. The first horse is a two-year-old Thoroughbred filly who presents with profuse hemorrhagic diarrhea. The bloody diarrhea began about three days ago. The fecal cultures were positive for *Salmonella* species. The horse also had a red tongue and rapid pulse. Conventional Western practitioners may diagnose the disease as *Salmonella* colitis, yet TCVM practitioners recognize an Excess Pattern because of red tongue, rapid pulse, young age and acute onset. The other horse, an eighteen-year-old Thoroughbred mare, presents with a twenty-one day history of bloody diarrhea. The fecal test was positive for *Salmonella* species, and the mare had a pale tongue and weak pulse. Just as in the first case, conventional Western practitioners diagnosed *Salmonella* colitis. The TCVM practitioners, however, diagnosed Spleen Qi Deficiency based upon her pale tongue, weak pulse, old age and chronic diarrhea.

Traditional Chinese Medical practitioners developed four diagnostic methods, the *si-zhen*, to accurately determine a Pattern of illness. *Si* and *zhen* are respectively translated as "four" and "diagnostic methods". *Si-zhen* includes four methods of obtaining clinical data: Inspecting, Hearing and Smelling, Inquiry and Palpation. From a Western sense, they refer to observation, auscultation and olfaction, interrogation, and palpation. These should not be used separately because they relate to and supplement one another. Clinically, a practitioner combines the four diagnostic methods to gain a comprehensive and systematic understanding of a disease condition and to make the correct diagnosis.

The principle behind the *Si-zhen* is the examination of the Exterior to reveal the condition of the body's Interior. This is based upon the understanding that the animal body, as an organic entity, may have regional pathological changes or Zang-Fu organ pathology which may affect the whole body or may become evident on the body surface. Thus, the Exterior signs may reflect the condition of the Zang-Fu organs. For example, redness and swelling of the eyes may indicate a Liver Heat Pattern.

Table 7.1: The four diagnostic methods

Si-zhen		Examination	Western Medicine Counterpart
Inspection	wang	• View the Tongue appearance • Observe the Shen • Observe the general body condition • View the hair coat appearance	Observation
Hearing Smelling	wen	• Listen to the voice quality • Listen to breathing • Listen to heart and lungs • Smell breath or body odor	Auscultation Olfaction
Inquiring	wen	• Question owner about medical history • Question owner about habits	Interrogation
Palpation	qie	• Feel the pulse • Palpate the Meridians • Palpate the shu and mu points	Palpation

Inspection

Wang Zhen

Inspecting is a method of diagnosis that involves observation of abnormal changes in the patient's Shen, tongue appearance, general condition, secretions and excretions. Each of the following elements should be closely observed: Shen, tongue, movement and posture, skin and hair appearance, body appearance, appetite and thirst, defecation and urination, and local regional appearance of eyes, ears, nose, lips, and limbs.

SHEN

The Shen or Spirit refers to the outward manifestations of the body's vital activities. By observing the animal's spirit, the veterinarian may get a rough idea of the overall condition and the severity of a disease. The state of the Shen is highly significant for the prognosis.

The presence or absence of spirit may be observed in the eyes, the ears and the mentation. When an animal has a normal spirit, the eyes glitter and reveal an inner vitality, the ears move nimbly in response to environmental stimuli, and the mind functions appropriately. The clinical appearance of Shen loss includes weariness, dull eyes, sluggishly responding eyes and ears, and drooped head and ears. If an animal is ill but has a normal Shen, the Zheng Qi is strong and the disease is mild with a good prognosis. A sick animal with no Shen has a Zheng Qi Deficiency; this indicates the presence of a severe disease with a bad prognosis.

Shen Summary

Normal Shen:	Loss of Shen:
• Glittering eyes	• Weariness
• Eyes have luster and vitality	• Dull eyes
• Nimble ears respond to environmental stimuli	• Sluggish eyes and ears
	• Drooping head and ears
• Zheng Qi is strong	• Often indicates Zheng Qi Deficiency
• Indicates a mild disease	• Indicates a severe disease
• Good prognosis for recovery	• Poor prognosis
• Good response to acupuncture or Chinese herbal treatment	• Poor response to acupuncture or Chinese herbal treatment

---

TONGUE

Evaluation of the tongue is a pillar of diagnosis because it is the basis of not only Pattern Identification and Treatment, but also prognosis. The observation of the tongue should include examination of the color and luster of the oral cavity, the mouth moisture, and the tongue shape and coating. This is known as the Tongue Diagnosis.

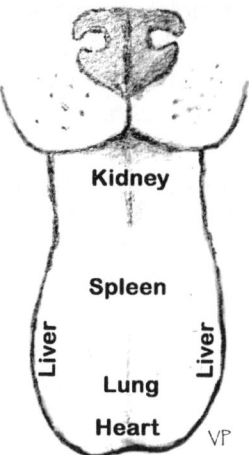

Figure 7.1: The regions of the tongue

The surface of the tongue is divided into several regions that correspond to individual Zang organs (Figure 7.1). The tip of the tongue is the realm of the Heart. The Lung resides just caudal to the tongue tip. The center of the tongue is the location of the Spleen. The Kidney is found at the very back of the tongue. The sides of the tongue are reserved for the Liver. Changes in any of these regions may give clues about which organs are involved in the disease.

Method of Examination

One should carefully evaluate the tongue, the internal surfaces of the lips, the gums, and the caruncula sublingualis. Compare all the relevant parts of the oral cavity before making the final decision about the tongue appearance. This is especially true in horses that always graze in the pasture. Some feeds such as grass may change the color of the tongue, so it is important to observe the lips, gums, and caruncula sublingualis in addition to the tongue itself. There should be moderate moisture on the ventral, inside surface of the lower lip. This is the first place to check the body fluid status in horses. In dogs, cats, and cattle, the first place to check the body fluid status is in the nostrils.

To examine the tongue of a horse, begin by placing the right hand on the halter to restrain the head. Use the index and middle fingers of the left hand to open the lips and to permit observation of the mucous membrane color and luster. Extend those two fingers into the oral cavity to feel the temperature and moisture of the mouth. Then open the mouth to observe the tongue and the caruncula sublingualis. Finally, take the tongue out of the mouth to observe the tongue body and the coating (Figure 7.2).

To examine the tongue of a dog, one can observe the tongue as the dog pants. Otherwise, one may begin by lifting the upper lip to evaluate the color and moisture of the mucous membranes. Open the mouth and observe the size, shape, and color of the tongue as it rests in the mouth. In addition, make note of the tongue coating quality as well as the presence of any ulcers, cracks, or other lesions. Avoid manipulations of the tongue itself as this may artificially alter the tongue appearance. When evaluating a dog with a pigmented tongue, such as the Chow Chow, use instead the mucous membrane color of the conjunctiva, the penis, or the vulva.

To examine the tongue of a cat, begin by restraining the head with one hand. The other hand may be used to retract the lips and observe the mucous membranes. Open the mouth and observe the appearance of the tongue and oral cavity. Upward pressure with a finger between the bones of the mandible can elevate the tongue and may facilitate observation of the structures under the tongue. Make note of the saliva quality, the tongue color, the tongue shape, the tongue coating, and the presence of any lesions. A fractious cat may provide a quick view of the oral cavity when hissing or yowling.

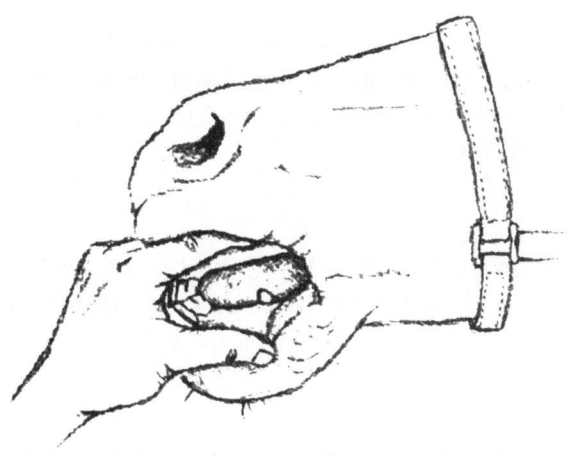

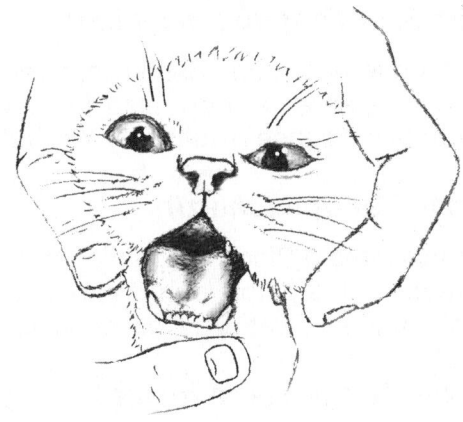

Figure 7.2: Equine oral exam

Figure 7.3: Feline oral exam

The Tongue Color

Normal Color

The normal tongue color is light-red or slightly yellow-red with a luster like a peach flower. It varies with the different seasons becoming slightly red in hot seasons or slightly pale-red in cold seasons. It also varies with the different species. The canine and feline tongue is brighter and redder than the equine one.

Abnormal Color

When there is a disease condition, the tongue may be pale, red, dark-red, purple, or yellow.

Pale Tongue (she bai)

The tongue is less red than normal. This indicates a Deficiency Pattern of either Blood or Qi. Usually, the Qi Deficiency Pattern has a slightly wet and swollen tongue, but a Blood Deficiency Pattern has a dry tongue. General weakness or immunodeficiency may accompany a Qi Deficiency Pattern, and anemia or general weakness may occur with a Blood Deficiency Pattern.

Red Tongue (she hong)

The tongue is bright red or is more red than normal. This indicates a Heat Pattern. A red tongue with a coating indicates an Excess Heat Pattern, which may be seen in cases of infection, inflammation, or fever. A red tongue with no coating indicates a Deficient Heat Pattern, which may be seen in cases with chronic inflammation or infection. A red tongue tip indicates a Heart Heat Pattern, while red sides of the tongue indicate a Liver Heat Pattern.

Deep-Red Tongue (she jiang)

The tongue is a shade darker than red. This indicates a more severe Heat Pattern. This tongue appearance may also be seen when extreme Heat injures Yin or when an exogenous disease results in a Yin Deficiency Pattern.

Purple Tongue (she zi)

This indicates a Blood Stagnation and Pain Pattern, which may be related to either Cold or Heat. A blue-purple and dry tongue indicates a Heat Pattern while a pale-purple and moist tongue indicates a Cold condition.

Yellow Tongue (she huang)

This indicates a Damp Pattern mostly related to the accumulation of Damp-Heat in the Liver. A tongue that is bright yellow, like a citrus peel, indicates an Excess Heat Pattern of the Liver. Acute hepatitis and cholestasis (Gall Bladder Stagnation) both produce Excess Heat Patterns of the Liver. When the tongue is a lusterless yellow, like smoke stains, a Cold-Damp Pattern is present such as those found in cases with chronic liver problems.

Death Color (jue she)

This is the typically blue-black or purple-black color that may be visible when the animal is near death.

The Tongue Coating

The residual "Dampness", which is left over from the Spleen and Stomach's digestion, reaches upwards to form the coating of the tongue. Therefore, the tongue coating reflects the state of the Spleen and Stomach function. Normally, the tongue should have a very thin and white, green, or slightly yellow coating with adequate moisture to indicate that the Spleen/Stomach is digesting food properly.

Normal Coating

The tongue of healthy animals should have a very thin and green, white, or slightly yellow coating with proper moisture.

Abnormal Coating

When there is a disease condition, the tongue coating color may be white, yellow, or grey-black and the consistency may be too thick, wet or dry.

White Coating (bai tai)

This often refers to an Exterior Pattern or a Cold Pattern. A thin, white coating indicates an Exterior Pattern as may be found in the early stages of a respiratory infection. A thick, white coating indicates a Cold Pattern.

Yellow Coating (huang tai)

This indicates a Heat Pattern, which is often found during the course of infection and inflammation. The intensity of the color reflects the severity: the deeper yellow the coating, the more severe the Heat Pattern. A mild Heat Pattern has a light yellow coating while a severe Heat Pattern has a deep yellow coating.

Grey-Black Coating (hui hei tai)

This may indicate a Heat Pattern, a Cold-Damp Pattern, or a Deficiency Cold Pattern. A dry, gray-black coating indicates an Extreme Heat Pattern or a Yin Deficiency Pattern. A moist, grey-black coating indicates a Cold Pattern due to a Yang Deficiency.

Thick Coating and Thin Coating (bao tai and hou tai)

The thickness of the coating may be used to determine the progression and severity of a disease. *Bao tai*, the thin coating, indicates a normal condition or a superficial pattern. *Hou tai*, the thick coating, may indicate retention of Damp and Phlegm or Food in the Interior. Transformation of a thick coating into a thin coating denotes a good prognosis and a gradual elimination of pathogens. On the other hand, a thin coating that becomes a thick coating may suggest an aggravation of pathological conditions. If the coating becomes thicker after treatment, it often suggests that a wrong treatment may have been administered.

Wet Coating and Dry Coating (zao tai and tai run)

These coatings may be used to determine the condition of body fluid (Yin). The normal coating is moist and lustrous. A dry coating, *zao tai*, indicates an injury of body fluid due to extreme Heat. A wet coating (*tai run*), which is visible as excessive saliva or dribbling from the tongue, indicates Water-Damp retention.

Sticky Coating and Crusty Coating (tai ni and fu tai)

Tai ni, the sticky coating, is a glossy, grimy coat that is hard to scrub off. This indicates an accumulation of Phlegm and Damp or Food Stasis. *Fu tai*, the crusty coating, is a soft, loose, and thick crust on the tongue surface that is easily rubbed off. This indicates indigestion or retention of phlegm or food.

The Tongue Shape

A swollen but pale tongue indicates a Kidney Yang Deficiency Pattern. A swollen but deep red tongue refers to an Extreme Heat Pattern. The swollen and stiff tongue that occupies the entire space of the mouth indicates Heart Heat. The thin, pale tongue without elasticity often suggests a Qi or Blood Deficiency Pattern. A soft, pale tongue that is unable to return to the mouth or trembles when the tongue is held out indicates a very severe disease condition or severely Deficient Qi or Blood.

Table 7.2: TCVM or Western diagnosis associated with tongue appearance

Appearance		TCVM Diagnosis	Western Diagnosis
TONGUE COLOR	**Pale**	**Wet:** Qi Deficiency	Anemia, General weakness, Immunodeficiency
		Dry: Blood Deficiency	
	Red	Heat: Yin Deficiency or Excess Heat	Inflammatory diseases, Infections, Fever
		Tip: Heart Fire	
		Sides: Liver Heat/Fire	
	Deep Red	Heat with Yin Deficiency Severe Heat, Yin Deficiency	Dehydration, Chronic inflammation
	Purple	Qi or Blood Stagnation, Cold Pattern	Pain, Poor circulation, Heart failure
	Yellow	**Lusterless:** Damp, Spleen Deficiency	Liver problems, Chronic Gastrointestinal disorders
		Bright: Liver Damp-Heat	
TONGUE COATING	**White**	**Thin:** Exterior Pattern, Wind-Cold	Common Cold, Food retention, Indigestion, Chronic GI disorders
		Thick: Cold, Cold-Damp, Phlegm	
	Yellow	Heat, Excess Heat	Inflammatory diseases, Infections
	Grey-Black	**Dry:** Heat, Yin Deficiency	Chronic inflammatory diseases, Chronic illness, Renal failure
		Wet: Yang Deficiency, Cold	
	Dry	Yin Deficiency, Blood Deficiency	Dehydration
	Wet	Qi Deficiency, Yang Deficiency Damp-Cold, Water-Damp	General weakness, Water retention, Diarrhea, Edema
	Sticky	Phlegm, Damp, Food Stasis	Chronic GI disorders
	Crusty	Indigestion, Food retention, Phlegm	
TONGUE SHAPE	**Swollen**	**Pale:** Kidney Yang Deficiency	
		Red: Extreme Heat Pattern	
	Soft Small	**Since Birth:** Kidney Jing Deficiency	
		Pale: Qi or/and Blood Deficiency	
		Quivering: Internal Wind, Severe Deficiency of Qi/Yang/Blood	

BODY APPEARANCE

Observation of the body's appearance should include an evaluation of general strength and body condition. Generally speaking, if the Zang-Fu organs are normal, the body appears strong and heavy. However, in a pathological condition, strength and heaviness of an animal's body indicates an Excess Pattern or a Heat Pattern. Weakness and emaciation indicate a Deficiency Pattern or a Cold Pattern.

SKIN AND HAIR

Normally, an animal's skin is soft and elastic and the hair is groomed and lustrous. Depending upon the environment and weather conditions, animals usually change their hair coat twice a year.

Because the skin is physiologically and pathologically related to the Lung in TCVM, abnormal Lung function may cause many skin problems. For instance, skin contraction and piloerection indicate a Wind-Cold Pattern (Common Cold due to Wind Cold) due to the restraint of Wind-Cold in the Lung. Wind-Heat in the Lung causes itchy skin or urticaria.

The health of the hair and skin also depends upon Qi and Blood. Alopecia, coarse hair coats without luster, and dry, inelastic skin result from a Deficiency of Qi and Blood. If the skin is swollen, hot and painful, the edema is due to Heat-Toxin. Kidney-Spleen Yang Deficiency causes edema that appears as swollen skin which retains the marks from finger pressure.

MOVEMENT AND POSTURE

The movement and posture of animals varies between the different species.

Horse

Under normal conditions, a horse likes to stand for long periods of time while alternately resting each of the limbs. Typically, the horse will hold its head in an elevated position. Sometimes, he may lie down on the ground but will stand up whenever someone approaches. Deviations from these normal movements and postures may indicate various disease conditions.

If a horse suffers from abdominal pain, he may show such behaviors as alternating between standing up and lying down, rolling, pawing, kicking at or turning to look at his abdomen, grinding his teeth, or grimacing. Enterospasm and constipation may both cause abdominal pain. Enterospasm may be accompanied by diarrhea with loud sounds of intestinal peristalsis (borborygmi). A decrease in intestinal peristalsis and difficult defecation may accompany constipation.

If the signs of abdominal pain suddenly disappear and the horse demonstrates shortness of breath, excretion of gastric contents from nose, muscle quivering of the whole body, and profuse sweating, there may be a rupture of the stomach or diaphragm.

Observation of a head nod while the horse moves may provide insight into a horse's lameness. A nod of the head in a high position indicates pain in the scapular region. A head nod in the middle position indicates pain in the carpal region. A nod of the head in the low position indicates pain in the foot. Difficulty moving the front leg may indicate pain in the acupuncture point Qing-Feng.

At the walk and trot, the horse may be observed on long straight paths and on turns. The steps of opposite legs should be equidistant and smooth. The head may go down when a lame hind foot hits the ground, and the head may go up when a lame forefoot hits the ground. In addition, the level of the rump as seen from behind may reveal a hip drop of a lame leg.

Signs such as stiffness of the ears and neck, elevation of the third eyelids, and closed mouth may indicate tetanus. Stiffness of the neck and lumbar area as well as difficulty making a turn indicates arthritic pain.

Cattle

Normally, cattle rest in sternal recumbency but lean to one side or the other. Beads of sweat are evenly distributed on the planum nasale. The cattle will keep their nose clean by frequently licking their nostrils. Their ears move forwards and backwards in response to environmental stimuli. When someone approaches, they will usually stand up. Cattle rise by first elevating the hind end then standing in the front. Similarly, cattle lie down by first kneeling in the front and then sitting in the back. One may observe cattle at rest to bring up a bolus of feed, to chew it for a while then swallow it again. They ruminate regularly in this manner.

Signs such as frequent switching between standing and lying down, pawing or stomping, kicking the abdomen with a hind limb and turning the head towards the abdomen probably indicate abdominal pain. When suffering from pain in the urinary bladder, cattle may stand with a wider stance of the hind limbs, maintain a low lumbar position, and stamp on the ground. Standing with wider distance between the two front limbs (elbows may appear turned outward), frequently shifting foot position, and moving obliquely down a hill may indicate traumatic reticulopericarditis.

Dogs

Normally, dogs may rest by sitting, lying on their side, or lying in sternal recumbency. A resting dog will usually raise their head and rise to greet a person who enters the room. Unfamiliar people approaching the house often stimulate the dog to bark. A dog is usually awake during the day and sleeps at night with possible naps throughout the day. A healthy, athletic dog is usually willing and eager to run, jump, and play with other dogs or humans throughout the day. The gait should be smooth and even. Typically, the dog's eyes, nose and ears will follow sights, smells and sounds of interest.

Difficulty rising, lameness and a stiff gait may indicate arthritic conditions. Exercise intolerance and fainting during activity may indicate heart disease. Straining to urinate and frequent posturing to urinate may indicate disease of the urinary system. Sudden inability to walk in the hind legs may be due to intervertebral disc disease.

Cats

Cats may have active and rest periods throughout the day and night. When satisfied, they may purr, but when upset they may hiss and swipe with clawed paws. Often they will sit or lie in sternal recumbency while leaning to one side. A cat will often rub his face and body against the humans and objects that he encounters in his house. Quick movements will often catch their attention. Cats are agile and graceful, easily leaping to countertops and elevated surfaces. Cats will stalk, run and pounce on moving objects (toys) and will use their forepaws to bat them around. Outdoor cats may climb trees and catch small prey items. A cat will spend much time grooming himself with his rough tongue. Cats typically will bury their feces and urine.

Frequent posturing to urinate without urine production may indicate blockage of the urethra. Inappropriate urination outside of the litter box may indicate behavior problems or urinary tract disorders. Lethargy and an ungroomed appearance may indicate a systemic internal medicine problem

DRINKING AND EATING

Observations of changes in appetite and thirst and of the behaviors associated with drinking water and eating food are important for forming a TCVM diagnosis.

An increase in appetite may indicate a Stomach Excess Heat pattern. When the Stomach is hot, the animal tries to take in whatever it can in an attempt to cool down the Stomach. On the other hand, a loss of appetite may point to a Spleen Qi Deficiency, Stomach Food Stasis, Heat (febrile disease), or diseases of the oral cavity.

If horses or cattle prefer to eat fresh juicy grass instead of grain, they may suffer from Stomach Heat or Stomach Yin Deficiency. Similarly, a dog's desire to drink water or to eat watery food may be due to accumulation of Heat in the Stomach (Stomach Heat). However, a great desire to eat hay and grain along with decreased thirst or water intake points to a Spleen Cold-Damp Pattern or a Stomach Cold Pattern. Generally, a lack of thirst indicates a Cold-Damp Pattern, and a significant increase in water intake indicates a Yin Deficiency or Heat Pattern.

Table 7.3: Abnormalities associated with appetite and thirst

Clinical Sign	Diagnosis	Explanation
Ravenous Appetite	Stomach Heat Stomach Yin Deficiency	The Stomach is hot. The patient tries to consume anything that will cool down the stomach.
Loss of Appetite (Anorexia)	Spleen Qi Deficiency	The Spleen controls taste.
	Stomach Food Stasis or Stomach Qi Stagnation	The Stomach receives food.
	Heat	Global Heat (Fire) disrupts the Shen (Heart) consequently affecting typical behaviors such as eating and drinking.
	Diseases of the oral cavity	Local lesions generate Stagnation and block the Qi flow of the sense of taste.
Eating only fresh grass or raw, wet foods	Stomach Heat Stomach Yin Deficiency	Fluids (Yin) can help cool down the hot stomach.
Preference for hay, grain or dry food	Spleen Cold-Damp Pattern Stomach Cold	Dry food can help eliminate Excess Cold or Damp.
Lack of thirst	Cold-Damp Pattern	Decreased water intake helps to avoid extra Cold or Damp.
Polydipsia	Yin Deficiency	Extra water intake helps balance the Deficiency of Body Fluid (Yin).

FECES AND URINATION

Feces

The observation of the feces should include notation of quantity, color, smell, shape and texture. As an end product of digestion, feces may be another clue about the function of the digestive system and the body in general.

Normally, equine feces are shaped like kidney-shaped balls. The surface of the fecal-ball is moist and glitters. A horse produces a group of fecal balls that fall in a loose mound. Sometimes a fecal ball may break open when it falls to the ground revealing the fibrous appearance due to the undigested plant materials. The colors range around variations of green and yellow-green.

Cattle produce soft feces. It falls to the ground to form a mound with ripples or plies. The plant fibers may be visible in close examination of the pile. The coarseness of these fibers and the solidity of the pile may give some indication about the digestive function of the animal.

Dogs usually produce small piles of typically long, smooth and cylindrical fecal material. The color of the feces depends upon the diet of the dog; however, it typically appears as a shade of light to dark brown. The fecal quantity and diameter varies with body size of the dog.

Cats produce feces similar in appearance to dogs, formed brown cylinders. Typically though, a cat will bury the fecal material. The feces may contain hair due to hair ingestion while grooming.

An Excess Heat Pattern or Body Fluid Deficiency results in dry feces, while watery feces often results from a Deficient Cold Pattern. Coarse feces with undigested food and a sour smell or soft, watery feces may indicate a Spleen Qi Deficiency and indigestion. Soft, watery, or pasty feces with mucus or blood indicate an accumulation of Damp-Heat in the intestinal tract such as in enteritis or dysentery.

Table 7.4: Abnormalities associated with feces

Clinical Sign	Diagnosis	Explanation
Dry feces Constipation	Excess Heat Deficient Large Intestine Yin	Excess Heat consumes the Large Intestine's body fluids. Insufficiency of LI body fluid leads to dry feces or even constipation.
Watery or loose feces	Spleen Qi Deficiency Spleen Cold-Damp	Deficient Spleen Qi fails to transform and transport Gu Qi upward resulting in diarrhea.
Bloody diarrhea possibly with mucus	Damp-Heat	Heat damages blood vessels and leads to bleeding. The Damp combines with the Heat and leads to shedding of the mucosa.

Urine

Observation of the urine should include notations of quantity, frequency, color, clarity, and odor. As an end product of water metabolism, urine may provide clues about the function of the body in general.

Normal equine urine is turbid and yellow with a bad smell. Bovine urine is clear, colorless to slightly yellow, and almost without an odor. Canine urine should be clear and may be yellow to colorless. Feline urine, especially that of intact male cats, has a very distinctive, unpleasant odor and it should be clear yellow in color.

Red urine that is voided in a short stream indicates a Heat Pattern. Large amounts of clear, dilute urine reflect a Kidney Qi or Yang Deficiency (Cold Pattern). Urinary incontinence or leakage indicates a Kidney Qi Deficiency. Dribbling of urine or prolonged retention of urine in addition to the hunched back, rolled tail and abdominal pain indicates Damp-Heat accumulation in the Bladder and urinary stone formation. Bloody urine is due to trauma or to accumulation of Heat in the Bladder. Complete retention of urine indicates paralysis of the Bladder or Kidney Qi Deficiency.

Table 7.5: Abnormalities associated with urine

Clinical Sign	Diagnosis	Explanation
Red and short urination	Heat	Heat consumes body fluids and leads to short urination. Heat damages blood vessels and leads to red urine.
Urinary incontinence	Kidney Qi Deficiency	Deficient Kidney Qi fails to hold the bladder (front door) and this permits leakage.
Clear and long urination	Kidney Qi Deficiency Kidney Yang Deficiency Cold Pattern	Kidney Qi/Yang fails to separate the fluid (reabsorption) so this leads to long urination because more fluid goes to the bladder. The Cold freezes the Kidney Qi/Yang and tends to bring water leading to clear urine.
Bloody urine	Bladder Damp-Heat	Heat damages blood vessels and leads to bleeding, while Damp combines with Heat and leads to shedding of the mucosa.
Painful urination with dribbling	Bladder Damp-Heat Kidney/Bladder Stone	Damp-Heat or stones block Qi-flow and leads to dribbling and painful urination.
Urine Retention	Bladder paralysis	Qi is blocked and there is no connection between the bladder and Shen.

EYES

The eyes are part of a local region that is examined as part of the inspection process. Normally, the eyes are clear and glistening and the conjunctiva is pink, clear, and moist without discharge. The eye provides a window to view the function of the internal organs. The eyes as a whole are generally associated with the Liver. The pupil is associated with the Kidney Jing. The blood vessels inside the eyes are associated with Heart. The Spleen is associated with upper and lower eyelids.

One may perform the ocular examination in horses by holding the halter with one hand and using the other hand to manipulate the eyelids. The index and middle fingers push the upper eyelid upwards and the thumb pulls the lower lid downward. This provides a view of the horse's eye and ocular mucosa (Figure 7.5).

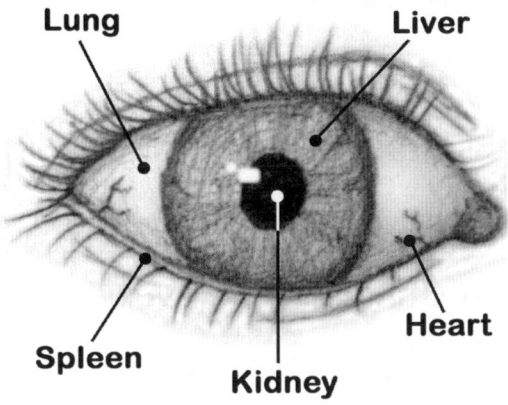

Figure 7.4: The general organ relationship to parts of the eye

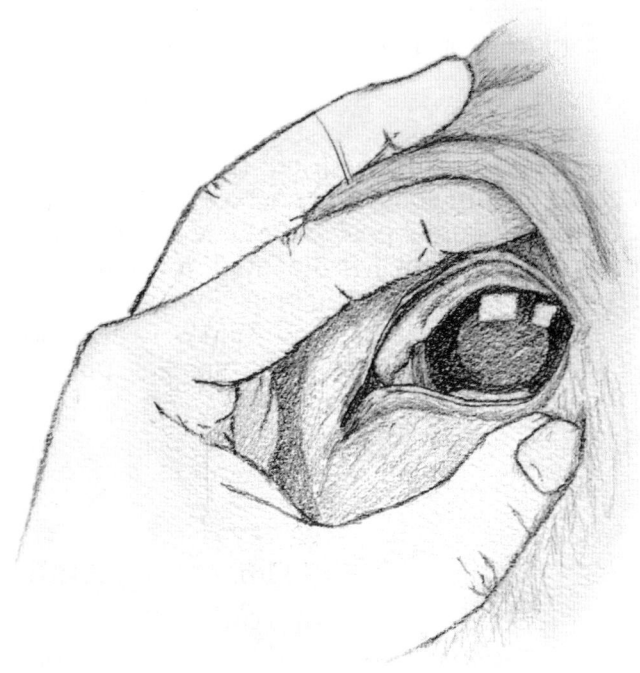

Figure 7.5: The equine ocular exam

Dull or cloudy eyes without luster indicate a Deficiency Pattern, especially a Zheng Qi Deficiency Pattern or Shen Loss. A deep red color of the blood vessels inside the eyes indicates a Heart Heat Pattern, but a pale corner or conjunctiva results with a Blood Deficiency Pattern. Red and swollen conjunctiva with watery or purulent ocular discharge occurs with a Liver Heat Pattern or with Liver Yang Rising. Elevated third eyelids may indicate tetanus. Drooping eyelids may be due to a Spleen Qi Deficiency. Chronic cataracts may indicate Kidney Jing Deficiency.

Table 7.6: Abnormalities associated with eyes

Clinical Signs	Diagnosis	Explanation
Dull or cloudy eyes	Shen Loss	The eye is the window of the Shen
Deep red blood vessels	Heart Heat	The Heart dominates the blood vessels.
Pale corner of eye or pale conjunctiva	Blood Deficiency	Deficient Blood fails to nourish the eyes.
Red and swollen conjunctiva	Liver Heat Liver Yang Rising	Liver Yang Rising becomes Liver Heat. Liver Heat rises and inflames the eyes.
Drooping eyelids	Spleen Qi Deficiency	Deficient Spleen Qi fails to hold the eyelid (muscle).
Cataracts	Kidney Jing Deficiency	Kidney Jing nourishes the pupil.

One may also examine the eyes using the Eight Diagrams. With this concept, the eyes are divided into eight portions or regions, and each one of the Eight Diagrams belongs to one of these regions. The most dorsal position relates to the Heart (fire) with the Spleen (earth) and Gall Bladder (wind) respectively located to the medial and lateral to it. The Liver (thunder) is located at the lateral canthus, and the Small and Large Intestines (pond) are located at the Medial canthus. The Kidney (water) lies in the most ventral aspect. The Lung (heaven) lies on the ventromedial portion, and the Stomach (mountain) relates to the ventrolateral portion.

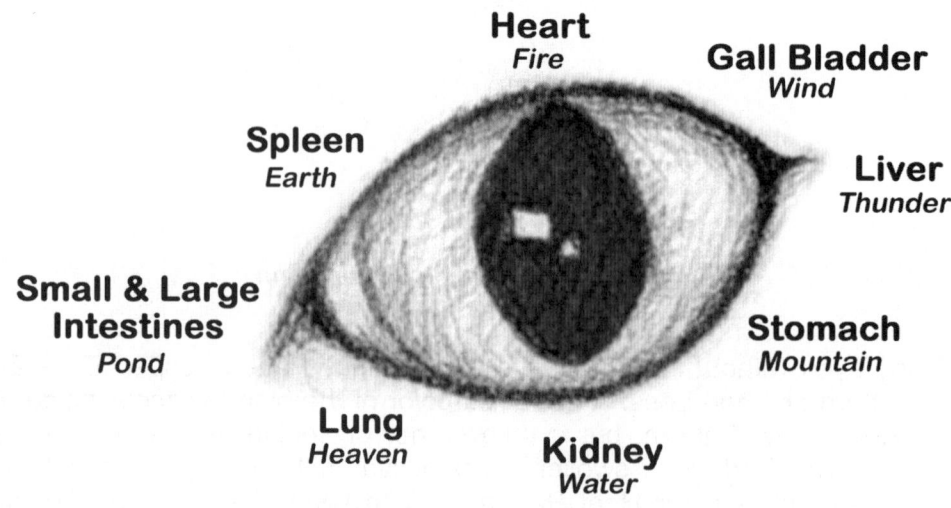

Figure 7.6: The eight regions of the eye (left eye)

EARS

If an animal is healthy, its ears appear erect and reactive to environmental stimuli. Drooping ears may indicate Qi Deficiency and fatigue. If the animal frightens easily and has hot ears (three or four of the examiner's fingers feel warm) there is accumulation of Heat in the Heart. If the blood vessels on the dorsal surface of the ears are distended and easily visible, the animal demonstrates an Exterior Heat Pattern. When the ears are cold (three or four fingers feel cool) and the blood vessels disappear, the animal suffers from an Exterior Cold condition. Malodorous, wet discharge from ears indicates a Gall Bladder Damp Heat Pattern.

Table 7.7: Abnormalities associated with ears

Clinical Signs	Diagnosis	Explanation
Hot ears	Heat Patterns	Heat flares up in the ears.
Hot ears and frightens easily	Heart Heat	Heart Heat disturbs the Shen, causing the patient to become easily frightened.
Distended blood vessels	Exterior Heat	Exterior Heat speeds up blood circulation in the ears.
Cold ears	Cold Patterns or Yang Deficiency	Cold freezes the circulation of Qi and Blood leading to cold ears. Yang Deficiency can generate Interior Cold.
Malodorous and wet discharge	Gallbladder Damp-Heat	Damp-Heat can follow the pathway of the GB Channels, spread around the ears and then into the ears.

NOSE

Normally, the nostrils will slightly expand and contract in rhythm with the breathing. In addition, the nostrils should be clean and moist.

Frequent sneezing with a clear, watery nasal discharge is due to a Wind-Cold Pattern. Widely flared nostrils with rapid breathing and a thick, yellow nasal discharge indicates a Lung Heat Pattern. Turbid discharge from both nostrils along with swelling of the maxillary lymph nodes points to adenitis. Turbid discharge from a single nostril indicates sinusitis.

Depigmentation of the planum nasale indicates a Lung Qi Deficiency because the Lung fails to distribute the Qi and blood to the nose. Crusting of the planum nasale indicates Lung Heat because the Lung Heat consumes the fluids and damages the skin.

Table 7.8: Abnormalities associated with the nose

Clinical Signs	Diagnosis	Explanation
Sneezing, watery nasal discharge	Wind-Cold Pattern	The Wei Qi tries to dispel the pathogen Wind-Cold which leads to sneezing. Cold tends to bring water which results in watery discharge.
Thick, yellow nasal discharge	Lung Heat	Heat damages blood vessels and consumes fluids, leading to thick and yellow discharge.
Turbid, mucoid nasal discharge	Sang-Huang (Sinusitis)	Heat flames local tissues, leading to mucoid and turbid discharge.
Depigmentation of planum nasale	Lung Qi Deficiency	The Lung fails to distribute the Qi and Blood to the nose.
Crusting of the planum nasale	Yin Deficiency or Lung Heat	A dry or crusty nose is the first sign of a Yin Deficiency. Lung Heat consumes the fluids and damages the skin.

LIPS

The lips of horses and cattle are usually quite nimble when eating food. If a horse raises the upper lip like a smile, it may indicate Stomach Qi Stagnation such as colic or enterospasm. If the lower lip droops and is unable to return its normal position, this is a Spleen Deficiency Pattern due to chronic indigestion or ageing.

Under normal conditions, the internal surface of lips is pale-red, moist and shiny. If the lips are very pale, they indicate Blood Deficiency Pattern. If they are too red and dry, they indicate Heat in the Spleen and Stomach, constipation, or Yin Deficiency.

Table 7.9: Abnormalities associated with the lips

Clinical Signs	Diagnosis	Explanation
Raising upper lip like a smile	Stomach Qi Stagnation; Colic	The lips are the orifice of the Spleen and Stomach. The animal tries to raise the upper lip to relieve Stomach Qi Stagnation or colic.
Drooping lower lip	Spleen Qi Deficiency or ageing	Deficient Spleen Qi fails to hold the low lip (muscle).
Pale lips	Qi Deficiency or Blood Deficiency	Deficient Qi or Blood fails to nourish lips.
Red and dry lips	Yin Deficiency or Heat Pattern	Yin Deficiency generates Interior Heat leading to red lips.

LIMBS

Observation of the limbs while standing and moving is an important part of diagnosing lameness. When standing, an animal will not support his body weight on the painful limb, so he may hold the leg in an unusual position. A horse may extend the leg forward, backward, inward or outward so that only the tip of the hoof contacts the ground. A dog may stand with the sore leg elevated off the ground.

It is also important to evaluate an animal in motion. Difficulty lifting and extending a limb when taking a step may indicate pain in the upper regions of the limb. A horse with pain in the lower regions of the limb (foot or pastern) will quickly raise the hoof whenever it strikes the ground.

Hearing and Smelling

Wen

The Chinese character wen means to hear and to smell. Hearing-Smelling is one of the four diagnostic methods.

Hearing

This diagnostic method describes the use of the auditory senses to identify the sounds of a patient's vocalizing, breathing, coughing, chewing and intestinal peristalsis.

VOICE

Generally speaking, healthy animals make various loud, clear vocalizations when they pursue a mate, call out to the group (e.g. herd, pack, flock) and cry out for their offspring. The voice is controlled by Zong-Qi. A strong, clear voice reflects normal Zong-Qi, Lung Qi, and Heart Qi.

Pathologic conditions may cause a change in the voice. A loud, coarse voice accompanies an Excess Pattern, but a weak, thin voice indicates a Deficiency Pattern. Moaning and groaning may indicate severe pain or a severe pathogenic condition.

Table 7.10: Abnormalities associated with the voice

Clinical Signs	Diagnosis	Explanation
Loud and coarse voice	Excess Pattern	A stronger and more excessive patient has a loud and coarse voice.
Weak and thin voice	Deficiency Pattern	A weaker and more deficient patient has a weak and thin voice.

BREATHING

An animal normally breathes evenly with no easily audible respiratory noises. If an animal meets a stranger or becomes frightened, the animal may make very loud and clear vocalization. The breathing becomes hoarse and loud with physical exertion.

A pathologically forceful and coarse respiratory noise indicates an Excess Pattern. Low, weak breathing sounds reflect a Deficiency Pattern. Asthma is characterized by superficial and rapid breathing. Forceful and long asthmatic breathing sounds indicate Excess Asthma, while feeble and short asthmatic breathing sounds indicate Deficiency Asthma.

Table 7.11: Abnormalities associated with breathing

Clinical Signs	Diagnosis	Explanation
Forceful and coarse respiratory noise	Excess Pattern	A stronger and more excessive patient has forceful and coarse breathing.
Low and weak breathing sound	Deficiency Pattern	A weaker and more deficient patient has weak and low breathing.
Forceful and long asthmatic breathing	Excess Asthma	A stronger and more excessive patient has forceful and long dyspnea.
Feeble and short asthmatic breathing	Deficiency Asthma	A weaker and more deficient patient has weak and feeble dyspnea.

COUGH

Generally, a healthy animal does not cough. Cough is an important result of Lung ascending-descending dysfunction, which then leads to upward perversion of Qi.

A forceful, loud cough indicates a Lung Excess Heat Pattern, but a feeble or weak cough indicates a Qi Deficiency Pattern. Cough with sputum is called a wet-cough, which reflects the Cold-Damp Pattern and Heat Pattern. Dry-cough, a cough without sputum, results from a Lung Yin Deficiency Pattern or Lung Heat. An acute cough in the daytime, Yang-cough, indicates a Lung Excess Heat Pattern and is easily cured. However, a cough at night (Yin-cough) is due to a Deficiency Cold Pattern of the Lung and is hard to treat. Deficient Lung Qi or Yin may cause a prolonged cough. A feeble cough or asthma that is much worse at night as compared to the daytime may result from a Deficiency of the Kidney and Lung due to overwork.

Table 7.12: Abnormalities associated with cough

Clinical Signs	Diagnosis	Explanation
Forceful, loud cough	Lung Excess Heat	A stronger and more excessive patient has forceful and coarse cough.
Feeble or weak cough	Qi Deficiency Pattern	A weaker and more deficient patient has weak and low cough.
Cough with sputum	Damp-Cold Pattern	Wei Qi tries to dispel the pathogens, leading to cough. Cold tends to bring water and Damp, leading to wet cough.
Cough without sputum	Yin Deficiency or Lung Heat	Yin Deficiency or Heat consumes fluids and leads to a dry cough.
An acute cough during the daytime	Lung Excess Heat	Excess and Heat both belong to Yang, thus the cough occurs during the Yang time (daytime).
Chronic cough only during the day	Lung Qi Deficiency	Both daytime and Lung Qi belong to Yang, so a Lung Qi Deficiency leads to a chronic cough during the daytime.
Chronic cough only during the night	Lung Yin Deficiency	Lung Yin and Night are both Yin, thus Lung Yin Deficiency leads to chronic cough at night.
Cough or asthma that is worse at night than during the day	Lung and Kidney Yang Qi Deficiency	Kidney Qi helps to pull Qi down from the Upper *Jiao* to the Lower *Jiao*. Night tends to be Cold, which can damage Yang. Thus, cough due to Lung and Kidney Yang Qi Deficiency is worse at night than during the daytime.

CHEWING

Under normal conditions, animals chew their food with a regular, clear and melodious sound. Careful and quiet chewing may indicate a toothache or loose tooth. Chewing without food is a common sign of pain in horses and cattle with acute enteritis, gastric distention, Lung pain, or Heart pain.

Table 7.13: Abnormalities associated with chewing

Clinical Signs	Diagnosis	Explanation
Careful and quiet chewing	Stomach Heat	Stomach Heat flames up to the gums, leading to toothaches, stomatitis and gingivitis.
Chewing without food	Stomach Qi Stagnation	The animal tries to relieve abdominal discomfort by continuing to chew even without food.

INTESTINAL SOUNDS

The intestinal sounds include the bubbling and gurgling noises that result from the propulsion of intestinal contents. Typically, the small intestinal sounds are like the flow of water and those of the large intestine are like distant thunder.

An increase in the volume of the intestinal sound indicates enterospasm and diarrhea due to Cold. A lack of or a decreased volume of the intestinal sound indicates Qi Stagnation of the gastrointestinal tract and constipation.

Table 7.14: Abnormalities associated with intestinal sounds

Clinical Signs	Diagnosis	Explanation
Increased gut sounds	Cold	The body tries to dispel Cold, leading to an increase in gut sounds.
Decreased gut sounds	Spleen Qi Deficiency or Qi Stagnation	Qi Stagnation causes impaction and food stasis, leading to a decrease in gut sounds. Spleen Qi Deficiency fails to move the digestive system.

Smelling

This diagnostic method differentiates the changes in odor of the mouth, nose and various secretions or excretions such as pus, feces and urine.

ODOR OF THE MOUTH

A healthy animal's mouth smells only like food, and it should not be malodorous. A sour-smelling mouth along with a yellow, greasy coating reflects a disturbance of the Stomach (Food Stasis) due to overfeeding or overeating. Accumulation of Heat in the Stomach results in a foul mouth odor. A bad smell similar to that of rotten fish indicates either a rotten oral ulcer due to Heart Fire or stomatitis due to Stomach Fire.

Table 7.15: Abnormalities associated with the oral cavity

Clinical Signs	Diagnosis	Explanation
Sour-smelling with a greasy, yellow coating	Food stasis	Food Stasis ferments and upsets the Stomach.
Foul mouth odor	Stomach Heat	Heat accumulates and steams the Stomach.
Bad smell like rotten fish	Heart Fire Stomach Fire	Heart or Stomach Fire flames up to the gums or tongue which leads to stomatitis or ulcers in the oral cavity.

ODOR OF THE NOSE

Grey-yellow, thick, malodorous nasal discharge indicates suppurative bronchitis (Lung Excess Heat). A thick yellow or yellow-white nasal discharge that smells like a dead body indicates suppurative pneumonia or pneumonia due to a foreign body (Lung Heat with Phlegm). Sticky, grey or yellow-white, malodorous nasal discharge from only one nostril indicates accumulation of pus in the paranasal sinuses.

Table 7.16: Abnormalities associated with nasal discharge odor

Clinical Signs	Diagnosis	Explanation
Grey-yellow, thick and malodorous discharge	Lung Excess Heat	Heat "cooks" fluids and flames up to the nose.
Thick yellow discharge with dead-body smell	Lung Heat with Phlegm	Heat "cooks" fluids to transform into phlegm, and it "cooks"/damages tissues to become "pus".
Sticky, grey and malodorous discharge from only one nostril	*Sang Huang* (pus in paranasal sinuses)	Heat "cooks" and damages local tissues and fluids to become pus.

PUS

Yellow, thick, turbid pus with a fetid smell indicates a Yang Pattern due to the accumulation of extreme Heat or Fire in the Interior. Grey-white, watery pus with a bad smell indicates a Yin Pattern due to the retention of the Xie Qi (Heat Toxin) and a Deficiency of Qi and Blood.

Table 7.17: Abnormalities associated with the odor of pus

Clinical Signs	Diagnosis	Explanation
Yellow, thick, turbid pus with fetid smell	Excess Heat/Fire Pattern or Yang Pattern	Heat or Fire "cooks" and damages local fluids and tissues to transform them into pus.
Grey-white, watery pus without foul odor	Combination of Qi-blood Deficiency and Heat Toxin	Deficiency of Qi and Blood results in no stench.

FECES

Normally, the fecal matter of animals has a certain unpleasant odor. Watery feces with no special smell is diarrhea due to a Spleen Qi Deficiency. Soft feces with a sour odor indicates overfeeding (Food Stasis). Foul smelling stools containing blood and mucous indicate a Damp-Heat Pattern or enteritis.

Table 7.18: Abnormalities associated with feces

Clinical Signs	Diagnosis	Explanation
Watery stool without odor	Spleen Qi Deficiency	Deficiency of Spleen Qi fails to ascend Gu Qi without a stench.
Sour and soft stool	Food stasis	Food stasis leads to loose stool with a sour smell from fermentation.
Foul smelling, bloody and mucoid stool	Damp-Heat	Heat damages blood vessels and leads to bleeding. Damp combines with the Heat and promotes mucosal shedding. Damp-Heat results in foul smelling feces.

URINE

Equine urine normally has a smell that irritates the nose. Small amounts of smelly, thick urine with blood indicate an Excess Heat Pattern. Large amounts of clear urine with no special smell indicate a Deficiency Cold Pattern.

Table 7.19: Abnormalities associated with urine

Clinical Signs	Diagnosis	Explanation
Small amount of smelly urine with blood	Excess Heat Pattern	Excess Heat makes urine smelly. Heat damages blood vessels and leads to bleeding.
Large amount of clear urine with no smell	Deficient Cold; Kidney Yang Deficiency	Deficiency results in odorless urine. A large amount of clear urine is due to a lack of Fire from Kidney Yang.

Inquiring

Wen

Inquiry or taking down the history is a very important part of the Traditional Chinese Veterinary diagnosis. The practitioner must question the animal's owner or breeder about the disease condition in order to understand the pathological processes. This may cover a wide range of topics which may include discussions of prior medical conditions or treatment, management, current health status, diet, and breeding history.

CURRENT CONDITION AND PREVIOUS TREATMENTS

It is important to inquire about the current disease occurrence. Ask about when the disease began and how it has changed over time. By understanding the time frame and transformation of the disease condition, one can stage the condition as initial, middle, or late in the disease process. Most cases in an early stage of a disease belong to an Exterior Pattern or an Excess Pattern. On the other hand, most of the cases in the late stage have an Interior Deficiency Pattern. If a disease occurs suddenly and involves the death of multiple animals, the condition may be due to infectious diseases or poisoning.

Information regarding the patient's appetite, feces, urine, abdominal pain, cough and behavior may also be obtained through questioning of the owner. This can help to define the current medical problem and to guide treatment.

If the patient has received treatment previously, knowledge of the previous diagnosis, treatment methods, and patient response to treatment can also help to determine the diagnosis and therapy of the current illness. In some cases, improper or prolonged previous treatment may have contributed to the current medical condition. Prolonged antibiotics or Cold herbal medications, which have a cooling effect, may cause a Yang or Qi Deficiency. Alternatively, steroids have a warming effect which can eventually impair the Yin. Similarly, extended use of Yang tonics can also cause a Yin Deficiency.

Vaccine history is also important. Vaccines help to prevent the occurrence of certain infectious diseases; however, immunization is a tool that must be used wisely and carefully. Over-vaccination can overwhelm the Wei Qi and eventually lead to Wei Qi Deficiency.

- Short course of a disease → Excess Pattern
- Long course of a Cold herbal medication → Yang or Qi Deficiency
- Long course of a Yang tonic → Yin Deficiency
- Long course of a Blood tonic → Stagnation
- Chronic steroids → Warming effect → Yin Deficiency
- Antibiotics → Cold effect → Yang or Qi Deficiency
- Over-vaccination → Wei Qi is overwhelmed → Wei Qi Deficiency
- Young animals → Tend towards Excess or Heat conditions
- Senior patients → Tends towards Deficiency or Cold conditions

DIETARY PROGRAMS

A TCVM practitioner should ask about the type, origin, quality and quantity of food that is fed daily. Learning about the owner's method of feeding may also be important. Gastrointestinal diseases such as abdominal pain, abdominal fullness and diarrhea may directly relate to the feeding program. Sudden changes in food, feeding too much, feeding too little, or providing contaminated (filth, mildew) food could cause gastrointestinal upset in most animals. Feeding horses with only dry grass for a long period of time may lead to disease. Animals require healthy, balanced diets that provide all their necessary nutrients.

MANAGEMENT

A TCVM practitioner should also ask about the conditions in which an animal is housed and how the animal is cared for on a day to day basis. This should include questions regarding the heating, ventilation, illumination, hygiene of the housing area and feed containers, grooming, exercise, and basic health care maintenance. The methods of preventing heatstroke are also important in hot climates.

For example, the common cold, rheumatic pain and Lung problems may develop if an animal resides for long periods in a cold environment such as a cold, damp stable or if exposed to sudden changes of weather.

ORIGIN OF THE PATIENT

An animal imported from a distant place may be susceptible to the environmental conditions and infectious diseases of the new location. In general, an animal that is relocated to a cold region from a warm district will catch Wind-Cold and will exhibit signs such as cough, asthma, and nasal discharge. If an animal moves to a warm district from a cold place, he may be susceptible to heatstroke or a Lung Heat Pattern.

MEDICAL HISTORY

The medical history may help practitioners understand the patient's illness. If a patient had suffered trauma, tetanus should be considered. Long term lameness and vomiting of food may indicate osteomalacia. Acute enteritis may transform into chronic enteritis. Long term steroid administration may cause Yin Deficiency, and prolonged antibiotic usage may lead to Qi or Yang Deficiency. Overvaccination may cause disorders of Qi or Blood as well.

BREEDING AND PREGNANCY

A Kidney Yang Deficiency Pattern may develop with too frequent breeding of a male animal. A pregnant animal may exhibit loss of appetite and swelling prior to parturition. During and after parturition, dystocia and retention of the placenta may occur. Before instituting a treatment regimen during pregnancy, it is important to be aware of what drugs and therapies are contraindicated.

Palpating

Qie

This is a method of diagnosis in which the veterinarian detects pathological conditions by using the sense of touch. Feeling and pressing various body parts of an animal may reveal some abnormalities or disease conditions. Palpation uses touch or physical manipulation to evaluate the pulse, the Meridians or acupoints and the state of the Body Fluids (Yin), the body temperature (Yang), and Qi Flow (local sensitivities).

FEELING THE PULSE (PULSE DIAGNOSIS)

Pulse diagnosis, *mai zhen*, is a diagnostic method in which the palpable changes of an arterial pulse reveal pathological conditions. Similar to tongue diagnosis, pulse diagnosis plays an important role in traditional Chinese veterinary diagnostics because it reflects the state of the Zang-Fu organs, Qi, and Blood.

Location and Method

The location of the pulse commonly used for pulse diagnosis varies between the species. Typically, the common carotid artery or the external maxillary artery is palpated in horses. The median caudal artery running in the midline of the ventral tail is the usual place to examine the pulse in cattle. The femoral artery is used in dogs, cats and pigs.

The common carotid artery is called *Shuang Fu Mai* in the equine TCVM classic text *Yuan Heng Liao Ma Ji* (*Yuan-Heng's Therapeutic Treatise of Horses, 1608*). *Mai* refers to artery and *Shuang Fu* is the location where one palpates the carotid artery. In this book, *Shuang Fu* is considered the sole location for pulse diagnosis in horses:

Shuang fu mai … is the gate of the sea of Qi, the pathway of the sea of Blood. As a human being enters and exits his house, Qi and Blood have to pass through their gate and pathway when they ascend and descend. Qi impels Blood into the head, and then Blood is distributed into the whole body and Five Zang and Six Fu organs. Deficiency, Excess, Cold and Heat are all manifested in *Shuan Fu*. Thus, *Shuan Fu* is the sole location for pulse diagnosis.

While performing a pulse diagnosis, it is important to maintain a quiet environment. If the patient has been working or exercising, let the animal rest until he is breathing evenly before feeling the pulse. During the procedure, the veterinarian should focus on the patient, keep breathing evenly, and feel the pulse carefully. Feeling the pulse should take no less than three minutes to complete.

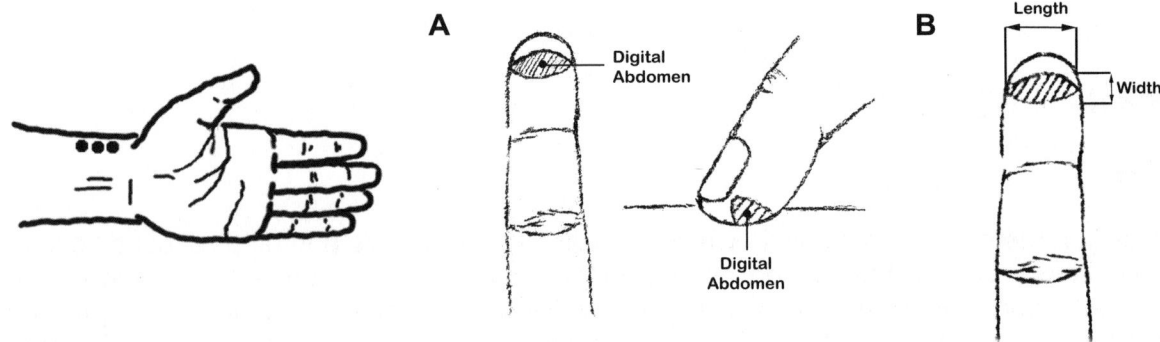

Figure 7.7: The human pulse   **Figure 7.8: The digital abdomen and finger measurements**

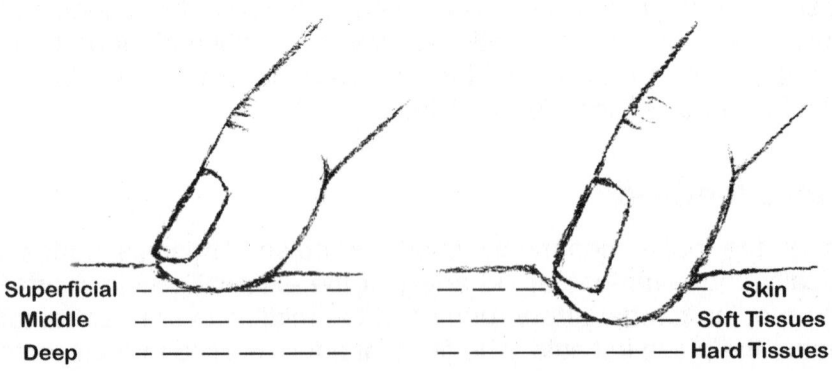

Figure 7.9: Finger forces during pulse palpation

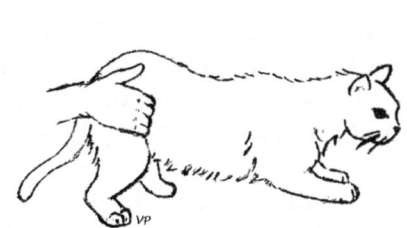

Figure 7.10: Pulse diagnosis in the cat

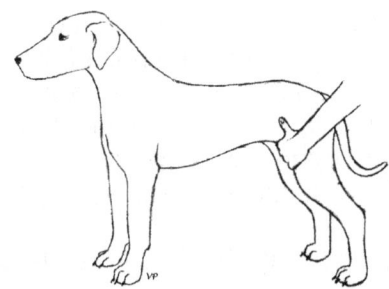

Figure 7.11: Pulse diagnosis in the dog

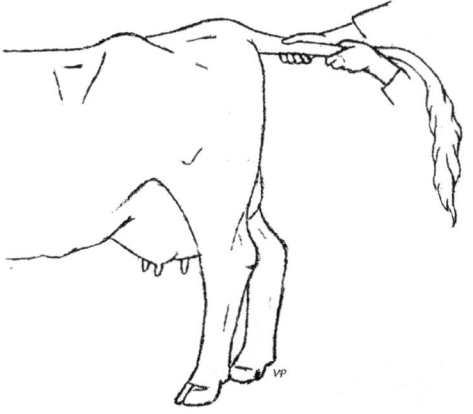

Figure 7.12: Pulse diagnosis in cattle

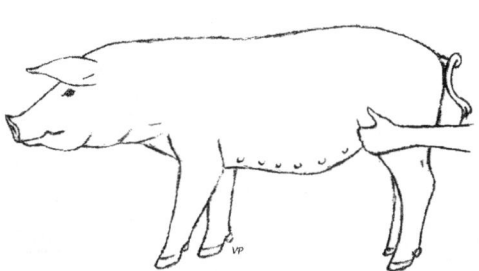

Figure 7.13: Pulse diagnosis in the pig

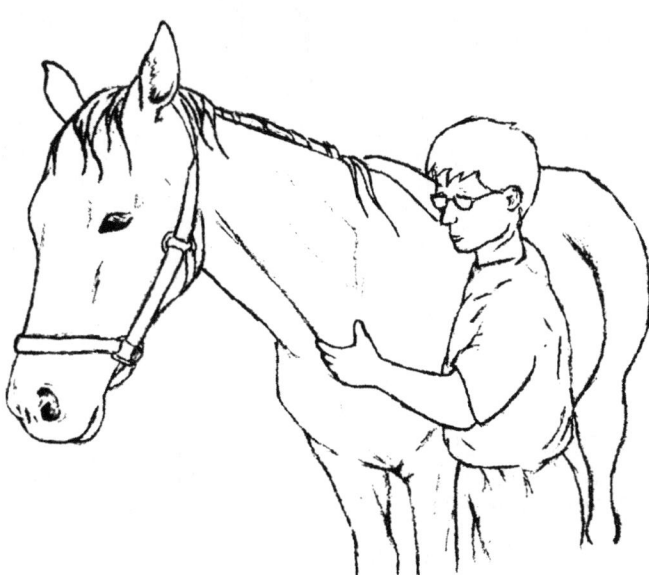

Figure 7.14: Pulse diagnosis in the horse

To feel the pulse of the common carotid artery in a horse, allow the horse to stand naturally with both front limbs at the same level. The veterinarian stands by the patient's cervical region and uses one hand to locate the three pulse levels (Figure 7.14). Use the index finger to locate the Upper or Feng location in the junction between the middle and lower 1/3 of the jugular groove. The middle finger is then used to feel the pulse of the Middle or Qi location. The ring finger locates the pulse of the Lower or Ming location.

The spacing that should be used between the fingers depends upon the length of the jugular groove. If the patient is tall and has a long jugular groove, one must separate the fingers accordingly. If the patient is short and has a short jugular groove, the three fingers are placed more closely to each other.

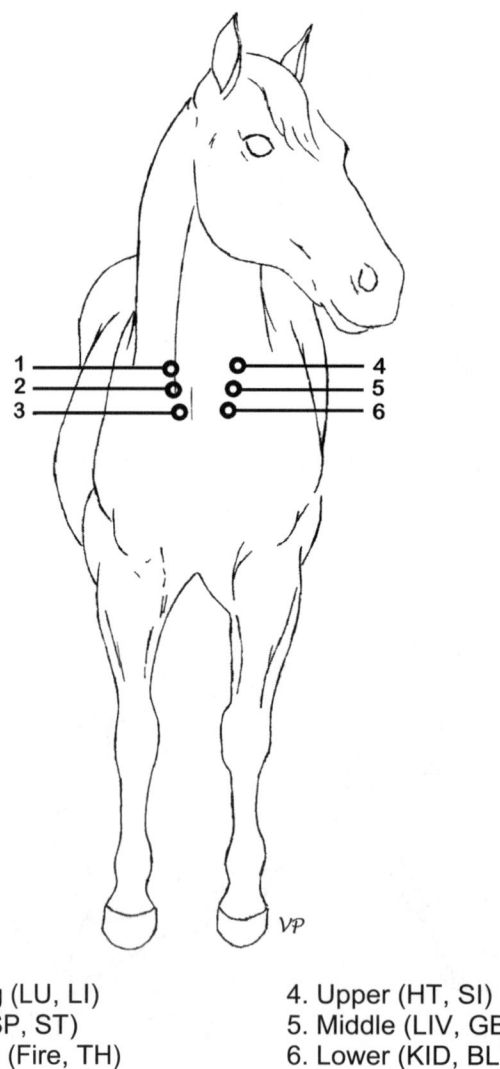

1. Feng (LU, LI)
2. Qi (SP, ST)
3. Ming (Fire, TH)

4. Upper (HT, SI)
5. Middle (LIV, GB)
6. Lower (KID, BL)

Figure 7.15: The three left and three right pulse locations

To feel the pulse in the tail of cattle, the veterinarian should raise the tail with one hand and use the other hand to feel the pulse (Figure 7.12). The index, middle, and ring fingers are pressed into the first three junctions of the ventral coccygeal vertebrae. Left and right do not matter for the pulse in cattle. This pulse is based upon the San-jiao. The first finger corresponds to the upper jiao (HT and LU). The middle finger relates to the middle jiao (SP and ST). The ring finger corresponds to the lower jiao (KID and LIV).

To feel the pulse in dogs, cats, and pigs, the animal should stand with the hind legs positioned at the same level (Figure 7.10, Figure 7.11, Figure 7.13). The veterinarian stands behind the animal and reaches around the cranial portion of the thigh to feel the pulses on the medial aspect of the legs. The index finger is placed on the upper position closest to the body wall. The middle and ring fingers rest more distally to locate the middle and lower pulses. Space the fingers proportionally to the size of the animal.

Except for the midline pulse in the tail (cattle), the pulses are bilateral. According to *Yuan Heng Liao Ma Ji* (*Yuan-Heng's Therapeutic Treatise of Horses*) published in 1608, the pulse on the right side is divided into San Guan (three positions): Feng, Qi, and Ming. The left side is divided into San Bu (three locations): Upper (Shang), Middle (Zhong) and Lower (Xia). Each of these locations respectively pertains to one of the Zang-Fu organs.

On the right side, the position *Feng* means Wind. This refers to the Lung because the Lung controls the body surface and is easily attacked by Wind. The position *Qi* indicates the Spleen since the Spleen is the Qi generator. *Ming* refers to *Ming Men*, indicating the Life Gate Fire or Kidney Yang. On the left side, the Upper location refers to the Heart and Small Intestines. The Middle location relates to the Liver and Gallbladder. The Lower location corresponds with the Kidney Yin.

Table 7.20: The relationship between the pulse positions and the Zang-Fu organs

	Left Side			Right Side		
	Upper Location	Middle Location	Lower* Location	Upper (Feng)	Middle (Qi)	Lower* (Ming)
Relevant Zang	Heart	Liver	Kidney Yin	Lung	Spleen	Kidney Yang
Relevant Fu	SI	GB	BL	LI	ST	TH

* Some sources list KID / BL in the low position of the left and PC / TH in that of the right.

Using these methods, the veterinarian may differentiate the pulses in terms of depth, speed, strength, shape and rhythm. The depth is determined by progressively pressing more firmly until the pulse becomes indistinct or obliterated. Normally the pulse is most forceful in the middle region. A pulse that is Full or too strong will be easily felt at all three depths. A pulse that is Weak may only be felt with superficial palpation because the pulse disappears with more forceful palpation. The width of the pulse is normally about two millimeters in humans and four to six millimeters in horses. A pulse that is too wide is a full pulse, and a pulse that is too narrow is a thin pulse. The normal length of the pulse in humans is three finger-widths. The pulse is too long if the pulse can be felt with a fourth finger, and it is too weak if it can be felt with less than three fingers. Naturally, though, the normal length in various species will of course vary with the size of the animal.

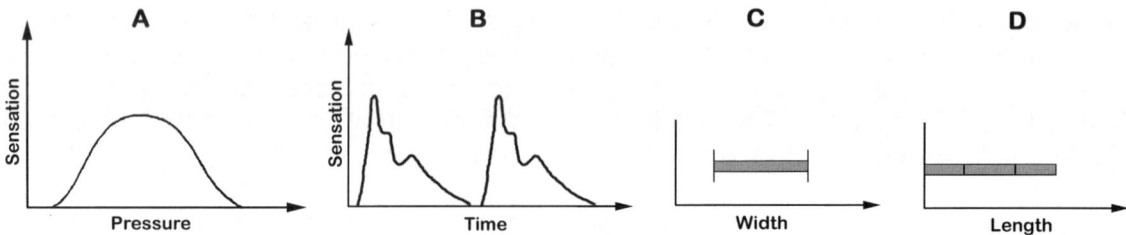

Figure 7.16: Diagrammatic view of the normal pulse qualities

In Figure 7.16, graph A illustrates how the normal pulse sensation initially grows stronger with increased pressure until it reaches a peak and then declines with additional pressure as the blood vessel is occluded. Graph B shows the pressure waves that pass by the fingers with time when feeling the arterial pulse. Graph C indicates the width of the pulse or perceived diameter of the artery (Figure 7.8 B). Graph D indicates the length of the pulse with each segment indicating one finger-length (Figure 7.8 B).

Normal Pulse

A normal pulse is even, forceful and persistent. It is neither superficial nor deep, neither fast nor slow. The normal pulse may, however, vary with climatic changes, sex, age and body physique.

Traditionally, the pulse rate is compared to the veterinarian's breathing. Within the span of a single breath of the veterinarian, horses have three heartbeats and cattle have four beats. In current times, though, the heart rate is typically counted using a watch. The normal heart rates are listed below.

Species	Heart Rate (beats/minute)
Dog	70-180
Cat	145-200
Horse	30-45
Cattle	40-60
Pig	60-90
Goat	70-90

The normal pulse may change during the four seasons. The pulse tends to be surging in summer, superficial in autumn, deep in winter, and string-taut in spring. A young animal's pulse tends to be rapid, but pulses of old and weak animals tend to be deficient. A corpulent animal tends to have a deep and forceful pulse, but an emaciated animal tends to have a superficial pulse. A pregnant animal often has a rolling or slippery pulse.

Abnormal Pulse

There are fifteen abnormal pulses commonly seen in animals.

Superficial or Floating Pulse (fu mai)

The superficial pulse can be easily felt with light finger pressure (Superficial Palpation), but it is easily obliterated by heavy pressure.

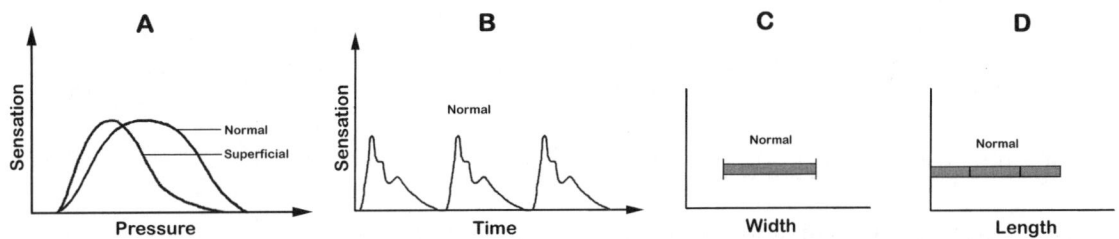

Clinically, this relates to an Exterior Pattern or the early stages of exogenous diseases due to Wind-Cold or Wind-Heat invasion.

- A superficial and forceful pulse indicates an Exterior Excess Pattern.
- A superficial and weak pulse indicates an Exterior Deficiency Pattern
- A superficial and rapid pulse indicates an Exterior Heat Pattern
- A superficial and slow pulse indicates an Exterior Cold Pattern
- A superficial, large and weak pulse indicates Outward Floating of Yang Qi

Deep or Sinking Pulse (chen mai)

This pulse cannot be felt with light pressure of the fingers. It can only be felt with heavy pressure (Deep Palpation).

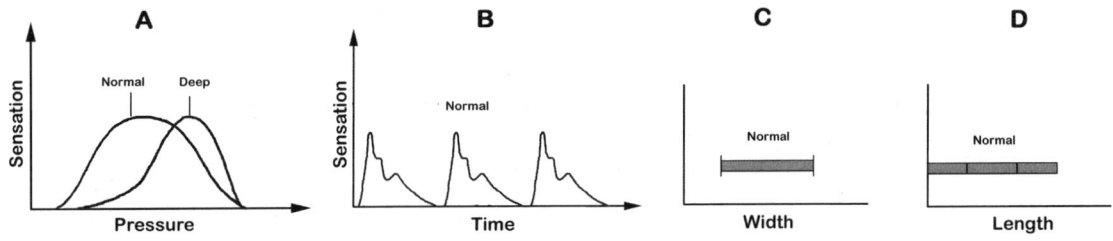

Clinically, this pulse relates to an Interior Pattern.

- A deep and forceful pulse indicates an Interior Excess Pattern.
- A deep and weak pulse indicates an Interior Deficiency Pattern.

Slow Pulse (chi mai)

The rate of this pulse is slower than normal. The TCVM practitioner will note less than three heartbeats of a horse or four beats in cattle for each breath of the veterinarian.

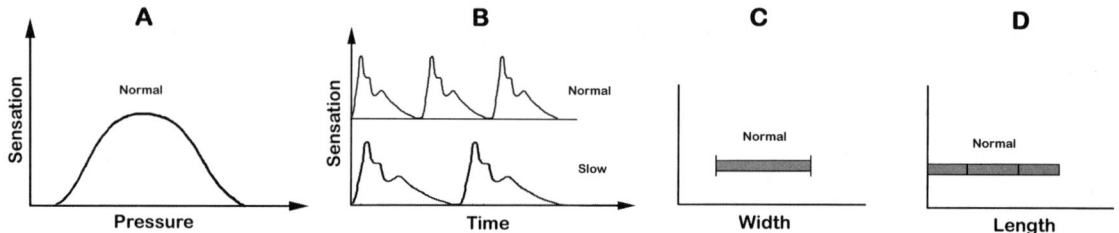

Clinically, this pulse indicates a Cold Pattern.

- A slow and forceful pulse indicates an Excess Cold Pattern.
- A slow and superficial pulse indicates an Exterior Cold Pattern.
- A slow and deep indicates an Interior Cold Pattern.

Rapid Pulse (shu mai)

The rate of this pulse is faster than normal. The TCVM practitioner will note more than four heartbeats of a horse or five beats in cattle for each breath of the veterinarian.

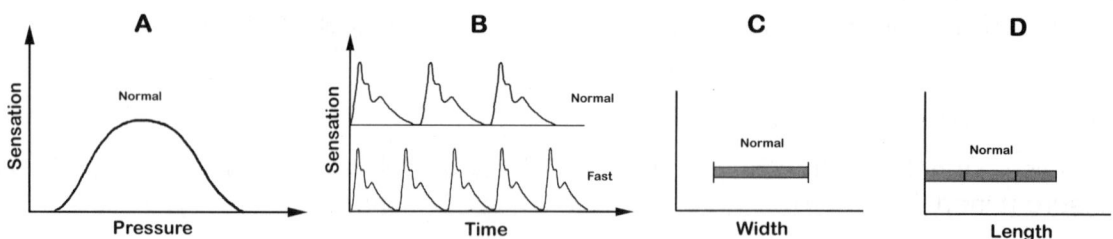

Clinically, this pulse indicates a Heat Pattern.

- A rapid and forceful pulse indicates an Excess Heat Pattern.
- A rapid and weak pulse indicates a Deficiency Heat Pattern.
- A rapid, weak and superficial pulse indicates an Outward Floating of Deficient Yang.

Deficient, Weak or Empty Pulse (xu mai)

The deficient pulse feels rather soft, weak and forceless at all three pressure levels (Superficial, Middle and Deep Palpation).

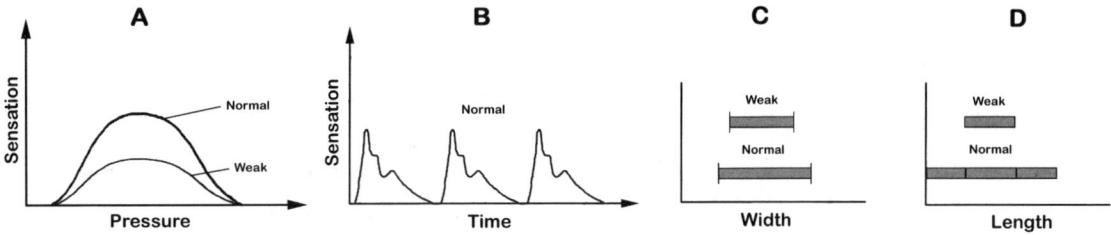

This pulse indicates a Deficiency Pattern of Qi or a Deficiency of both Qi and Blood.

Excessive, Full or Forceful Pulse (Shi mai)

This pulse feels very forceful at all three pressure levels (Superficial, Middle and Deep).

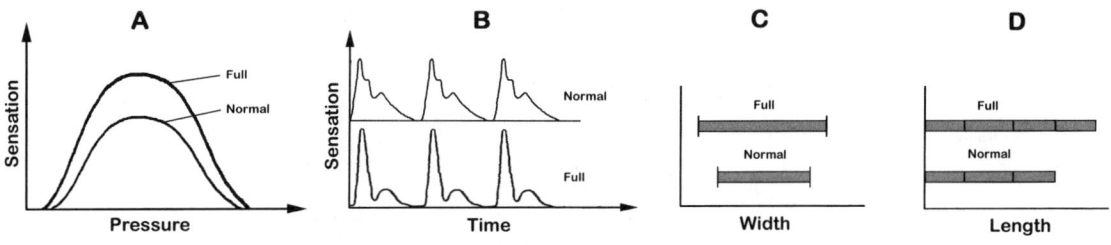

Clinically, this pulse indicates an Excess Pattern. This includes Stagnant Blood, constipation, and high fever.

Slippery or Rolling Pulse (hua mai)

The slippery pulse feels smooth, rounded, and slippery like pearls rolling on a dish.

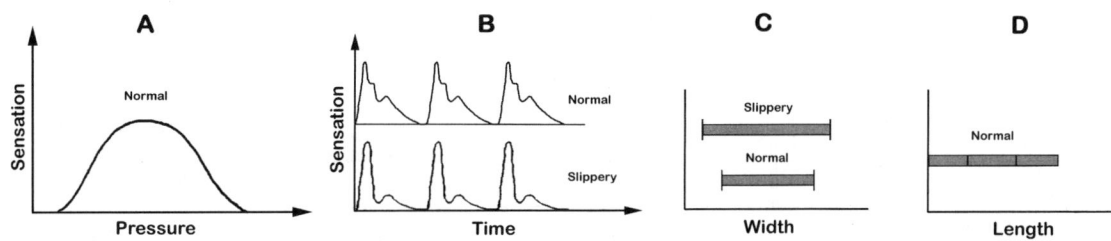

Clinically, this pulse indicates phlegm, accumulation of food in the Stomach or an Excess Heat Pattern. This pulse often occurs normally in pregnant animals.

Hesitant or Choppy Pulse (se mai)

The hesitant pulse feels rough and irregular like lightly scraping the surface of bamboo with a knife.

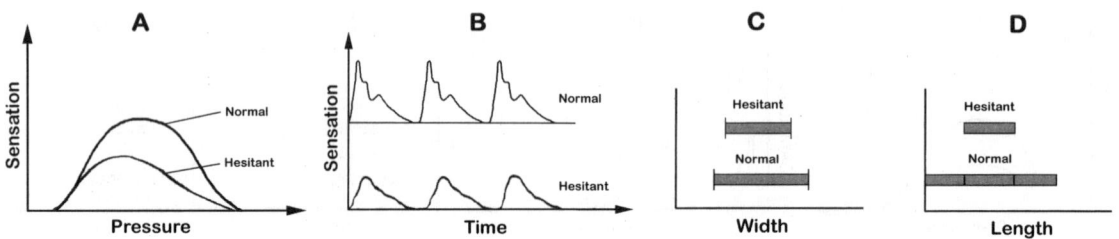

Clinically, this pulse indicates Stagnation of Qi or Blood, impairment of Essence or Deficiency of Yin.

Thready, Thin or Small Pulse (xi mai)

This pulse feels soft and weak like a fine thread, but it is very distinct and clear.

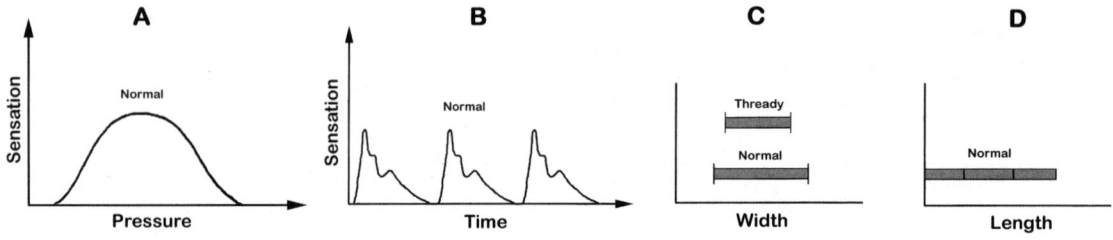

Clinically, this pulse indicates a Yin Deficiency Pattern or a Deficiency of Blood.

Wiry Pulse or String-taut (xuan mai)

The Wiry pulse feels taut, straight and long like pressing a string of a violin.

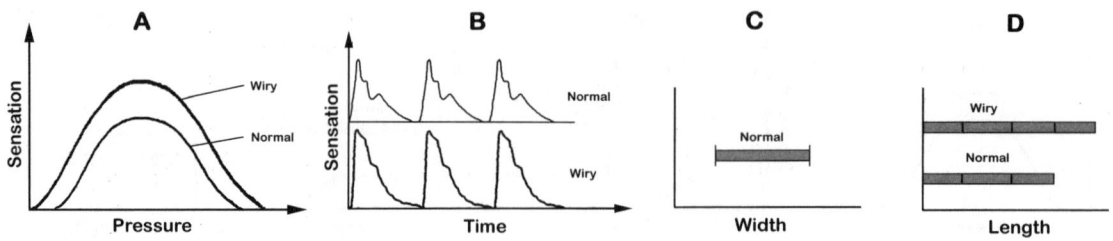

Clinically, this pulse indicates a disorder of the Liver, an Interior Wind Pattern, a Pain Pattern or a Phlegm Pattern.

Soft or Soggy Pulse (ru mai)

This pulse feels superficial, thready and forceless. It can be easily felt by a gentle touch (Superficial Palpation), but becomes indistinct with heavy pressure (Deep Palpation).

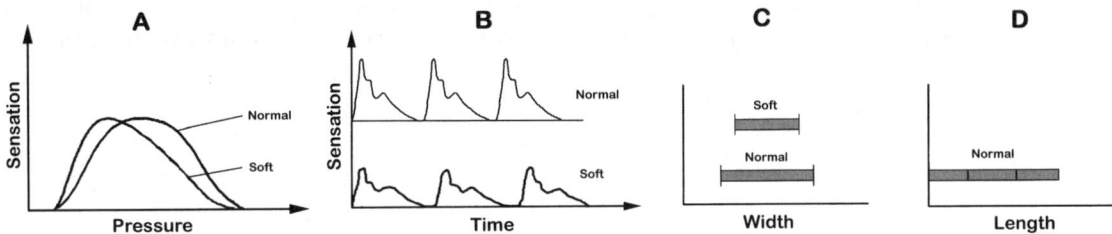

Clinically, this pulse indicates a Spleen Qi Deficiency Pattern or a Damp Pattern.

Abrupt or Hasty Pulse (cu mai)

The pulse feels hurried and rapid with irregularly missed beats. This pulse is illustrated in Figure 7.17.

Clinically, this pulse indicates Excess Yang Heat, Stagnation of Qi and Blood, heart disease or retention of phlegm or food.

Regularly Intermittent Pulse (dai mai)

The pulse is weak and slower than normal with missed beats at regular intervals. This pulse is illustrated in Figure 7.17Figure 1.1.

Clinically, this pulse indicates a weakness of the Zang-Fu organ's activities, a Pain Pattern or a traumatic incident.

Knotted Pulse (jie mai)

The pulse is slower than normal with missing beats at irregular intervals. This pulse is illustrated in Figure 7.17.

Clinically, this pulse indicates an Extreme Yin Pattern, accumulation of Cold, retention of Cold Phlegm or Stagnant Blood.

Unusual Pulse

The unusual pulse is called *guai mai* which can also be translated into "strange pulse". It usually refers to a critical clinical condition and often occurs when the patient is near death. This pulse is irregular, disordered, and about to stop. There are seven forms of the unusual pulse: sparrow-pecking pulse, leaky-roof pulse, stone-tapping pulse, rope-unwinding pulse, fish-swimming pulse, shrimp-jumping pulse, and boiling-water pulse.

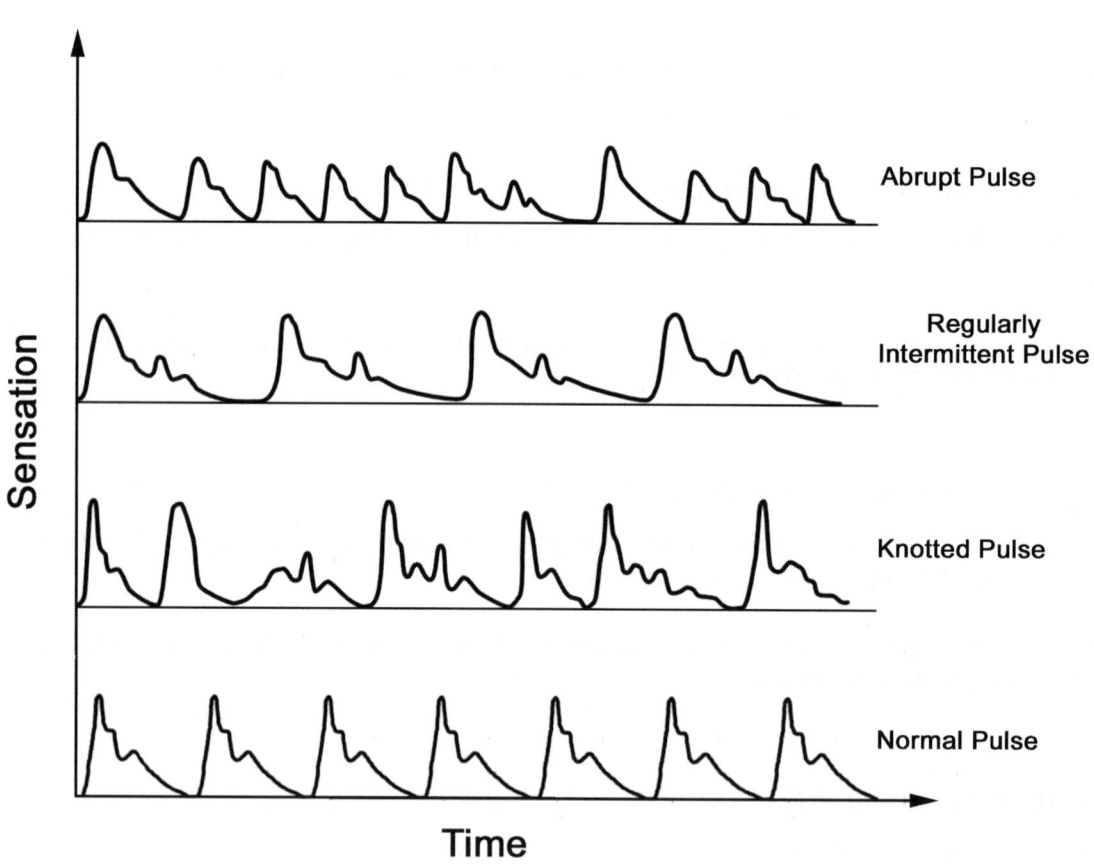

Figure 7.17: The Abrupt, Knotted and Regularly Intermittent Pulses

Table 7.21: The characteristics of the pulse types

Pulse Type	Depth or Force	Width	Length	Time
Floating Pulse (Superficial)	Superficial	Normal	Normal	Normal
Deep Pulse (Sinking)	Deep	Normal	Normal	Normal
Rapid Pulse	Normal	Normal	Normal	Increased Rate
Slow Pulse	Normal	Normal	Normal	Decreased Rate
Full Pulse (Excess)	Increased	Wide	Long	Rapid
Thready Pulse (Thin)	Normal	Narrow	Normal	Normal
Weak Pulse (Deficient)	Soft, Weak	Narrow	Short	Normal
Slippery Pulse (Rolling)	Increased	Wide	Normal	Rapid
Choppy Pulse (Hesitant)	Decreased	Narrow	Short	Decreased Rate
Soft Pulse (Soggy)	Superficial	Narrow	Normal	Decreased Rate
Wiry Pulse (String-taut)	Increased	Normal	Long	Increased Rate
Knotted Pulse	Normal	Normal	Normal	Slow Missed beats, Irregular intervals
Intermittent Pulse	Weak	Normal	Normal	Slow Missed beats, Regular intervals
Abrupt Pulse	Normal	Normal	Normal	Rapid Irregular pauses

Table 7.22: Descriptions of the various pulse types

Pulse Type	Description	Significance
Floating Pulse	Easily palpated with light pressure but easily obliterated by heavy pressure	The early stage of exogenous diseases due to invasion of Wind-Cold and Wind-Heat
Deep Pulse	Cannot be felt with light pressure. Felt only with heavy pressure.	Interior Pattern
Rapid Pulse	The rate is faster than normal	Heat Pattern
Slow Pulse	The rate is slower than normal	Cold Pattern
Full Pulse	Very forceful with all three palpation depths.	Excess Pattern; Stagnant Blood; Constipation; High Fever
Thin Pulse	Soft and weak like a fine thread but very distinct and clear.	Yin Deficiency Pattern; Deficiency of Blood
Weak Pulse	Soft, weak and forceless at all levels	Deficiency Pattern of Qi; Deficiency of Qi and Blood
Slippery Pulse	Smooth, rounded, and slippery like pearls rolling on a dish.	Phlegm; Accumulation of Food in the Stomach; Excess Heat Pattern; Normal during pregnancy (or after drinking alcohol or taking some pharmaceutical agents)
Choppy Pulse	Rough / Irregular like scraping bamboo surface lightly with a knife	Stagnation of Qi and/or Blood; Impairment of Essence and Deficiency of Yin
Soft Pulse	Superficial, Thready, Forceless. Easily felt with superficial palpation but indistinct on deep palpation	Deficiency of Spleen Qi; Damp Pattern
Wiry Pulse	Taut, straight, and long like pressing a string of a violin	Disorder of the Liver; Interior Wind Pattern; Pain Pattern; Phlegm Pattern

Table 7.23: Patterns associated with various pulses

Pulse Type		Pattern
Floating Pulse	Forceful	Exterior Excess Pattern
	Weak	Exterior Deficiency Pattern
	Rapid	Exterior Heat Pattern
	Slow	Exterior Cold Pattern
	Large/Weak	Outward floating of Deficient Yang Qi
Deep Pulse	Forceful	Interior Excess Pattern
	Weak	Interior Deficiency Pattern
Rapid Pulse	Forceful	Excess Heat Pattern
	Weak	Deficiency Heat Pattern
	Weak/Superficial	Outward Floating of Deficient Yang
Slow Pulse	Forceful	Excess Cold Pattern
	Superficial	Exterior Cold Pattern
	Deep	Interior Cold Pattern
Full Pulse		Excess Pattern Stagnant Blood Constipation High Fever
Thin Pulse		Yin Deficiency Pattern Deficiency of Blood
Weak Pulse		Deficiency Pattern of Qi Deficiency of Qi and Blood
Slippery Pulse		Phlegm Accumulation of Food in the Stomach Excess Heat Pattern Physiological during pregnancy
Choppy Pulse		Stagnation of Qi and/or Blood Impairment of Essence and Deficiency of Yin
Soft Pulse		Deficiency of Spleen Qi Damp Pattern
Wiry Pulse		Disorder of the Liver Interior Wind Pattern Pain Pattern Phlegm Pattern

PALPATION OF THE MERIDIANS AND ACUPOINTS

TCVM practitioners can identify a disorder in the body by feeling for sensitive acupoints or Meridian pathways. The back-Shu (Association) points and front-Mu (Alarm) points are special acupoints where the Zang-Fu organ Qi is distributed. Sensitivity to palpation of these areas relates to imbalances within the corresponding Meridians or internal organs. For example, tenderness at BL-13 may indicate a Lung problem, and sensitivity at CV-12 indicates a Stomach disorder.

The back-Shu and front-Mu points may be used in combination. One may wonder how to differentiate local back pain from sensitivity at a back-Shu point related to a Zang-Fu organ. This can be difficult, but it may be partially resolved by palpating the related front-Mu point when sensitivity is noted at a back-Shu point. If both the back-Shu and front-Mu points are sensitive, one might feel more confident that the related organ is unbalanced.

Zang-Fu	Back-Shu Points	Front-Mu Points
LU	BL-13	LU-1
PC	BL-14	CV-17
HT	BL-15	CV-14
LIV	BL-18	LIV-14
GB	BL-19	GB-24
SP	BL-20	LIV-13
ST	BL-21	CV-12
TH	BL-22	CV-5
KID	BL-23	GB-25
LI	BL-25	ST-25
SI	BL-27	CV-4
BL	BL-28	CV-3

In horses, one can use a pen or needle cap to palpate or "scan" specific pathways on the body surface to evaluate lameness. Sensitivity during the scanning can indicate the location of soreness. From a Western perspective, musculoskeletal or neurological disorders are the typical causes of lameness. In TCVM, lameness is mainly considered a sign of pain which results from Stagnation of Qi-Blood. Evaluation using a TCVM approach will not provide a specific diagnosis, but it can help determine which body regions are involved in the lameness.

The results of this examination may be used to determine the treatment strategy. Performing the scan for sensitive points before and after each acupuncture treatment can help the practitioner evaluate the clinical progress and success of therapy.

Table 7.24: Diagnostic acupuncture points for front limb lameness in horses

Points	Shoulder Pain	Carpal Pain	Tendon Pain	Fetlock Pain	Hoof Pain
LI-18					++
TH-16				++	
SI-16			++	+	
Knee Point		++			
TH-15			++		
BL-13		+			++
GB-21	+				
LI-15	++				
LI-16	++			+	
LI-17		++			
TH-14	++				
SI-9	++				
Yan Zhou	++				
SI-10	+				
PC-1					++
BL-14		+	+		
BL-15			+		++
BL-16					
BL-17			+		
BL-18			+		
BL-19			+		
BL22		+			
BL-25		+		+ Opposite	+
BL-27					+

Table 7.25: Diagnostic acupuncture points for front limb lameness in horses

Points	Coxofemoral	Stifle	Hock
Coxa Hip Point	+		
BL-54	+		
Lu-Gu	+		
GB-29, GB-30	+		
Shen Shu, Shen Peng, Shen Jiao	+		
ST-10		+	
Dan Tian		+	
BL-36, BL-37, BL-38		+	
Yang Ling		+	
BL-20, BL-21, BL-22		+	
Coxa Hock point			+
BL-35			+
BL-39 a/b			+
BL-17, BL-18, BL-19			+
GB-20, GB-21, BL-10	+		+

PALPATION OF BODY REGIONS

Evaluating the Body Fluids (Yin), Yang (Temperature), Qi Flow (Sensitivities)

The Mouth

While observing the mouth color, a veterinarian can feel the temperature in the oral cavity. Under normal conditions, the mouth feels mildly warm and moist. Coldness in the oral cavity indicates a Cold Pattern, and a hot mouth indicates a Heat Pattern. A hot, dry mouth indicates Interior Heat and Impairment of Yin.

The Nose

A veterinarian may place the palm of a hand on the anterior end of the nose to feel the temperature of the skin and the exhaled air. Normally these areas are mildly warm and moist. A hot nose indicates a Heat Pattern while a cold nose indicates a Cold Pattern.

The Ear

During the physical exam, a practitioner may wrap a hand around the ears to evaluate the temperature. A healthy animal has a warm ear base but a cool ear tip. The two fingers close to the ear base should feel warm, but the distal two fingers should feel cooler. If both ear base and tip are hot, this reflects a Heat Pattern. If both the ear base and tip are cold, this indicates a Cold Pattern.

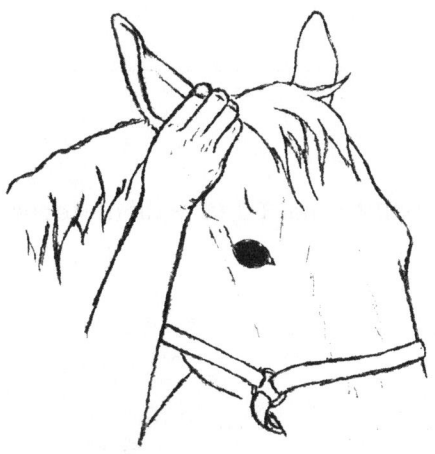

Figure 7.18: Examination of the ear

The Body Surface and Limbs

Under normal conditions, the body surface and the four limbs are neither too hot nor too cold. A hot body surface and limbs indicate a Heat Pattern; however, a cold body surface and limbs indicate a Cold Pattern. If the ends of the limbs are icy, the Yang Qi is very deficient.

The Throat and its Surroundings

A veterinarian may palpate the outside of the throat to detect sensitivities, swellings and temperature changes. A hot, painful, swollen throat region indicates adenitis or laryngitis.

The Thorax and Abdomen

Pain or cough in response to pressure on the thoracic wall of horses indicates pain in the Lung or pleuropneumonia. A painful response to pressure along the cranioventral thoracic wall in cattle may indicate traumatic pericarditis. If palpation of the flank region reveals a feeling of tightness, elasticity and fullness without encountering hard structures, this indicates gas distention. If the abdominal cavity feels hard and full, this indicates food distention. Fluctuation of abdomen, like pressing a bag of water, indicates ascites.

Application of TCVM Diagnostics in Practice

Making an accurate diagnosis requires collection of a complete clinical history and analysis of all the clinical data using the TCVM diagnostic systems. The best way to gather all the pertinent data is to integrate all four diagnostic methods and record the findings in the patient's permanent record. Medical records are as important in TCVM practice as in conventional Western medical practice. Some may find custom designed examination forms, such as the two examples below, to be helpful when collecting TCVM patient information.

Date: _____   Name: _____ _____
                                              Last   First

Small Animal TCVM Patient Record

PATIENT IDENTIFICATION

Patient Name: _____   Breed: _____   Weight: _____

                                     DOB: _____   Sex: F FS M MC

Address:

_____   Telephone: _____

_____   E-mail: _____

VISIT INFORMATION

Major Complaint: _____

	Yang (Heat)	Yin (Cold)
Preference:	☐ Shade or cool locations (concrete / tile)	☐ Sun or warm locations (carpet)
Personality:	☐ Hyperactive, outgoing, confident, strong (Fire/Wood)	☐ Quiet, timid, less confident (Earth/Water)
Diet:	☐ Dry food, hot food (chicken, mutton, deer meat)	☐ Iced food or drink, cold food (fish, tofu)
Thirst:	☐ Thirsty	☐ Less Thirsty
Appetite:	☐ Good or ravenous	☐ Good or finicky
Feces:	☐ Dry or bloody or malodorous	☐ Loose or diarrhea
Urine:	☐ Short stream or malodorous or bloody	☐ Long stream or urinary leakage
Medications:	☐ Steroids, Yang / Qi tonic herbs	☐ Antibiotic, Heat-clearing / Yin tonic herbs
Age:	☐ Young	☐ Old
Disease Course:	☐ Short	☐ Long
Vaccinations:	☐ Acute disease following vaccination	☐ Chronic disease following excessive or frequent vaccination
Predisposition:	☐ Yang Excess, Heat pattern, Yin Deficiency, Blood deficiency, Liver Yang Rising	☐ Yang Deficiency, Yin Excess, Cold Pattern, Qi Deficiency, Qi Stagnation, Blood Stagnation

HEAT CONDITION:	☐ 4 or more Yang signs **(Excess Heat)**	☐ 2 or less Yin signs **(Yin Deficiency)**
COLD CONDITION:	☐ 2 or less Yang signs **(Yang / Qi Deficiency)**	☐ 4 or more Yin signs **(Excess Cold)**
COMBINATION:	☐ 3 or more signs	☐ 3 or more signs

Personality

	Wood	Fire	Earth	Metal	Water
Yang / Yin type:	☐ Yang	☐ Yang	☐ Yin	☐ Yang/Yin	☐ Yin
Interactions:	☐ Aggressive (bossy)	☐ Very friendly	☐ OK with everyone	☐ OK; aloof (confident)	☐ Timid; not confident (runs away)
Greeting strangers:	☐ Barks or attacks	☐ Wags tail warmly	☐ Slow reaction	☐ Does not care	☐ Runs away
Patience:	☐ No	☐ No	☐ Yes	☐ Yes	☐ Yes
Excitability:	☐ Yes	☐ Easily	☐ Slow	☐ No	☐ No
Reaction to needling:	☐ Cooperative	☐ Highly sensitive	☐ No problems	☐ Cooperative	☐ Sensitive
Others:	☐ Irritable	☐ Vocal	☐ Mellow; laid-back	☐ Follows the rules	☐ Insecure (fear)

Point Sensitivity

Zang-Fu	Back-Shu Points	Front-Mu Points
LU	☐ BL-13	☐ LU-1
PC	☐ BL-14	☐ CV-17
HT	☐ BL-15	☐ CV-14
LIV	☐ BL-18	☐ LIV-14
GB	☐ BL-19	☐ GB-24
SP	☐ BL-20	☐ LIV-13
ST	☐ BL-21	☐ CV-12
TH	☐ BL-22	☐ CV-5
KID	☐ BL-23	☐ GB-25
LI	☐ BL-25	☐ ST-25
SI	☐ BL-27	☐ CV-4
BL	☐ BL-28	☐ CV-3

Diagnostic Test Results

Radiograph or Ultrasound: _____
_____

CBC / Biochemical Panel: _____
_____

Other Tests: _____
_____

Figure 7.19: Small animal medical record page 2 of 4

Physical Exam

Shen:	☐ Great	☐ Good	☐ OK	☐ Disturbance	☐ Loss
Tongue color:	☐ Pale	☐ Red	☐ Yellow	☐ Deep Red	☐ Purple
Tongue coat:	☐ Pale	☐ Dark	☐ Yellow	☐ Thin	☐ Thick ☐ Greasy
Tongue moisture:	☐ Dry	☐ Wet	☐ Small	☐ Swollen	

Pulse:	☐ Floating	☐ Deep	☐ Fast	☐ Slow	☐ Forceful ☐ Weak
	☐ Thin	☐ Slippery	☐ Choppy	☐ Soft	☐ Wiry
Hair / Skin:	☐ Wet	☐ Dry	☐ Alopecia	☐ Malodorous	☐ Dandruff
	☐ Pruritus	☐ Hot	☐ Cold	☐ Poor follicle	
Ears:	☐ Hot	☐ Cold	☐ Red	☐ Scratching	☐ Alopecia ☐ Other
Discharge:		☐ with odor	☐ with blood	☐ with pus	☐ Other
Eyes:	☐ Red	☐ Pale	☐ Yellow	☐ Itchy	☐ Dry ☐ Swollen
Discharge:		☐ thick	☐ watery	☐ purulent	☐ Other
Nose:	☐ Wet	☐ Dry	☐ Crusting	☐ Depigmentation	☐ Hot ☐ Cold
Discharge:		☐ clear	☐ thick	☐ bloody	☐ purulent ☐ Other
Gums:	☐ Pale	☐ Red	☐ Swollen	☐ Foul odor	☐ Bloody
Lips:	☐ Pale	☐ Red	☐ Purple	☐ Ulcers	
Oral cavity:	☐ Dry	☐ Wet	☐ Ulcers	☐ Foul odor	☐ Hot ☐ Cold
Water intake:	☐ Normal	☐ No thirst	☐ Increased	☐ Decreased	
Food intake:	☐ Normal	☐ Finicky	☐ Poor	☐ Ravenous	
Voice:	☐ Loud	☐ Weak			
Cough:	☐ Dry	☐ Wet	☐ Loud	☐ Worse at night	☐ Weak
	☐ Daytime	☐ Nighttime			
Respiration:	☐ Heavy	☐ Strong	☐ Superficial	☐ Weak	
Feces:	☐ Loose	☐ Watery	☐ Dry	☐ Constipation	
	☐ Bloody	☐ Mucous	☐ Incontinent	☐ Malodorous	
Urination:	☐ Long	☐ Short	☐ Incontinent	☐ Malodorous	☐ Bloody
Exercise:	☐ Too much	☐ Too little	☐ Intolerance		
Sleep:	☐ Too much	☐ Too little	☐ Vocalizes or wakes up the owner at night		
	☐ Soft bed	☐ Hard bed	☐ Muscle jerking during sleep		
Vomiting:	☐ Frequent	☐ Sporadic	☐ With undigested food		
	☐ Much	☐ Little	☐ Just after eating		
Stiffness:	☐ Acute	☐ Chronic			
Worse:		☐ in morning	☐ in evening	☐ with cold	☐ with heat
		☐ with damp	☐ after walk	☐ before walk	
Massage:		☐ Likes	☐ Dislikes		

Figure 7.20: Small animal medical record page 3 of 4

Diagnosis

☐ Exterior   ☐ Interior   ☐ Cold   ☐ Heat

☐ EXCESS
- ☐ Wind-Cold   ☐ Wind-Heat   ☐ Heat-Toxin
- ☐ Damp-Heat   ☐ Cold-Damp   ☐ Phlegm
- ☐ Qi Stagnation   ☐ Blood Stagnation   ☐ Food Stasis
- ☐ Impaction   ☐ Stones   ☐ Trauma

☐ DEFICIENCY

Lung	☐ Yin	☐ Yang	☐ Qi
Heart	☐ Yin	☐ Yang	☐ Qi	☐ Blood
Spleen	☐ Yin	☐ Yang	☐ Qi	☐ Blood
Liver	☐ Yin			☐ Blood
Kidney	☐ Yin	☐ Yang	☐ Qi	☐ Jing

Treatment

Acupuncture: _____
_____

Herbs: _____
_____

Exercise: _____
_____

Massage: _____
_____

Other: _____
_____
_____

Visit Comments

_____
_____
_____
_____
_____

Figure 7.21: Small animal medical record page 4 of 4

Date: _____   Name: _____ _____
                                      Last   First

Large Animal TCVM Patient Record

PATIENT IDENTIFICATION

Patient Name: _____   Breed: _____   Color: _____

                                              DOB: _____   Sex: F   M   Intact: Y | N

Address:

_____   Telephone: _____

_____   E-mail: _____

VISIT INFORMATION

Major Complaint: _____

	Yang (Heat)		Yin (Cold)
Preference:	☐ Shade or cool locations	☐	Sun or warm locations
Personality:	☐ Hyperactive, outgoing, confident, strong (Fire/Wood)	☐	Quiet, timid, less confident (Earth/Water)
Diet:	☐ Warm food (oats and sweet feed)	☐	Green grass
Thirst:	☐ Thirsty	☐	Less Thirsty
Appetite:	☐ Good or ravenous	☐	Good or finicky
Feces:	☐ Dry or bloody or malodorous	☐	Loose or diarrhea
Urine:	☐ Short stream or malodorous or bloody	☐	Long stream or urinary leakage
Medications:	☐ Steroids, Yang / Qi tonic herbs	☐	Antibiotic, Heat-clearing / Yin tonic herbs
Age:	☐ Young	☐	Old
Disease Course:	☐ Short	☐	Long
Vaccinations:	☐ Acute disease following vaccination	☐	Chronic disease following excessive or frequent vaccination
Predisposition:	☐ Yang Excess, Heat pattern, Yin Deficiency, Blood deficiency, Liver Yang Rising	☐	Yang Deficiency, Yin Excess, Cold Pattern, Qi Deficiency, Qi Stagnation, Blood Stagnation

HEAT CONDITION:	☐ 4 or more Yang signs **(Excess Heat)**	☐	2 or less Yin signs **(Yin Deficiency)**
COLD CONDITION:	☐ 2 or less Yang signs **(Yang / Qi Deficiency)**	☐	4 or more Yin signs **(Excess Cold)**
COMBINATION:	☐ 3 or more signs	☐	3 or more signs

Figure 7.22: Large animal medical record page 1 of 4

Personality

	Wood	Fire	Earth	Metal	Water
Yang / Yin type:	☐ Yang	☐ Yang	☐ Yin	☐ Yang/Yin	☐ Yin
Interactions:	☐ Aggressive (bossy)	☐ Very friendly	☐ OK with everyone	☐ OK; aloof (confident)	☐ Timid; not confident (runs away)
Intraexam behavior:	☐ Takes charge	☐ Plays	☐ Easy going	☐ Cooperates	☐ Cautious or runs away
Patience:	☐ No	☐ No	☐ Yes	☐ Yes	☐ Yes
Excitability:	☐ Yes	☐ Easily	☐ Slow	☐ No	☐ No
Reaction to needling:	☐ Cooperative	☐ Highly sensitive	☐ No problems	☐ Cooperative	☐ Sensitive
Others:	☐ Irritable	☐ Vocal	☐ Mellow; laid-back	☐ Follows the rules	☐ Insecure (fear)

Lameness Exam

Diagnostic Point Sensitivity

	LI-18	LI-17	Knee Point	LI-15	LI-16	TH-16	SI-16	TH-15	SI-9	TH-14	PC-1
Left											
Right											

	BL-13	BL-14	BL-15	BL-18	BL-19	BL-20	BL-21	BL-22	BL-23	BL-25	BL-26	BL-27
Left												
Right												

	BL-54	Lu Gu	GB-29	Hip Point	Hock Point	Dan Tian	ST-10	BL-37	BL-38	BL-35	BL-39
Left											
Right											

Diagnostic Test Results

Radiograph or Ultrasound: _____
_____

CBC / Biochemical Panel: _____
_____

Other Tests: _____
_____

Figure 7.23: Large animal medical record page 2 of 4

Physical Exam

Shen:	☐ Great	☐ Good	☐ OK	☐ Disturbance	☐ Loss
Tongue color:	☐ Pale	☐ Red	☐ Yellow	☐ Deep Red	☐ Purple
Tongue coat:	☐ Pale	☐ Dark	☐ Yellow	☐ Thin	☐ Thick	☐ Greasy
Tongue moisture:	☐ Dry	☐ Wet	☐ Small	☐ Swollen		
Pulse:	☐ Floating	☐ Deep	☐ Fast	☐ Slow	☐ Forceful	☐ Weak
	☐ Thin	☐ Slippery	☐ Choppy	☐ Soft	☐ Wiry	
Hair / Skin:	☐ Wet	☐ Dry	☐ Alopecia	☐ Malodorous	☐ Dandruff	
	☐ Pruritus	☐ Hot	☐ Cold	☐ Poor follicle		
Ears:	☐ Hot	☐ Cold	☐ Other			
Eyes:	☐ Red	☐ Pale	☐ Yellow	☐ Itchy	☐ Dry	☐ Swollen
Discharge:	☐ thick	☐ watery	☐ purulent	☐ Other		
Nose:	☐ Wet	☐ Dry	☐ Crusting	☐ Depigmentation	☐ Hot	☐ Cold
Discharge:	☐ clear	☐ thick	☐ bloody	☐ purulent	☐ Other	
Gums:	☐ Pale	☐ Red	☐ Swollen	☐ Foul odor	☐ Bloody	
Lips:	☐ Pale	☐ Red	☐ Purple	☐ Ulcers		
Oral cavity:	☐ Dry	☐ Wet	☐ Ulcers	☐ Foul odor	☐ Hot	☐ Cold
Water intake:	☐ Normal	☐ No thirst	☐ Increased	☐ Decreased		
Food intake:	☐ Normal	☐ Finicky	☐ Poor	☐ Ravenous		
Voice:	☐ Loud	☐ Weak				
Cough:	☐ Dry	☐ Wet	☐ Loud	☐ Worse at night	☐ Weak	
	☐ Daytime	☐ Nighttime				
Respiration:	☐ Heavy	☐ Strong	☐ Superficial	☐ Weak		
Feces:	☐ Loose	☐ Watery	☐ Dry	☐ Constipation		
	☐ Bloody	☐ Mucous	☐ Incontinent	☐ Malodorous		
Urination:	☐ Long	☐ Short	☐ Incontinent	☐ Malodorous	☐ Bloody	
Training or Work:	☐ Too much	☐ Too little	☐ Intolerance			
Stiffness:	☐ Acute	☐ Chronic				
Worse:	☐ in morning	☐ in evening	☐ with cold	☐ with heat		
	☐ with damp	☐ after walk	☐ before walk			
Massage:	☐ Likes	☐ Dislikes				

Figure 7.24: Large animal medical record page 3 of 4

Diagnosis

☐ Exterior ☐ Interior ☐ Cold ☐ Heat

☐ EXCESS ☐ Wind-Cold ☐ Wind-Heat ☐ Heat-Toxin

☐ Damp-Heat ☐ Cold-Damp ☐ Phlegm

☐ Qi Stagnation ☐ Blood Stagnation ☐ Food Stasis

☐ Impaction ☐ Stones ☐ Trauma

☐ DEFICIENCY

Lung	☐ Yin	☐ Yang	☐ Qi	
Heart	☐ Yin	☐ Yang	☐ Qi	☐ Blood
Spleen	☐ Yin	☐ Yang	☐ Qi	☐ Blood
Liver	☐ Yin			☐ Blood
Kidney	☐ Yin	☐ Yang	☐ Qi	☐ Jing

☐ LAMENESS ☐ Shoulder ☐ Carpal ☐ Fetlock ☐ Back

☐ Coxofemoral ☐ Stifle ☐ Hock ☐ Foot

Treatment

Acupuncture: _____

_____

Herbs: _____

_____

Exercise: _____

_____

Massage: _____

_____

Other: _____

_____

_____

Visit Comments

_____
_____
_____
_____

Figure 7.25: Large animal medical record page 4 of 4

Self Test

Question 7.1: A red tongue indicates:

    a. Cold
    b. Heat
    c. Wind
    d. Damp
    e. Dryness

Question 7.2: A yellow coating indicates:

    a. Qi Deficiency
    b. Blood Deficiency
    c. Yin Deficiency
    d. Excess Heat
    e. Qi Stagnation

Question 7.3: A slow pulse indicates:

    a. Excess Heat
    b. Yang Deficiency
    c. Damp-Heat
    d. Wind-Heat
    e. Deficiency Heat

Question 7.4: A rapid pulse and red tongue indicate:

    a. Blood Deficiency
    b. Qi Deficiency
    c. Yin Deficiency
    d. Yang Deficiency
    e. Excess Cold

Question 7.5: A malodorous, wet discharge from ears indicates:

    a. Blood Deficiency
    b. Yin Deficiency
    c. Excess Cold
    d. Wind Heat
    e. Damp Heat

Question 7.6: Dandruff indicates:

    a. Blood Deficiency
    b. Qi Deficiency
    c. Yang Deficiency
    d. Excess Cold
    e. Damp-Cold

Question 7.7: Halitosis indicates:

    a. Deficiency Blood
    b. Excess Cold
    c. Exterior Cold
    d. Exterior Heat
    e. Excess Heat

An eighteen year old Thoroughbred mare has had chronic diarrhea for three months. She is a mellow and laid-back mare. According to her owner, her appetite seems poor and she has had significant weight loss. Physical exam reveals a pale tongue, a weak pulse and low Shen. She appears emaciated. Her stool is loose without odor or blood. Historically, she has had intermittent bouts of watery diarrhea. Dietary changes including switching to different hays, cutting down on grain and administering enzymes have not improved the diarrhea.

Question 7.8: What is the TCVM diagnosis for this mare?

    a. Heart Qi Deficiency
    b. Lung Qi Deficiency
    c. Spleen Qi Deficiency
    d. Liver Qi Deficiency
    e. Kidney Qi Deficiency

CHAPTER EIGHT

DIAGNOSTIC SYSTEMS AND PATTERN DIFFERENTIATION

> The physician who is attending a patient … has to
> know the cause of the ailment before he can cure it.
>
> – Mo-tze, *Ethical and Political Works*

An accurate TCVM diagnosis forms the basis of appropriate treatment selection, whether the therapy involves various acupuncture methods or Chinese herbal medicines. The TCVM diagnostic system is known as *Bian Zheng* or Pattern differentiation. Observation of the patient's condition, which includes noting the quality of the Shen, tongue and pulse, allows a veterinarian to determine a TCVM Pattern. Having discussed the diagnostic methods in Chapter 7, the next step is to learn how to use various diagnostic systems to interpret the clinical information and to identify the Pattern. There are five steps to developing a TCVM diagnosis and treatment plan.

1. Clinical Data Collection: Use the four diagnostic methods (inspecting, hearing and smelling, inquiring, and palpating) for this step. Tongue and pulse diagnoses are especially important.

2. Naming the Disease: The disease name is often the same as the major complaint. For example, the disease name may be diarrhea, colic, bleeding, cough, or asthma.

3. Pattern Differentiation: This step is the most important because the treatment plan depends on it. The systems commonly used to differentiate the Pattern of disease include the Eight Principles, the Zang-Fu Syndromes, the Six Channels, the Four Stages, the San-jiao Patterns, the Pathogen Patterns, Qi-Blood-Body Fluid Patterns and the Meridian Patterns.

4. Treatment Strategy: This step is based upon the Pattern differentiation. Determine the appropriate treatment principle according to the Pattern identified in the previous step. Use tonification for a Deficiency Pattern, and use sedation for an Excess Pattern. Cold Patterns require warming acupuncture techniques or hot herbs, but Heat Patterns need cooling acupuncture techniques or cool herbs.

5. Selection of Treatment: Choose treatments that correspond with the treatment principle determined in the 4th step. For example, GV-14 and Coptis *Huang Lian* have a cooling effect and may be used for a Heat Pattern

Table 8.1: Three examples of the five-step TCVM diagnostic method

1ST STEP Clinical Data	2ND STEP Disease Name	3RD STEP Pattern Differentiation	4TH STEP Treatment Strategy	5TH STEP Treatment Selection
CASE 1: Diarrhea Rapid pulse Red tongue	Diarrhea	Heat Pattern	Clear Heat	Coptis *Huang Lian* LI-11, ST-44, ST-36
CASE 2: Diarrhea Weak pulse Pale tongue	Diarrhea	Qi Deficiency Pattern	Tonify Qi	Ginseng *Ren Shen* BL-21, BL-20, ST-36
CASE 3: Anorexia Weak pulse Pale tongue	Anorexia	Qi Deficiency Pattern	Tonify Qi	Ginseng *Ren Shen* BL-21, BL-20, ST-36

Case 1 and Case 2 both have the same name. They are both called diarrhea because that is the major complaint; however, they are not the same Pattern.

Case 1 is a Heat Pattern because of the rapid pulse and the red tongue. Thus, in this case the treatment strategy is to clear the Heat. Coptis *Huang Lian* can clear Heat in the Stomach and Heart. One may use the acupuncture points LI-11 and ST-44 to clear Heat while using ST-36 to strengthen the Spleen and Stomach and to stop the diarrhea.

Case 2 is diagnosed as a Qi Deficiency Pattern because of the weak pulse and pale tongue. Thus, its treatment strategy is to tonify Qi. Ginseng *Ren Shen* is a Qi tonic herbal medicine. BL-20 and BL-21 can tonify the Qi of the Spleen and Stomach.

As demonstrated, different treatments are given in case 1 and 2 even though each is named diarrhea because they each have a totally different diagnosis (Pattern). This is called "tong-bing-yi-zhi (TBYZ)", which means that different treatments are given for the same disease.

Case 3 is considered anorexia; however, it is also diagnosed as a Qi Deficiency Pattern just like Case 2 because of the tongue and pulse qualities. Since they have the same Pattern, the treatment strategy and treatment methods are totally the same despite the differences in their names. This is called "yi-bing-tong-zhi (YBTZ)", which means that the same treatments are given for different diseases.

The reason TBYZ and YBTZ occur is because the TCVM approaches are based on the Pattern, not the disease. TCVM practitioners focus on diagnosing the Pattern because this will form the basis of their treatment. It is evident how crucial the Pattern Differentiation (the 3rd step) is in Traditional Chinese Veterinary Medicine.

Table 8.2: An overview of the eight TCVM diagnostic systems

TCVM Diagnosis	Brief Introduction	Application
Eight Principles	The foundation of pattern differentiation. Four pairs, six root patterns: Exterior — Interior Heat — Cold Excess — Deficiency Yang — Yin	Foundation of TCVM diagnosis Any disease
Zang-Fu Syndromes	Each Zang-Fu organ has a Deficiency or Excess or Heat/Cold Pattern. LU / LI PC / TH HT / SI KID / BL SP / ST LIV / GB	Internal Medicine, Chronic illness, General weakness, Geriatric diseases
Six Channel Patterns (Six Phases)	Tai-yang Tai-yin Yang-ming Shao-yin Shao-yang Jue-yin	Exogenous diseases, Chronic inflammatory diseases, A disease with initial cold signs
Four Stages (Four Levels)	Four stages of disease progression: Wei (Defense) Qi Ying (Nutrient) Xue (Blood)	Exogenous diseases, Infectious diseases, Any disease starting with fever
San-Jiao Patterns (Triple Heater Patterns)	Upper Jiao (Heart and Lung) Middle Jiao (Spleen and Stomach) Lower Jiao (Kidney and Liver)	Water metabolism disorders Diseases due to Damp-Heat
Pathogen Patterns	Exogenous pathogens: Wind Dampness Cold Dryness Summer Heat Fire Endogenous pathogens: Hungry Overwork Overfeeding Underwork Emotional stress Others: Trauma Stagnation Phlegm Contusion Falling down	Exogenous diseases Any disease related to emotional stress
Qi-Blood-Body Fluid Patterns	Qi Blood Body Fluid	Chronic internal diseases Endocrine disorders
Meridian Patterns	Twelve Regular Channels Eight Extra Channels	Musculoskeletal problems Meridian therapy

How does one differentiate a TCVM Pattern? This is possible by using one or more of the eight diagnostic systems for Pattern Differentiation. A brief introduction to these systems is listed in Table 8.2. The Eight Principles become the foundation and guidelines of TCVM diagnosis. The Zang-Fu Syndromes form the core. The Four Stages, Six Channels, and Pathogen Patterns are usually used for the diseases caused by exogenous pathogens. The San-jiao Pattern system is often used for water metabolism disorders and diseases caused by Damp-Heat. Qi-Blood-Body Fluid Patterns can be used for endocrine disorders and other chronic illnesses. The Meridian Patterns are used for musculoskeletal problems.

Eight Principles

Six Roots

There are four pairs in this diagnostic system: 1) Exterior and Interior; 2) Heat and Cold; 3) Excess and Deficiency; and 4) Yang and Yin. The fourth pair, Yang and Yin, is often used for the category based on the Yin-Yang theory (Table 8.3). In other words, Exterior, Heat, and Excess belong to Yang, while Interior, Cold and Deficiency belong to Yin. Thus, the basic patterns of Eight Principles are Exterior, Interior, Heat, Cold, Excess and Deficiency. These six patterns are sometimes called the Six Root Patterns (*Liu Gen Zheng*).

Table 8.3: Eight Principles and Six Root Patterns

1ST PAIR PATTERNS	Exterior	Interior
2ND PAIR PATTERNS	Heat	Cold
3RD PAIR PATTERNS	Excess	Deficiency
CATEGORY	Yang	Yin

1. Exterior Pattern and Interior Pattern

This pattern pair is used to determine the location of a disease and the depth of the affected area. From a TCVM perspective, the Exterior refers to the skin, hair, muscles and the space between them as well as the superficial portion of the Meridians and Collaterals. The Interior refers to the Zang-Fu organs.

The Exterior Pattern can be further divided into four sub-patterns: Exterior Heat, Exterior Cold, Exterior Excess and Exterior Deficiency (Table 8.5).

Table 8.4: Differentiation of Exterior and Interior Patterns

Pair	Location	Signs
Exterior	Superficial Skin, hair, muscles Meridian pathways	• Early stage of disease • External attack of exogenous pathogens • Sudden onset of symptoms • A short course • Fever • Aversion to cold (contrary piloerection) • Cold shivers • Tongue: Thin coating • Pulse: Floating (superficial)
Interior	Internal organs	• Later disease stage due to exogenous pathogens • Internal emotional stress • Improper training or feeding program • A long course • Tongue: Thick coating or no coating • Pulse: Deep

Table 8.5: Differentiation and treatment of the four Exterior Patterns

Pattern	Differentiation	Treatment Strategy	Acupoints	Herbal Examples and Formula
Exterior Cold	Clear nasal discharge Severe cold shivering Tongue: Pale Coating: Thin Pulse: Slow	Clear Wind-Cold	BL-10, GB-20 GV-16 Tian-men	Cinnamon *Gui Zhi* *Gui Zhi Tang*
Exterior Heat	Thick nasal discharge Cough Tongue: Red Coating: Thin Pulse: Rapid	Clear Wind-Heat	LI-4, LU-5, LI-11	Mentha *Bo He* *Yin Qiao San*
Exterior Excess	No sweating Fever Tongue: Red Pulse: Forceful	Clear the Exterior	GV-14, LI-11 *Er Jian* (Ear Tip)	Ephedra *Ma Huang* *Ma Huang Tang*
Exterior Deficiency	Sweating General weakness Tongue: Pale Pulse: Weak, floating	Tonify Qi, Clear the Exterior	LU-7 TH-5 *Da Feng Men*	Astragalus *Huang Qi* Ledebouriella *Fang Feng* *Yu Ping Feng San*

2. Cold Pattern and Heat Pattern

The Cold and Heat Patterns are used to determine the nature or property of a disease. A Cold Pattern can be divided into Exterior Cold and Interior Cold. Exterior Cold is discussed in Table 8.5. Interior Cold can be further divided into Excess Cold and Deficiency Cold. The Excess Cold Pattern is often caused by the direct invasion of Cold such as drinking ice water. Pathogenic Wind-Cold can also invade the body thus resulting in an Excess Cold Pattern. The Deficiency Cold Pattern is often caused by a Yang Deficiency.

The Heat Pattern is divided into Exterior Heat and Interior Heat. The Interior Heat is then divided into Excess and Deficiency Heat Patterns (Table 8.8). Excess Heat is mainly caused by the invasion of Wind-Heat, Summer Heat, or Dryness-Heat. It is sometimes caused by the Stagnation of food, which turns into Heat in the Stomach. Less frequently, Excess Heat develops as a result of transformation from the external attack of Wind-Cold. On the other hand, Deficiency Heat is due to the Yin Deficiency that arises during a prolonged course of a disease or during the later stages of a febrile disease.

3. Deficiency Pattern and Excess Pattern

The Deficiency and Excess Patterns are used to determine strength of the Zheng Qi (the body's resistance to diseases) and the presence or absence of pathogens. A Deficiency of Zheng Qi resulting from overwork, loss of blood, or chronic illness, often causes the Deficiency Pattern. There are four types of Deficiency Patterns: Qi, Blood, Yin and Yang Deficiency Pattern. The general symptoms of a Deficiency Pattern may include dry or burned hair, emaciation, lassitude, exercise intolerance, limb or back weakness, general weakness, pale tongue, no coating, and weak pulse. The differentiation of these four Deficiency Patterns is summarized in Table 8.6. The Qi Deficiency Pattern is related to the Lung, Heart, Spleen and Kidney. The Blood Deficiency Pattern is related to the Liver, Spleen and Heart. A Yin Deficiency Pattern is similar to a Deficiency Heat Pattern (Table 8.8), and a Yang Deficiency Pattern is similar to a Deficiency Cold Pattern (Table 8.8).

The Excess Pattern is characterized by the presence of pathogens. The pathogens include the six exogenous Xie Qi: Wind, Cold, Dampness, Summer Heat, Dryness and Fire/Heat. The pathogens can also include secondary pathological products such as food stasis, blood stagnation and phlegm. The Excess Patterns often present as hyperfunctional states. The signs include high fever, rapid breath, hyper-excitation, abdominal fullness or pain, constipation, a red or deep red tongue, a thick tongue coating and an excessive or surging pulse.

4. Yin and Yang

The categories of Yin and Yang within the Eight Principles have two meanings. In a general sense, Yin and Yang are used to guide and summarize the three other pairs of Principles. Exterior, Heat and Excess Pattern belong to the category of Yang, while Interior, Cold and Deficiency Pattern belong to the category of Yin. In a special sense, Yin and Yang are also used in conditions of depletion or collapse. In this case, they are called Yin Pattern and Yang Pattern separately.

Yin Pattern and Yang Pattern

The Yin Pattern refers to the clinical signs of chronic illness, coldness, inactivity, weakness, and depression or to the inward and downward nature of a condition that results from a Deficiency of the Zheng Qi and retention of the Xie Qi. As a matter of fact, it is a consolidation of the Cold Pattern and the Deficiency Pattern. Its primary manifestations include dry hair, emaciation, listlessness, preference for lying down, cold trunk and limbs, shivering, watery saliva, loose feces, large amounts of clear urine, pale mouth and tongue, white and wet tongue coating, and slow and weak pulse. A Yin Pattern following surgical or traumatic diseases may include such signs as swelling without pain or heat and watery pus without a foul smell.

The Yang Pattern refers to clinical signs that include acute, febrile, active, excited, hyperfunctional or hypermetabolic states or the outward and upward nature of a condition. This results from the hyperactivity of Yang Qi in the body and excessive pathogenic Heat. In fact, the Yang Pattern includes the Heat Pattern and the Excess Pattern. Its primary manifestations are hyper-excitation, restlessness, fever, excessive thirst, rapid breathing, hot trunk and limbs, oral ulcers, constipation, scanty and concentrated urine, red and dry mouth and tongue, dry and yellow tongue coating, and surging pulse. A Yang Pattern following surgical or traumatic diseases may include such signs as red, hot, painful swellings and thick, malodorous pus.

Yin Collapse and Yang Collapse

Yin or Yang Collapse simply indicates an extremely severe state of a Deficiency Pattern. It also implies a complete separation of Yin and Yang from each other, and it is often followed by death.

Yin Collapse is caused by the further aggravation of a Yin Deficiency Pattern. This may occur when there is severe vomiting and diarrhea or a great loss of Blood and high fever with excessive sweating (sweat loss). Hyper-excitation, restlessness, profuse and sticky sweating, warm nose and ears, excessive thirst, shortness of breath, dry and red mouth or tongue, and weak pulse may accompany Yin Collapse.

Yang Collapse results from the further aggravation of a Yang Deficiency by profuse sweating, severe diarrhea, or a great loss of Blood. Listlessness, depression, muscle fasciculations or shivering, profuse and watery sweating, cool ears and nose, no thirst, weak respiration, pale or green-purple mouth and tongue with moisture, and very weak pulse may accompany Yang Collapse.

Summary

In summary, the Exterior and Interior Patterns are used to differentiate the location of a disease. The Heat and Cold Patterns are used to differentiate the nature or properties of a disease. The Excess and Deficiency Patterns can determine the strength or weakness of the Zheng Qi and identify the existence of Xie Qi.

Table 8.6: Differentiation of Deficiency Patterns

Pattern	Differentiation	Treatment Strategy	Treatment
Qi Deficiency	• Spontaneous sweating • Short of breath or cough • Loss of appetite • Loose stool • Exercise intolerance • Prolapse of uterus or rectum • Frequent urination • Infertility or incontinence • Tongue: Pale, wet • Pulse: Weak	Tonify Qi	ST-36, CV-4, CV-6, CV-17 *Si Jun Zi Tang* (Four Gentlemen)
Blood Deficiency	• Dull eyes • Easily frightened • Weakness in tendons • Crack lines in the hoof wall • Tongue: Pale, dry • Pulse: Thready, soft	Nourish Blood	SP-10, SP-6, BL-17 *Si Wu Tang* (Four Substances)
Yin Deficiency	Similar to Deficiency Heat Pattern (Table 8.8)		
Yang Deficiency	Similar to Deficiency Cold Pattern (Table 8.8)		

Table 8.7: Summary of the three pattern pairs of the Six Roots

Pattern	Six Roots	Involvement	Characteristics
1st Pair	Exterior	Skin, hair, muscles and the superficial portion of the Meridians and Collaterals	The location of a disease
	Interior	The Zang-Fu organs	
2nd Pair	Heat	Caused by Pathogenic Heat/Fire. Major signs include fever, inflammation, infection, red tongue, fast pulse	The nature of a disease
	Cold	Caused by Cold/Damp Pathogen. Major signs include coldness, purple or pale tongue, slow pulse	
3rd Pair	Excess	Six exogenous Pathogens (Wind, Damp, Cold, Heat, Dryness, Summer Heat), pain, constipation, stagnation, phlegm, acute injury	The conflict between Zheng Qi and Xie Qi
	Deficiency	Weakness of Zheng Qi. Qi Deficiency, Blood Deficiency, Yin Deficiency, Yang Deficiency	

Table 8.8: Differentiation of the Cold and Heat Patterns

Primary Pattern		Sub-Pattern	Signs	Treatment Strategy Acupoints Herbal formula
Cold	Exterior Cold		Same as Table 8.5	
	Interior Cold	Excess Cold	• Cold ear and nose • Cold limbs • Loud intestinal peristalsis • Colic • Tongue: Purple, wet • Pulse: Deep, slow	Warm the Interior, Disperse Cold GV-4, BL-21, BL-20 (Moxibustion) *Gui Xin San*
		Deficiency Cold	• Cold nose and ears • Cold trunk and limbs • Lassitude • Loss of appetite • Diarrhea with undigested food • Edema or clear long urination • Tongue: Pale purple, • Coating: Thin or none • Pulse: Deep, slow, weak	Tonify and Warm the Interior, Disperse Cold GV-3, *Bai Hui*, BL-36 (Moxibustion) *Li Zhong Tang*
Heat	Exterior Heat		Same as Table 8.5	
	Interior Heat	Excess Heat	• Fever • Hot nose and ears • Rapid respiration • Dry feces • Scanty and dark urine • Thirsty • Tongue: Red, dry • Coating: Yellow • Pulse: Rapid and surging	Clear Heat LI-4, LI-11, LI-20, GV-14 *Huan Lian Jie Du Tang*
		Deficiency Heat	• Weariness • Prolonged low fever or afternoon fever • Dry and small feces • Scanty dark urine • Tongue: Red, dry • Coating: Less or none • Pulse: Thready, rapid	Nourish Yin, Clear Heat KID-3, SP-6, KID-7 *Zhi Bai Di Huang Tang*

Table 8.9: Differentiation between Excess (*Shi*) Pattern and Deficiency (*Xu*) Pattern

Parameter	Excessive Signs	Deficient Signs
Course of illness	Acute (or new)	Chronic (prolonged)
Constitution	Strong (mostly)	Must have weakness
Age	< 6 years	> 10 years
Appearance	Hyperactive	Depression
Voice	Loud	Weak
Massage or Touch Preference	No	Yes
Fever	High (>2° F)	Low (<1.5° F) or no fever
Cold Shivers	No change after warming	Alleviated with warming
Tongue Color	Purple or red	Pale or red
Tongue Coating	Thick	None or Little
Pulse	Forceful	Weak
Nodule or Enlargement	Yes	No
Excess Pattern	4 or more excess signs	—
Deficiency Pattern	—	4 or more deficient signs
Excess with Deficiency Pattern	2 or more excess signs + 2 or more deficient signs	

Zang-Fu Patterns

This system is also known as "Pattern Identification according to the Zang-Fu Organs". Because it is based on the pathological manifestations and physiological functions of the Zang-Fu organs, Zang-Fu Pattern identification is used to analyze the clinical data and to determine the location, nature and Pattern of a Zang-Fu organ's disease.

The Zang-Fu Patterns originated from the *Huang Di Nei Jing* (*Yellow Emperor's Internal Classic*) published in the Warring States period (475 to 221 BC). Later, TCM practitioners during the Han, Jin, Sui and Tang dynasties further developed these patterns. *Zhu Bing Yuan Hou Lun* (*General Treatise on Etiology and Symptomology of Disease*), which was written by Chao Yuan-Fang and published in 610 AD, described 1,739 different types of Zang-Fu Patterns. *Zhong Zang Jing* (*Treasury Classic*) recorded the well-known Hua Tuo's TCM diagnostic system.

Regardless of the complexity of the clinical signs or the variability of the Patterns, the mechanisms of a disease are attributed to one of the Zang-Fu Organs. For instance, one may identify a Yin Deficiency Pattern according to the Eight Principles, but this is related to the Heart, Lung, Kidney, Liver or Spleen. To get the best treatment results, an exact organ should be identified as the primarily affected system by using the Zang-Fu Pattern Identification method.

Zang-Fu Pattern identification works well together with the Eight Principles in order to form a TCVM diagnosis. In general, the Eight Principles (Six Roots) may first classify a disease as either an Excess or a Deficiency Pattern. The Pattern is then further associated with one of the Zang-Fu organs. This produces a useful diagnosis that will form the foundation of the subsequent treatment plan.

CLINICAL SKETCH: A thirteen-year-old, spayed, female German Shepherd named "Max" was diagnosed with spondylosis at L7-S1 and right hip dysplasia based on radiographic findings. She had shown weakness of her back as well as rear limb lameness and weakness for three years. She became worse recently. Her tongue was pale and wet. Her pulse was very weak, slow and deep. She preferred to sleep in warm places such as carpet, and she loved massage. Using the Eight Principles, the preference for warmth, the chronic nature of the illness, the weak pulse and the pale tongue identify Max's condition as a Yang Deficiency. Further investigation is needed to develop a better treatment plan; thus, the next step requires identification of the Zang-Fu organ involved. Because the Kidney controls the bones and because the lower back is the house of the Kidney, the Kidney is considered the major organ associated with Max's disease. Thus, the final diagnosis for Max is Kidney Yang Deficiency (Figure 8.1).

The Zang-Fu syndromes form the core of TCVM diagnosis. Even though there are twelve organs, the most significant of these are the five Yin organs. This is sometimes known as the Five systems as based upon the Five Elements. These five systems are the Heart, Lung, Spleen, Liver, and Kidney systems.

Heart System: Cardiovascular, Central Nervous System, mental

Lung System: Respiratory, skin, immune

Spleen System: Alimentary tract, immune, muscular, endocrine and metabolic

Liver System: Hepatobiliary, eyes, endocrine, metabolic, ligaments and tendons, hooves/paws

Kidney System: Reproductive, renal, bone and joints, endocrine, and metabolic

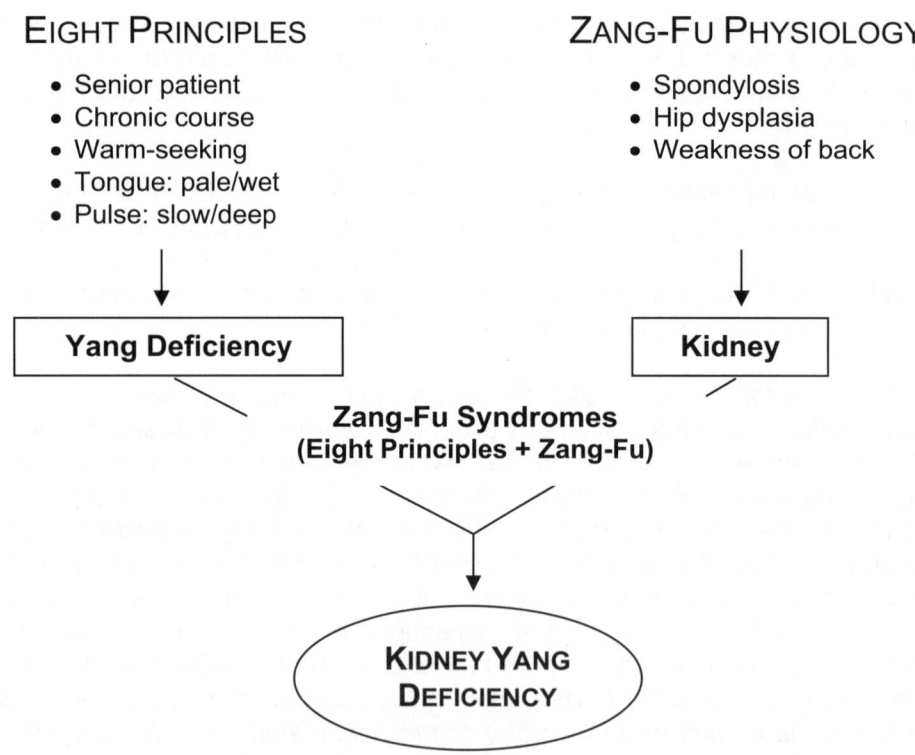

Figure 8.1: Eight Principles and Zang-Fu Patterns in TCVM Diagnosis

PATTERNS OF THE HEART AND SMALL INTESTINE

The Heart rules the whole body, governs blood circulation, houses the Shen and controls sweating. Pathological changes of the Heart will be associated with those physiological activities. Since the Small Intestine (SI) is the "husband" (Yang organ) of the Heart and belongs to the Fire system, Small Intestine pathology is also discussed along with the Heart pathology.

Eight Principles	Zang-Fu Syndromes (Pattern)
Deficiency	Heart Qi Deficiency
	Heart Yang Deficiency
	Heart Blood Deficiency
	Heart Yin Deficiency
Excess	Extreme Heart Heat
	Phlegm Obstructing Mind
	Phlegm-Fire Disturbing Heart
	Heart Blood Stagnation
	Colic due to Small Intestine Cold

Excess Patterns

1. Extreme Heart Heat

Etiology

This may occur when the Six Excessive Qi invade the body and accumulate in the Interior where they turn into Heat or Fire in the Heart. It may also happen when herbal medicines that tonify Yang Qi are incorrectly administered.

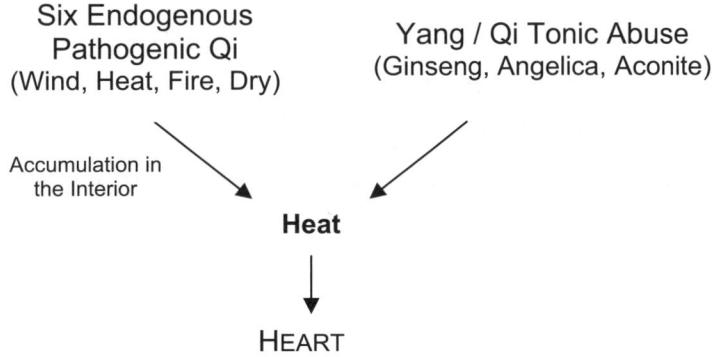

Clinical Signs

In general, Extreme Heart Heat may produce the following signs:

- High fever
- Profuse sweating
- Rapid breathing
- Excessive thirst and drinking
- Mental restlessness

- Dry feces
- Scanty, dark urine or bloody urine
- Dry mouth or stomatitis
- Deep red mouth and tongue
- Surging and rapid pulse

TCVM Diagnosis and Analysis

This is an Excess Heat Pattern; therefore, a high fever, rapid breathing, a deep red tongue, and a surging, rapid pulse are characteristic of this condition. As Heat tends to consume the body fluids (Yin), Excess Heat results in thirst, dry feces, scanty urine and dry mouth. Stomatitis arises when the Heat flares up.

Because the Heart controls sweating and houses the Shen (Mind), Excessive Heat in the Heart tend to cause excessive secretion of sweat and to disturb the Shen. For this reason, profuse sweating and restlessness are also common clinical signs. Heart Heat easily transfers into the Small Intestines where it affects the water metabolism during the separation process and leads to dark, bloody urine.

Treatment Principles

- Eliminate Heart Fire
- Calm the Shen
- Nourish Yin
- Promote urination

The principle of eliminating Heart Fire/Heat directly addresses the underlying Heat Pattern. Calming the Shen relieves the secondary Shen disturbance due to Heat/Fire. Similarly, nourishing Yin can benefit body fluids which may be damaged by the excess Heat. By promoting urination, it is possible to drain some of the Heat.

Acupuncture Treatment*

Clear Heart Fire: *Xiong Tang*, HT-3, HT-9 (HA), SI-1 (HA), LI-11, ST-39

Nourish Yin: SP-6, KID-3, BL-15, HT-7

Calm Shen: *An Shen*, PC-6, PC-7, HT-5, HT-6, HT-7, BL15

*Note: HA indicates hemoacupuncture. Moxa indicates moxibustion. EA indicates electroacupuncture

Chinese Herb Examples

Eliminate Heart Fire:	Coptis	*Huang Lian*
	Gardenia	*Zhi Zi*
	Forsythia	*Lian Qiao*
	Bambusa	*Zhu Ye*
Calm Shen:	Polygala	*Yuan Zhi*
	Zizyphus	*Suan Zao Ren*
	Biota	*Bai Zi Ren*
	Schisandra	*Wu Wei Zi*
Nourish Heart Yin:	Rehmannia	*Sheng Di Huang*
	Ophiopogon	*Mai Men Dong*
	Lily	*Bai He*
	Scrophularia	*Xuan Shen*
	Glehnia	*Sha Shen*
	Asparagus	*Tian Men Dong*
Promote urination:	Lophatherum	*Dan Zhu Ye*
	Akebia	*Mu Tong*
	Talcum	*Hua Shi*

Herbal Formula Example

Xi Xin San (Clearing Heart Powder)

2. Phlegm-Fire Disturbing Heart (Wind Pattern due to Heart Heat)

Etiology

This occurs when the first Pattern, Extreme Heart Heat, becomes worse or when the Qi and Blood become stagnant for long periods of time. They transform into Fire, which boils off the Body Fluid and leaves phlegm behind to disturb the Shen.

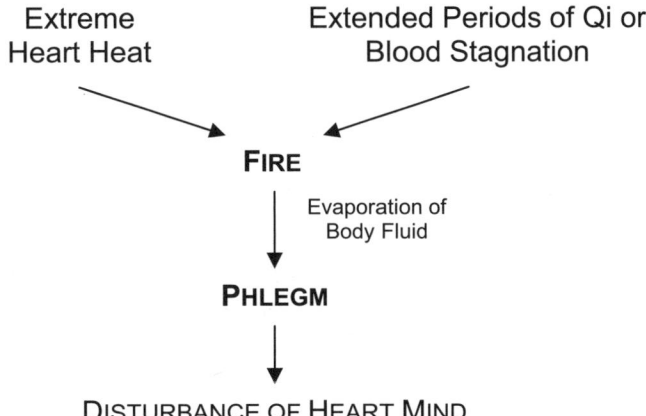

Clinical Signs

The Phlegm-Fire Heart Disturbance Pattern may produce the following signs:

- Easily frightened
- Aimless running
- Slippery and rapid pulse
- Yellow, greasy coating
- Quickly eating then immediately stopping eating
- Biting its own thorax or knee (Self-mutilation)
- Aggressively attacking humans or animals
- Deep red mouth and tongue

TCVM Diagnosis and Analysis

This is a Heart Excess Fire/Heat Pattern with the addition of Heat Phlegm. Heat Phlegm disturbs the Shen. As a result, the clinical signs include various neurologic and behavioral abnormalities such as aimless running, startling easily, quickly starting and ceasing to eat, self-mutilation and aggressive behavior.

Due to the Heart Fire/Heat, the pulse is rapid, the tongue is deep red, and the coating of tongue is yellow. A slippery pulse and a greasy coating of the tongue reflect the Phlegm.

Treatment Principles

- Eliminate the Heart Fire and Phlegm
- Calm the Shen (Mind)
- Open the orifice

Eliminating the Heart Fire and Phlegm directly manages the underlying cause. Calming the Shen is used to address the major clinical signs. Opening the orifice of the Heart wakes up the Shen and smoothes the Heart Channel to facilitate Phlegm removal.

Acupuncture Treatment

Clear Heart Fire:	*Xiong Tang*, HT-3, HT-9 (HA), SI-1 (HA), LI-11, ST-39
Transform Phlegm:	ST-40, BL20/21, SP-1, PC-5
Calm Shen:	*An Shen*, PC-6, PC-7, HT-5, HT-6, HT-7, BL15
Open the Orifice:	GV-26, CV-8 (moxa), LU-11, *Da Feng Men*

Chinese Herb Examples

Eliminate Heart Fire:	See above	
Calm Heart Mind	See above	
Eliminate Heat Phlegm:	Fritillaria	*Bei Mu*
	Arisaema	*Tian Nan Xing*
	Bambusa	*Zhu Ru*
Open the Orifice:	Musk	*She Xiang*
	Borneol	*Bing Pian*

Herbal Formula Examples

There are two options available. The first herbal formula, *Zhu Sha San* (Cinnabar Powder), is used for mild symptoms. The second formula, *Zhen Xin San* (Calming-Heart Powder), is used for severe signs.

3. Heart Blood Stagnation

Etiology

Blood Stagnation may result from Heat or overexercise which injures Blood Vessels or by Cold or Qi Deficiency which slows the circulation of the Blood.

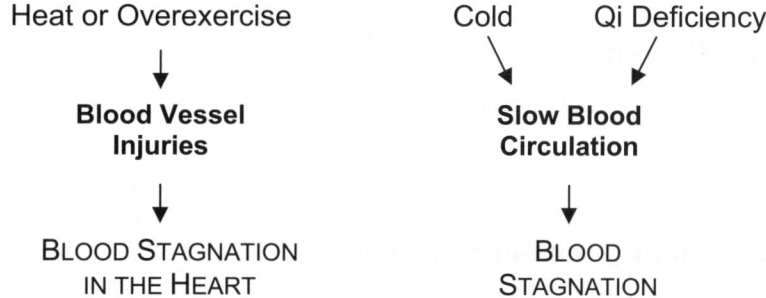

Clinical Signs

In general, the signs of Heart Blood Stagnation may include the following:

- Lameness
- Palpitations
- Shortness of breath
- Chest pain (sensitive to palpation of the chest)
- Irregular and tight pulse
- Purple tongue with petechiae

TCVM Diagnosis and Analysis

This Pattern is Blood Stagnation in the Heart. The chest pain, lameness and purple tongue with petechiae all reflect the presence of Blood Stagnation. Blood Stagnation can block the Heart Qi which leads to palpitations, shortness of breath and irregular pulses.

Treatment Principles

- Activate Blood
- Disperse Stagnation
- Promote the flow of Qi to stop pain

Acupuncture Treatment

Activate Blood; Disperse Stagnation: *Xiong Tang*, BL-14, BL-15, BL-17, HT-9, SI-1

Move Qi to stop pain: LI-11, LI-4, ST-36, BL-60, LIV-3

Chinese Herb Examples

Activate Blood:	Ligusticum	*Chuan Xiong*
	Angelica	*Dang Gui*
	Olibanum	*Ru Xiang*
	Myrrh	*Mo Yao*
	Salvia	*Dan Shen*

Promote Qi Flow:	Citrus	*Chen Pi*
	Citrus	*Qing Pi*
	Magnolia	*Hou Po*
	Aurantium	*Zhi Ke*
	Fennel	*Hui Xiang*
	Areca	*Bing Lang*

Herbal Formula Example

Xue Fu Zhu Yu Tang (Blood Mansion Stagnation Powder)

4. Phlegm Obstructing the Mind (Shen)

Etiology

This may develop when there is Cold-Damp in the Channel (Meridian) which hinders the Qi flow. This prevents effective distribution of Water-Damp; thus, Water-Damp condenses in the Channel and becomes Phlegm. This causes obstruction of the Heart Mind, which disturbs the mental activities.

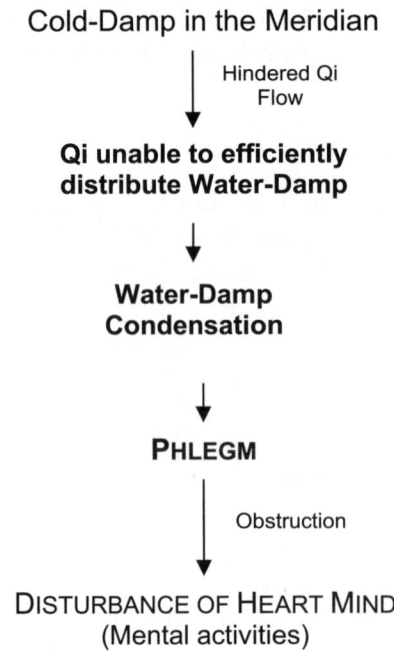

Clinical Signs

In general, Phlegm Obstructing the Mind may produce the following signs:

- Foamy saliva
- Disorientation
- Slow and slippery pulse

- Mental depression or dullness
- Pale mouth with a white, sticky coating
- Ataxia or uncoordinated movements like a drunkard
- Sudden collapse and coma

TCVM Diagnosis and Analysis

This condition is due to obstruction of the Heart by Cold Phlegm. This blocks or mists the Shen. Consequently, the patient displays mental dullness (depression), disorientation, ataxia, sudden collapse or coma. The slippery pulse, foamy saliva and sticky coating are indications of Phlegm. A slow pulse and pale tongue with a white coating indicate Cold.

Treatment Principles

- Eliminate Cold Phlegm
- Open the Orifice

Acupuncture Treatment

Warm Cold: *Bai Hui*, GV-4 (moxa)

Transform Phlegm: ST-40, BL20/21, SP-1, PC-5

Open the Orifice: GV-26, CV-8 (moxa), LU-11, *Da Feng Men*

Chinese Herb Examples

Eliminate Cold Phlegm: Pinellia   *Ban Xia*
                         Arisaema   *Tian Nan Xing*
                         Typhonium   *Bai Fu Zi*

Open the Orifice: See above

Herbal Formula Examples

Er-Chen Tang Modification (Two-old-Herbs Powder)

5. Colic due to Small Intestine Cold

Etiology

Pathogenic Cold enters the body through sudden changes of weather, prolonged exposure to cold wind and water, or drinking profuse quantities of cold water. The Cold enters the Small Intestine where it obstructs the flow of Qi and causes colic.

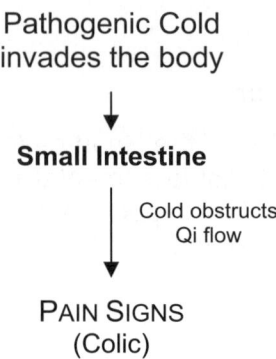

Pathogenic Cold
invades the body

↓

Small Intestine

Cold obstructs
Qi flow

↓

PAIN SIGNS
(Colic)

Clinical Signs

This Pattern may involve enterospasm or diarrhea due to Cold. The signs of colic associated with Small Intestine Cold may include the following:

- Cold nose and ears
- Cold shivers
- Slow and deep pulse
- Diarrhea
- Pale and purple tongue
- Loud sound of intestinal peristalsis
- Abdominal pain (a horse alternately lies down and stands up, looks at the abdomen, etc.)

TCVM Diagnosis and Analysis

This Pattern is Cold Stagnation in the Small Intestines. Cold ears and nose, cold shivers, a pale purple tongue and a slow deep pulse are all Cold signs. Cold slows the Qi Flow and subsequently causes blockage in the Small Intestine. Since it is said that "where there is blockage, there must be pain", abdominal pain occurs as a result of Cold. As the body's Yang Qi fights and expels the Cold, loud gut sounds and diarrhea may occur.

Treatment Principles

- Warm the Middle-Jiao and Expel Cold
- Activate Blood and Promote Qi Flow

The Small Intestines are located in the Middle Jiao; thus, warming the Middle-Jiao can warm the Small Intestines and dispel the Cold. Activating Blood and promoting Qi Flow improves the circulation of Qi and Blood and relieves the pain.

Acupuncture Treatment

Warm Middle-Jiao and Eliminate Cold: *Bai Hui*, GV-3, GV-4, CV-8, CV-12 (moxa)

Activate Blood and Promote Qi Flow: LIV-3, LI-11, LI-10, ST-36, ST-39

Chinese Herb Examples

Warm the Middle-Jiao and Eliminate Cold:	Cinnamon	*Rou Gui*
	Ginger	*Gan Jiang*
	Evodia	*Wu Zhu Yu*
	Atractylodes	*Cang Zhu*
	Dahurian Angelica	*Bai Zhi*
	Asarum	*Xi Xin*
Activate Blood:	Curcuma	*Yu Jin*
	Angelica	*Dang Gui*
	Moutan	*Mu Dan Pi*
	Paeonia	*Chi Shao Yao*
Promote Qi Flow:	Citrus	*Chen Pi*
	Aurantium	*Zhi Shi*
	Magnolia	*Hou Po*
	Cyperus	*Xiang Fu*

Herbal Formula Example

Ju Pi San (Tangerine-Peel Powder)

Deficiency Patterns

There are four Deficiency Patterns for the Heart. Since there are numerous similarities between the Heart Qi and Heart Yang Deficiency Patterns as well as between the Heart Blood and Yin Deficiency Patterns, these two groups are listed together.

1. Heart Qi Deficiency and Heart Yang Deficiency

Etiology

This may be due to the gradual decline of the Heart Qi associated with a long illness or old age or to the damage of Heart Qi or Yang with an abrupt severe sweating and diarrhea. Heart Yang Deficiency is a more severe condition that progresses from a Heart Qi Deficiency. Heart Yang Collapse is a further procession of a Heart Yang Deficiency.

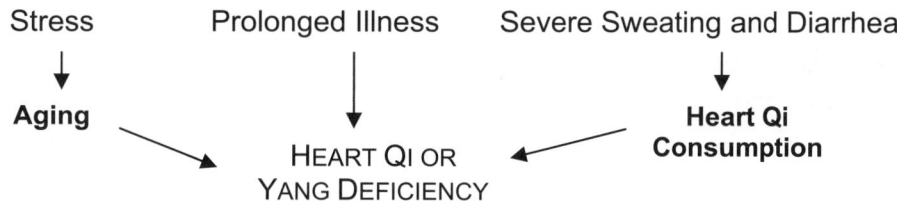

Clinical Signs

In general, Heart Qi and Yang Deficiencies may produce the following signs:

- Shortness of breath or palpitations
- Spontaneous sweating
- Increased severity of signs with movement
- Weak pulse or irregularly / regularly intermittent pulse
- Pale or purple tongue

TCVM Diagnosis and Analysis

These signs are consistent with a Heart Qi or Yang Deficiency Pattern. Shortness of breath, palpitations, a weak pulse and a pale tongue reflect a Qi Deficiency. Because deficient Heart Qi fails to control sweating, this condition may lead to spontaneous sweating. This occurs during the daytime especially because the day belongs to Yang. Movement consumes Qi and can exasperate the clinical signs. When Yang is deficient, there is a decrease in the internal warming system, thus it generates a state of internal Cold, which is evidenced by a purple tongue.

Clinical Differentiation

From a clinical perspective, a Heart Yang Deficiency is similar to a Heart Qi Deficiency with Cold signs.

Heart Qi Deficiency:	Listlessness, lassitude Pale tongue with white coating
Heart Yang Deficiency:	Coolness of ears, nose, trunk and limbs Feeble breathing Pale or purple tongue Weak pulse
Heart Yang Collapse:	Disappearance of pulse or coma

Treatment Principles

Heart Qi Deficiency:
- Tonify Heart Qi
- Calm the Mind

Heart Yang Deficiency:
- Warm Heart Yang
- Calm the Mind

Heart Yang Collapse:
- Resuscitation of Yang from collapse

Acupuncture Treatment

Heart Qi Tonic:	CV-14, CV-6, CV-17, PC-6, ST-36
Heart Yang Tonic:	*Bai Hui*, GV-4, GV-14, GV-20 (moxa), CV-4, CV-14
Yang Resuscitation:	GV-26, *Wei Jian* (tail tip, HA), CV-8 (moxa)
Calm Shen:	*An Shen*, PC-6, PC-7, HT-5, HT-6, HT-7, BL-15

Chinese Herb Examples

Tonify Heart Qi:	Codonopsis	*Dang Shen*
	Astragalus root	*Huang Qi*
	Ginseng	*Ren Shen*
Warm Heart Yang:	Aconite	*Fu Zi*
	Cinnamon	*Rou Gui*
	Cinnamon	*Gui Zhi*
	Ginger	*Gan Jiang*
Calm the Mind (Shen):	Polygala	*Yuan Zhi*
	Zizyphus	*Suan Zao Ren*
	Biota	*Bai Zi Ren*
	Schisandra	*Wu Wei Zi*

Herbal Formulas

Heart Qi Deficiency:
- *Yang Xin Tang* (Tonifying-Heart Powder)

Heart Yang Deficiency:
- *Bao Yuan Tang* (Protecting Heart Powder)

Heart Yang Collapse:
- *Shen Fu Tang* (Ginseng Aconite Decoction)

2. Heart Blood Deficiency and Heart Yin Deficiency

Etiology

This may occur when there is a weak body constitution, a traumatic Blood loss, a prolonged disease or a post-parturition condition. Heart Blood and Yin mutually support and nourish each other. A Heart Blood Deficiency can transform into a Heart Yin Deficiency or a Yin Deficiency may become a Blood Deficiency.

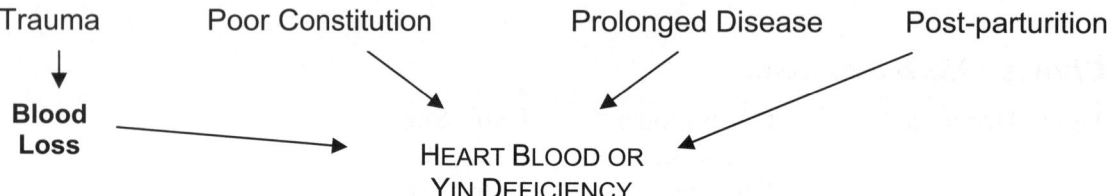

Clinical Signs

In general, Heart Blood and Yin Deficiencies may produce the following signs:
- Palpitations
- Restlessness
- Easily frightened

TCVM Diagnosis and Analysis

These signs are typical of a Heart Blood or Heart Yin Deficiency Pattern. Palpitations reflect a Heart Deficiency in general. Because both Heart Blood and Yin nourish the Shen, a Deficiency of either Heart Blood or Heart Yin deprives the Shen of nourishment. Consequently, the animal becomes restless and will frighten easily.

Clinical Differentiation

Heart Blood Deficiency: Pale mouth and tongue
Thready and weak pulse

Heart Yin Deficiency: Prolonged low fever or afternoon fever
Night sweating or restlessness at night
Dry, red mouth and tongue
Ulcer on the tongue
Thready and rapid pulse

Treatment Principles

Heart Blood Deficiency:
- Nourish Heart Blood
- Calm Shen

Heart Yin Deficiency:
- Nourish Heart Yin
- Calm Shen

Acupuncture Treatment

Heart Blood Tonic: BL-15, BL-17, SP-6, SP-10, ST-36, HT-7

Heart Yin Tonic: KID-3, KID-6, BL-17, PC-6, HT-7

Calm Shen: PC-6, PC-7, HT-5, HT-6, HT-7, BL-15

Chinese Herb Examples

Nourish the Heart Blood:	Angelica	*Dang Gui*
	Rehmannia	*Shu Di Huang*
	Polygonum	*He Shou Wu*
	Paeonia	*Bai Shao Yao*
Nourish Heart Yin:	Rehmannia	*Sheng Di Huang*
	Ophiopogon	*Mai Men Dong*
	Lily	*Bai He*
	Scrophularia	*Xuan Shen*
	Glehnia	*Sha Shen*
	Asparagus	*Tian Men Dong*
Calm the Mind (Shen):	Polygala	*Yuan Zhi*
	Zizyphus	*Suan Zao Ren*
	Biota	*Bai Zi Ren*
	Schisandra	*Wu Wei Zi*

Herbal Formula Examples

Heart Blood Deficiency:
- *Gui Pi Tang* (Heart & Spleen Tonic Powder)

Heart Yin Deficiency:
- *Bu Xin Dan* (Nourishing-Heart Powder)

Summary

There are four Heart Deficiency Patterns and four Excess Heart Patterns. Congestive heart failure, behavioral problems (Shen disturbance), hypertension, cardiac arrhythmia, Mitral Valvular Insufficiency Complex, and Cardiomyopathy Complex may be differentiated and treated based upon those Patterns.

Patterns Associated with Major Cardiovascular Diseases

Congestive Heart Failure Complex:
1. Obstruction of Heart by Blood Stasis
2. Phlegm Obstruction of the Orifices
3. Accumulation of Yin Cold
4. Deficiency of Heart and Kidney Yin
5. Deficiency of Qi and Yin
6. Exhaustion of Yang Qi

Hypertension Patterns:
1. Deficiency of Yin and Profusion of Yang
2. Profusion of Liver Fire
3. Obstruction by Phlegm Dampness
4. Deficiency of Both Yin and Yang

Cardiac Arrhythmia (Palpitation) Patterns:
1. Deficiency of Heart and Gallbladder Qi
2. Deficiency of Heart Blood
3. Deficiency of Yin with Upflaming of Fire
4. Deficiency of Heart Yang
5. Oppression of the Heart by Water and Phlegm-Fluid
6. Obstruction of the Heart by Blood Stasis

Mitral Valvular Insufficiency Complex:
(Evolving Progressive Syndrome)

1. Heart Blood Deficiency
2. Heart Qi Deficiency
3. Heart Yin Deficiency
4. Heart Yang Deficiency
5. Phlegm Obstructing the Orifices
6. Heat in the Heart
7. Chest Bi-Obstruction of Qi in the Chest

Cardiomyopathy Complex:
(Evolving Progressive Syndrome)

1. Emotional Stress, Hereditary Cardiac Weakness
2. Spleen Qi deficient
3. Heart Blood deficient
4. Palpitations
5. Heart Yin deficient
6. Heart Qi deficient
7. Lung Damp
8. Qi deficient

PATTERNS OF LUNG AND LARGE INTESTINE

The Lung dominates Qi and respiration, regulates the water pathway, and controls the body surface. The pathological changes of the Lung affect those physiological activities. Since the Large Intestine belongs to the Metal system and is the "husband" (Yang) organ of the Lung, Large Intestine pathology is also discussed along with Lung pathology.

Eight Principles	Zang-Fu Syndromes (Pattern)
Deficiency	Lung Qi Deficiency
	Lung Yin Deficiency
	Lung Yin & Qi Deficiency
	Lung Qi & Kidney Qi Deficiency
Excess	Invasion of Lung by Wind Cold
	Invasion of Lung by Wind Heat
	Dryness-Heat Impairing Lung
	Cough and Asthma due to Lung Heat
	Large Intestine Food Accumulation
	Large Intestine Damp-Heat
	Diarrhea due to Large Intestine Cold

Excess Patterns

1. Invasion of Lung by Wind Cold

Etiology

The Wind-Cold invades the Lung via the Lung Channel. It then impairs the ascending and descending functions of the Lung.

Clinical Signs

The clinical signs of Wind Cold invasion of the Lung may include the following:

- Cough or sometimes asthma
- Worse cough with exposure to cold and less coughing while warm
- Sneezing, nasal obstruction, watery nasal discharge
- Aversion to cold
- Pale purple tongue with a thin white coating
- Superficial (floating) pulse

TCVM Diagnosis and Analysis

This Pattern is considered a Wind Cold or Exterior Cold Pattern. It may occur during the course of the common cold, acute bronchitis or chronic bronchitis. The cough and asthma indicate Lung involvement in this condition. Nasal congestion results from Wind-Cold obstruction of the entryway (nasal passages) into the Lung system. When the Wei Qi tries to expel the Pathogens, sneezing and nasal discharge develop. If the Cold Pathogen combines with Damp, the nasal discharge will have a watery consistency. Both the pale purple tongue with a thin white coating and the floating, slow pulse reflect the presence of a Wind-Cold Pattern.

Treatment Principles

- Disperse Wind-Cold
- Eliminate phlegm and Stop cough

Dispersing the Wind-Cold will treat the underlying cause of disease. Since it is said that "where there is cough, there must be Phlegm", transformation of the Phlegm can stop the cough.

Acupuncture Treatment

Disperse Wind-Cold: LU-7, LI-1, GB-20, BL-10, BL-12

Eliminate phlegm and stop cough: ST-40, BL-13, *Ding Chuan*, CV-22

Chinese Herb Examples

Disperse Wind-Cold:	Ephedra	*Ma Huang*
	Cinnamon	*Gui Zi*
	Schizonepeta	*Jing Jie*
	Ledebouriella	*Fang Feng*
Eliminate phlegm and stop cough:	Pinellia	*Ban Xia*
	Citrus	*Chen Pi*
	Apricot	*Xing Ren*
	Aster	*Zi Wan*

Herbal Formula Example

Zhi Sou San (Cough-stopping Powder)

2. Invasion of Lung by Wind-Heat

Etiology

Wind Heat invades the Lung via the Lung Channel and nasal passages, and then it impairs the ascending and descending functions of the Lung.

Clinical Signs

The signs of Lung Wind Heat invasion may include the following:

- Cough
- Yellow, thick nasal discharge
- Swollen, painful throat
- Fever with warm nose and ears
- Red tongue with white or yellow, thin coating
- Rapid and superficial pulse

TCVM Diagnosis and Analysis

This is a type of Wind-Heat Pattern which may occur during the course of Influenza, acute bronchitis or pharyngolaryngitis. Wind-Heat may lead to obstruction which can impair the ascending and descending functions of the Lung. This leads to coughing and nasal discharge. Since Heat tends to damage blood vessels, the nasal discharge will be bloody or yellow. Heat also tends to dry up fluids so the nasal discharge will be thick. The Wind-Heat Pathogen follows the Lung Channel to the throat, which is called the gate of the Lung system because it is the starting place of the Lung Channel's External Branch. A rapid, superficial pulse and a red tongue with thin coating both reflect a Wind-Heat condition.

Treatment Principles

- Clear Wind-Heat
- Open the body surface to benefit the Lung

The principle of clearing the Wind-Heat is intended to treat the underlined cause. Opening the surface can benefit the Lung's ascending and descending functions and relieve the secondary problems such as cough or asthma.

Acupuncture Treatment

Disperse Wind-Heat: LI-4, LI-11, LU 10, GV-14, GB-20, BL-12

Open the surface to benefit Lung: LU-6, LU-7, BL-13

Chinese Herb Examples

Eliminate Wind-Heat:

Bupleurum	Chai Hu
Mentha	Bo He
Chrysanthemum	Ju Hua
Arctium	Niu Bang Zi
Forsythia	Lian Qiao

Open the surface to benefit Lung: Platycodon   Jie Geng

Herbal Formula Example

Yin Qiao San (Lonicera-Forsythia Powder)

1. With serious fever add:	Gardenia	*Zhi Zi*
	Scutellaria	*Huang Qin*
	Gypsum	*Shi Gao*
2. With a sore, swollen throat add:	Isatis	*Ban Lan Gen*
	Belamcanda	*She Gan*
3. With thirst add:	Trichosanthes	*Tian Hua Fen*

3. Dryness-Heat Impairing Lung

Etiology

Wind-Dryness-Heat invades the Lung Channel and enters the Lung where it impairs the ascending and descending function of the Lung.

Clinical Signs

The signs of Dryness-Heat impairing the Lung may include the following:

- Dry cough without sputum
- Dry skin and hair, dry mouth
- Thirst
- Fever or aversion to cold
- Red tongue with thin or thick coating
- Superficial or thready and rapid pulse

TCVM Diagnosis

This is Exterior Dryness-Heat in the Lung system. This may occur during the course of the common cold or acute bronchitis. Coughing occurs because the Pathogen impairs the ascending and descending function of the Lung. The Pathogens Dryness and Heat tend to damage body fluids (Yin) and consequently lead to dry cough, dry skin, and thirst. The fever, red tongue, thick tongue coating, rapid pulse all indicate a Heat condition. Since this illness is still in the Exterior stage, the pulse feels superficial.

Treatment Principles

- Moisten the Lung
- Eliminate Dryness-Heat

Acupuncture Treatment

Eliminate Dryness-Heat and Moisten Lung: BL-13, LU-7, KID-3, KID-7, KID-6

Chinese Herb Examples

Eliminate Dryness-Heat and Moisten the Lung:	Mulberry	*Sang Ye*
	Eriobotrya	*Pi Pa Ye*
	Phragmites	*Lu Gen*
	Anemarrhena	*Zhi Mu*
	Asparagus	*Tian Men Dong*

Herbal Formula Example

Qing Zao Jiu Fei Tang (Eliminating-Lung-Dryness Powder)

4. Cough and Asthma due to Lung Heat

Etiology

Wind-Heat (or Wind-Cold that transforms into Wind-Heat) invades the Lung via the Lung Meridian. Within the Lung, it transforms into Heat which impairs the ascending and descending functions of the Lung.

Clinical Signs

The common signs of a Lung Heat Pattern may include the following:

- Cough with loud and clear sound, rapid breath
- Yellow, thick, malodorous nasal discharge
- Sore, swollen throat
- Dry feces, scanty urine, thirst and much drinking
- Deep red mouth with dry and yellow coating
- Surging and rapid pulse

TCVM Diagnosis and Analysis

This is an Interior Lung Heat Pattern. This Pattern may occur during the course of acute bronchopneumonia, pharyngolaryngitis, or suppurative pneumonia. The Pathogen impairs the ascending and descending functions of the Lung which leads to coughing. A yellow, thick nasal discharge, a sore throat, a deep red tongue with a yellow coating, and a surging, rapid pulse indicate a Heat Pattern. Because Heat tends to consume body fluids, dry feces, scanty urine, thirst may occur in Heat conditions.

Treatment Principles

- Eliminate Lung Heat
- Transform phlegm
- Stop cough and asthma

Acupuncture Treatment

Clear Lung Heat and Transform phlegm: LU-5, LU-6, LU-7, ST-40, LI-11, PC-5

Stop Cough and asthma: CV-22 (*Tian Tu*), *Ding Chuan*, LU-7, BL-13

Chinese Herb Examples

Eliminate Lung Heat:
Scutellaria	*Huang Qin*	
Gardenia	*Zhi Zi*	
Gypsum	*Shi Gao*	
Trichosanthes	*Tian Hua Fen*	

Eliminate Heat Phlegm:
Trichosanthes	*Gua Lou*
Fritillaria	*Bei Mu*
Bamboo shavings	*Zhu Ru*

Stop cough and asthma:
Apricot	*Xing Ren*
Ephedra	*Ma Huang*
Aristolochia	*Ma Dou Ling*
Aster	*Zi wan*

Herbal Formula Example

Qing Fei San (Clearing-Lung Powder)

5. Large Intestine Food Accumulation

Etiology

The Pattern may occur when an animal overeats subsequent to a period of starvation. In addition, sudden changes in the food, failure to drink water for a long time, or failure of older animals to thoroughly masticate food may lead to this condition.

Clinical Signs

This may occur during the course of constipation and may include the following:

- Constipation
- Halitosis
- Deep red tongue
- Yellow, thick tongue coating
- Abdominal fullness and pain (Turning the head to observe the abdomen; alternately standing up and lying down)
- Deep, surging pulse

TCVM Diagnosis and Analysis

This is a type of Large Intestine Interior Excess Pattern. It may occur during the course of impaction or constipation. Constipation, halitosis, or a thick tongue coating can indicate the presence of Food Accumulation. Food accumulation obstructs Qi flow and results in abdominal fullness and pain. A long-term obstruction of Qi flow (Stagnation) may transform into Heat, which leads to a deep red tongue with yellow coating and surging pulse.

Treatment Principles

- Purge accumulation from the intestines
- Promote Qi flow to stop pain

Acupuncture Treatment

Purge intestinal accumulation: ST-37, ST-25, GV-1, BL-21, SP-15

Promote Qi Flow to stop pain: ST-36, CV-12, LI-4, LIV-3

Chinese Herb Examples

Purge intestinal accumulation:	Rheum	*Da Huang*
Promote Qi flow:	Aurantium	*Zhi Shi*
	Magnolia	*Hou Po*
	Citrus	*Qing Pi*
	Cyperus	*Xiang Fu*

Herbal Formula Example

Da Cheng Qi Tang (Drastic-Purgative Powder)

6. Large Intestine Damp-Heat

Etiology

This condition may occur with invasion of Damp-Heat, eating dirty, contaminated, rancid food or ingestion of poisonous substances.

Clinical Signs

This Pattern may occur during the course of acute gastroenteritis and dysentery. The following signs may be observed:

- Fever
- Abdominal pain
- Dysentery with foul smell
- Bloody, mucoid feces
- Dry mouth

- Thirst
- Scanty urine
- Red and yellow tongue
- Yellow, greasy or dry tongue coating
- Slippery and rapid pulse

TCVM Diagnosis and Analysis

This is a Large Intestine Damp Heat Pattern which may occur during the course of acute gastroenteritis or dysentery. Fever, bloody feces, a red tongue with a yellow coating and a rapid pulse indicate the pathogen Heat. Heat tends to damage body fluids (Yin) and to cause dry mouth, thirst, and scanty urine. Mucoid feces, a yellow-colored tongue, a greasy tongue coating and a slippery pulse indicate the pathogen Damp. The combination of Damp and Heat can cause a Qi Flow blockage in the Large Intestines which leads to abdominal pain and dysentery. A foul odor of the feces indicates an Excess (Damp-Heat) condition.

Treatment Principles

- Eliminate Heat and Damp
- Activate Blood and promote Qi flow

Acupuncture Treatment

Eliminate Heat and Damp: ST-44, LI-11, SP-6, *Wei Jian, Qu Chi*

Activate blood and promote Qi flow: LIV-3, ST-36

Chinese Herb Examples

Eliminate Heat and Damp in the Large Intestine:	Pulsatilla	*Bai Tou Weng*
	Coptis	*Huang Lian*
	Phellodendron	*Huang Bai*
	Sophora	*Ku Shen*
Activate Blood:	Curcuma	*Yu Jin*
	Angelica	*Dang Gui*
	Moutan	*Mu Dan Pi*
	Paeonia	*Bai Shao Yao*

Herbal Formula Example

Yu Jin San (Curcuma Powder)

7. Diarrhea due to Large Intestine Cold

Etiology

This condition occurs due to invasion of Wind-Cold into the body or to over-eating of cold food or water.

Clinical Signs

This Pattern may occur during the course of intestinal catarrh. Some of the common signs include the following:

- Abdominal pain
- Abundant and clear urine
- Purple tongue
- White and greasy coating

- Cold nose and ears
- Loud intestinal peristalsis sounds
- Diarrhea (without ball-form in horses)
- Alternately normal and watery feces
- Deep and slow pulse

TCVM Diagnosis and Analysis

This is a Large Intestine Cold Pattern. A purple tongue, a white, greasy tongue coating, cold nose and ears, and a deep, slow pulse all indicate the Pathogen Cold. Cold tends to obstruct Qi flow which leads to abdominal pain. Cold also tends to hold Water-Damp which leads to a long stream of clear urine. As the body's Yang Qi tries to expel the Cold pathogen, it may secondarily cause watery diarrhea and an increase in the gut sounds.

Treatment Principles

- Warm the Middle-Jiao
- Eliminate Cold
- Eliminate Damp and excrete Water

Acupuncture Treatment

Warm the Middle-jiao and eliminate Cold: *Bai Hui*, GV-3, GV-4, CV-6 (moxa), SP-15

Eliminate Damp and excrete water: SP-6, SP-9

Chinese Herb Examples

Warm the Middle-Jiao and eliminate Cold:	Cinnamomum	*Rou Gui*
	Ginger	*Gan Jiang*
Excrete Damp and Water:	Poria	*Fu Ling*
	Polyporous	*Zhu Ling*

Herbal Formula Example

Wei Ling San (Stomach-poria Powder)

Deficiency Patterns

1. Lung Qi Deficiency

Etiology

Overwork and chronic illness (Spleen or Kidney Qi Deficiency) may eventually lead to Lung Qi Deficiency.

Clinical Signs

Some common signs of a Lung Qi Deficiency Pattern include the following:

- Reoccurring common colds
- Weak pulse
- Pale tongue
- Aversion to cold and wind
- Emaciation and lassitude
- Obvious groove along the costal arch (Heaves Line)
- Chronic clear nasal discharge
- Spontaneous sweating, especially during the day
- Weak, chronic cough or asthma that worsens with movement

TCVM Diagnosis and Analysis

This is a typical Lung Qi Deficiency Pattern. This condition may occur during the course of chronic bronchitis or chronic pulmonary emphysema.

When Lung Qi is deficient, it fails to perform its normal ascending and descending function which leads to the weak, chronic cough of asthma. Since movement or exercise requires Qi, activity draws upon the already deficient Qi source and makes the cough or asthma worse. The deficient Lung fails to controls the body surface, thus spontaneous sweating and reoccurring common colds are seen. Since the deficient Lung Qi fails to warm the body surface, the patient shows aversion to Cold and Wind. The "Heaves line" is a typical sign of severe Lung Qi Deficiency. When the Lung Qi is deficient, it tends to consume the Spleen Qi in a process known as "the deficient Child steals its mother's Qi". For this reason, emaciation and lassitude occur with Lung Qi deficiencies. The pale tongue and the weak pulse both reflect deficient Qi.

Treatment Principles

- Tonify Lung Qi
- Stop cough and asthma

Acupuncture Treatment

Lung Qi Tonic: CV-17, CV-6, *Bai Hui*, BL-13, LU-9
Stop cough and asthma: CV-22, LU-7, BL-13, *Ding Chuan*

Chinese Herb Examples

Lung Qi Tonic:	Codonopsis	*Dang Shen*
	Pseudostellaria	*Tai Zi Shen*
	Astragalus	*Huang Qi*
Stop cough and asthma:	Apricot	*Xing Ren*
	Ephedra	*Ma Huang*
	Aster	*Zi wan*

Herbal Formula Example

Bu Fei San (Tonifying-Lung Powder)

2. Lung Yin Deficiency

Etiology

Prolonged fever or illness, excessive sexual activities, and improper management (diet, work, and exercise) can all lead to Lung Yin Deficiency.

Clinical Signs

The signs of Lung Yin Deficiency Pattern may include the following:

- Sweating at night
- Thready and rapid pulse
- Red tongue
- Little to no tongue coating
- Dry mouth, nose, and hair coat
- Sticky, thick nasal discharge
- Cough or asthma that is worse at night than day
- Prolonged low fever or late afternoon fever
- Dry cough without sputum

TCVM Diagnosis and Analysis

This is Lung Yin Deficiency Pattern. This condition may occur during the course of chronic bronchitis or of some infectious diseases such as tuberculosis. Because the Lung Yin is deficient, there are insufficient body fluids to moisten the body. Thus, a dry cough, dry mouth, dry nose, and dry hair coat may result. As the night belongs to Yin and the Yin is deficient, sweating occurs at night and the cough/asthma worsens at night. When Yin is deficient, a false Heat occurs due to the decrease in the body's cooling source, and this leads to a prolonged low fever.

In addition, a Lung Yin Deficiency tends to cause a Kidney Yin Deficiency. This process is known as "the Mother's illness transmitted to the Child". The Kidney dominates the late afternoon (5 to 7 pm); thus, a fever occurs in the late afternoon when the Lung Yin is deficient. A red tongue with no coating and a thready, rapid pulse are indications of a Yin Deficiency.

Treatment Principles

- Nourish Yin
- Moisten the Lung

Acupuncture Treatment

Yin Tonic: KID-3, KID-6, BL-13, SP-6, SP-9, SP-10

Stop cough and asthma: CV-22 (*Tian Tu*), Ding Chuan, LU-7, BL-13

Chinese Herb Examples

Yin Tonic Herbs:	Lilium	*Bai He*
	Glehnia	*Sha Shen*
	Asparagus	*Tian Men Dong*
	Ophiopogon	*Mai Men Dong*
	Rehmannia	*Sheng Di Huang*
	Polygonatum	*Yu Zhu*

Stop cough and asthma:	Apricot	*Xing Ren*
	Ephedra	*Ma Huang*
	Aster	*Zi wan*

Herbal Formula Example

Bai He Gu Jin Tang (Lily Combination Powder)

3. Lung Yin and Qi Deficiency

Etiology

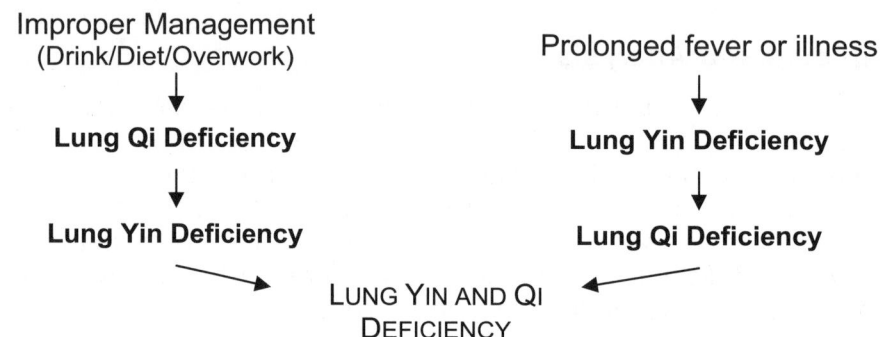

Clinical Signs

A Lung Yin and Qi Deficiency may include the following signs:

- Exercise intolerance
- Chronic cough
- Dry hair coat or dandruff
- Chronic nasal discharge and congestion
- Dry or wet mouth and pale or red tongue
- Thready and rapid or weak and deep pulse

TCVM Diagnosis and Analysis

This is a combination of a Lung Qi Deficiency and a Lung Yin Deficiency. This condition may arise when either a Lung Qi Deficiency or a Lung Yin Deficiency become worse. The clinical signs can be mixed. For example, the animal may have various combinations of a red, dry tongue (Yin Deficiency) with a deep, weak pulse (Qi Deficiency) or a red tongue with a rapid pulse (Yin Deficiency) or a wet tongue with a weak pulse (Qi Deficiency).

Treatment Principles

- Nourish Yin and Moisten the Lung
- Tonify Lung Qi
- Stop cough and asthma

Acupuncture Treatment

Yin Tonic:	KID-3, KID-6, BL-13, SP-6, SP-9, SP-10
Lung Qi Tonic:	CV-17, LU-9, CV-6, ST-36
Stop cough and asthma:	CV-22 (*Tian Tu*), *Ding Chuan*, LU-7

Chinese Herb Examples

Yin Tonic Herbs:	Lilium	*Bai He*
	Glehnia	*Sha Shen*
	Asparagus	*Tian Men Dong*
	Ophiopogon	*Mai Men Dong*
	Rehmannia	*Sheng Di Huang*
	Polygonatum	*Yu Zhu*

Stop cough and asthma:	Apricot	*Xing Ren*
	Ephedra	*Ma Huang*
	Aster	*Zi wan*

Herbal Formula Example

Bai He Gu Jin Tang (Lily Combination Powder) and *Bu Fei San* (Tonifying-Lung Powder)

4. Lung Qi and Kidney Qi Deficiency

Etiology

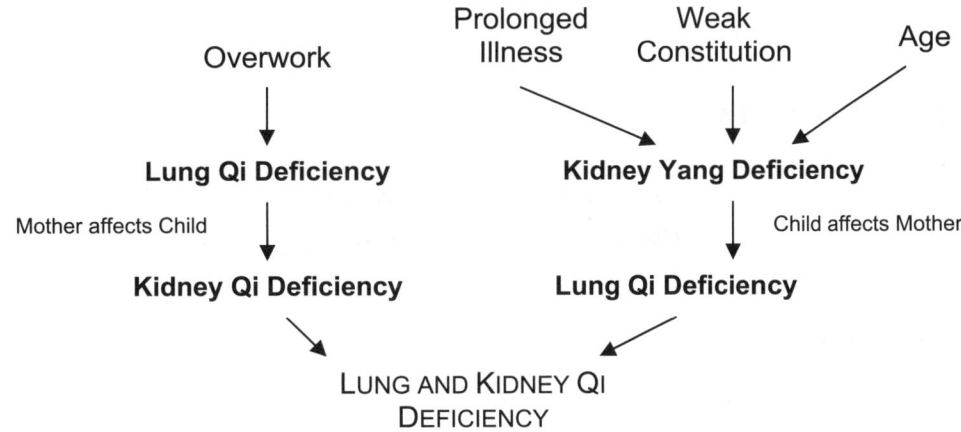

Clinical Signs

A Lung and Kidney Qi Deficiency may include the following signs:

- Lethargy and fatigue
- Cold limbs and trunk
- Prolonged cough or asthma
- Pale, swollen tongue
- Deficient and feeble pulse
- Rapid, weak breaths, worse with movement
- Chronic dyspnea, shortness of breath
- Difficult inhalation and exhalation, but it may be easier to inhale than to exhale or to exhale than to inhale

TCVM Diagnosis and Analysis

This is a combination of a Lung Qi Deficiency and a Kidney Qi Deficiency. The Qi Deficiency leads to lethargy, fatigue, a pale tongue and a feeble pulse. Deficient Qi fails to warm the body and leads to Yang Deficiency. For this reason, the limbs and trunk are cold and the tongue is swollen.

Normal breathing requires coordination between the Lung and the Kidney. The Lung dominates Qi and controls the inhalation and exhalation. The Kidney "grasps or receives" the Qi and helps the Lung inhale Qi. The Lung is the "Mother" of the Kidney, so a chronic Lung Qi Deficiency can lead to a Kidney Qi Deficiency. Deficient Kidney Qi fails to help the Lung with its respiratory functions, thus resulting in chronic dyspnea or prolonged asthma.

Treatment Principles

- Tonify Lung Qi
- Tonify Kidney Qi

Acupuncture Treatment

Lung Qi Tonic: CV-17, BL-13, LU-9

Kidney Qi Tonic: CV-4, CV-6; BL 23, Shen-Shu

Benefit Kidney Qi Reception: CV-17, CV-6, LU-7

Chinese Herb Examples

Lung and Kidney Qi Tonic: Gecko   *Ge Jie*

                               Schisandra *Wu Wei Zi*

                               Psoralea   *Bu Gu Zhi*

Herbal Formula Example

Ren Shen Ge Jie San (Ginseng-Gecko Powder)

Patterns Associated with Major Respiratory Diseases

Asthma (Heaves):
1. Invasion of Lungs by Wind-Cold
2. Phlegm-Heat Accumulation in Lung
3. Deficiency of Lung Qi
4. Deficiency of Lung and Kidney Qi

Nasal Congestion and Discharge:
1. Invasion of Lungs by Wind-Cold
2. Invasion of Lungs by Wind-Heat
3. Spleen and stomach Damp-Heat
4. Lung Qi Deficiency
5. Lung Yin Deficiency

Rhinitis:
1. Wind-Cold
2. Wind-Heat
3. Qi-Blood Stagnation
4. Stomach Damp-Heat
5. Lung Qi Deficiency
6. Lung Yin Deficiency
7. Kidney Yin Deficiency

Sinusitis:
1. Wind-Cold
2. Wind Heat
3. Heat-toxin
4. Stagnation
5. Damp-Heat

Nasal Bleeding:
1. Lung and Stomach Heat
2. Liver Yang Rising
3. Spleen Qi Deficiency
4. Lung Yin Deficiency

Pneumonia:
1. Wind-Heat in the Lung
2. Lung Extreme Heat
3. Lung Qi Deficiency
4. Lung Yin Deficiency

Acute Bronchitis:
1. Wind-Cold Cough
2. Wind-Heat Cough

Chronic Bronchitis:
1. Lung Qi Deficiency Cough
2. Lung Yin Deficiency Cough
3. Spleen-Lung Deficiency Cough

Acute Laryngitis:
1. Wind Cold
2. Wind Heat

Chronic Laryngitis
1. Lung Heat
2. Lung Yin Deficiency
3. Blood Stagnation
4. Phlegm Stagnation
5. Lung-Spleen Qi Deficiency

Sore Throat:
1. Invasion of Lungs by Wind-Heat
2. Excess Lung and Stomach Heat
3. Depletion of Lung and Kidney Yin

PATTERNS OF SPLEEN AND STOMACH

Spleen Qi transports and transforms food and water, and it should always rise. Stomach Qi receives, ripens and rots the food/drink, and it should always go down. The Spleen favors dryness and fragrance. Any Damp such as a rainy or damp environment will damage the Spleen Qi. Considering that Earth is the child of Fire, Spleen Qi requires fire to "cook" and to digest food; however, cold damages the Spleen Yang (warming capacity). Cold and Damp are the worst problems that the Spleen may encounter, and they greatly impair the Spleen's function.

Some Spleen Patterns may be the result of Spleen disorders combined with other organ diseases:

1. Spleen-Lung Qi Deficiency or Spleen disorders which lead to Lung disorders (Child to Mother)

2. Spleen Yang Deficiency with Kidney Yang Deficiency

3. Spleen Qi Deficiency with Heart Blood Deficiency

4. Disharmony between Liver and Spleen

Eight Principles	Zang-Fu Syndromes (Pattern)
Deficiency	Spleen Qi Deficiency
	Spleen Qi Sinking
	Spleen Not Controlling Blood
	Spleen Yang Deficiency
	Stomach Yin Deficiency
Excess	Accumulation of Cold-Damp in Spleen
	Accumulation of Damp-Heat in Spleen
	Stomach Cold Pattern
	Stomach Heat Pattern
	Stomach Food Retention

Excess Patterns

1. Accumulation of Cold-Damp in Spleen

Etiology

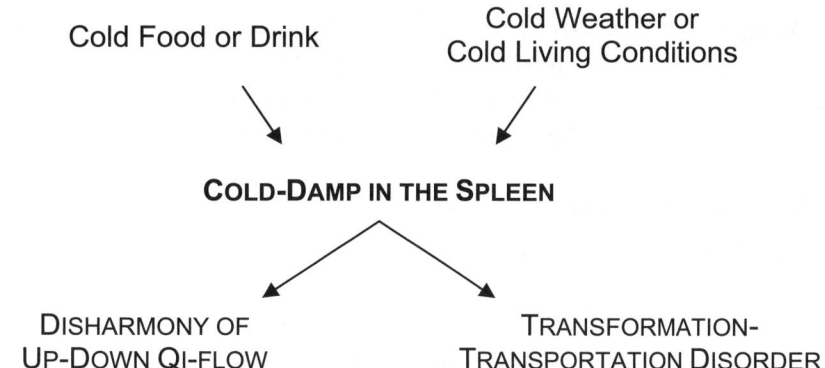

Cold Food or Drink   Cold Weather or Cold Living Conditions

COLD-DAMP IN THE SPLEEN

DISHARMONY OF UP-DOWN QI-FLOW   TRANSFORMATION-TRANSPORTATION DISORDER

Clinical Signs

Cold-Damp Accumulation in the Spleen may produce the following signs:

- Lassitude
- Loss of appetite
- Loose stool

- No thirst
- Swelling
- White, greasy tongue coating
- Soft, slow pulse

TCVM Diagnosis and Analysis

This Pattern is caused by an accumulation of Cold and Damp in the Spleen. The Pathogens Cold and Damp tend to obstruct the Qi flow of the Spleen leading to lassitude, loss of appetite, and loose stool. A lack of thirst, swelling, a white, greasy tongue coating, and a soft, slow pulse reflect the presence of Cold and Damp.

Treatment Strategy

- Warm the Middle-Jiao to dispel Cold
- Eliminate Damp

Acupuncture Treatment

Warm middle jiao to disperse Cold: *Bai Hui*, GV-4, ST-25 (moxa)

Transform Damp: CV-9, *Fen Shui* (horse), SP-6, SP-9, ST-36

Chinese Herb Examples

Warm the Middle-Jiao and eliminate Cold:	Cinnamon	*Rou Gui*
	Dry Ginger	*Gan Jiang*
	Galanga	*Gao Liang Jiang*
	Evodia	*Wu Zhu Yu*
Eliminate Damp:	Poria	*Fu Ling*
	Alisma	*Ze Xie*
	Polyporus	*Zhu Ling*
	Plantago	*Che Qian Zi*

Herbal Formula Example

Wei Ling San (Stomach Poria Powder)

2. Accumulation of Damp-Heat in the Spleen

Etiology

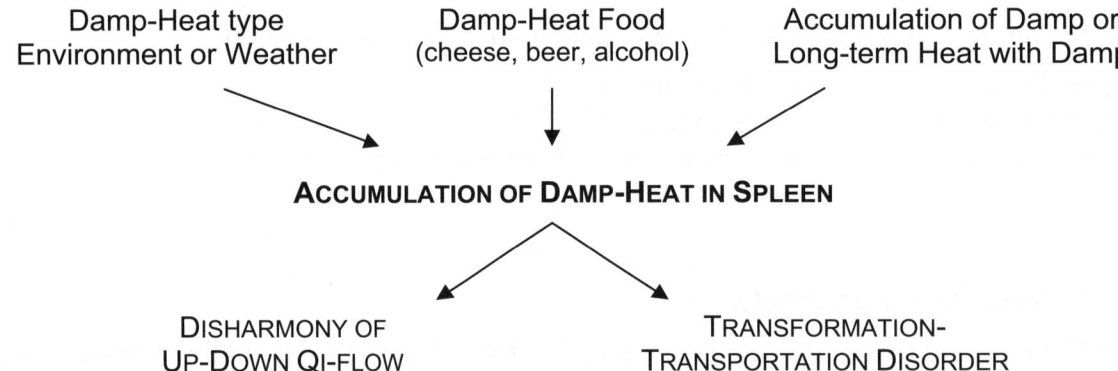

Clinical Signs

Damp-Heat Accumulation in the Spleen may produce the following signs:

- Lassitude
- Weariness
- Loss of appetite
- Yellow or red tongue
- Yellow and short urination
- Thick, greasy, yellow tongue coating
- Soft, rapid pulse
- Loose stool with a foul odor

TCVM Diagnosis and Analysis

This condition is caused by the accumulation of Damp and Heat in the Spleen. The accumulation of Damp-Heat in the Spleen may occur during the course of chronic indigestion or acute indigestion or as a secondary problem to enteritis.

Damp tends to obstruct the Spleen Qi Flow leading to lassitude, weariness, loss of appetite and loose stool. Heat is consistent with inflammation, thus the stool has a foul odor. A short, yellow urine stream, a red tongue, a yellow tongue coating and a rapid pulse are indications of Heat, but a yellow tongue, a greasy tongue coating, and a soft pulse indicate Damp.

Treatment Strategies

Damp-Heat in the Spleen: Eliminate Heat and Damp

Acupuncture Treatment

Clear Damp-Heat: SP-9, SP-6, LI-11, BL-18, BL-20

Chinese Herb Examples

Clear Damp-Heat: Coptis   *Huang Lian*
                   Phellodendron *Huang Bai*
                   Scutellaria   *Huang Qin*
                   Gardenia   *Zhi Zi*

Herbal Formula Example

Huang Lian Jie Du Tang (Coptis Detoxifying Powder)

3. Stomach Cold Pattern

Etiology and Clinical Signs

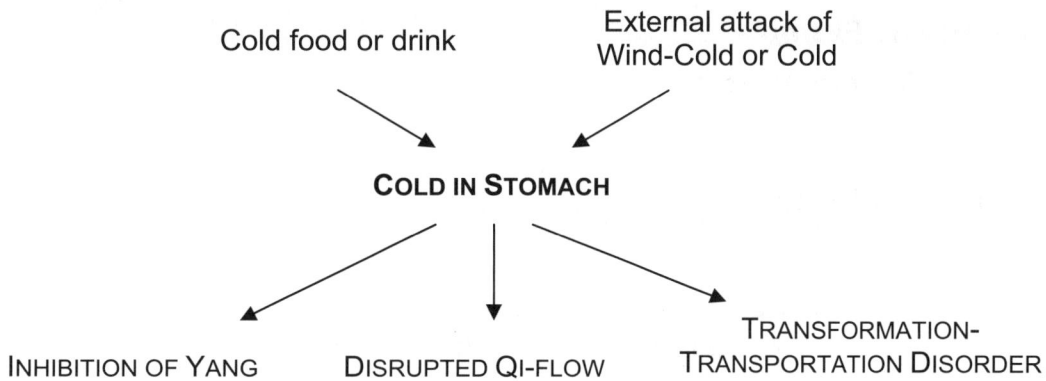

Clinical Signs

A Stomach Cold Pattern may produce the following signs:

- Coldness of lips and mouth
- Aversion to cold
- Abdominal pain, colic
- Loss of appetite
- Loose stool
- Too much saliva
- Long, clear urination
- Pale, purple tongue with white, greasy coating
- Deep, slow pulse
- Increase in intestinal peristalsis (loud gut sounds)

TCVM Diagnosis and Analysis

This is a Stomach Cold Pattern. Cold in the Interior (Stomach) leads to coldness of the body surface (lips and mouth) and aversion to cold. Cold slows down and blocks the Qi flow of the Stomach which leads to Stomach Qi Stagnation and abdominal pain (colic). The Stomach fails to receive food which causes the appetite loss. The Yang Qi tries to dispel the pathogen Cold resulting in loud gut sounds and loose stool. Cold tends to carry water, leading to excess saliva and long, clear urine streams. A pale, purple tongue; a white, greasy tongue coating; and a deep, slow pulse reflect a Cold Pattern.

Treatment Principles

* Warm the Middle-jiao to dispel Cold
* Regulate the Stomach to move Qi

Acupuncture Treatment

Warm Middle-jiao to disperse Cold: *Bai Hui*, GV-4 (moxa)

Regulate Stomach to move Qi: ST-36, LI-10, BL-21

Chinese Herb Examples

Regulate the Stomach to move Qi: Citrus   *Chen Pi*

     Pinellia   *Ban Xia*

Warm the Middle-jiao to dispel Cold: Cardamon   *Sha Ren*

     Cluster   *Bai Dou Kou*

Herbal Formula Example

Gui Xin San (Cinnamon Powder)

4. Stomach Heat Pattern

Etiology

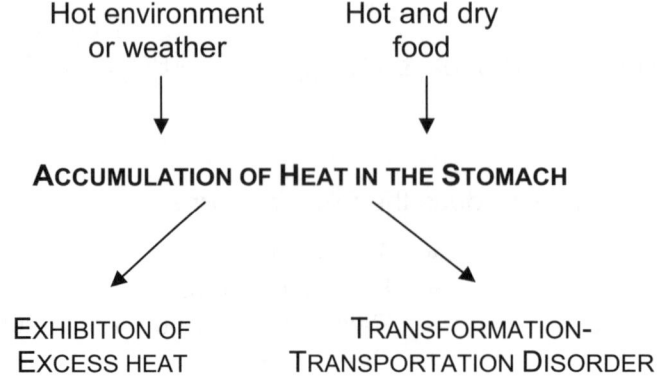

Hot environment or weather   Hot and dry food

ACCUMULATION OF HEAT IN THE STOMACH

EXHIBITION OF EXCESS HEAT   TRANSFORMATION-TRANSPORTATION DISORDER

Clinical Signs

A Stomach Heat Pattern may produce the following signs:

- Hot lips and mouth
- Bad smell from mouth
- Thirsty
- Red tongue
- Dry nose or dry feces
- Yellow tongue coating
- Surging, rapid pulse
- Loss of appetite or ravenous appetite

TCVM Diagnosis and Analysis

This is a Stomach Heat Pattern. The accumulation of Heat in the Stomach results in hot lips and mouth as well as a bad odor from the mouth. The Stomach fails to receive food, which can lead to a loss of appetite or to a ravenous appetite. The animal keeps eating and drinking in an attempt to cool down the Stomach. Heat tends to consume the body fluids leading to a dry nose and dry feces. A red tongue, a yellow tongue coating, and a surging, rapid pulse reflect a Heat Pattern.

Treatment Strategies

- Clear the Stomach Heat/Fire
- Generate Body Fluid to stop thirst

Acupuncture Treatment

Clear Stomach Fire: *Shan Gen*, *Yu Tang*, ST-45 (HA)

Body Fluid Tonic: KID-3, SP-6, SP-9

Chinese Herb Examples

Clear the Stomach Fire:

Gypsum	*Shi Gao*
Anemarrhena	*Zhi Mu*
Lophatherum	*Dan Zhu Ye*
Coptis	*Huang Lian*

Generate Body Fluid to stop thirst:

Phragmites	*Lu Gen*
Trichosanthes	*Tian Hua Fen*
Glehnia	*Sha Shen*

Herbal Formula Example

Bai Hu Tang (White-Tiger Powder)

5. Stomach Food Retention

Etiology

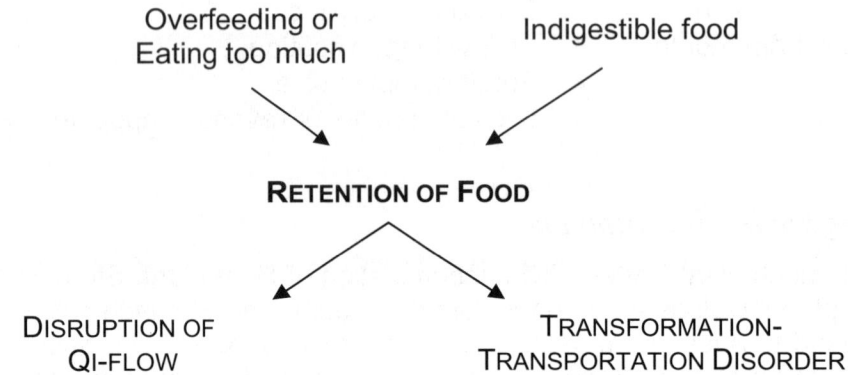

Clinical Signs

Stomach Food Retention may produce the following signs:

- Abdominal pain (colic)
- No appetite
- Loose or dry stool

- Red, dry tongue
- Thick, greasy tongue coating
- Slippery pulse

TCVM Diagnosis and Analysis

Food stasis (food retention) in the Stomach blocks Qi Flow which leads to abdominal pain (colic). Because the Stomach has no room to receive food, the animal suffers a loss of appetite. If the retained food stagnates for an extended time, it may then transform into Heat. This results in dry feces and a red, dry tongue. Loose stool develops as the Yang Qi tries to dispel the food stasis. A thick, greasy coating and a slippery pulse reflect Food Stasis.

Treatment Strategies

- Promote digestion and resolve stagnated food
- Purge accumulation from the intestines

Acupuncture Treatment

Horse:

Yu Tang	Promote appetite and clear food stasis
Guan Yuan Shu (BL-21)	Promote gastrointestinal motility
BL-20	Strengthen Spleen
Mi Jiao Gan	Promote appetite
ST-36	Regulate Middle-jiao, general tonic

Dog or Cat:

Shan Gen	Promote appetite and clear food stasis
GV-1	Regulate Spleen and Stomach
GV-6	Regulate middle jiao
BL-21	Strengthen Spleen
BL-20	Strengthen Stomach
ST-36	Tonify Spleen and Stomach

Chinese Herb Examples

Promote digestion:	Hawthorn	*Shan Zha*
	Medicated leaven	*Shen Qu*
	Germinated barley	*Mai Ya*
	Radish	*Lai Fu Zi*
Resolve stagnated food:	Saussurea	*Mu Xiang*
	Magnolia	*Hou Po*
	Aurantium	*Zhi Shi*
	Areca	*Bing Lang*
Purge accumulation from the intestines:	Rhubarb	*Da Huang*
	Mirabilite	*Mang Xiao*
	Rush-cherry seed	*Yu Li Ren*

Herbal Formula Examples

There are two Chinese herbal formulas. *Qu Mai San* is recommended for horses and cattle. *Bao He Wan* is recommended for dogs and cats.

Deficiency Patterns

1. Spleen Qi Deficiency

Etiology

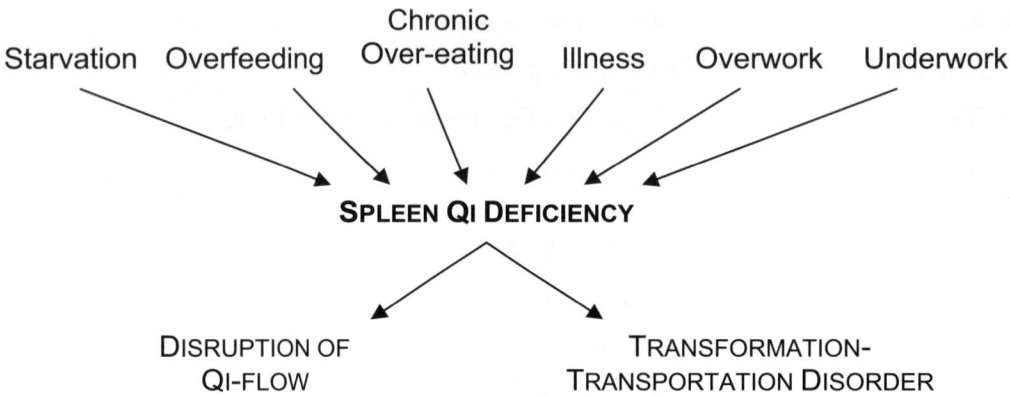

Clinical Signs

A Spleen Qi Deficiency may produce the following signs:

- Loss of appetite
- Loose stool
- Lassitude, fatigue
- Weak pulse
- Poor quality of hair follicles
- Dry and yellow hair coat
- Pale tongue
- Emaciation, loss of body weight

TCVM Diagnosis and Analysis

When the Spleen Qi is deficient, taste is lost resulting in a loss of appetite. Deficient Spleen Qi fails to transport and transform food and to direct the *Gu Qi* (nutrients) upward. The nutrients go downward instead and cause loose stool. Furthermore, Qi and Blood lack their source of regeneration. As a result, the limbs, muscles, and hair follicles lack nourishment, which results in fatigue, emaciation, and poor hair follicle quality. The pale tongue and weak pulse reflect a Qi Deficiency.

Treatment Strategies

- Tonify Qi
- Strengthen the Spleen

Acupuncture Treatment

Spleen Qi Tonic: ST-36, BL-20/21, CV-6, SP-9, SP-1

Chinese Herb Examples

Tonify Qi and Strengthen the Spleen:

Codonopsis	*Dang Shen*
Atractylodes	*Bai Zhu*
Diascorea	*Shan Yao*
Poria	*Fu ling*

Herbal Formula Example

Shen Ling Bai Zhu San (Ginseng and Atractylodes Combination Powder)

2. Spleen Qi Sinking

Etiology

Prolonged period of Spleen
Qi Deficiency

↓

SPLEEN FAILS TO HOLD THE
INTERNAL ORGANS

Clinical Signs

This condition has Spleen Qi Deficiency signs plus the following signs:

• Prolonged diarrhea
• Prolapse of anus or rectum
• Prolapse of vagina or uterus
• Dribbling or dripping urine

TCVM Diagnosis and Analysis

This condition occurs when a Spleen Qi Deficiency becomes worse. Deficient Spleen Qi fails to hold the internal organs, which leads to anal, rectal, vaginal or uterine prolapse. Prolonged Spleen Qi Deficiency may affect the Qi Flow (*Qi-hua*) of the Kidney thus resulting in dribbling urine. When deficient Spleen Qi is sinking, the associated diarrhea may be more severe.

Treatment Strategies

• Tonify and strengthen the Spleen Qi
• Raise the Spleen Qi

Acupuncture Treatment

Spleen Qi Tonic: BL-20/21, CV-6, SP-9, ST-36

Raising Spleen Qi: GV-1, *Gang Tui*, GV-20

Chinese Herb Examples

Raise Spleen Qi: Bupleurum   *Chai Hu*
                          Cimicifuga   *Sheng Ma*

Herbal Formula Example

Bu Zhong Yi Qi Tang (Central Qi Tonic Powder)

3. Spleen Yang Deficiency

Etiology

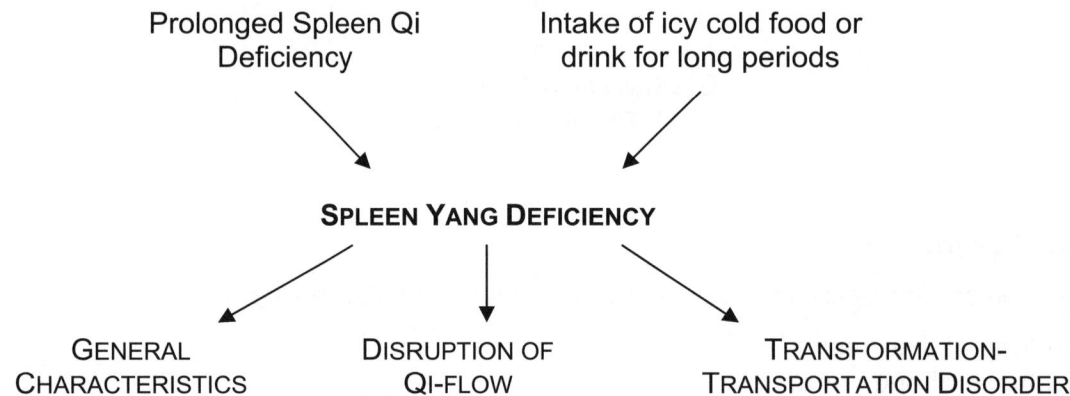

Clinical Signs

A Spleen Yang Deficiency can cause the following signs:

- Cold trunk and ears
- Warm-seeking
- Abdominal pain (Colic)

- Poor appetite, loose stool
- Excessive moisture in mouth
- Pale, purple tongue
- Slow, weak pulse

TCVM Diagnosis and Analysis

This is Spleen Yang Deficiency Pattern. Deficient Yang fails to warm the body; thus, the body surface is cold, and the patient seeks warm places to rest. Yang Deficiency generates Interior Cold which blocks Qi Flow and leads to abdominal pain. Since a Spleen Qi Deficiency is a part of a Spleen Yang Deficiency, the clinical signs include poor appetite and loose stool. Because a deficient Spleen fails to transform Water-Damp and Cold tends to hold water, a Spleen Yang Deficiency results in excess moisture in the mouth. A pale, purple tongue and a slow, weak pulse reflect a Yang Deficiency.

Treatment Strategies

- Warm the Middle-jiao to dispel Cold
- Tonify Qi to strengthen the Spleen

Acupuncture Treatment

Spleen Qi Tonic: BL-20/21, SP-6, CV-6, SP-9

Warm Middle-jiao to disperse cold: *Bai Hui*, GV-4 and CV-8 (Moxa)

Chinese Herb Examples

Warm the Middle-jiao to dispel Cold

Cinnamon	*Rui Gui*
Dry Ginger	*Gan Jiang*
Evodia	*Wu Zhu Yu*

Tonify Qi and Strengthen the Spleen:

Codonopsis	*Dang Shen*
Atractylodes	*Bai Zhu*
Diascorea	*Shan Yao*

Herbal Formula Example

Li Zhong Tang (Warming Middle Powder)

4. Spleen Not Controlling Blood

Etiology

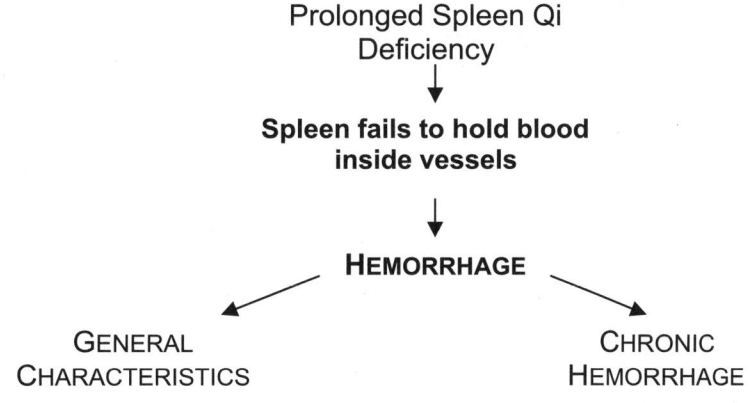

Clinical Signs

Spleen's failure to hold blood can result in the following signs:

- Feeble pulse
- Bloody feces, color
- Bloody urine
- Bloody spots under skin
- Hemorrhage is dark and chronic
- Very pale or white tongue
- General signs of Spleen Qi Deficiency

TCVM Diagnosis and Analysis

Spleen Qi Deficiency can progress to this condition. Severely Deficient Spleen Qi fails to hold blood inside vessels and leads to chronic hemorrhage. The very pale tongue and feeble pulse reflect a severe Spleen Qi Deficiency.

Treatment Strategies

- Tonify Qi
- Strengthen the Spleen
- Stop bleeding

Acupuncture Treatment

Spleen Qi Tonic: BL-20/21, SP-6, CV-6, SP-9

Stop hemorrhage: *Duan Xue* (horse), *Tian Ping* (dog)

Chinese Herb Examples

Stop Bleeding: Agrimony   *Xian He Cao*
                   Cat-tail pollen   *Pu Huang*
                   Bletilla   *Bai Ji*

Herbal Formula Example

Gui Pi Tang (Heart and Spleen Tonic Powder)

5. Stomach Yin Deficiency

Etiology

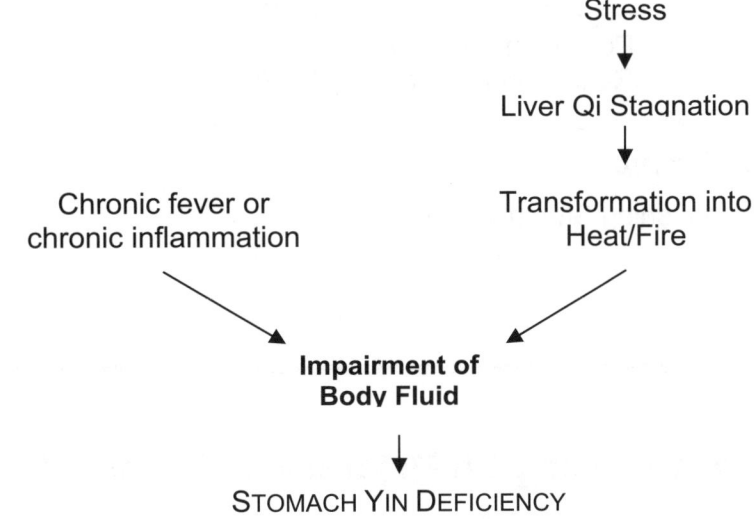

Stress
↓
Liver Qi Stagnation
↓
Transformation into Heat/Fire

Chronic fever or chronic inflammation

Impairment of Body Fluid
↓
STOMACH YIN DEFICIENCY

Clinical Signs

A Stomach Yin Deficiency can result in the following signs:

- Thirsty
- Dry nose and mouth
- Dry, small feces
- Red tongue
- Ravenous or poor appetite
- Less or no tongue coating
- Thready, rapid pulse
- Cool-seeking behavior

TCVM Diagnosis and Analysis

This is a Stomach Yin Deficiency Pattern. Deficient Stomach Yin may cause a relatively hyper Stomach Yang which leads to a ravenous appetite, or it may fail to support Stomach Yang which leads a to poor appetite. Yin Deficiency results in insufficient body fluids and leads to thirst, dry nose, dry mouth, and small, dry feces. Cool-seeking behaviors, a red tongue, no tongue coating, and a thready, rapid pulse reflect Yin Deficiency.

Treatment Strategies

- Nourish Stomach Yin

Acupuncture Treatment

Stomach Yin Tonic: KID-3, SP-6, SP-9, SP-10, CV-12

Chinese Herb Examples

Nourish Stomach Yin:
	Glehnia	*Bei Sha Shen*
	Dendrobium	*Shi Hu*
	Asparagus	*Tian Men Dong*
	Polygonatum	*Yu Zhu*
	Rehmannia	*Sheng Di Huang*

Herbal Formula Example

Yang Wei Tang (Nourishing Stomach Powder)

Patterns Associated with Major Gastrointestinal Diseases

Megaesophagus:
1. Stomach Heat
2. Stomach Cold
3. Phlegm
4. Qi Deficiency
5. Yin Deficiency

Constipation:
1. Heat Pattern
2. Cold Pattern
3. Food Stasis
4. Yin Deficiency
5. Qi and Yin Deficiency

Parvovirus Infection:
1. Heat Toxin
2. Damp Heat
3. Blood Stagnation
4. Yin Deficiency
5. Qi and Yin Deficiency

Vomiting:
1. Exogenous Pathogens disrupt ST
2. Food Stagnation obstructs Stomach
3. Disruption of Stomach by Liver Qi
4. Spleen and Stomach Deficiency Cold
5. Deficiency of Stomach Yin

Megacolon:
1. Qi Deficiency
2. Yin Deficiency
3. Qi and Yin Deficiency

Anorexia:
1. Stomach Cold
2. Stomach Heat
3. Spleen Deficiency
4. Food Stagnation

Diarrhea:
1. Cold
2. Heat
3. Food Stasis
4. Spleen Deficiency
5. Kidney Deficiency
6. Diarrhea In Foal
7. Liver Stagnation
8. Allergic Diarrhea
9. Dysentery

Inflammatory Bowel Disease:
1. Heat Toxin
2. Damp Heat
3. Yin Deficiency
4. Qi Deficiency

PATTERNS OF THE LIVER AND GALLBLADDER

The Liver is the General. It enjoys the free flow of Qi, but it is easily stressed by any emotional or medicinal challenge. The Liver stores blood, adjusts the blood volume, and controls the ligaments and tendons.

Eight Principles	Zang-Fu Syndromes (Pattern)
Deficiency	Liver Blood Deficiency
	Liver Yin Deficiency
	Internal Wind due to Liver Blood Deficiency
	Internal Wind due to Liver Yin Deficiency
Excess	Liver Fire Blazing Upwards
	Liver Damp Heat
	Extreme Heat Generating Liver-Wind
	Retention of Cold in the Liver Meridian

Excess Patterns

1. Liver Fire Blazing Upwards

Etiology

Stagnation of Liver Qi may transform into Liver Heat or Liver Fire. Alternatively, Wind-Heat can enter the Liver via the Channel and result in Liver Heat/Fire. Liver Fire Blazing Upwards may manifest as an acute course of conjunctivitis/keratitis, nebula, and uveitis.

Clinical Signs

- Epistaxis
- Red tongue
- Weak vision
- Ocular discharge
- Wiry and rapid pulse
- Redness, swelling, and pain of the eyes
- Difficulty in opening the eyes
- Dry feces or constipation
- Thick, dark yellow urine
- Corneal opacity or nebula

TCVM Diagnosis and Analysis

This is a type of Liver Heat/Fire Pattern. The eyes are the orifice of the Liver. Liver Fire rises up to the eyes and leads to ophthalmic conditions. In addition, excessive Liver Fire tends to counter-control (insult) the Lung and cause nasal bleeding. Excessive Liver Fire (Wood) may also over-control the digestive system (Earth) and consume the gastrointestinal fluid, which leads to dry feces or constipation. When excessive Liver Fire affects its "Mother" organ, the Kidney, it results in thick, dark urine. In this case the "illness of Child is transferred into its Mother". A red tongue and a wiry, rapid pulse reflect the presence of Liver Fire.

Treatment Strategies

- Clear Liver Fire
- Brighten the eyes and dispel the nebula

Acupuncture Treatment

Clear Liver Fire: LIV-2, GB-34

Brighten the eyes: GB-1, *Tai Yang*, ST-1, GB-37, BL-1

Chinese Herb Examples

Clear the Liver Fire:

Gentian	*Long Dan Cao*
Scutellaria	*Huang Qin*
Gardenia	*Zhi Zi*
Prunella	*Xia Ku Cao*
Chrysanthemum	*Ju Hua*

Disperse Wind:

Ledebouriella	*Fang Geng*
Schizonepeta	*Jing Jie*
Cicada	*Chan Tui*
Tribulus	*Ci Ji Li*

Brighten the eyes and
dispel the nebula:

Haliotis	*Shi Jue Ming*
Celosia	*Qing Xiang Zi*
Cicada	*Chan Tui*

Herbal Formula Example

Long Dan Xie Gan Tang (Gentian Combination Powder)

1. With acute conjunctivitis add:

Chrysanthemum	*Ju Hua*
Cassia	*Jue Ming Zi*

2. With turbid urine add:

Lysimachia	*Jin Qian Cao*
Polygonum	*Bian Xu*

2. Liver Damp-Heat

Etiology

There are two methods by which Damp-Heat develops in the Liver. 1) Prolonged Liver Qi Stagnation develops into Liver Heat. Combination of Damp with the Liver Heat results in Damp-Heat in the Liver. 2) Damp-Heat invades the body and then the Damp and Heat accumulates in the Liver.

Clinical Signs

This condition may occur during the course of vaginitis, scrotitis, prostatitis or hepatitis. The signs may include the following:

- Jaundice
- Scanty, dark or thick yellow urine
- Vaginal itching
- Swollen, hot, painful scrotum

- Yellow vaginal discharge with foul odor
- Swollen or painful prostate
- Red or yellow tongue
- Yellow and greasy tongue coating
- Wiry and rapid pulse

TCVM Diagnosis and Analysis

This condition is due to Damp-Heat in the Liver and Gall Bladder. The Pathogen Damp-Heat forces excessive bile distribution to the body surface, which leads to jaundice. The Damp-Heat in the Liver affects its "Mother" organ (Kidney) resulting in dark, thick urine. A red or yellow tongue, a yellow, greasy tongue coating, and wiry, rapid pulse reflect the Damp-Heat in the Liver.

The Damp-Heat follows the Liver Channel to the genital areas and is responsible for vaginal itching or a swollen, hot scrotum. In addition, the Liver regulates the Ren and Chong Channels and maintains the Qi flow of the uterus and prostate, so Damp-Heat in the Liver can result in vaginal discharge and prostatic swelling.

Treatment Strategies

- Clear Damp-Heat in the Liver

Acupuncture Treatment

Transform Damp-Heat: GB-34, GB-40, GB-41, BL-19, LI-11, SP-9

Chinese Herb Examples

Clear Liver Heat:
Gentian	*Long Dan Cao*
Gardenia	*Zhi Zi*
Phellodendron	*Huang Bai*
Artemisia	*Yin Chen Hao*
Plantago	*Che Qian Zi*
Talc	*Hua Shi*

Herbal Formula Example

Yin Chen San Plus (Artemisia Powder)

3. Extreme Heat Generating Liver-Wind

Etiology

Heat enters the body and becomes Extreme Heat in the Interior. It then generates Internal Wind, also known as Liver Wind.

Clinical Signs

The signs of Extreme Heat Generating Liver-Wind may include the following:

- High fever
- Rigidity of the neck
- Opisthotonos
- Coma

- Convulsions or tremors of the limbs
- Running into walls or circling
- Red tongue
- Wiry and rapid pulse

TCVM Diagnosis and Analysis

This is a Liver Wind condition due to Extreme Heat. This may be seen with high fever and infectious diseases. *Plain Questions* states that "Extreme Heat generates Wind". Thus, Extreme Heat results in Internal Wind. Signs of Internal Wind include rigidity of the neck, convulsions or tremors of the limbs, circling, running into walls, or even opisthotonos or coma. The red tongue and wiry, rapid pulse indicate the presence of Liver Heat.

Treatment Strategies

- Clear Heat
- Vanquish Wind to resolve convulsion

Acupuncture Treatment

Vanquish Wind to resolve convulsion: GB-20, LIV-3, BL-17, SP-10, GB-41, GB-34

Clear Heat: Jing-well points (HA), GV-14, LI-4, LIV-2

Chinese Herb Examples

Clear Heat:	Gypsum	*Shi Gao*
	Anemarrhena	*Zhi Mu*
	Chrysanthemum	*Ju Hua*
	Gentian	*Long Dan Cao*
Vanquish Wind to resolve convulsion:	Antelope	*Ling Yang Jiao*
	Uncaria	*Gou Teng*
	Earthworm	*Di Long*
	Batryticated silkworm	*Jiang Can*
	Scorpion	*Quan Xie*
	Centipede	*Wu Gong*

Herbal Formula Example

Ling Yang Gou Teng Tang (Uncaria Combination Powder)

4. Retention of Cold in the Liver Meridian

Etiology

Cold invades the body, and the Cold is retained in the Liver. The Coldness is then distributed along the Liver Channels. This results in Blood Stagnation of the testicles or prostate, which forms a swelling or mass.

Clinical Signs

- Hind limb stiffness
- Cold nose and ears
- Purple and wet tongue
- Deep pulse
- Swollen, cold scrotum and testis
- Swollen or painful prostate
- Infertility due to Coldness in uterus
- Cold trunk and limbs

TCVM Diagnosis and Analysis

This is a Liver Meridian Cold Pattern. It occurs with testicular hyperplasia, chronic prostatitis, or prostatic enlargement. The pathogen Cold follows the Liver Channel to the genital areas where it blocks the Qi flow of the testis, prostate and uterus which leads to cold, swollen testis, prostate and uterus (infertility) and hind limb stiffness. A cold body surface, purple tongue, and deep, slow pulse reflect a Cold Pattern.

Treatment Strategies

- Warm the Liver to dispel Cold
- Move Qi to resolve Stagnation

Acupuncture Treatment

Warm Liver to dispel Cold: LIV-14, LIV-8, LIV-3 (moxa)

Move Qi to resolve Stagnation: LIV-1, LIV-3, GB-34, LIV-5

Chinese Herb Examples

Warm the Liver to dispel Cold:

Fennel	*Hui Xiang* (Foeniculum)
Cinnamon	*Rou Gui*
Dry ginger	*Gan Jiang*

Move Qi Flow to resolve Stagnation:

Saussurea	*Mu Xiang*
Magnolia	*Hou Po*
Aurantium	*Zhi Shi* (Immature bitter orange peel)
Melia	*Chuan Lian Zi*

Herbal Formula Example

Hui Xiang San (Foeniculum Powder)

Deficiency Patterns

There are four major Liver Deficiency Patterns. Liver Blood Deficiency often leads to Liver Yin Deficiency while Liver Yin Deficiency may also cause Liver Blood Deficiency. Both Liver Blood and Yin Deficiency share some common clinical signs. Severe Liver Blood and Yin Deficiency may generate internal Wind.

1. Liver Blood Deficiency and Liver Yin Deficiency

Etiology

There are two ways that this Pattern occurs. 1) A Deficiency of the Spleen and Stomach Qi results in a failure to make enough Blood. 2) A Deficiency of the Kidney fails to nourish the Liver.

This Pattern may be associated with night blindness, chronic ocular inflammation, anemia, and keratoconjunctivitis sicca (KCS).

Clinical Signs

In general, Liver Blood and Yin Deficiencies may produce the following signs:
- Dry eyes
- Weak sight, especially at night

Liver Blood Deficiency: Dry or cracked paws or hooves
Dandruff (odorless)
Recumbence or lethargy
Pale tongue
Wiry and thready pulse

Liver Yin Deficiency: Red eyes
Tearing, watery eyes
Slightly swollen eyelids
Nebula or corneal opacity
Red mouth with scanty fluid
Thready, wiry and rapid pulse

TCVM Diagnosis and Analysis

This condition represents a Liver Blood or Yin Deficiency. The eyes require nourishment by Liver Yin and Blood; thus, a Deficiency of either Liver Yin or Blood can lead to dry eyes or weak sight. Since the hooves, paws and hair coat require nourishment by Liver Blood, a Liver Blood Deficiency can result in cracked paws or hooves and dandruff. In addition, a Deficiency of Blood tends to cause Qi Deficiency, which may appear as recumbence and lethargy. A Liver Yin Deficiency tends to cause Liver Yang Rising which can lead to red eyes, tearing, swollen eyelids and nebula.

A pale tongue reflects a Blood Deficiency. A red, dry tongue and a thready, rapid pulse indicate a Liver Yin Deficiency.

Treatment Strategies

Liver Blood Deficiency:
- Nourish Liver Blood

Liver Yin Deficiency:
- Nourish Liver Yin

Acupuncture Treatment

Liver Blood Deficiency: BL-18, SP-10, BL-17, SP-6
Liver Yin Deficiency: LIV-3, BL-18, BL-23, KID-3, SP-6

Chinese Herb Examples

Nourish Liver Blood:	Angelica	*Dang Gui*
	Paeonia	*Bai Shao Yao*
Clear the eyes and dispel nebula:	Haliotis	*Shi Jue Ming*
	Celosia	*Qing Xiang Zi*
	Cicada	*Chan Tui*
Nourish the Kidney and Liver:	Prepared rehmannia	*Shu Di Huang*
	Cistanche	*Rou Cong Rong*
	Dodder seed	*Tu Si Zi*
	Lycium	*Gou Qi Zi*
	Cornus fruit	*Shan Zhu Yu*

Herbal Formula Examples

Liver Blood Deficiency:
- *Si Wu Tang* (Four Substance Powder)

Liver Yin Deficiency:
- *Liu Wei Di Huang Wan* (Rehmannia Six Powder)

1. With serious fever add:	Anemarrhena	*Zhi Mu*
	Phellodendron	*Huang Bai*
2. With poor sight add:	Lycium	*Gou Qi Zi*
	Chrysanthemum	*Ju Hua*
3. With asthma add:	Schisandra	*Wu Wei Zi*

2. Deficient Liver Blood Wind and Deficient Liver Yin Wind

Etiology

Prolonged illness leads to loss of Blood and Body Fluid. This results in a Deficiency of Liver Blood or Yin. If this Deficiency lasts for a long time a Wind Pattern results.

This Pattern may be associated with the later stages of a febrile disease, profuse loss of Blood or Body Fluid, hypocalcemia, and hypomagnesemia.

Clinical Signs

In general, Liver Blood and Yin Deficient Wind may produce the following signs:
- Numbness of limbs
- Muscular tremors and convulsions

Deficient Liver Blood causing Wind: Dandruff
Pale tongue
Weak and thready pulse

Deficient Liver Yin causing Wind: Liver Yang Rising Wind
Prolonged low fever
Night sweating
Red and dry tongue with no coating
Weak and thready pulse

TCVM Diagnosis and Analysis

This condition is a Liver Blood (or Yin) Deficiency, which generates Internal Wind. The Liver controls the *Jin* (sinews, fascia, ligaments, tendons), which requires nourishment by the Liver Yin (or Blood). Deficient Liver Yin (or Blood) fails to nourish the *Jin*, which leads to contraction of the *Jin*. As a consequence, clinical signs such as numbness of limbs, convulsions, tremors and seizures may occur.

Treatment Strategies

Deficient Liver Blood Causing Wind:
- Nourish Liver Blood
- Clear Internal Wind

Deficient Liver Yin Causing Wind:
- Nourish Liver Yin
- Clear Internal Wind

Acupuncture Treatment

Clear Internal wind:	GB-20, GB-34, *Da Feng Men*, SP-10
Liver Blood tonic:	BL-18, SP-10, BL-17, SP-6
Liver Yin tonic:	BL-18, BL-23, KID-3, LIV-3, SP-6

Chinese Herb Examples

Nourish Liver Blood:	See above	
Nourish Liver Yin:	See above	
Clear Internal Wind:	Draconis	*Long Gu* (Dragon's bone)
	Oyster shell	*Mu Li*
	Magnetite	*Ci Shi*
	Lumbricus	*Di Long* (Earthworm)
	Uncaria	*Gou Teng* (Stem with hooks)
	Bombyx	*Jiang Can* (Batryticated silkworm)
	Antelope	*Ling Yang Jiao*

Herbal Formula Example

Deficient Liver Blood Causing Wind:
- *Tian Ma San* (Gastrodia Powder)

Deficient Liver Yin Causing Wind:
- *Da Ding Feng Zhu*

Patterns Associated with Hepatic Diseases

Hepatic Lipidosis:
1. Damp Phlegm with Qi Deficiency
2. Damp Phlegm with Heat
3. Damp Phlegm with Yin Deficiency
4. Damp Phlegm with Blood Stagnation

Hepatitis and Necrosis:
1. Liver Qi Stagnation
2. Damp-Heat at the Liver
3. Blood Stagnation
4. Liver Yin Deficiency
5. Qi and Blood Deficiency

Ascites:
1. Damp/water retention
2. Blood Stagnation and Water retention
3. Spleen Deficiency and Qi Stagnation
4. Spleen/Kidney Yang Deficiency
5. Liver/Kidney Yin Deficiency

Hepatomegaly/Cirrhosis:
1. Liver Blood Stasis with Damp-Heat
2. Liver Blood Stasis with Qi Deficiency
3. Liver Blood Stasis with Qi and Blood Deficiency
4. Liver Blood Stasis with Yin Deficiency
5. Liver Blood Stasis with Yang Deficiency

PATTERNS OF KIDNEY AND BLADDER

The Kidney is the root of prenatal life. It stores Jing, controls water metabolism, dominates the bones and marrow, and controls urination and defecation. The Kidney is almost always deficient if there is a problem. Thus, the Kidney Jing should always be stored or conserved. The Bladder is the storage place for urine. The Bladder is almost always in Excess if there is a problem.

The Kidney and Bladder Patterns include diseases such as urinary incontinence, renal failure, disc disease, arthritis, geriatric diseases, and infertility. Any chronic diseases may eventually lead to Kidney Deficiency.

Eight Principles	Zang-Fu Syndromes (Pattern)
Deficiency	Kidney Yang Deficiency
	Kidney Qi Not Firm
	Kidney Failing to Receive Qi
	Edema due to Kidney Yang Deficiency
	Kidney Yin Deficiency
	Kidney Jing Deficiency
Excess	Bladder Damp-Heat

Excess Pattern

Bladder Damp-Heat

Etiology

This Pattern occurs when Damp-Heat invades the body and accumulates in the Bladder.

Clinical Signs

The signs of this Pattern may include the following:

- Frequent and urgent urination
- Difficult urination
- Posturing to urinate, but no urine
- Dribbling scanty urine with pain
- Turbid or bloody urine with foul odor
- Fine stones or crystals in urine
- Red tongue with yellow and greasy coating
- Forceful and rapid pulse

TCVM Diagnosis and Analysis

This is a Bladder Damp-Heat Pattern associated with cystitis, urethritis, urolithiasis or acute nephritis. The pathogen Damp-Heat blocks the Qi flow of Bladder and urethra resulting in difficult urination, posturing to urinate, and painful dribbling of urine. The Heat boils off the body fluids, leading to scanty urine, urinary stones or crystals. Heat also damages blood vessels, which leads to bloody urine. Frequent and urgent urination occur as the body tries to get rid of the pathogen. The turbid urine, greasy tongue coating and soft pulse indicate Damp. A red tongue and a rapid pulse reflect Heat conditions.

Treatment Strategies

- Eliminate Heat
- Excrete Damp

Acupuncture Treatment

Clear Damp-Heat in Bladder: *Wei Jian* (Tip of the Tail), BL-39, SP-6, BL-40

Chinese Herb Examples

Elimination of Damp-Heat:

Gardenia	*Zhi Zi*
Rhubarb	*Da Huang*
Akebia	*Mu Tong*
Dianthus	*Qu Mai*
Plantago	*Che Qian Zi*
Polygonum	*Bian Xu*
Pyrrosia	*Shi Wei*
Talc	*Hua Shi*
Lygodium	*Hai Jin Sha*

Herbal Formula Example

Ba Zheng San (Eight Righteous Powder)

1. With urinary tract stones add:

Lysimachia	*Jin Qian Cao*
Lygodium	*Hai Jin Sha*

2. With bloody urine add:

Imperata	*Bai Mao Gen*
Cephalanoplos	*Xiao Ji*

Deficiency Patterns

1. Kidney Yang Deficiency

Etiology

Prolonged illness, overwork, weak constitution, and age may contribute to a Kidney Yang Deficiency. This Pattern may be associated with prolonged illness, weakness, rheumatism, infertility, and osteomalacia.

Clinical Signs

The signs of Kidney Yang Deficiency may include the following:

- Aversion to cold
- Cold back, limbs and ears
- Impotence
- Inability to conceive
- Pale, wet, swollen tongue

- Weakness of rear limbs or lumbosacral area
- Difficulty standing up or lying down
- Decreased sexual function
- Inability to return ejaculated penis
- Deep, slow and weak pulse

TCVM Diagnosis and Analysis

Kidney Yang originates from the Ming Men Fire (Life Gate of Fire). Ageing, long-term exposure to cold and chronic illness can debilitate the Ming Men Fire and lead to Kidney Yang Deficiency. Thus, the animal develops aversion to cold and has cold limbs, ears and back.

Since the Kidney is the source of reproductive capacity, deficient Kidney Yang leads to impotence and infertility. Also, Kidney Yang controls the bones and lower back (house of the Kidney) so Deficiency leads to lumbar pain and pronounced hind limb weakness. A pale, wet, swollen tongue and deep, slow, weak pulse reflect Yang Deficiency.

Treatment Strategies

- Tonify Kidney Yang.

Acupuncture Treatment

Kidney Yang Tonic: *Bai Hui*, GV-4, GV-20, GV-14, CV-6, CV-4 (moxa)

Chinese Herb Examples

Tonify the Kidney Yang:
Cistanche	Rou Cong Rong
Morinda	Ba Ji Tian
Psoralea	Bu Gu Zhi
Aconite	Fu Zi
Cinnamon	Rou Gui

Herbal Formula Example

Shen Qi Wan (*Jin Gui Shen Qi Wan*)

2. Kidney Qi Not Firm

Etiology

Prolonged illness, overwork, weak constitution and age all may lead to a Kidney Qi Deficiency.

Clinical Signs

The signs of this Pattern may include the following:

- Deep and weak pulse
- Fatigue, lassitude
- Clear, frequent urination
- Dribbling urine
- Urinary Incontinence

- Rectal incontinence
- Early fetus loss or abortion
- Spermatorrhea or involuntary emission
- Pale tongue with white and thin coating
- Weakness of back and knees

TCVM Diagnosis and Analysis

This is a Kidney Qi Deficiency Pattern which may be seen with urinary incontinence. The Kidney dominates the lower back and the knees. Signs of Kidney Qi Deficiency include weak back and knees, fatigue and lassitude. In addition, the Kidney controls the "front door" (bladder/urethral sphincter) and the "back door" (anal sphincter). Kidney Qi Deficiency leads to urinary incontinence and/or rectal incontinence. As the Kidney controls the reproductive activities, a Kidney Qi Deficiency results in early embryonic loss, abortion, or involuntary emission. Frequent voiding of clear urine, a pale tongue, and a deep, weak pulse reflects a Qi Deficiency.

Treatment Strategies

- Tonify Kidney Qi
- Consolidate the Kidney

Acupuncture Treatment

| Kidney Qi Tonic: | CV-4, CV-6, BL-23, Shen Shu |
| Consolidate the Kidney: | SP-6, Ba Jiao, Yan Chi |

Chinese Herb Examples

Tonify Kidney Qi	Psoralea	Bu Gu Zhi
	Morinda	Ba Ji Tian
Consolidate the Kidney:	Mantis egg-case	Sang Piao Xiao
	Black cardamon	Yi Zhi Ren
	Raspberry fruit	Fu Pen Zi
	Euryale seed	Qian shi

Herbal Formula Example

There are two commonly used herbal formulas: 1) Suo Quan Wan for urinary continence and 2) Jin Suo Gu Jing Wan for emission and urinary incontinence.

3. Kidney Failing to Grasp Qi

Etiology

Prolonged illness, overwork, a weak constitution and age may all lead to Kidney Yang Deficiency, which results in Kidney Qi and Lung Qi Deficiency.

Clinical Signs

The signs of this Pattern may include the following:

- Shortness of breath
- Prolonged cough
- Chronic asthma or heaves
- Pale tongue
- Lethargy

- Rapid and weak breath, worse if moving
- Weakness of hind limbs and back
- Spontaneous sweating
- Deficient and feeble pulse
- Difficult inhalation or exhalation

TCVM Diagnosis and Analysis

This is a Kidney and Lung Qi Deficiency Pattern. Chronic bronchitis, chronic pulmonary emphysema, and chronic obstructive pulmonary disorder (COPD) may be associated with this pattern. The Lung is the Master of Qi, and the Kidney is the Root of Qi. The respiratory function of the Lung requires the Kidney to grasp (pull down) the Qi, thus a Kidney Qi Deficiency can cause respiratory disorders such as shortness of breath, difficult inhalation or exhalation, chronic heaves, or rapid and weak breathing. Considering that this is a Qi Deficiency, all the clinical signs become worse with movement. Because the Kidney controls the lower back and stifles, Kidney Qi Deficiency leads to weakness of the hind limbs and back. Spontaneous sweating is a sign of Lung Qi Deficiency as it controls the open-close mechanism of the skin pores. Lethargy, a pale tongue, and a deficient, feeble pulse reflect a Qi Deficiency.

Treatment Strategies

- Tonify Kidney Qi
- Benefit Kidney Qi grasping

Acupuncture Treatment

Kidney Qi Tonic:	CV-4, CV-6, BL-23, *Shen Shu*
Benefit Kidney Qi grasping:	CV-17, CV-6, LU-7, *Ding Chuan*

Chinese Herb Examples

Tonify Kidney Qi:	See above	
Kidney Qi Deficiency:	Gecko	*Ge Jie*
	Schisandra	*Wu Wei Zi*
	Psoralea	*Bu Gu Zhi*

Herbal Formula Example

Ren Shen Ge Jie San (Ginseng-Gecko Powder)

4. Kidney and Heart Yang Deficiency

Etiology

Same as Kidney Yang Deficiency

Clinical Signs

The signs of this Pattern may include the following:

- Cold limbs and trunk
- Heat-seeking behavior
- Deep and weak pulse
- Ascites or swollen scrotum
- Heart failure, fluid in the lungs, and cough
- Possible cough and asthma
- Pale, swollen tongue with a white coating
- Edema, especially the hind limbs

TCVM Diagnosis and Analysis

This is a Kidney and Heart Yang Deficiency Pattern. A Yang Deficiency leads to cold limbs and trunk, heat-seeking behavior, a pale, swollen tongue, and a deep, weak pulse. The Kidney is the Gate of Water, and the Heart is the force that propels Blood circulation for the whole body. Thus, a Kidney and Heart Yang Deficiency can cause edema, ascites, heart failure, and fluids in the Lung.

Treatment Strategies

- Tonify Kidney and Heart Yang
- Excrete Water-Damp

Acupuncture Treatment

KID and HT Yang Tonic: GV-3, GV-4, *Bai Hui*, CV-17, CV-4, CV-6, HT-7, BL-14, *Shen Shu*
Excrete Water Damp: ST-40, SP-6, SP-9

Chinese Herb Examples

Tonify Kidney Yang: See above

Excrete Water-Damp:
Polyporus	*Zhu Ling*
Poria	*Fu Ling*
Plantago	*Che Qian Zi*
Alisma	*Ze Xie*

Herbal Formula Example

Zhen Wu Tang modification

5. Kidney Yin Deficiency

Etiology

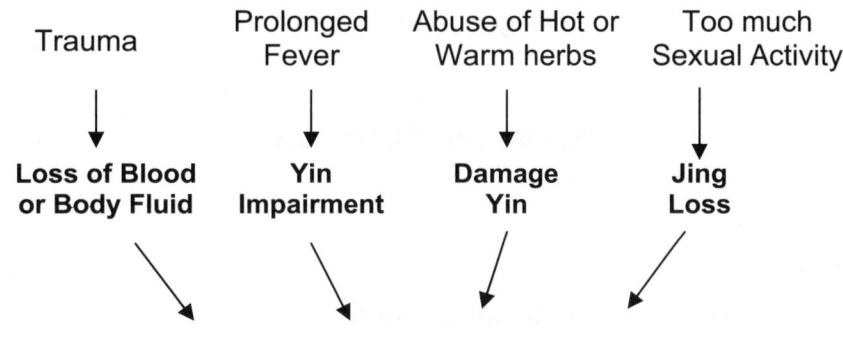

Clinical Signs

The signs of this Pattern may include the following:

- Dry feces
- Involuntary emission
- Infertility
- Weak sight
- Thready, rapid pulse

- Abnormal nighttime behavior or nightmares
- Spontaneous sweating at night
- Weakness of the back and rear limbs
- Lower degree of fever in the afternoon
- Dry, red tongue with little coating

TCVM Diagnosis and Analysis

The Kidney Yin Deficiency Pattern may accompany prolonged illness, weakness, chronic anemia, and infertility. It may occur during some chronic infectious diseases. The Kidney controls the back and stifles, thus a weak Kidney leads to weakness of the back and rear limbs. The Kidney also controls reproductive functions, so a deficient Kidney leads to involuntary emission or infertility. Abnormal nighttime behavior (disturbed sleep pattern), low grade afternoon fevers, dry feces, a dry and red tongue, decreased tongue coating, and a thready, rapid pulse can indicate a Yin Deficiency.

Acupuncture Treatment

Kidney Yin Tonic: KID-3, KID-6, BL-23, SP-6

Chinese Herb Examples

Kidney Yin Tonic: Rehmannia   *Shu Di Huang*
                      Ligustrum   *Nu Zhen Zi*
                      Tortoise plastron   *Gui Ban*
                      Cornus   *Shan Zhu Yu*
                      Polygonum   *He Shou Wu*
                      Lycium   *Gou Qi Zi*

Herbal Formula Example

Liu Wei Di Huang Wan (Rehmannia Six Powder)

6. Kidney Jing Deficiency

Etiology

Congenital Weakness

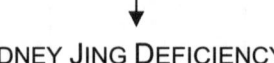

KIDNEY JING DEFICIENCY

Clinical Signs

The signs of this Pattern may include the following:

- Early ageing
- Red or pale tongue
- Weak pulse
- Slow growth
- Skeletal maldevelopment
- Dull reaction to any stimulus
- General weakness

TCVM Diagnosis and Analysis

This is Kidney Jing Deficiency Pattern. The Kidney Jing is the solid form of Primary Qi (Source Qi, Yuan Qi). Primary Qi is the initial energy that stimulates the body's growth and development, thus a Kidney Jing Deficiency leads to slow growth and maldevelopment. As a result, the animal may experience early ageing, dull reactions to stimuli, general weakness and weak pulses. In addition, the Kidney Jing is the origin of both Kidney Yin and Kidney Yang, so a deficient Kidney Jing can result in Kidney Yin Deficiency (red tongue) or Kidney Yang Deficiency (pale tongue).

Treatment Strategies

- Tonify Kidney Jing

Acupuncture Treatment

Jing Tonic: KID-3, KID-7, BL-23, BL-20, ST-36, SP-6

Chinese Herb Examples

Tonify Kidney Jing: Epimedium   *Yin Yang Huo*
                       Polygonum   *He Shou Wu*

Herbal Formula

Sheng Jing San (Epimedium Powder)

Patterns Associated with Major Urinary Tract Diseases

Cystitis/Lower Urinary Tract Disease:
1. Heat Dribbling (*re-lin*)
2. Stone Dribbling (*Shi-lin*)
3. Blood Dribbling (*xue-lin*)
4. Turbid Dribbling (*gao-lin*)
5. Stagnation Dribbling (*qi-lin*)
6. Deficiency Dribbling (*lao-lin*)

Nephritis:
1. Damp Heat
2. Spleen-Kidney Yang Deficiency
3. Liver-Kidney Yin Deficiency

Renal Failure:
1. Kidney Qi Deficiency
2. Kidney Yang Deficiency
3. Kidney Yin Deficiency
4. Kidney Qi/Yin Deficiency
5. Kidney Jing Deficiency

Kidney or Bladder Stones:
1. Damp Heat
2. Stagnation of Phlegm
3. Qi Deficiency

Urinary Incontinence:
1. Kidney Qi Deficiency
2. Kidney-Spleen Yang Deficiency
3. Kidney Qi and Yin Deficiency

Six Channels Patterns

Liu Jing Bian Zhen

Liu Jing Bian Zhen, known as the Six Channel Patterns, Six Meridian Patterns or Six Phases, is one of the earliest approaches of pattern-identification. It is an important diagnostic method in Traditional Chinese Medicine (TCM) clinical practice, especially when applied to exogenous diseases. Zhang Zhongjing developed this approach around the third century. He wrote a detailed description of his diagnostic system in the book *Shang Han Za Bing Lun* (*Treatise of Cold-Induced Disorders and Miscellaneous Diseases*) which was published in 220 AD. The system was originally designed for people who suffered from exogenous diseases. Since that time, it has been widely used in TCM diagnosis of exogenous and endogenous diseases for both humans and animals.

Yin and Yang are sub-classified into three Yang types and three Yin types. Yang includes Tai-yang, Yang-ming and Shao-yang. Yin includes Tai-yin, Shao-yin and Jue-yin. Each Yang or Yin sub-classification represents two Meridians. For instance, Yang-ming includes the Large Intestine Meridian and the Stomach Meridian, and Shao-yin refers to both the Kidney and Heart Meridians. This diagnostic system recognizes a total of six channels: three Yang channels and three Yin channels (Table 8.10).

When the exogenous pathogenic factors (Xie-Qi, pathogens) invade the body, the six channels either fight against the Xie Qi or suffer affliction due to the pathogens. The disorders are summarized into the Six Channel Patterns, which include the Tai-yang, Yang-ming, Shao-yang, Tai-yin, Shao-yin and Jue-yin Patterns. The first three, as Yang Patterns, represent conditions in which the body's resistance to disease (Zheng-Qi) is strong. In the last three (Yin) Patterns, the Zheng Qi is weak.

Table 8.10: The Six Channels (The three Yang and the three Yin)

Yang Meridians	Yin Meridians
Tai-yang	Tai-yin
Shao-yang	Shao-yin
Yang-ming	Jue-yin

TAI-YANG PATTERN

This Pattern is often seen at the initial stage of exogenous diseases. It affects the body on a superficial level and is thus associated with two Exterior Patterns. The Tai-yang Pattern is divided into Invasion of Tai-yang by Cold and Invasion of Tai-yang by Wind based upon the relative strengths of the Zheng Qi and the Xie Qi. The Invasion of Tai Yang by Cold is an Exterior Excess Pattern, and the Invasion of Tai Yang by Wind is an Exterior Deficiency Pattern.

Common clinical signs of Tai-yang Patterns may include the following:

- Fever
- Cough
- Depression
- Decreased appetite
- Watery nasal discharges
- Nasal obstruction
- Sneezing
- White, thin tongue coating
- Superficial pulse
- Cold or hot ears and nose
- Swollen and painful joints
- Lameness
- Aversion to cold (Cold shivers, tight skin, contrary piloerection)

1. Invasion of Tai-Yang by Cold

Clinical Signs

- Aversion to cold
- Fever
- No sweating
- Cough
- Asthma
- Superficial and forceful pulse

Treatment Principles

- Induce perspiration and diaphoresis
- Disperse the Lung and stop cough

Acupoints

BL-10, *Tai Yang*

Herbal Formula

Ma Huang Tang (Ephedra Powder)

2. Invasion of Tai-Yang by Wind

Clinical Signs

- Aversion to wind
- Fever (mild)
- Sweating
- Weak and superficial pulse
- This Pattern is often seen in old or weak animals

Treatment Principles

- Relieve the skin-muscles and dispel Wind
- Regulate Ying (Nutrient) system and Wei (Defensive) System

Acupoints

GB-20, LI-4

Herbal Formula

Gui Zhi Tang (Cinnamon-Twig Powder)

SHAO-YANG PATTERN

This Pattern affects the body in a manner that is neither superficial nor deep. It exists on a level between the Exterior and the Interior; therefore, it is a half Exterior and half Interior Pattern.

Common clinical signs of Shao-yang Patterns may include the following:

In general:	Prolonged low fever
	Alternating chills and fever
With fever present:	Nose and ears are too warm
	Loss of appetite
	No cold shivers
	Depression is not as severe
With chills present:	Depression
	Cool nose and ears
	Cold shivers
	Contrary piloerection

Treatment Principles

- Mediate and regulate the Shao-yang Channel

Acupoints

GB-20, *Er Jian* (ear tip), BL-10, TH-5, TH-10

Herbal Formula

Xiao Chai Hu Tang (Minor-Bupleurum Powder)

YANG-MING PATTERN

This Pattern affects the body on a deep level and is thus associated with two Internal Patterns. The Yang-ming Pattern is divided into the Yang-ming Channel Pattern and the Yang-ming Fu Pattern.

1. Yang-Ming Channel Pattern

Clinical Signs

- Fever
- Sweating
- Rapid respiration
- Thirst and much drinking
- Dry, yellow and thick tongue coating
- Surging and rapid pulse

Treatment Principles

- Eliminate Heat
- Generate Body Fluid

Acupoints

ST-44, *Wei Jian* (tail tip), CV-12, BL-20, GB-34

Herbal Formula

Bai Hu Tang (White Tiger Powder)

2. Yang-Ming Fu Pattern

Clinical Signs

- Fever
- Sweating
- Scanty, dark urine
- Constipation
- Aversion to heat, but no aversion to cold
- Dry feces with small ball-shape
- Difficulty discharging feces
- Deep and forceful pulse

Treatment Principles

- Eliminate Heat
- Purge accumulation from the intestines

Acupoints

ST-25, LI-10, ST-37, BL-21

Herbal Formula

Da Cheng Qi Tang (Drastic-Purgative Powder)

TAI-YIN PATTERN

This Pattern affects the body at the level of the Spleen-Stomach and it has the properties of Deficiency and Cold.

Common clinical signs of Tai-yin Patterns may include the following:

- Abdominal pain or fullness
- Cold nose and ears
- Watery feces
- White tongue coating
- Thready and slow pulse

Treatment Principles

- Warm the Middle-Jiao
- Eliminate Cold

Acupoints

Moxa at CV-4, CV-6, GV-3, GV-4, ST-36

Herbal Formula

Li Zhong Tang (Regulating the Middle Powder)

SHAO-YIN PATTERN

The Shao-yin Pattern is divided into the Shao-yin Deficient Cold and the Shao-yin Deficient Heat Pattern. The internal organs Heart and Kidney are associated with a Shao-yin Pattern.

1. Shao-Yin Deficient Cold Pattern

Clinical Signs

- Aversion to cold
- Pale purple tongue
- Lethargy, exercise intolerance, fatigue
- Cold nose, ears and limbs
- Deep and slow pulse

Treatment Principles

- Revive Yang for resuscitation

Acupoints

Bai Hui, GV-4, *Shen Shu* (moxibustion), KID-3, GV-26

Herbal Formula

Si Ni Tang (Cold-Limbs Powder)

2. Shao-Yin Deficient Heat Pattern

Clinical Signs

- Dry mouth
- Painful throat
- Restlessness at night
- Deep red mouth
- Thready and rapid pulse

Treatment Principles

- Nourish Yin
- Eliminate Heat

Acupoints

KID-3, SP-6, PC-6

Herbal Formula

Da Bu Yin Wan (Great Yin Tonic Powder)

JUE-YIN PATTERN

This Pattern is often seen in the final stages of exogenous diseases when the Zheng Qi is exhausted. The Jue-yin Pattern is divided into the Cold Jue Pattern, the Heat Jue Pattern, and the Ascaris Jue Pattern.

1. Cold Jue Pattern

Clinical Signs

- Cold, clammy limbs
- No fever
- Aversion to cold
- Pale mouth and tongue
- Thready and feeble pulse

Treatment Principles

- Revive Yang for resuscitation

Acupoints

Bai Hui, GV-4, *Shen Shu* (moxibustion), KID-3, GV-26

Herbal Formula

Si Ni Tang (Cold-Limbs Decoction)

2. Heat Jue Pattern

Clinical Signs

- Cold, clammy limbs
- Aversion to heat
- Scanty and dark urination.
- Red or yellow and dry tongue

Treatment Principles

- Eliminate Heat
- Regulate Yin

Acupoints

ST-44, *Wei Jian* (tail tip), CV-12, BL-20, GB-34

Herbal Formula

Bai Hu Tang (White-Tiger Decoction)

3. Ascaris Jue Pattern

Clinical Signs

- Yellow eyes and mouth
- Thirst and drinking
- Alternately cold and warm limbs
- Acute abdominal pain due to ascarids
- Vomiting ascarids

Treatment Principles

- Regulate Cold and Heat
- Mediate the Stomach
- Eliminate the ascarids.

Herbal Formula

Wu Mei Wan (Mume Pill)

Concurrent Patterns

Not only may diseases develop with each of the Six Channel Patterns individually, but also two or more Patterns may merge together in some disease states. A concurrent Pattern develops when one Channel Pattern appears before a previous one has yet been cured. A concurrent disease occurs when two Patterns have a simultaneous onset.

1. Concurrent Tai-Yang Shao-Yang Pattern

Before the Tai-yang Pattern has been cured, the Xie Qi invades into Shao-yang and causes a Shao-yang Pattern.

Clinical Signs

Tai-Yang: Cough
Sneezing or nasal obstruction
Depression
Swollen and painful joints

Shao-Yang: Alternating chills and fever

Treatment Principles

- Eliminate the Xie Qi from both Tai-yang and Shao-yang

Acupoints

TH-5, Tai-yang, GB-20, LU-10, LU-7

Herbal Formula

Chai Hu Gui Zhi Tang (Bupleurum-Cinnamomum Powder)

2. Concurrent Shao-Yang Yang-Ming Pattern

This occurs with the simultaneous development of Shao-yang and Yang-ming Patterns.

Clinical Signs

Yang-Ming: Weak intestinal peristalsis sounds
Dry feces with small ball-shape

Shao-Yang: Alternating chills and fever

Treatment Principles

- Eliminate the Xie Qi from both Shao-yang and Yang-ming

Acupoints

TH-5, GB-20, ST-44, *Wei Jian*, ST-37, BL-21

Herbal Formula

Da Chai Hu Tang (Major-Bupleurum Decoction)

3. Concurrent Disease of Tai-yang and Yang-ming

This occurs with simultaneous development of the Tai-yang and Yang-ming Patterns.

Clinical Signs

Yang-Ming: Weak intestinal peristalsis sounds
                    Dry feces
                    Dry mouth

Tai-Yang: Aversion to cold
                    Cold shivers
                    Fever
                    Cough

Treatment Principles

To eliminate both Exterior and Interior

Acupoints

Tai Yang, BL-10, *Er Jian*, ST-37, GV-1, SP-10, TH-5

Herbal Formula

Fang Feng Tong Sheng San (Ledebouriella Combination Powder)

Transformation of the Six Channel Patterns

Transformation of Six Channel Patterns refers to the process of development or change that occurs when one Pattern transforms into another. There are three forms: Regular Transformation, Transformation by Skipping Channels, and Direct Attack.

1. Regular Transformation

The exogenous diseases transform from the Exterior into the Interior by passing from one channel to another. This occurs in the following sequence.

Tai-Yang → Shao-Yang → Yang-Ming → Tai-Yin → Shao-Yin → Jue-Yin

2. Transformation by Skipping Meridians

It is possible for the transformation to skip one or more Channels rather than progressing through the whole sequence. For instance, a Tai-Yang Pattern transforms into a Yang-Ming Pattern, a Tai-Yin Pattern or a Shao-Yin Pattern.

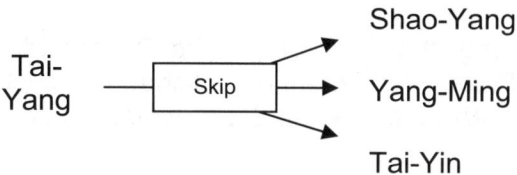

3. Direct Attack

The Xie-Qi directly invades into the three Yin Meridians without going through the three Yang Meridians. In this way, it is possible to directly cause the three Yin Meridian Patterns: Tai-yin Pattern, Shao-yin Pattern and Jue-yin Pattern. When there is direct attack of Tai-Yin, the Tai-Yin Pattern occurs at the initial stage of exogenous disease.

Four Stages

Wei Qi Ying Xue Patterns

Wei Qi Ying Xue Bian Zheng, the Four Stages, is Pattern Identification According to Defense, Qi, Nutrient and Blood. Ye Tianshi established this system and described it his book, *Wai Gan Wen Re Pian* (*Treatise on Exogenous Epidemic Fevers*), which was published in 1746.

This system is recommended for use when the initial symptoms of disease include acute febrile conditions (Excess Heat). Wei Qi Ying Xue can identify the Patterns of acute febrile diseases which are commonly seen in veterinary practice. Acute febrile diseases usually occur when the Zheng Qi is not strong enough to prevent the Xie Qi from invading the body. These diseases are characterized by their abrupt onset of symptoms, by their tendency to injure Yin, Body Fluid and Blood, and by their frequent changes.

In addition to generalizing the clinical appearance of febrile diseases, the Defense, Qi, Nutrient and Blood represent four different stages of a disease's pathological development. They measure the depth and severity of a disease. The most superficial is the Defense Stage. The next level is the Qi Stage, and deeper still is the Nutrient Stage. The deepest level is the Blood Stage. Defense and Qi Patterns are mild and superficial, but Nutrient and Blood Patterns are deep and severe.

Table 8.11: The four stages (four levels) of an illness

Stage	Level		Location
1	*Wei*	Defense	Superficial, Body surface: Muscle and Joints
2	*Qi*		Internal organs: Lung, Stomach, Large Intestine
3	*Ying*	Nutrient	CNS, Shen, Heart, Pericardium
4	*Xue*	Blood	Hemorrhage

WEI STAGE

Defense Stage Pattern

Etiology

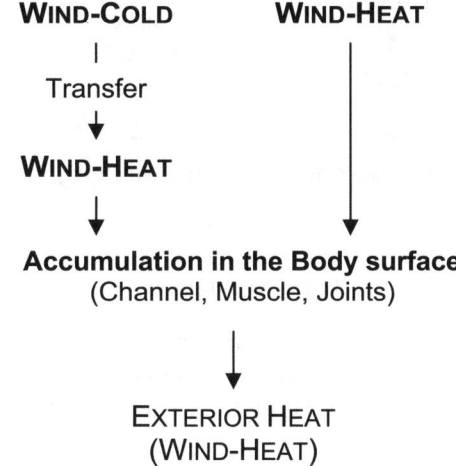

WIND-COLD   **WIND-HEAT**
|
Transfer
↓
WIND-HEAT
↓

Accumulation in the Body surface
(Channel, Muscle, Joints)

↓

EXTERIOR HEAT
(WIND-HEAT)

Clinical Signs

Signs related to the initial stages of acute febrile diseases (Exterior Pattern).

- Severe fever
- Slight aversion to Cold
- Cough
- Slightly red/dry tongue
- Thin and yellow tongue coating
- Floating and rapid pulse

Treatment Principles

- Relieve Exterior
- Clear Heat

Acupoints

Regular points: GV-14, LI-4, LI-11, LU-5

Hemoacupuncture: *Er Jian* (ear tip), *Wei Jian* (tail tip)

Herbal Formula

Yin Qiao San

QI STAGE
Etiology

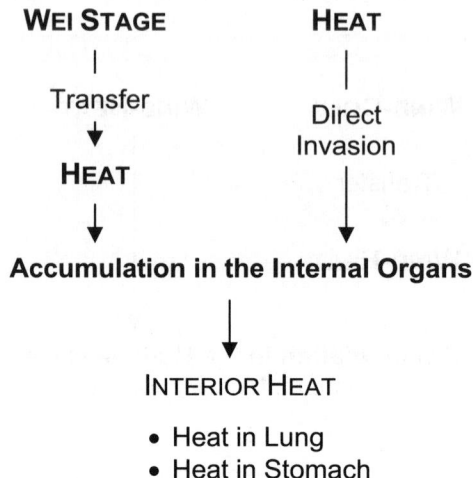

1. **Retention of Heat in the Lung**

Clinical Signs

- Fever
- Rapid breath
- Cough

- Bright red /dry tongue
- Dry and yellow tongue coating
- Surging and rapid pulse

Treatment Principles

- Clear Lung Heat and resolve phlegm
- Stop cough or asthma

Acupoints

LI-4, LI-11, LU-5, LU-10, CV-22, *Ding Chuan*

Herbal Formula

Qing Qi Hua Tan Tang

2. Retention of Heat in the Stomach

Clinical Signs

The clinical signs are similar to the Yang-Ming Channel Pattern.

- Fever
- Sweating
- Thirst
- Increased drinking

- Bright red tongue and very dry (mouth odor)
- Dry and yellow tongue coating
- Surging and forceful pulse
- Point sensitivity at BL-21 and CV-12

Treatment Principles

- Eliminate Heat
- Generate Body Fluid

Acupoints

ST-44, *Shan Gen*, ST-45, Kid-3, SP-6, BL-21, *Wei Jian* (tail tip)

Herbal Formula

Bai Hu Tang (White-Tiger Decoction)

3. Retention of Heat in the Intestinal Tract

Clinical Signs

The clinical signs are similar to the Yang-Ming Fu Pattern.

- Fever
- Dry feces or constipation
- Impaction
- Abdominal pain, colic

- Scanty and dark urine
- Deep red and very dry tongue
- Yellow and thick tongue coating
- Forceful pulse

Treatment Principles

- Purge the intestines
- Eliminate Heat
- Generate Body Fluid
- Nourish Yin

Acupoints

ST-37, ST-25, BL-21, ST-36, GV-1

Herbal Formula

Da Cheng Qi Tang

YING STAGE

Nutrient Stage Pattern

Etiology

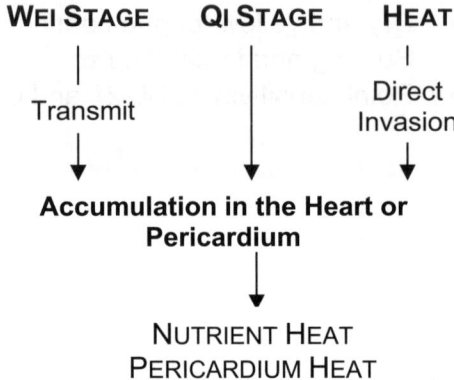

WEI STAGE	QI STAGE	HEAT
Transmit		Direct Invasion

Accumulation in the Heart or Pericardium

NUTRIENT HEAT
PERICARDIUM HEAT

1. Nutrient Heat

Clinical Signs

- Deep red tongue
- Restlessness
- Rapid breath, asthma
- Petechiae or macules in the skin or mucosa
- Thready and rapid pulse
- Prolonged high fever (especially at night)

Treatment Principles

- Eliminate Heat from Nutrient Stage and detoxify
- Nourish Yin

Acupoints

PC-6, HT-7, HT-9, SI-1, BL-15, BL-14, GV-14, *Wei Jian*

Herbal Formula

Qing Ying Tang

2. Pericardium Heat

Clinical Signs

- High fever
- Coma
- Delirium or dementia
- Seizure
- Deep-red tongue
- Rapid pulse

Treatment Principles

- Clear the Heart
- Open the orifice

Acupoints

GV-26, KID-1, PC-6, TH-5, HT-7, LI-11, GV-14

Herbal Formula

Qing Gong Tang (Clearing-Pericardium Decoction)

BLOOD STAGE

Etiology

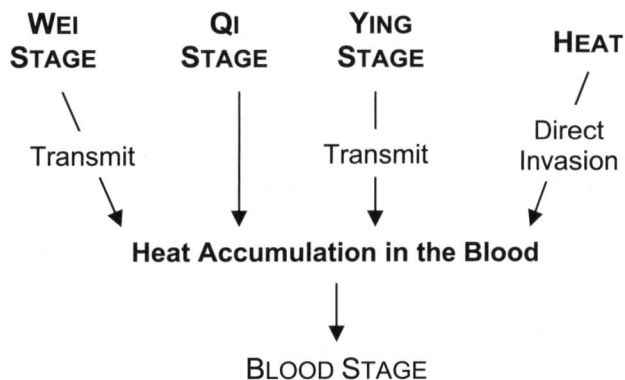

- Blood Heat causing Hemorrhage
- Liver Heat causing Wind
- Blood Heat Impairing Yin

1. Blood Heat Causing Hemorrhage

Clinical Signs

- Fever
- Coma
- Dark deep-red tongue
- Rapid pulse

- Various forms of Hemorrhage:
- Blood spots in mucosa or skin
- Rash
- Bloody urine or feces

Treatment Principles

- Eliminate Heat and detoxify
- Cool Blood
- Eliminate Stagnation

Acupoints

Duan Xue, Tian Ping, LI-11, LI-4, GV-14, BL-17, BL-18, SP-10

Herbal Formula

Xi Jiao Di Huang Tang

2. Liver Heat Causing Wind

Clinical Signs

- High fever
- Rigidity of neck and back
- Seizure or convulsions
- Dark deep-red tongue
- Wiry or string-taut and rapid pulse

Treatment Principles

- Eliminate Heart
- Clear the Liver
- Clear Wind
- Resolve seizure

Acupoints

GB-20, LIV-3, GV-20, GV-1, SP-10, LI-11, HT-7, KID-3

Herbal Formula

Ling Yang Gou Teng Tang

3. Blood Heat Impairing Yin

Clinical Signs

- Prolonged low fever
- Fatigue, lassitude
- Dry feces or short urination
- Red and dry tongue, crack lines
- No tongue coating or peeled off
- Thready, weak and rapid pulse

Treatment Principles

- Eliminate Heat
- Nourish Yin

Acupoints

KID-3, KID-6, BL-23, *Shen Shu*, SP-6, SP-10, BL-17, LI-11, GV-14

Herbal Formula

Qing Hao Bie Jia Tang

Disease Viewed with Four TCVM Systems

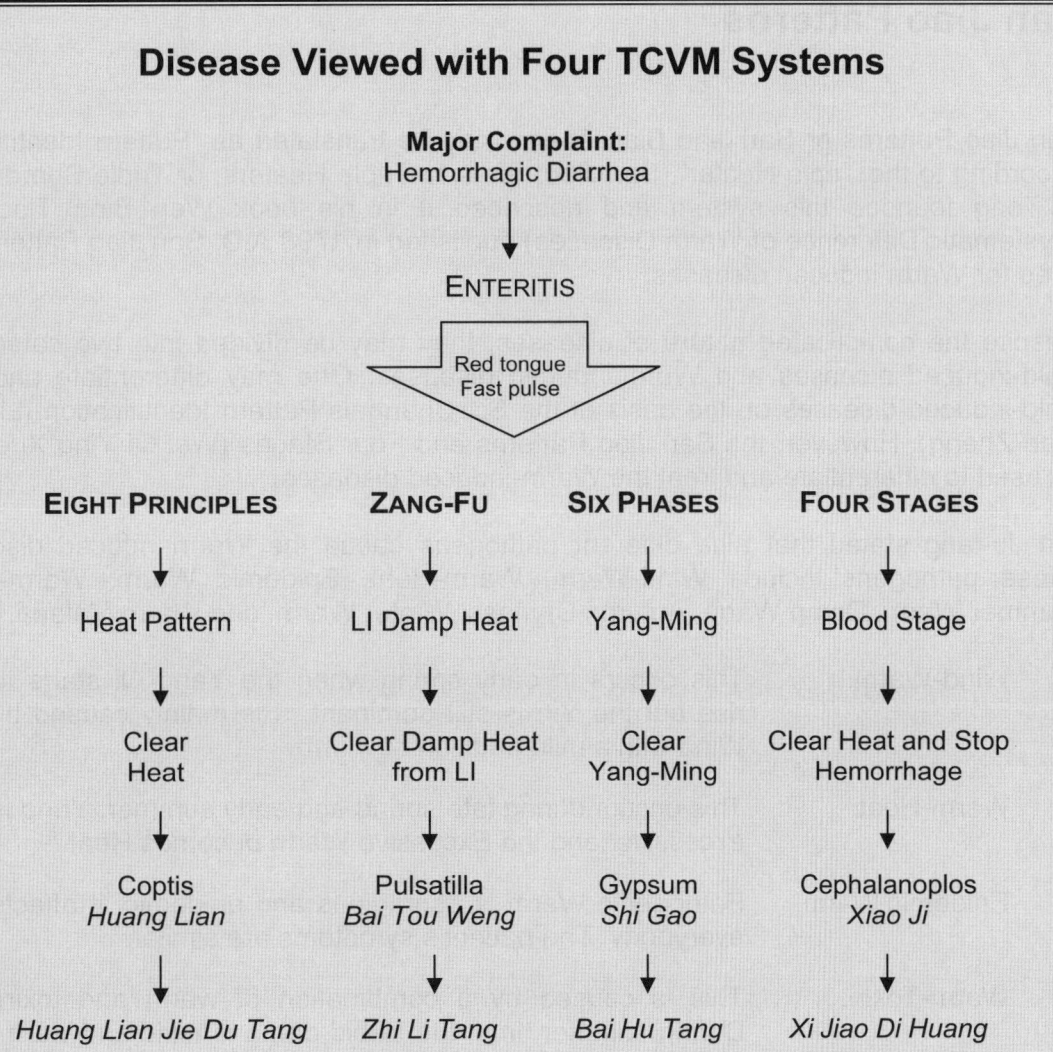

Major Complaint:
Hemorrhagic Diarrhea

↓

ENTERITIS

Red tongue
Fast pulse

EIGHT PRINCIPLES	ZANG-FU	SIX PHASES	FOUR STAGES
↓	↓	↓	↓
Heat Pattern	LI Damp Heat	Yang-Ming	Blood Stage
↓	↓	↓	↓
Clear Heat	Clear Damp Heat from LI	Clear Yang-Ming	Clear Heat and Stop Hemorrhage
↓	↓	↓	↓
Coptis *Huang Lian*	Pulsatilla *Bai Tou Weng*	Gypsum *Shi Gao*	Cephalanoplos *Xiao Ji*
↓	↓	↓	↓
Huang Lian Jie Du Tang	*Zhi Li Tang*	*Bai Hu Tang*	*Xi Jiao Di Huang*

The same disease may have different Patterns when using the various diagnostic systems. Based on the Eight Principles system, this disease is diagnosed as Excess Heat and the treatment principle is to clear the Excess and Heat. In this case, the formula *Huang Lian Jie Du Tang* may be used for generalized, whole-body Excess Heat.

The Zang-Fu Pattern system characterizes this disease as Large Intestine Damp Heat. This gives a practitioner a specific location of the pathogens Damp and Heat. Thus, the herbal formula *Zhi Li Tang* is a good treatment choice because it specifically clears Damp Heat from the Large Intestines.

This disease has a Yang Ming Pattern with the Six Phases system because the pathogen Heat invades the Yang Ming phase. *Bai Hu Tang* clears Heat from Yang Ming.

The Four Stages system identifies this disease as Blood Heat because the Heat is located in the level of Blood. *Xi Jiao Di Huang Tang* may be used to cool the Blood and stop the hemorrhage.

San Jiao Patterns

San Jiao Patterns or San Jiao Bian Zheng may be translated as "Pattern Identification according to the Triple Heater". San Jiao refers to Triple Heaters, or Triple Burners. Wu Ju-Tong founded this system and described it in his book Wen Bing Tiao Bian (Systematic Difference of Warm Diseases) published in 1798 A.D. San Jiao Patterns are used for Warm-induced diseases.

Despite the complicated nature of diseases, they may be divided into two categories: Cold-induced diseases and Warm-induced diseases. One may differentiate and treat Cold-induced diseases on the basis of the Six Channels Pattern Identification (Liu Jing Bian Zheng). However, the San Jiao Patterns and Four Stages (Wei Qi Ying Xue) may be used to differentiate and treat the Warm-induced diseases.

Wu Ju-tang stated that nine different pathogens cause the Warm-induced diseases. These pathogens include Wind-Warm, Warm-Heat, Epidemic Warm, Warm-Toxin, Summer Warm, Damp Warm, Autumn Dryness, Winter Warm, and Warm Malaria.

Wind-Warm:	This occurs in early spring when the Yang Qi starts to rise but the Yin is still dominant. It is mainly caused by Wind with a mild addition of Warm.
Warm-Heat:	This occurs during late spring and early summer. Yang is excessive, and the Excessive Warm becomes Heat.
Epidemic Warm:	Pathogenic Warm is contagious and epidemic; it affects everybody. The patient's symptoms are similar.
Warm-Toxin:	This is caused by a combination of warm and toxin. During summer time, the turbid damp is toxic and warm, and tends to become Warm-Toxin.
Summer Warm:	This occurs in the summertime. During the summer period, Heat often combines with Damp. Thus, Heat, with a minor addition of Damp, causes Summer Warm.
Damp Warm:	This occurs in late summer and early autumn when Damp and Heat combine. It is predominantly caused by Damp with minor portion of Heat.
Autumn Dryness:	This occurs in autumn when Dryness is dominant.
Winter Warm:	Normally, Winter time should be cold. If the Winter is warm, Yin fails to conceal Yang. The now-revealed Yang becomes Warm.
Warm Malaria:	When Yin is damaged at the first place, deficient Yin fails to cool the body. Thus, the pathogen warm tends to lead malaria in the Summer time.

Wu Ju-tong's writing compares the San-jiao Patterns with the Six Channel Patterns:

> The pathogens invade the body through the pores of the skin in the Cold-Induced Diseases (Six Channels Patterns). The symptoms start from the lower to the upper. The lower is the foot Tai-yang Bladder Channel. The Bladder Channel is Water. The Qi of Water is Cold. Thus, the Cold-induced disease originates from Tai-yang.

> The pathogens invade the body from the mouth and nose in the Warm-induced Diseases (San-jiao Patterns). The symptoms start from the upper to the lower. The nose is connected with the Lung. The hand Tai-yin Lung Channel belongs to Metal. The Qi of Fire is Warm. Imbalanced Fire over-controls Metal (Fire tends to melt Metal). Thus, the Warm-induced disease starts at the Lung.

The Cold-induced diseases are diagnosed using the Six Channels system. With the Cold diseases, the signs begin at the lowest part and move upward. This means that the disease originates in Tai-Yang. This may be understandable considering that the foot Tai-yang is the Bladder Channel, which belongs to the Water element and is associated with Cold. Also, Cold induced diseases affect the bladder because the bladder is Yang and Cold diseases affect Yang first.

On the other hand, the Warm-induced diseases are diagnosed using the San-Jiao Patterns. With the Warm diseases, the signs begin at the upper level of the body and move to the lower portions. The disease starts at the Lung. The nose, the entryway for the pathogens, connects with the Lung, which is the highest organ. The Lung and the hand Tai-yin (Lung Channel) belong to the Metal element. The Qi of the invading Warm pathogen belongs to the Fire element. When the Fire is excessive (for example during summer time), it tends to over-control the Metal (the Lung), thus disease results in the Lung. So, Warm induced diseases affect the nose first because Warm affects/controls Metal (lung) and the nose is the opening to the Lung.

UPPER JIAO PATTERNS

The Warm-induced diseases start at the nose, which is connected with the Lung. Two transformations may occur following the affliction of the Lung. These include a shift of an illness into the Middle Jiao (normal transfer) or into the Pericardium (counter-transfer).

Tai-yin Warm Diseases

1. Warm affects the Lung

Etiology

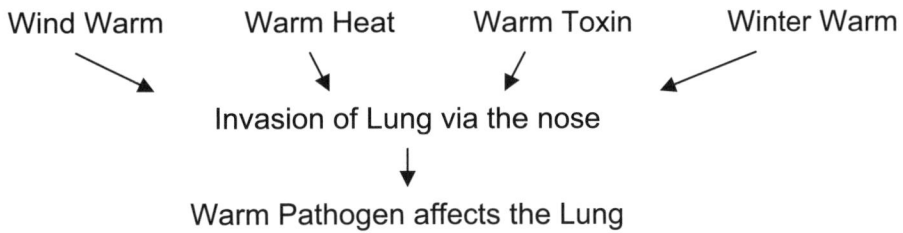

Wind Warm   Warm Heat   Warm Toxin   Winter Warm

Invasion of Lung via the nose

Warm Pathogen affects the Lung

Clinical Signs

- Mild fever
- Sweating
- Red tongue
- Fast Pulse

- Fever that is worse in early afternoon
- Slightly dislikes Wind-Cold
- Thirsty or coughing without thirst
- Headache (dislikes being touched on the head)

Acupoints

GV-14, LI-11, LI-4, BL-10, BL-12

Herbal Formula

Sang Ju Yin

2. Summer Warm affects the Lung

Etiology

Summer Warm

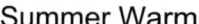

Invasion of Lung via
the nose

Summer Warm in the Lung

Clinical Signs

- Occurs in the summer
- Polydipsia
- Sweating too much
- Red tongue

- Begins with headaches, general body aches, fever or dislike of cold
- Forceful and fast pulse on the right, but normal on the left

Acupoints

LU-5, LU-10, *Wei Jian, Er Jian, Xiong Tang*

Herbal Formula

Xiang Ru San

3. Phlegm Heat stagnates in the Lung

Etiology

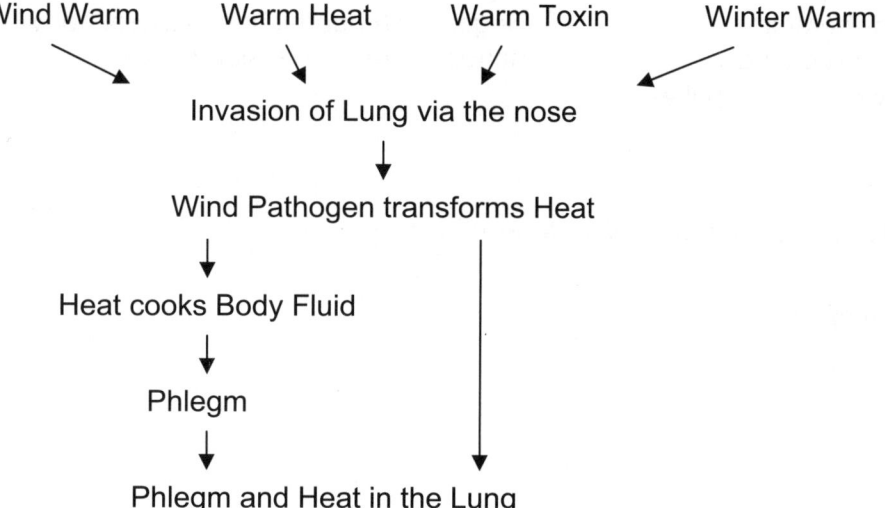

Wind Warm   Warm Heat   Warm Toxin   Winter Warm

Invasion of Lung via the nose

Wind Pathogen transforms Heat

Heat cooks Body Fluid

Phlegm

Phlegm and Heat in the Lung

Clinical Signs

- High fever
- Sweating
- Thirsty
- Red tongue
- Dislikes heat (seeks cool places)
- Dyspnea or productive cough (spitting phlegm)
- Yellow tongue coating:
- Forceful and fast pulse

Acupoints

LU-5, LU-10, GV-14, BL-13, PC-5

Herbal Formula

Qing Qi Hua Tan Tang

4. Damp Warm affects the Lung

Etiology

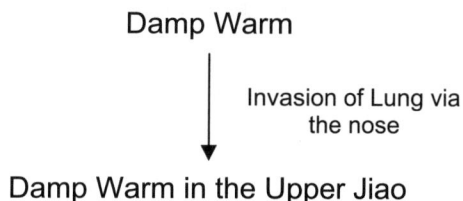

Damp Warm

Invasion of Lung via
the nose

Damp Warm in the Upper Jiao

Clinical Signs

- Lack of thirst
- No sweating
- Chest discomfort
- Yellow or red tongue
- Choppy or thready pulse

- Occurs in late summer or early fall
- High fever that is worse in the afternoon
- Begins with headaches, general body aches, fever or aversion to cold

Acupoints

LU-5, LU-10, *Wei Jian* and *Er Jian*, *Xiong Tang*

Herbal Formula

Sang Ren Tang

Counter-transferring into the Pericardium

Etiology

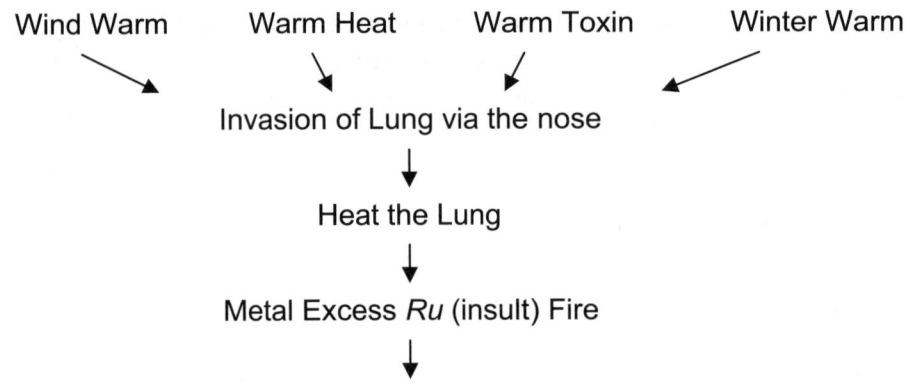

Wind Warm   Warm Heat   Warm Toxin   Winter Warm

Invasion of Lung via the nose

↓

Heat the Lung

↓

Metal Excess *Ru* (insult) Fire

↓

Heat Counter-transferring into Pericardium

Clinical Signs

- Cold extremities
- Deep red tongue
- Fast pulse

- Dyspnea, possibly with phlegm in the throat
- Sudden onset of aggressive behavior
- Sudden loss of consciousness

Acupoints

PC-9, PC-6, TH-5, SI-1

Herbal Formulas

An Gong Niu Huang Wan

MIDDLE JIAO PATTERNS

Yang-ming Warm Diseases

1. Dryness and Excess of Yang Ming

Etiology

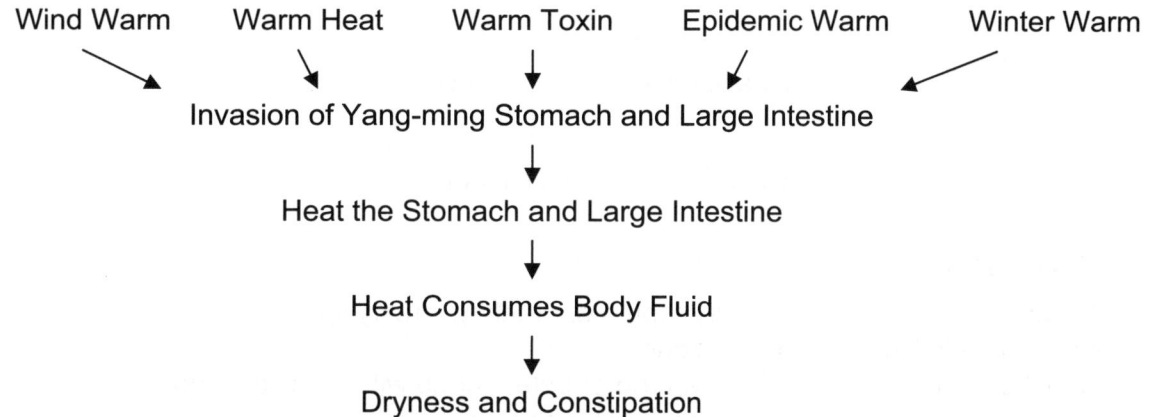

Wind Warm   Warm Heat   Warm Toxin   Epidemic Warm   Winter Warm

Invasion of Yang-ming Stomach and Large Intestine

Heat the Stomach and Large Intestine

Heat Consumes Body Fluid

Dryness and Constipation

Clinical Signs

- Short urination
- Dyspnea
- Difficult defecation

- Dislikes heat (cold-seeking)
- Red or deep red tongue
- Fast or forceful pulse

Acupoints

ST-44, LI-4, LI-10, ST-25, ST-37, BL-25

Herbal Formulas

Da Cheng Qi Tang

2. Body Fluid Deficiency of Yang Ming

Etiology

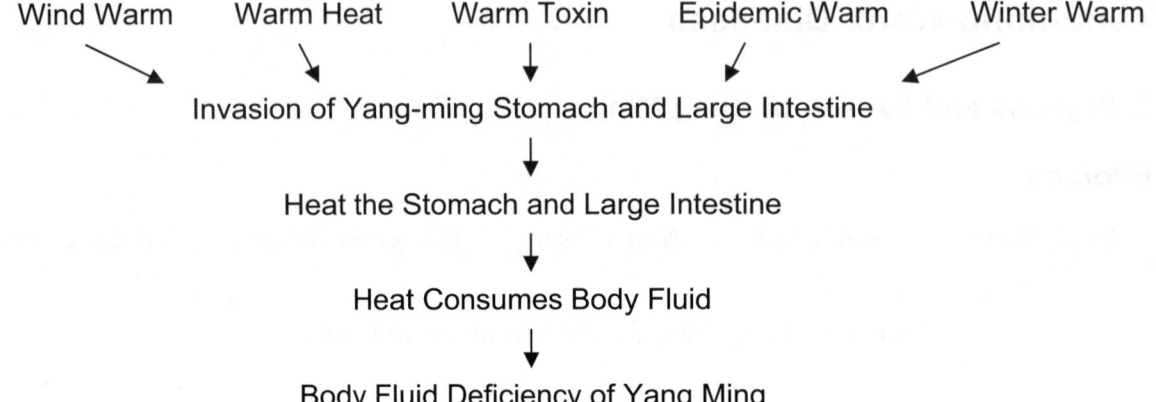

Wind Warm   Warm Heat   Warm Toxin   Epidemic Warm   Winter Warm

Invasion of Yang-ming Stomach and Large Intestine

Heat the Stomach and Large Intestine

Heat Consumes Body Fluid

Body Fluid Deficiency of Yang Ming

Clinical Signs

- Fever
- Abdominal fullness
- Constipation
- Thirsty

- Dry mouth or cracked, crusty lips
- Fatigue
- Deep red or pale tongue with black coating
- Deep and weak pulse

Acupoints

ST-36, BL-21, BL-20, CV-6, KID-3, SP-6, GV-1 and ST-37

Herbal Formula

Zeng Ye Tang

Damp enters the Middle Jiao

1. Heat-Damp in the Middle Jiao

Etiology

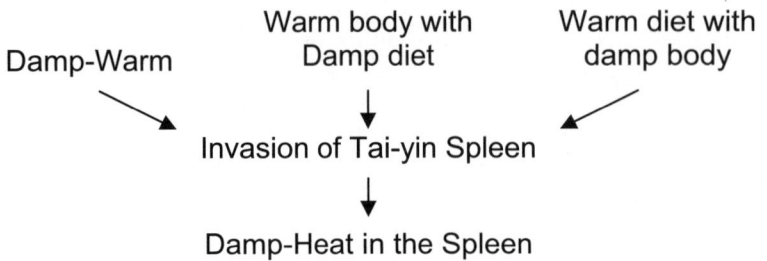

Damp-Warm   Warm body with Damp diet   Warm diet with damp body

Invasion of Tai-yin Spleen

Damp-Heat in the Spleen

Clinical Signs

- Fever
- Abdominal fullness
- Nausea or vomiting
- Red urine
- Malodorous and bloody diarrhea
- Fatigue
- Pale tongue with a greasy, yellow coating
- Fast pulse

Acupoints

ST-44, *Wei Jian*, SP-6, SP-9, SP-10

Herbal Formula

Da Xiang Lian Wan

2. Cold-Damp in the Middle Jiao

Etiology

Cold-Damp from diet or environment

↓

Cold Damp in the Spleen

Clinical Signs

- Coldness of the limbs
- Abdominal fullness
- Loose stool
- Anorexia or vomiting
- Fatigue
- General body soreness
- Pale tongue with white, greasy coating
- Unclear (Feeble) pulse

Acupoints

SP-6, SP-9, BL-20, CV-6, CV-4, GV-3, GV-4, *Bai Hui*, SP-15

Herbal Formulas

Li Zhong Tang

LOWER JIAO PATTERNS

Liver-Kidney Yin Deficiency

Etiology

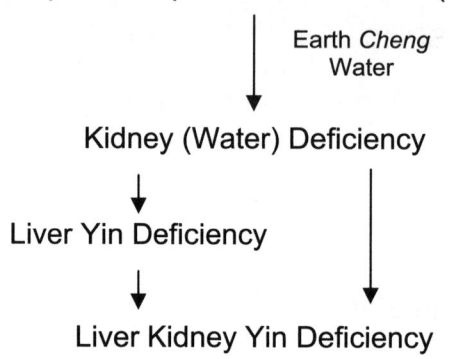

Damp in the Spleen and Stomach (Earth)

Earth *Cheng*
Water

Kidney (Water) Deficiency

Liver Yin Deficiency

Liver Kidney Yin Deficiency

Clinical Signs

- Fever
- Thirsty
- Deafness
- Dry eyes
- Depression

- Warm pads / palms and cooler dorsal paws / back of hands
- Dry mouth
- Crack lines in the tongue
- Deep red tongue with no coating or a peeled coating
- Thready and weak pulse

Acupoints

KID-3, KID-7, KID-10, LIV-3, LIV-8, BL-23, BL-18

Herbal Formula

Liu Wei Di Huang Wan

Spleen-Kidney Yang Deficiency

Etiology

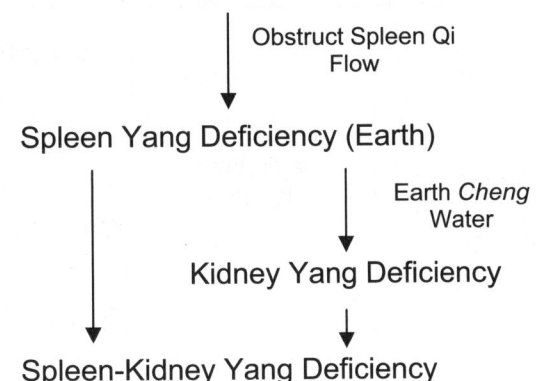

Damp in the Spleen (Damp is the Yin Factor)

Obstruct Spleen Qi Flow

Spleen Yang Deficiency (Earth)

Earth *Cheng* Water

Kidney Yang Deficiency

Spleen-Kidney Yang Deficiency

Clinical Signs

- General body ache
- Fatigue
- Heat-seeking
- Depression
- Edema in the limbs or abdominal areas
- Numb or weak back and/or rear limbs
- Pale and swollen tongue
- Deep, weak and slow pulse

Acupoints

GV-4, GV-3, *Bai Hui*, CV-4, ST-36, BL-20, *Shen Shu*

Herbal Formula

Shi Pi Yin

Table 8.12: The Upper, Middle and Lower Jiao Patterns

San Jiao	Location	Types	Sub-Types
Upper Jiao Patterns	Throat to chest Lung Pericardium Heart	Tai-yin Warm diseases	Warm affects the Lung
			Phlegm Heat stagnates in the Lung
			Damp Warm affects the Lung
			Summer Warm affects the Lung
		Counter-transferring into the Pericardium	
Middle Jiao Patterns	Chest to umbilicus Spleen Stomach	Yang-ming Warm Diseases	Dryness and Excess of Yang Ming
			Body Fluid Deficiency of Yang Ming
		Damp enters the Middle Jiao	Heat-Damp in the Middle Jiao
			Cold-Damp in the Middle Jiao
Lower Jiao Patterns	Umbilicus to pubis Kidney Liver	Liver-Kidney Yin Deficiency	
		Spleen-Kidney Yang Deficiency	

Pathogen Patterns

As discussed in Chapter 6, there are numerous factors that may impair the Yin-Yang equilibrium and may result in disease. These factors are known as the pathogens or the causes of a disease. Thus, disease may be due to the following: 1) the exogenous factors; 2) the internal etiologic factors; 3) the secondary factors; 4) the other factors. The major exogenous factors are the Six Pathogens: Wind, Cold, Summer Heat, Damp, Dryness, and Fire/Heat. The major internal etiological factors include the seven emotional states and the quality of the animal husbandry programs. The secondary factors include Blood Stagnation, Qi Stagnation, Phlegm, Stones and Food Stasis. The others include trauma, parasites, poisoning, iatrogenic factors and congenital factors.

Chen Yan (Song Dynasty) wrote about three types of Pathogenic Patterns. In his book *San Yin Ji Yi Bing Zheng Fang Lun* (*Discussion of Illnesses, Patterns, Formulas Related to Unification of Three Etiologies*), published in 1174 A.D., he describes the Three Etiologies as External, Internal, and Non-internal/Non-external. External Etiology refers to the Six Pathogens. Internal Etiology refers to the seven forms of emotion. The final one refers to disorders of diet or exercise programs.

Etiology	Description
External	Six Pathogens
Internal	Seven Emotion Patterns
Non-Internal Non-External	Feeding or Management Disorders (Disorders of Animal Husbandry)

SIX PATHOGENS PATTERNS

The Six Pathogens include Wind, Cold, Summer Heat, Damp, Dryness, and Fire. These Pathogens have several important characteristics:

1. They are related to the seasons. Wind often occurs in the spring. Cold occurs more often in the winter. Fire affects the body more often in the summer. Dryness occurs more frequently in the fall.

2. Pathogens may invade the body in combinations of two or more. For example, Wind often combines with Cold or Heat and becomes Wind-Cold or Wind-Heat. The combination of Damp and Heat is called Damp-Heat. The combination of Pathogens is also related to the seasons (Table 8.13).

3. The Pathogen combinations also depend upon the constitutional conditions. If Damp invades a Yang body (Heat), it may become Damp-Heat.

4. The pathological changes of the Six Pathogens are based on the constitutional conditions. For example, if the body is Yang, a pathogen tends to transform into Fire after it invades the body. If the body is Yin, a pathogen tends to transform into Cold.

Table 8.13: Pathogen relationship to the seasons and each other

Season	Dominant Pathogen	Combines with
Spring	Wind	Cold, Damp, Fire / Heat
Summer	Heat / Fire	Wind, Summer Heat, Damp, Cold
Later Summer	Damp Summer Heat	Wind, Heat
Fall	Dryness	Wind, Cold, Fire / Heat
Winter	Cold	Wind, Damp

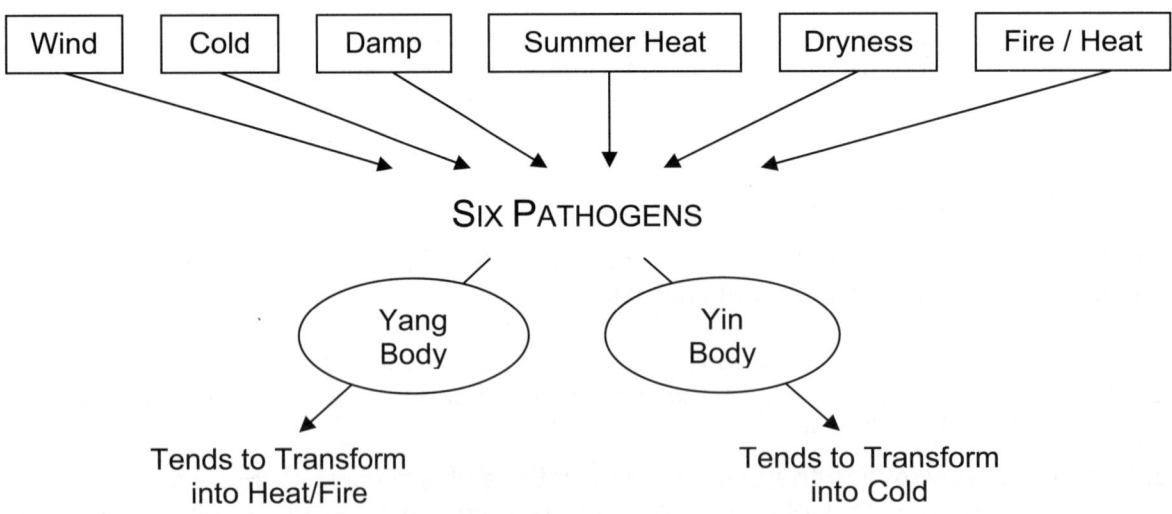

Figure 8.2: Six Pathogen effects in the body

Wind Patterns

Wind is the master pathogen. It penetrates everywhere and goes anywhere. An old TCVM maxim says "There is no place where Wind can not reach". Wind often brings other pathogens to invade the body and cause a disease. Wind is a light pathogen, and it often affects the upper parts or superficial portions of the body.

Wind Form	Effect in Body
Exogenous Wind	Wind affects body surface
	Wind stays in the muscle
	Wind attacks the Channels
	Wind obstructs the joints
Combination with other Pathogens	Wind-Cold
	Wind-Heat
	Wind-Dryness
	Wind-Cold-Damp
Internal Wind	Extreme Heat
	Liver Yang Rising
	Liver Blood Deficiency
	Liver Yin Deficiency

EXOGENOUS WIND

1. Wind affects body surface

Etiology

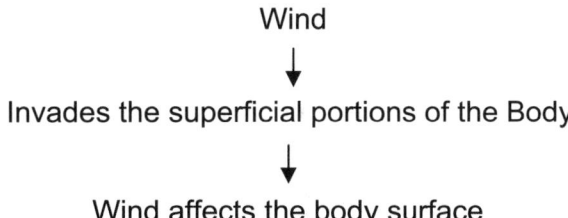

Clinical Signs

- Fever
- Aversion to wind
- Slightly coughing
- Headache

- Sweating or slight sweating
- Itching sensation in the throat
- Slightly thin white tongue coating
- Superficial and slow pulse

Acupoints

GB-20, BL-10, BL-12, LI-4

Herbal Formula

Jing Fang Bai Du San

2. Wind stays in the muscle

Etiology

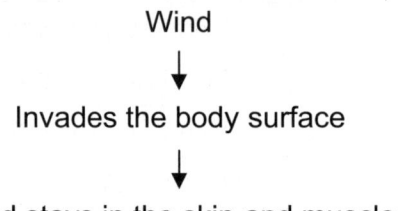

Wind
↓
Invades the body surface
↓
Wind stays in the skin and muscles

Clinical Signs

- Skin itching
- Skin rash
- Wheals or urticaria
- Sudden onset of skin lesions on head or neck
- Slightly pale or red or normal tongue
- Superficial or floating pulse

Acupoints

GB-20, BL-10, SP-10

Herbal Formula

Wai Feng San (External Wind Formula)

3. Wind attacks the Channels

Etiology

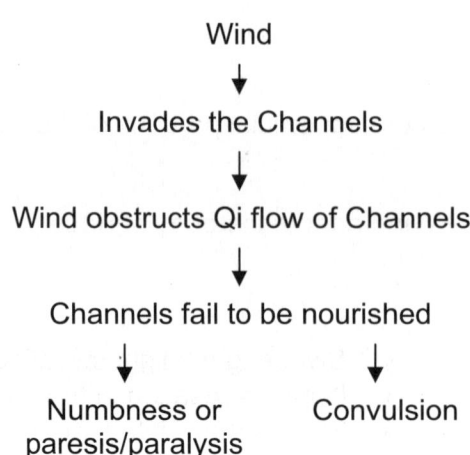

Wind
↓
Invades the Channels
↓
Wind obstructs Qi flow of Channels
↓
Channels fail to be nourished
↓   ↓
Numbness or   Convulsion
paresis/paralysis

Clinical Signs

- Numb
- Tight pulse
- Limb paresis
- Sudden onset of convulsions (tetanus)
- Slightly pale or red tongue
- Acute onset of facial paralysis

Acupoints

GB-20, BL-10, SP-10, LIV-3, *Da Feng Men*, *Bai Hui*

Herbal Formula

Ding Xian Wan

4. Wind Obstructs in the Joints

Etiology

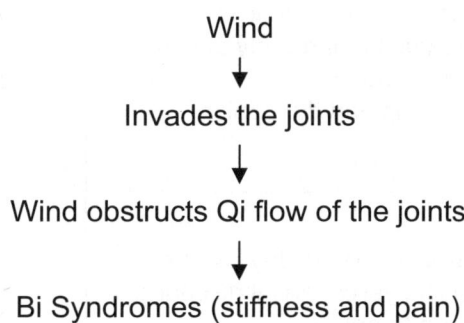

Wind
↓
Invades the joints
↓
Wind obstructs Qi flow of the joints
↓
Bi Syndromes (stiffness and pain)

Clinical Signs

- Rapid onset
- Meridian and joint pain
- Superficial (floating) pulse
- Changes from place to place ("pain wanders")
- Slight thin pale tongue coating
- Pain worsens when exposed to wind

Acupoints

GB-20, BL-17, SP-10, LIV-3, plus local points around the joints, SP-21 if pain in all joints

Herbal Formula

Fang Feng Tang

COMBINATION WITH OTHER PATHOGENS

1. *Wind-Cold*: Occurs in the common cold
2. *Wind-Heat*: Occurs in the common cold, in influenza, and in the early stages of warm diseases
3. *Wind-Dryness*: Occurs in dry environmental conditions such as the desert.
4. *Wind-Cold-Damp*

Common Wind Patterns	Clinical Signs	Acupoints	Herbal Formula
Wind-Cold	• Acute onset • Greater than 3-day course • Clear nasal discharge • Headache and body aches • Pale tongue • Floating and tight pulse	BL-10 GB-20 LI-4 BL-12	*Xiao Qing Long Tang*
Wind-Heat	• Greater than 7-day course • Thick, yellow nasal discharge • Sore throat • Cough • Thirst • Red tongue • Fast pulse	GV-14 LI-4 LI-11	*Yin Qiao San*
Wind-Dryness	• Greater than 7-day course • Bloody nasal discharge • Cough • Dry lips or mouth • Red tongue • Fast pulse	GV-14 LI-4 LU-9	*Sang Ju Yin*
Wind-Cold-Damp	• Sore joints and muscles • Stiffness • Bi syndromes	Local points (Moxibustion)	*Du Huo Ji Sheng Tang*

INTERNAL WIND

Internal Wind refers to seizures or convulsions, which are generated by disorders of the interior due to Extreme Heat, Liver Yang Rising, Liver Blood Deficiency or Liver Yin Deficiency.

Internal Wind Patterns	Clinical Signs	Acupoints	Herbal Formula
Extreme Heat	• High fever • Convulsion • Red tongue • Thick yellow coating • Fast and forceful pulse	*Shen Tang* GV-14	*An Gong Niu Huang Wan*
Liver Yang Rising	• The wood type constitution • Irritable • Hyperactive • Red eyes • Hypertension • Purple or red tongue • Wiry pulse	LIV-3 GB-34 GB-43	*Jue Ming San*
Liver Blood Deficiency	• Anemia • Dry hair or dandruff • Pale tongue • Weak and thready pulse • Chronic seizures	SP-10 BL-17 GB-20	*Bu Xue Xi Feng San*
Liver Yin Deficiency	• Dry nose and mouth • Seizure at night or late afternoon • Chronic seizure • Red tongue • Weak and thready pulse	KID-3 LIV-3 KID-10	*Yang Yin Xi Feng San*

Cold Patterns

Cold is a Yin pathogen. It tends to damage the Yang of the body and results in Yang Deficiency. Cold obstructs the Qi flow and leads to Qi Stagnation and secondary Blood Stagnation.

EXTERNAL COLD PATTERNS

External Cold Patterns	Clinical Signs	Acupoints	Herbal Formula
Exterior Cold	<ul><li>No sweating</li><li>Aversion to coldness</li><li>Shivering</li><li>Headache</li><li>Body ache</li><li>Pale and greasy tongue coating</li><li>Floating and tight pulse</li></ul>	BL-10 GB-20 BL-12 *Da Feng Men*	*Ma Huang Tang*
Cold in the Channels	<ul><li>Pain in joints</li><li>Difficulty in movement</li><li>Pain exacerbated by cold or massage</li><li>Purple tongue</li><li>Tight and wiry pulse</li></ul>	*Bai Hui* (Moxa) GV-4 SP-21 Local points	*Xiao Huo Luo Dan*
Direct attack of the Middle	<ul><li>Abdominal pain (colic)</li><li>Diarrhea</li><li>Vomiting</li><li>Coldness of nose or limbs</li><li>Pale tongue with white coating</li><li>Weak or deep pulse</li></ul>	CV-12 CV-4 GV-4 SP-15	*Ju Pi San*

INTERNAL COLD PATTERNS

Internal Cold refers to coldness originating in the Interior due to Yang Deficiency.

Internal Cold Patterns	Clinical Signs	Acupoints	Herbal Formula
Spleen Yang Deficiency	<ul><li>Colic</li><li>Anorexia</li><li>Diarrhea</li><li>Pale tongue</li><li>Deep, weak pulse</li><li>Cold extremities and ears</li></ul>	*Bai Hui* GV-4 CV-6 (Moxibustion)	*Li Zhong Tang*
Kidney Yang Deficiency	<ul><li>Coldness</li><li>Infertility</li><li>Urinary incontinence</li><li>Weak back or hind limbs</li><li>Pale, swollen tongue</li><li>Deep and weak pulse</li></ul>	*Bai Hui* GV-3 GV-4 *Shen Shu* (Moxibustion)	*Jin Gui Shen Qi Wan*

Summer Heat Patterns

Summer Heat Patterns most often occur in the summer. Summer Heat can invade the body alone or can combine with Damp-Heat or Cold-Damp.

Summer Heat Patterns	Clinical Signs	Acupoints	Herbal Formula
Summer Heat in the Lung and Stomach	• Fever • Thirst • Cough without phlegm • Slightly white, greasy tongue • Slipper and fast pulse	Er Jian Xiong Tang Lu-5	Cang Zhu Bai Hu Tang
Summer Heat Scorching Yang Ming	• Fever • Headache • Restlessness • Dyspnea • Sweating • Polydipsia • Forceful pulse • Coma	Xiong Tang ST-44 ST-45	Huang Lian Bai Hu Tang
Summer Heat with Damp-Heat	• Fever • Not thirsty • Malodorous and watery diarrhea • Short, red urination • Red tongue • Yellow, greasy tongue coat • Fast pulse	Wei Jian Shen Tang SP-6 ST-44	Lian Po Yin
Summer Heat with Cold-Damp	• Fever • Body ache • Non sweat • Tying-up • Restlessness • Pale and greasy coating	Tai Yang Wei Jian SP-6	Huo Po Xia Ling Tang
Summer Heat Damaging Body Fluid and Qi	• Steaming fever • Spontaneous sweat • Polydipsia • Fatigue • Heaviness of head • Weak and forceless pulse	ST-36 GV-14 SP-6 KID-3	Ren Shen Bai Hu Tang

Damp Patterns

Damp Patterns occur in the late summer or during rainy, high-humidity seasons. Damp is heavy and tends to obstruct Qi flow, especially the Spleen Qi flow. Damp also tends to be sticky; it is difficult to remove after it invades the body.

Damp Patterns	Clinical Signs	Acupoints	Herbal Formula
Damp affects Exterior	• Heaviness of head • Fever • Non-sweating (Anhidrosis) • General body soreness • Fatigue • Thin and white tongue • Floating and choppy pulse	LI-4 LI-10 SP-6	*Huo Po Xia Ling Tang*
Damp invades Skin	• Blister or ulcer on the skin • Eczema • Yellow discharge from skin lesions • Itching	SP-6 SP-9 Local points	*Er Miao San* (Topical application)
Damp stagnates in Joints	• Bi syndrome • Stiffness worse than pain • Pain relief with heat and dryness • Pain worse with cold-damp • Pain worse with weather changes • Greasy, pale coating • Soft, choppy pulse	SP-6 SP-9 ST-37 Local points	*Yi Yi Ren San*
Damp stagnates in the Interior	• Anorexia • Abdominal fullness or pain • Loose stool • Fatigue • White and greasy tongue • Slow and choppy pulse	ST-36 SP-6 BL-20	*Wei Cang He*

Dryness Patterns

The Pathogen Dryness dominates in the fall. Dryness tends to consume Body Fluid.

Dryness Patterns	Clinical Signs	Acupoints	Herbal Formula
Warm Dryness affects Exterior	• Fever • A little sweat • Dry nose and throat • Cough with less phlegm • Red tongue with white coating • Fast pulse on the right	BL-10 LU-9 LU-7 LI-4 KID-6	Sang Ju Yin
Cool Dryness affects Exterior	• Headache • Non-sweat • Nasal congestion • Dry throat • Dry lips • Cough with clear phlegm • White coating • Slow pulse	BL-10 LU-9 GV-20 KID-6	Zhi Sou San

Fire / Heat Patterns

Fire and Heat are similar. Fire is extreme Heat while Heat is a mild form of Fire. Fire/Heat is a Yang pathogen and tends to damage Yin. Fire/Heat tends to force blood out of the vessels and leads to hemorrhage. Any other pathogen including Wind, Cold, Dryness, Summer Heat and Damp may transform into Fire or Heat.

Fire Patterns	Clinical Signs	Acupoints	Herbal Formula
Excess Fire	• Fever • Sore throat • Polydipsia • Gingivitis • Bitter sensation in the mouth • Hyperactive • Dribbling urination • Red tongue with yellow coating • Fast and forceful pulse	GV-14 LI-4 Xiong Tang Shen Tang	Bai Hu Tang
Deficiency Fire	• Mild fever • Five-palm fever* • Insomnia • Red tongue • Thready and fast pulse	KID-3 BL-23 SP-6	Liu Wei Di Huang San

* Note: The Five Palms include two hand palms (around PC-8), two foot palms (around KID-1) and chest (around CV-17).

SEVEN EMOTIONAL PATTERNS

Joy (*Xi*), anger (*Nu*), melancholy (*You*), thinking (*Si*), sorrow/sadness/grief (*Bei*), fear (*Kong*), scare/fright/panic (*Jing*) are the seven mental emotional activities. Normal Qi flow of the physiological and psychological functions requires a small quantity of each of these emotions. However, Excess of these emotional factors can lead to Zang-Fu organ disorders. Excess may occur if the emotional experience is too strong. Deficiency may occur if an imbalanced emotional state lasts for too long. Some emotional factors affect only one Zang-Fu organ, while others affect several organs. For example, too much anger affects the Liver but excessive melancholy (*you*) can affect the Spleen and Lung.

Pin-Yin	Seven Emotions	Expression	Zang-Fu Organ Damaged
xi	Joy	Laughing	Heart
nu	Anger	Anger	Liver
you	Melancholy		Spleen, Lung
kong	Fear	Groaning	Kidney
si	Thinking Sympathy Worrying	Singing	Spleen
bei	Sorrow Sadness Grief	Crying	Lung
jing	Scared Frightened Panic		Heart, Liver, Gall Bladder, Stomach

1. Heart Joy Damage Pattern

Etiology

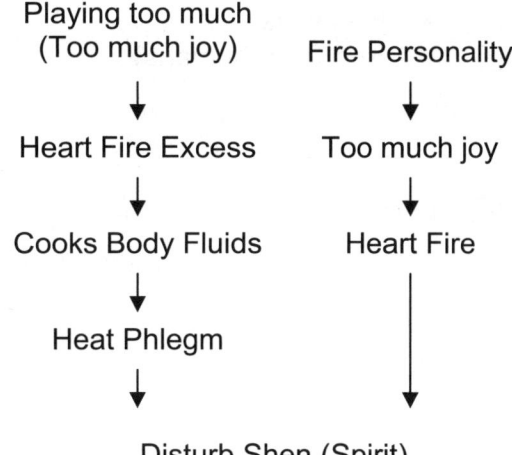

Playing too much (Too much joy) → Heart Fire Excess → Cooks Body Fluids → Heat Phlegm → Disturb Shen (Spirit)

Fire Personality → Too much joy → Heart Fire → Disturb Shen (Spirit)

Clinical Signs

- Loss of focus, easily distracted
- Restlessness
- Disorientation
- Abnormal behavior (barking at night)
- Unclear speech (humans)
- Non-stop smile (humans)

Acupoints

HT-7, PC-6, *An Shen*, BL-44 and BL-15

Herbal Formula

Modified *Tian Wang Bu Xin Dan* (Shen Calmer)

2. Liver Anger Damage Pattern

Etiology

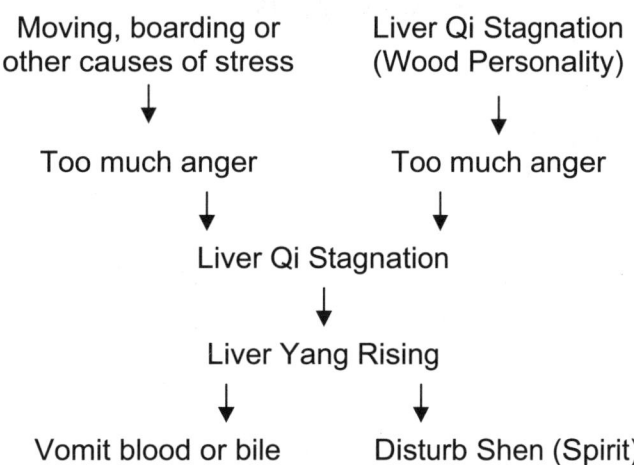

Moving, boarding or other causes of stress → Too much anger

Liver Qi Stagnation (Wood Personality) → Too much anger

Liver Qi Stagnation → Liver Yang Rising → Vomit blood or bile / Disturb Shen (Spirit)

Clinical Signs

- Irritability
- Impatience
- Hyperactivity
- Anxiety (panting in dog)
- Losing temper very easily
- Vomiting with blood or bile
- Red eyes
- Red face (humans)

Acupoints

LIV-3, GB-34, BL-18, BL-47, BL-48

Herbal Formula

Chai Hu Shu Gan Wan

3. Melancholy Damage Pattern

Etiology

Too much melancholy, depression
or unhappiness

↓

Obstruction of Qi Flow of Spleen and Lung

↓   ↓

Lung Qi Stagnation   Spleen Qi Stagnation

Clinical Signs

- Depression, melancholy
- Shortness of breath
- Dyspnea
- Fatigue
- Abdominal fullness
- Pressure in the chest
- Choppy pulse

Acupoints

BL-42, BL-49, CV-17, ST-36

Herbal Formula

Yue Ju Wan

4. Kidney Fear Damage Pattern

Etiology

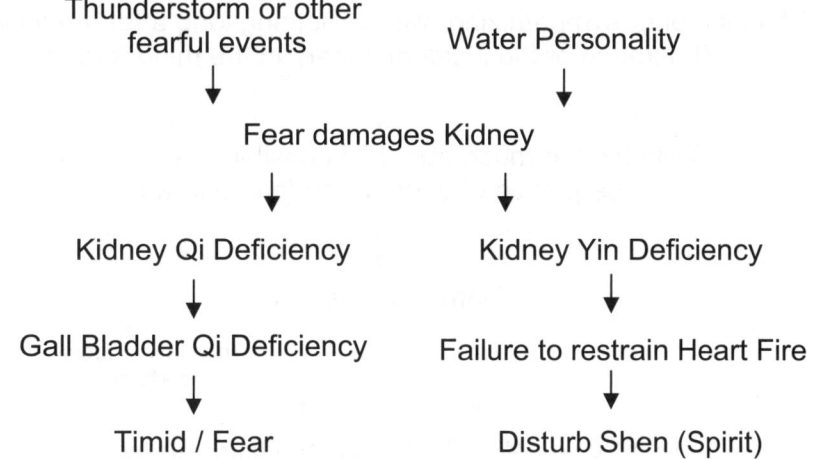

Clinical Signs

- Thunderstorm phobia
- Fear biting or fear kicking
- Insecure (separation anxiety)

- Fear of loud noises (fireworks, gun shot)
- Fear of strange events or strangers
- Hiding or running away in the exam room

Acupoints

BL-52, KID-3, *Shen Shu*, *Bai Hui*

Herbal Formula

You Gui Wan with *Bu Xin Dan*

5. Spleen Thinking Damage Pattern

Etiology

Thinking of or sympathizing with something long after the incident
(The image of the incident lingers in the mind forever)

↓

Thinking too much about all possible outcomes or
sequence of events with failure to act

↓

Damage Spleen Qi

The Child affects
the Mother

Spleen Qi Deficiency   Shen Disturbance

Clinical Signs

- Loss of appetite
- Fatigue
- Loss of body weight
- Muscle atrophy
- Forgetful, absentminded
- Palpitations

Acupoints

ST-36, BL-49, BL-20, HT-7

Herbal Formula

Wei Chang He (Happy Earth Powder)

6. Lung Grief Damage Pattern

Etiology

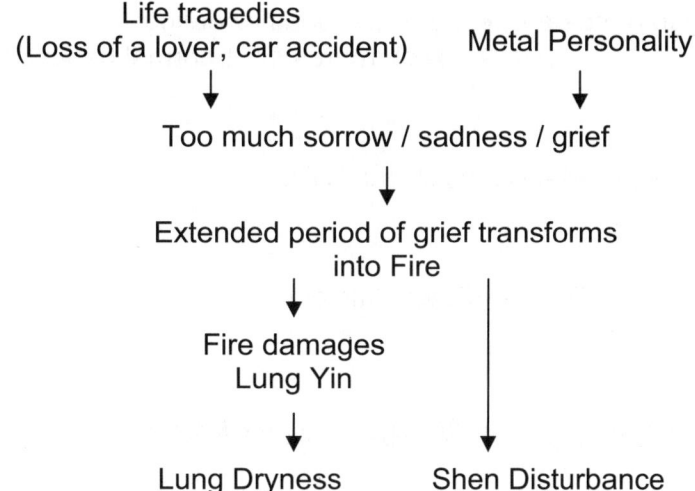

Life tragedies
(Loss of a lover, car accident)   Metal Personality

↓   ↓

Too much sorrow / sadness / grief

↓

Extended period of grief transforms
into Fire

↓

Fire damages
Lung Yin

↓

Lung Dryness   Shen Disturbance

Clinical Signs

- Easily saddened
- Crying a lot
- Dry skin or hair coat

- Depression
- Aloofness
- Cough or dyspnea

Acupoints

BL-42, BL-13, LU-9, CV-17

Herbal Formula

Gan Mai Da Zao Tang

7. Fright Damage Pattern

Etiology

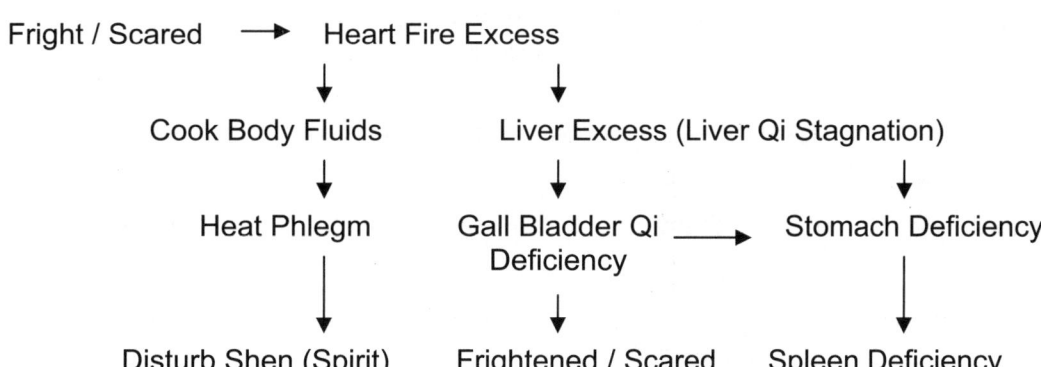

Fright / Scared ⟶ Heart Fire Excess

↓   ↓

Cook Body Fluids   Liver Excess (Liver Qi Stagnation)

↓   ↓   ↓

Heat Phlegm   Gall Bladder Qi ⟶ Stomach Deficiency
                Deficiency

↓   ↓   ↓

Disturb Shen (Spirit)   Frightened / Scared   Spleen Deficiency

Clinical Signs

- Anxiety
- Restlessness
- Easily frightened or scared
- Fatigue
- Panic during frightening events (losing one's mind)
- Dyspnea
- Spontaneous sweating
- Nightmares or abnormal behavior at the night

Acupoints

HT-7, PC-6, *An Shen*, BL-44, BL49, BL-50, HT-6

Herbal Formula

Modified *Tian Wang Bu Xin Wan* (Shen Calmer)

DISORDERS OF FEEDING AND MANAGEMENT PROGRAMS

> In the past ... people understood the principles of Yin-Yang, and kept its equilibrium. They ate a balanced diet. They got up and went to bed at the regular hours. They avoided overworking. Consequently, they maintained well-being of body and mind. Thus, it is not surprising that they lived over one hundred years without aging. These days, however, people have not followed the principles of lifestyle. They drink wine like water. They work excessively. They have too much sex. Consequently, they drain their Jing, and deplete Qi. ...They get up and go to bed irregularly. Thus, they are aging in their fifties and die soon after.
>
> – *Su Wen* (*General Questions*)

1. Overfeeding

Companion animals depend on their owners for food. The quantity of food provided should be appropriate to their nutritional requirements. Overfeeding, especially after periods of starvation (as seen in stray animals), will impair Spleen and Stomach function and result in sour regurgitation, abdominal distention and loss of appetite.

Etiology

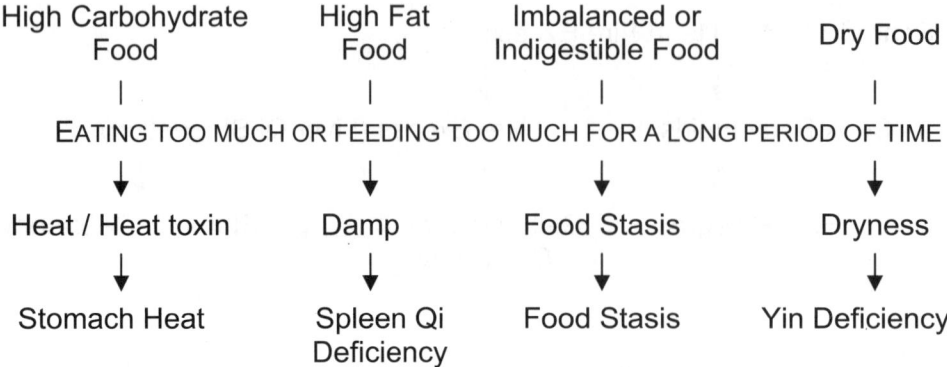

Clinical Signs

- Obesity
- Diabetes
- Anorexia
- Nausea or vomiting
- Fatigue
- Loose stool

Acupoints

ST-36, LI-10, GB-34, BL-21

Herbal Formula

Qu Mai San

2. Malnutrition

Because of a poor diet or lack of food, an animal does not take in adequate nutrition. In the long run, a poor diet leads to malnutrition, weight loss, slow growth of a young animal, and weariness.

Etiology

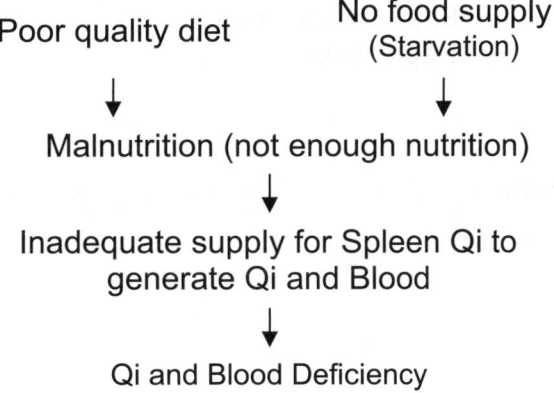

Clinical Signs

- Depression
- Pale tongue
- Weak pulse
- Loss of body weight
- General weakness
- Slow growth and development

Acupoints

ST-36, LI-10, BL-20, BL-21

Herbal Formula

Ba Zhen Tang

3. Overworking (Performance, training work, physical exercise)

Overwork or prolonged work will consume the Body Fluid and Qi. In the long run, overwork leads to Qi Deficiency.

Etiology

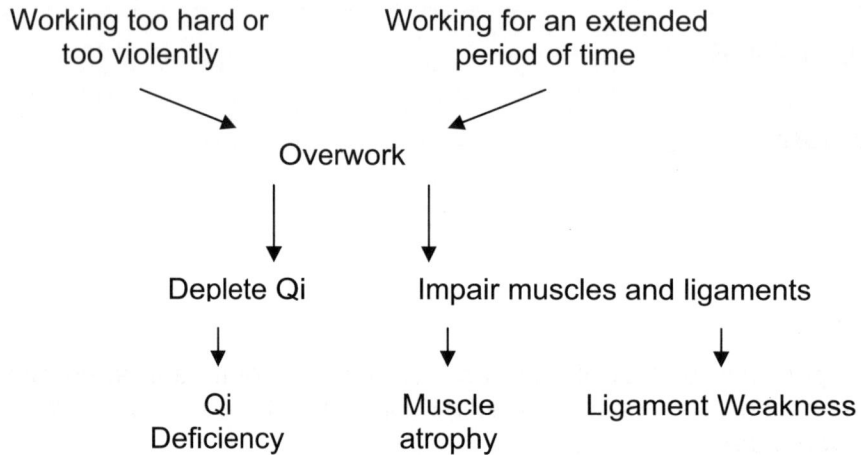

Clinical Signs

- Shortness of breath
- Fatigue
- Exercise intolerance
- Depression

Acupoints

ST-36, CV-4, CV-6, *Bai Hui*

Herbal Formula

Si Jun Zi Tang

4. Underworking or Lack of Physical Exercise

Regular physical exercise is very important to maintain free flow of Qi and Blood. A normal amount of training or work is also necessary for the competitive animals to maintain an athletic level of Qi and Blood.

Underwork indicates an extended period with insufficient physical exercise or training. Underwork can obstruct the circulation of Qi and Blood and affect the function of the Spleen and Stomach. As a result, the animal may experience a loss of appetite, weakness of limbs, and shortness of breath upon physical exertion. If a male breeding animal lacks physical exercise, the vital activity of the sperm will decrease. If a female breeding animal lacks physical exercise for a long time, she will become obese and infertile.

Etiology

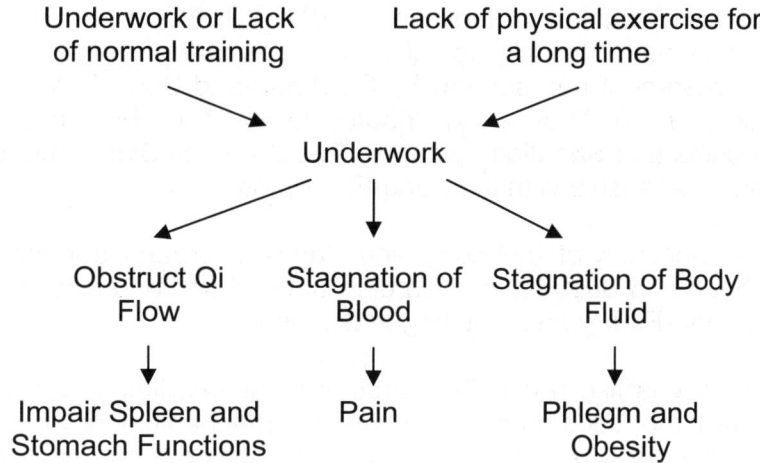

Clinical Signs

- General body soreness
- Obesity

- Loss of appetite
- Fatigue
- Exercise intolerance

Acupoints

ST-36, LI-10, BL-20, BL-21, ST-40, CV-6

Herbal Formula

Wei Ling San

Qi, Blood and Body Fluid Patterns

In Traditional Chinese Veterinary Medicine (TCVM), Qi, Blood and Body Fluid are the fundamental substances for the physiological activities of the Zang-Fu organs. Zang-Fu organs require nourishment and support by Qi, Blood and Body Fluid, which arise from the food Essence (Gu Qi). They are distributed to the Zang-Fu organs and the entire body by the Meridians and San Jiao systems. Therefore, Qi, Blood and Body Fluid have an interdependent relationship with the Zang-Fu organs.

The physiological functions of the body and Zang-Fu organs depend on the normal activities of Qi, Blood and Body Fluid. Disorders of Qi, Blood and Body Fluid may lead to imbalance of the Zang-Fu organs, resulting in disease.

Imagine that the body is like a car. The structural tissues, limbs, and Zang-Fu organs may be considered the car's frame and various mechanical devices. Something is missing, however, because this car will not start. In addition to the basic structure (body, tires, steering wheel) and engine, a car requires oil, gas, and water in order to operate. Similarly, the body requires adequate quantities of Qi, Blood and Body Fluid before it will function properly.

Based in the Zang-Fu and Eight Principle systems, the Patterns of Qi, Blood and Body Fluid provide a method to analyze the pathological changes of these fundamental substances. There is some overlap between these patterns and the Zang-Fu patterns.

Pattern	Form
Qi Pattern	Qi Deficiency
	Qi Sinking
	Qi Stagnation
	Rebellious Qi
Blood Pattern	Blood Deficiency
	Blood Stagnation
	Blood Heat
	Blood Cold
	Hemorrhage
Combination of Qi and Blood Patterns	Qi Stagnation and Blood Stasis
	Qi Deficiency and Blood Stagnation
	Dual Deficiency of Qi and Blood
	Deficient Qi failing to hold Blood
	Qi Deserting with Blood
Body Fluid Pattern	Body Fluid Deficiency
	Retention of Water
	Phlegm

Qi Patterns

Qi plays a very important role in the body. Problems develop if there is an imbalance or disruption of the normal Qi quantity or flow. Qi may exist in four pathologic states within the body: Deficiency, Stagnation, Rebellious, or Sinking (Collapsed)

Qi Deficiency

Qi Deficiency refers to weakness or reduction of the Zang-Fu organs. For example, if the Spleen Qi is too weak to digest and absorb the food and nutrients, it suffers from a Spleen Qi Deficiency. Every Zang-Fu organ can experience Qi Deficiency except the Liver. Only the Liver will never become Qi Deficient. Liver Qi will stagnate when an imbalance exists. However, the Gall Bladder Qi can become deficient and subsequently lead to fear and timidity.

Etiology

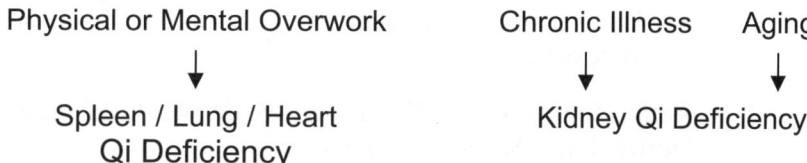

Clinical Signs

There are five general signs of Qi Deficiency:

- Weak pulse
- Pale tongue
- Fatigue or exercise intolerance
- Weakness in body and spirit (physical or mental exhaustion)
- Shortness of breath, dyspnea

Types

Heart Qi Deficiency:
- Palpitations
- Shortness of breath
- Spontaneous sweating (worse if moving)
- Irregularly or regularly intermittent pulse
- Easily frightened

Acupuncture points: HT-7, BL-15, CV-17, PC-6, LU-7
Herbal formula: *Yang Xin Tang*

Kidney Qi Deficiency:
- Arthritis (Bi syndrome)
- Weakness or pain in the lower back or rear limbs
- Urinary or fecal incontinence
- Deafness
- Infertility

Acupuncture points: BL-23, *Bai Hui*, CV-4/6, KID-3, *Shen Shu*
Herbal formula: *Shen Qi Wan*

Lung Qi Deficiency:
- Weak, chronic cough or asthma (worse with movement)
- Appearance of an obvious groove (heaves line) along the rib arch in horses
- Constant recurrence of the common cold
- Spontaneous sweating
- Occurs in the course of chronic bronchitis or chronic pulmonary emphysema.

Acupuncture points: LU-9, BL-13, CV-17, ST-36, *Ding Chuan*
Herbal formula: *Bu Fei San*

Spleen Qi Deficiency:
- Poor appetite
- Diarrhea
- Weight loss, difficulty in gaining body weight, or muscular atrophy
- Fatigue, limb weakness
- Hemorrhage, edema or prolapse of anus
- Occurs in the course of poor absorption or chronic indigestion

Acupuncture points: ST-36, CV-6, CV-4, BL-20, GV-1, SP-3
Herbal formula: *Si Jun Zi Tang*

Qi Stagnation

When Qi does not flow freely, there must be Stagnation. Qi Stagnation refers to blockage or obstruction of the Qi Flow. The major sign of Qi Stagnation is pain. Qi Stagnation can occur in the body surface, muscles, joints, Channels or internal organs. However, Qi Stagnation of the Channels and stagnation of Liver Qi, Stomach Qi or Large Intestine are the most common forms seen in practice. Qi Stagnation of the Channels is the major pathogenic pathway of the Channel disorders, which are addressed in the Channel Patterns section of Chapter 8.

Etiology

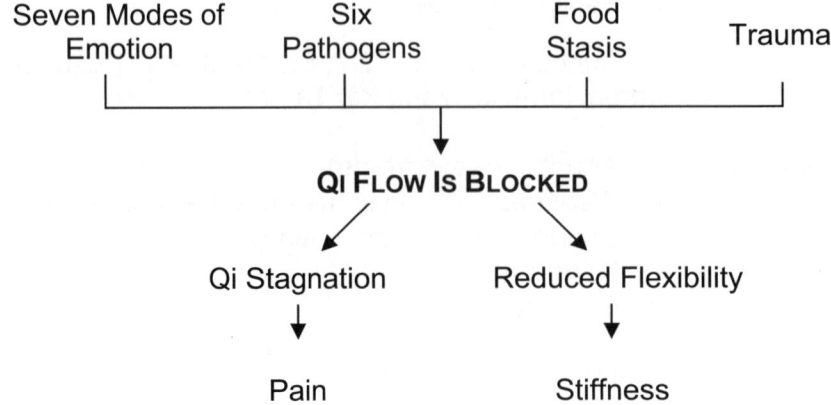

Types

Liver Qi Stagnation:

- Hyperactivity
- Emotional stress
- Depression
- Anger
- Nervous
- Hypertension
- Hypochondriac tension or pain

Acupuncture points: LIV-3, LIV-4, GB-34, GB-39, TH-1
Herbal formula: *Xiao Yao San*

Stomach Qi Stagnation:

- Stomachache
- Vomiting
- Nausea

Acupuncture points: CV-12, BL-21, GB-34, ST-36, ST-25
Herbal formula: *Qu Mai San*

Large Intestine Stagnation:

- Impaction
- Constipation
- Gaseous colic

Acupuncture points: ST-37, ST-36, ST-25, BL-25
Herbal formula: *Da Cheng Qi Tang*

Rebellious Qi

Rebellious Qi refers to Qi that is moving in the wrong direction or moving in an excessive way. There are two basic forms of normal Qi Flow: ascending ($\uparrow$) and descending ($\downarrow$). The normal direction of Qi Flow varies from organ to organ. Physiologically, the Stomach Qi is always descending while Spleen Qi is always ascending. The Heart Qi should descend while the Liver Qi should ascend. The Kidney Qi should descend. The Lung is only organ that may be ascending (for expiration) and descending (for inspiration).

Table 8.14: The Directions of Organ Qi Flow

Organ	Normal Qi Direction	Pathological Qi Direction	Signs of Abnormal Qi Flow
Stomach	$\downarrow$	$\uparrow$	Nausea, Vomiting, Hiccup, Belching
Spleen	$\uparrow$	$\downarrow$	Diarrhea, Prolapse
Heart	$\downarrow$	$\uparrow$	Restlessness, Anxiety, Insomnia
Liver	$\uparrow$	$\uparrow\uparrow$ (excessive)	Hypertension, Irritability, Hyperactivity, Red face
Kidney	$\downarrow$	$\uparrow$	Inspiratory asthma
Lung	$\downarrow\uparrow$	Abnormal	Cough, Asthma, Dyspnea

Etiology

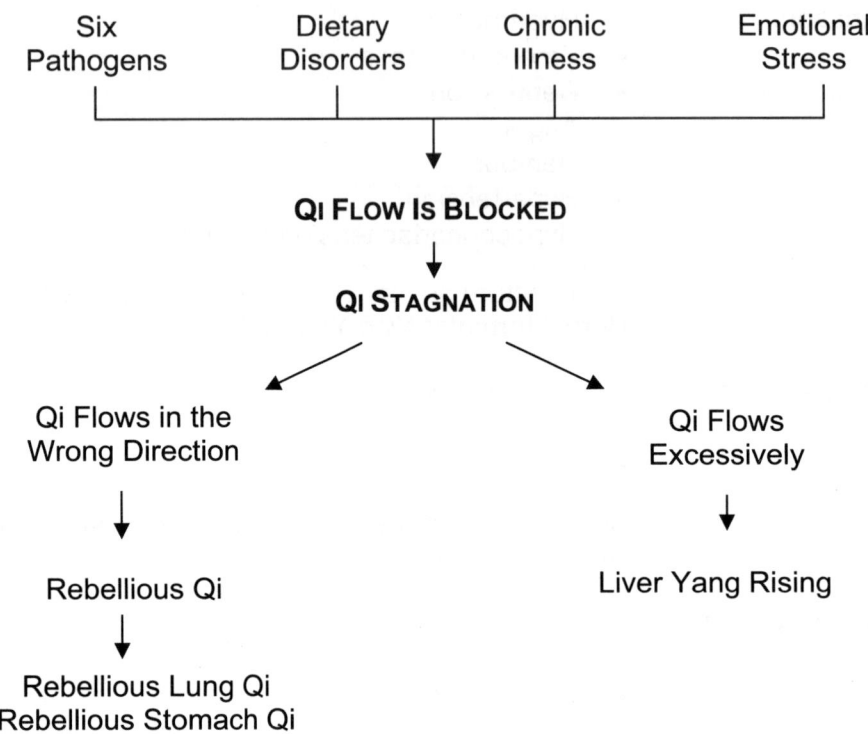

Types

Rebellious Stomach Qi:
- Hiccups
- Nausea
- Vomiting

Acupuncture points: ST-36, GB-34, PC-6, CV-12, CV-13
Herbal formula: *Cheng Xiang San*

Rebellious Lung Qi:
- Cough
- Asthma

Acupuncture points: BL-13, *Ding Chuan*, CV-22, LU-7
Herbal formula: *Su Zi Jiang Qi Tang*

Liver Yang Rising:
- Hyperactivity
- Irritability
- Headache
- Convulsion or seizure
- Red eyes
- Red face
- Vomiting of bile or blood
- Hypertension

Acupuncture points: GB-34, LIV-3, GB-20
Herbal formula: *Tian Ma Gou Teng Yin*

Sinking (Prolapsed) Qi

The inability of the Middle Qi (Zhong Qi) to hold the organs in their normal place which results in such problems as rectal or uterine prolapse.

Etiology

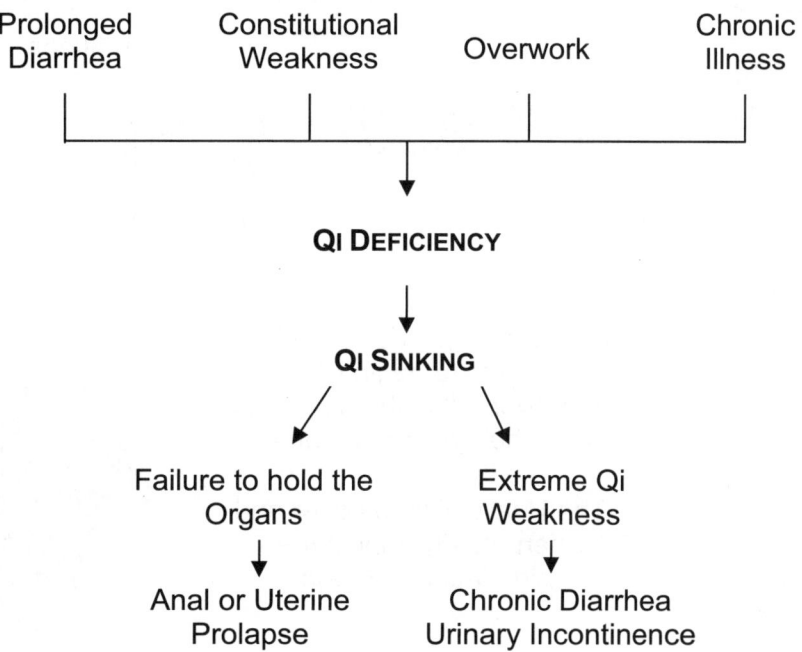

Clinical Signs

- Chronic diarrhea
- Urinary incontinence
- Prolapsed organs, such as rectum, uterus
- Drooping of lower lip
- Prolapse of lower eyelids

Acupoints

ST-36, GV-1, CV-1, *Gang Tui*, GV-20

Herbal Formula

Bu Zhong Yi Qi Tang

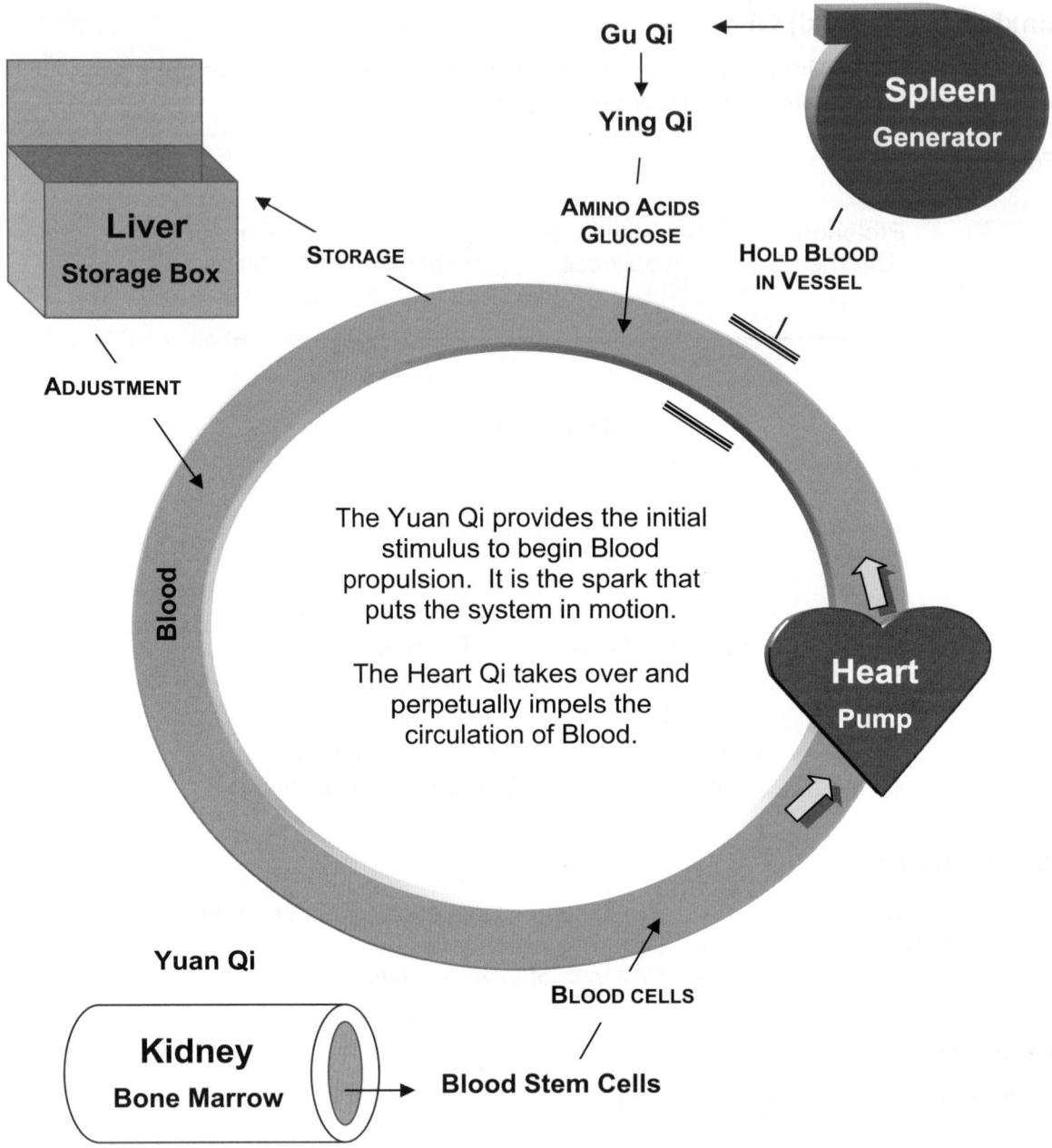

Figure 8.3: The relationship of Kidney, Liver, Spleen and Heart to Blood

BLOOD PATTERNS

Blood circulates through the body to nourish the hair coat, skin, muscles, bones, and internal organs. Blood is associated with the Spleen, Heart, Liver and Kidney. The Heart impels the Blood to move. The Spleen and Kidney help to generate Blood. The Spleen also holds blood inside the vessels. The Liver stores Blood and adjusts its volume. Impairment of the Blood Circulation results in disease. Blood may exist in five pathologic states within the body: Deficiency, Stagnation, Heat, Cold or Hemorrhage.

Blood Deficiency

There are three types of Blood Deficiency: Liver Blood Deficiency, Heart Blood Deficiency and Spleen-Heart Blood Deficiency.

Etiology

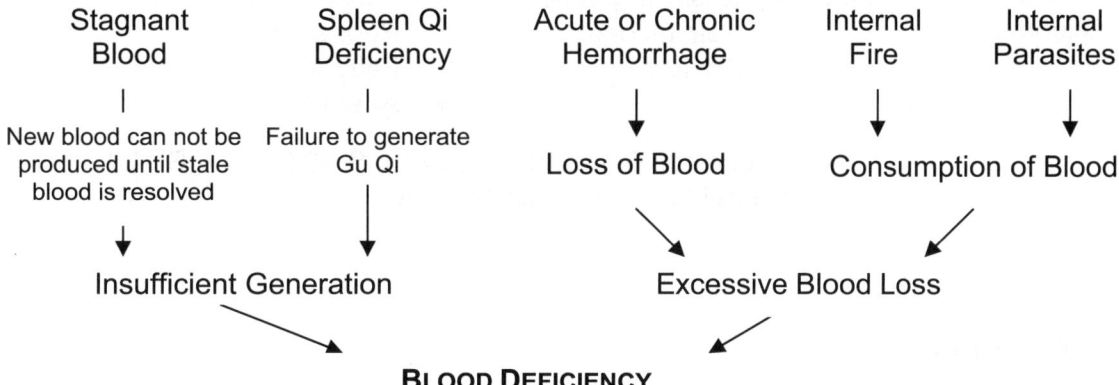

Clinical Signs

- Dizziness upon standing
- Dry hair coat or dandruff
- Cold extremities
- Subject to chills
- Thready pulse

- Poor growth of hooves (horse) or nails (dog/cat)
- Pale complexion (lips and tongue)
- Cracked line on hooves or paws
- General weakness or deficiency

Acupoints

BL-17, SP-10, ST-36

Herbal Formula

Si Wu Tang (Four Substances)

Types

Liver Blood Deficiency:
- Crack lines in the hoof or paws
- Weakness of tendons/ligaments
- Dry skin or hair coat
- Dry eyes

Acupoints: LIV-3, BL-17, BL-18, SP-10, SP-6
Herbal formula: *Si Wu Tang* (Four Substances)

Heart Blood Deficiency:
- Easily frightened
- Dull eyes
- Palpitations
- Restlessness
- Anxiety
- Anemic

Acupoints: BL-15, BL-17, PC-6, HT-7, SP-10, *An Shen*
Herbal formula: *Tian Wang Bu Xin Dan*

Heart and Spleen Blood Deficiency:
- Easily frightened
- Palpitations
- Anxiety
- Loose stool
- Poor appetite
- Fatigue
- Anemic

Acupoints: BL-15, BL-17, SP-6, ST-36, HT-7, BL-20
Herbal formula: *Ba Zhen Tang*

Blood Stagnation

Qi Stagnation may lead to Blood Stagnation, and Blood Stagnation can increase the severity of the Qi Stagnation. Severe Blood Stagnation results in Blood Stasis, which may form a mass or enlargement.

Blood Stagnation is a substantial stagnation in which there may be a mass or swelling present. The pain is localized, and the pain is more severe than the distension. The tongue appears purple or has purple spots.

Qi Stagnation is a non-substantial stagnation in which there is no swelling or the swelling quickly disappears. The pain moves; it comes and goes. The distension is more severe than pain. The tongue appears normal or slightly purple.

Etiology

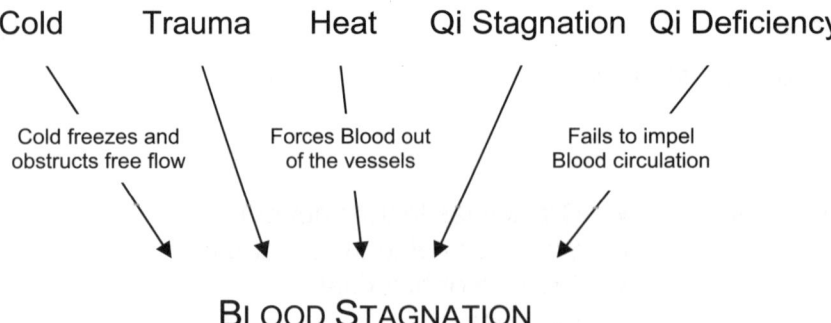

Clinical Signs

- Lumps
- Cysts
- Bruising
- Sharp stabbing pains

Acupoints

LIV-3, SP-10, and local points

Herbal Formula

Sheng Tong Zhu Yu Tang

Blood Heat

Etiology

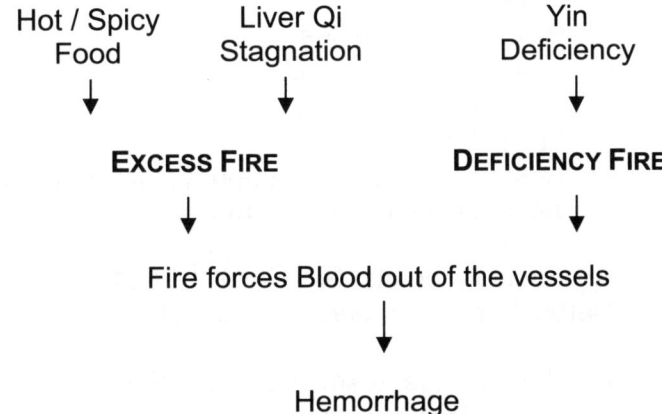

Hot / Spicy Food	Liver Qi Stagnation	Yin Deficiency

EXCESS FIRE   **DEFICIENCY FIRE**

Fire forces Blood out of the vessels

Hemorrhage

Clinical Signs

- Hives
- Rashes
- Dry skin
- Fast pulse
- Dry, red eye lids
- Red tongue
- Hemorrhage: a large amount of fresh, red blood without evidence of trauma

Acupoints

SP-10, LI-4, LI-11

Herbal Formula

Xi Jiao Di Huang Tang

Bleeding

There are three causes of bleeding: Excess Heat, Qi Deficiency and Deficient Heat.

Qi Deficiency:
- Chronic hemorrhage, small amounts with dark color
- General weakness
- Exercise intolerance
- Weak pulse
- Pale tongue

Acupuncture points: SP-10, BL-17, ST-36, CV-6
Herbal formula: *Gui Pi Tang*

Excess Heat:
- Fever
- Hives or skin rashes
- Inflammation or infection
- Red tongue with yellow coating
- Full pulse
- Hemorrhage: a large amount of fresh, red blood without evidence of trauma

Acupuncture points: SP-10, LI-4, LI-11
Herbal formula: *Xi Jiao Di Huang Tang*

Deficiency Heat:
- Hemorrhage: a small amount of fresh, dark blood
- Lower degree of fever
- Chronic inflammation or infection
- Red and dry tongue
- Thready and fast pulse

Acupuncture points: GV-14, KID-3, KID-6, HT-7
Herbal formula: *Xi Xian Cao San*

Blood Cold

Etiology

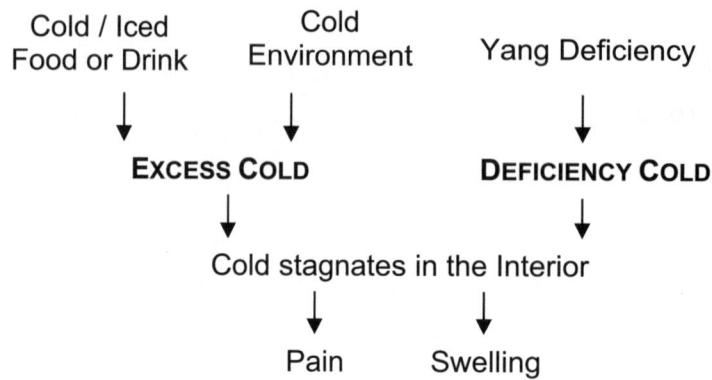

Clinical Signs

- Abdominal pain
- Hernia
- Pale purple tongue
- Slow, deep and choppy pulse

- Swelling, mass or enlargement
- Pain worsens when exposed to cold
- Pain relief when exposed to Heat
- Coldness in the limbs, nose and ears

Acupoints

BL-17, *Bai Hui*, SP-10, CV-6 and CV-17 using Moxibustion

Herbal Formula

Si Ni Tang

DUAL PATTERNS OF QI AND BLOOD

There is a close relationship between Qi and Blood. Qi, as Gu Qi (Food Qi), creates Blood. The Heart Qi provides the power to propel the circulation of Blood around the body. Spleen Qi also holds Blood inside the blood vessels to prevent hemorrhage. Thus, Qi is the general or commander of Blood. On the other hand, Blood carries and transports Qi. Blood also stores Qi. Thus, Blood is called the Mother of Qi.

Pathologic states of Qi and Blood also affect each other. Stagnant Qi can lead to Blood Stasis. Deficient Qi fails to generate Blood and leads to Blood Deficiency. Thus, various combinations of Qi and Blood pathology often occur in practice. There are five dual patterns of Qi and Blood pathology.

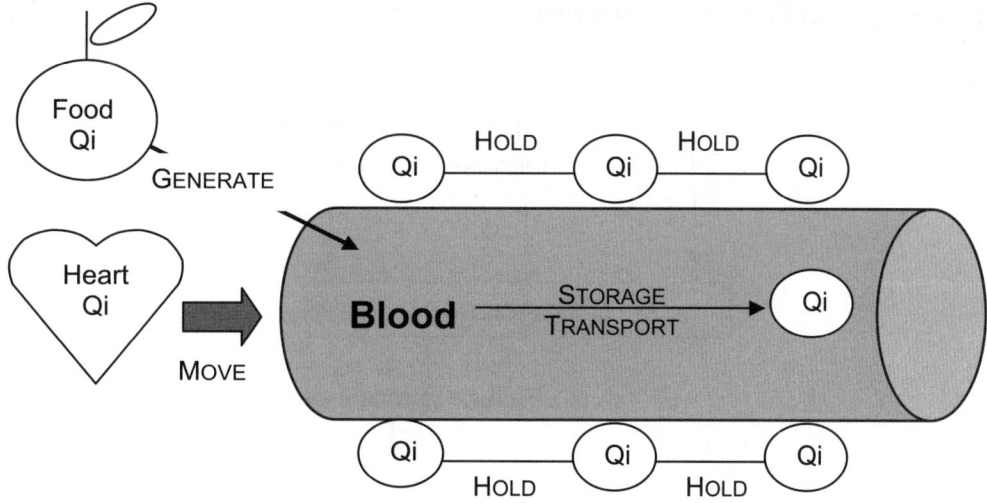

Figure 8.4: The relationship of Qi and Blood

Qi Stagnation and Blood Stasis

Etiology

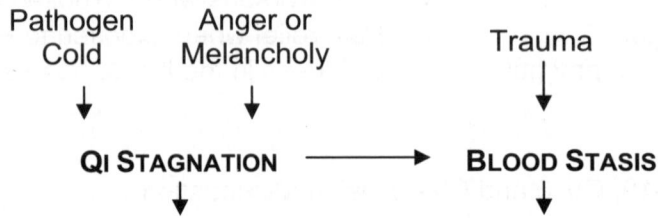

Pathogen Cold	Anger or Melancholy		Trauma
↓	↓		↓
QI STAGNATION	→	**BLOOD STASIS**	↓
↓			↓

Qi Stagnation and Blood Stasis

Clinical Signs

- Hyperactivity
- Irritability
- Hernia
- Mass or enlargement

- Dislikes massage on the chest or flank
- Distension of breast
- Deep red or dark tongue
- Choppy pulse

Acupoints

LIV-3, ST-36, GB-34, ST-44, *Shen Tang*, ST-45, *Wei Jian*

Herbal Formula

Ding Tong San

Qi Deficiency and Blood Stagnation

Etiology

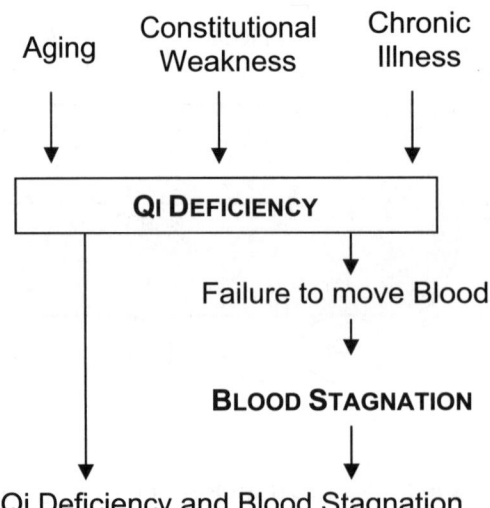

Aging   Constitutional Weakness   Chronic Illness

↓   ↓   ↓

QI DEFICIENCY

Failure to move Blood

↓

BLOOD STAGNATION

↓

Qi Deficiency and Blood Stagnation

Clinical Signs

- General weakness
- Fatigue
- Short of breath
- Mass or enlargement
- Dislikes massage of the distended areas
- Distension of breast
- Deep red or dark tongue
- Weak and choppy pulse

Acupoints

CV-4, CV-6, BL-20, LIV-3, ST-36

Herbal Formula

Tao Hong Si Wu Tang plus *Si Jun Zi Tang*

Dual Deficiency of Qi and Blood

Etiology

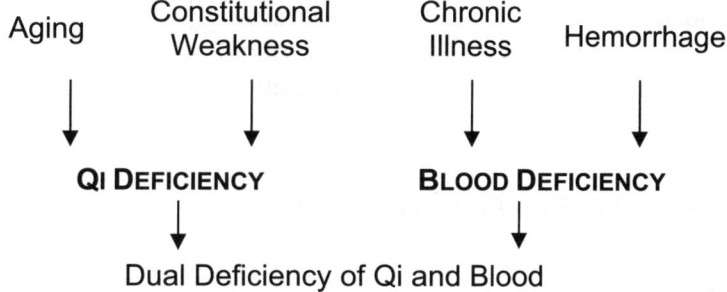

Clinical Signs

- General weakness
- Fatigue
- Palpitation
- Insomnia
- Pale and dry tongue
- Short of breath
- Spontaneous sweat
- Pale complexion
- Poor growth of nails/hooves
- Feeble pulse

Acupoints

BL-17, KID-3, SP-6, BL-20, CV-4, CV-6, ST-36, LI-10

Herbal Formula

Ba Zhen Tang

Deficient Qi Failing to hold Blood

Etiology

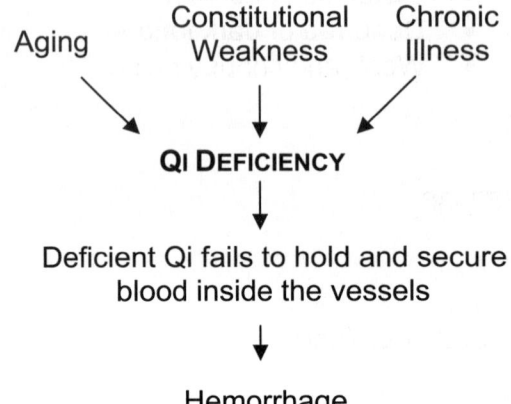

Aging   Constitutional Weakness   Chronic Illness

QI DEFICIENCY

Deficient Qi fails to hold and secure blood inside the vessels

Hemorrhage

Clinical Signs

- Fatigue or exercise intolerance
- Short of breath
- General weakness
- Pale tongue

- Weak and deep pulse
- Any internal chronic hemorrhage:
- Hematuria
- Hematochezia
- Epistaxis

Acupoints

SP-10, BL-17, ST-36, CV-6, *Tian Peng*, *Duan Xue*

Herbal Formula

Gui Pi Tang

Qi Deserting with Blood

Etiology

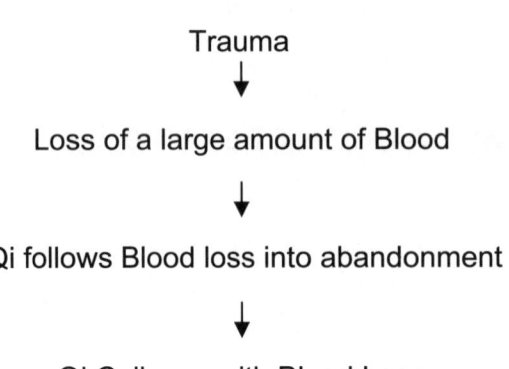

Trauma

Loss of a large amount of Blood

Qi follows Blood loss into abandonment

Qi Collapse with Blood Loss

Clinical Signs

- Blood loss
- Anemia
- Sweat
- Dyspnea
- Lower blood pressure
- Coldness at the extremities
- Coma
- White tongue
- Feeble or disappearing pulse

Acupoints

GV-26, PC-6 through TH-5, KID-1

Herbal Formula

Dang Gui Bu Xue Tang

BODY FLUID PATTERNS

Body Fluid (Jin-Ye) is the collective term for fluids inside the body. These fluids originate from food and drink. The Spleen, Lung, Stomach, Small Intestine, Bladder and San-jiao (Triple Heater) are involved with separation, distribution, and excretion of the Body Fluids. The "clean" or "pure" parts are removed from the fluids and are distributed upwards to moisten the body. The "dirty" or "turbid" parts are likewise separated and transported downwards where they will be excreted from the body.

The San-jiao is a water passage system that is associated with all stages of water metabolism. The San-jiao is divided into three portions: Upper-jiao, Middle-jiao and Lower-Jiao.

Disorders of water metabolism can lead to Body Fluid Pathology. This includes Body Fluid Deficiency, Retention of Water and Phlegm.

WHOLE BODY SURFACE

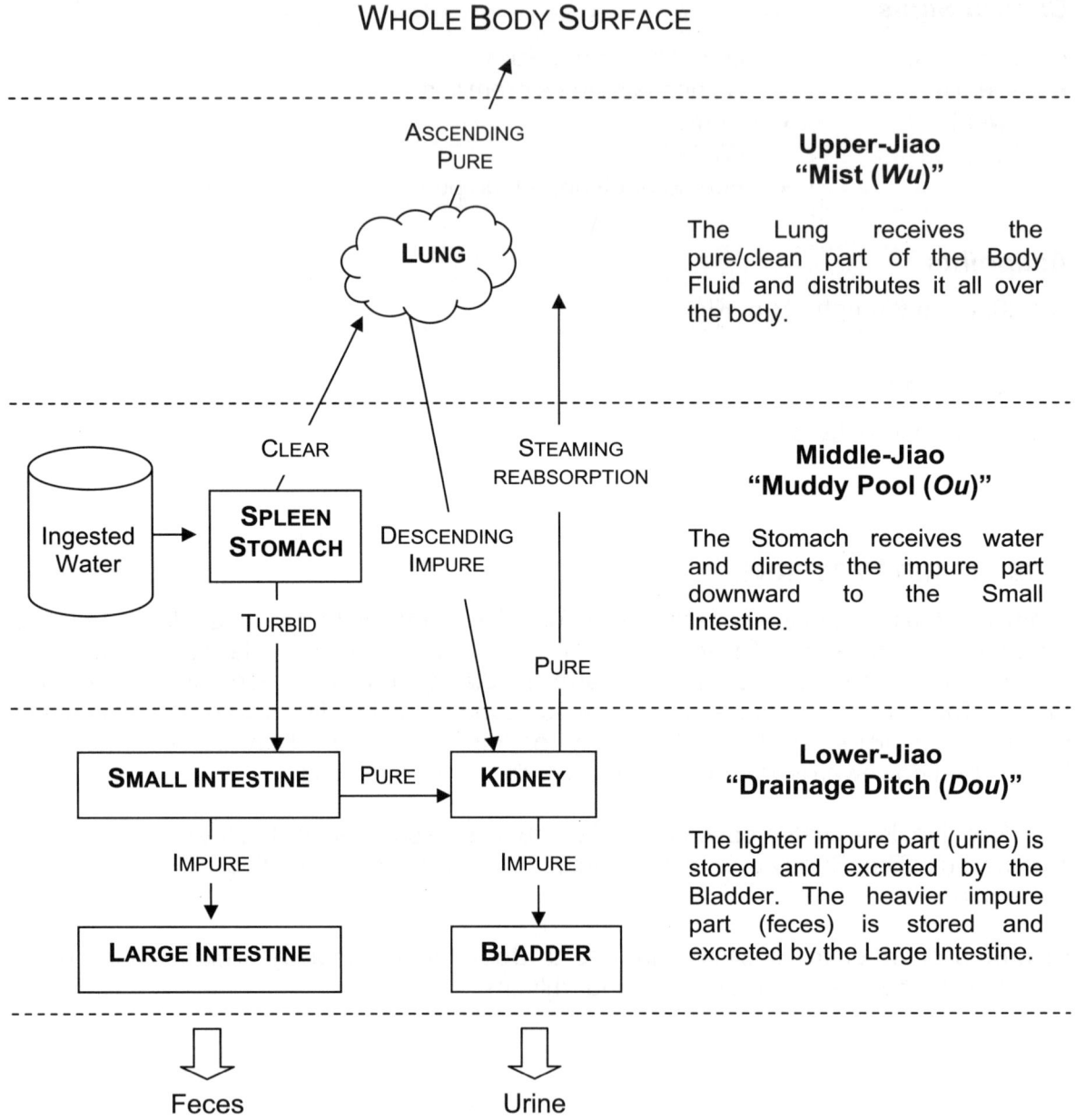

ASCENDING
PURE

LUNG

**Upper-Jiao
"Mist (*Wu*)"**

The Lung receives the pure/clean part of the Body Fluid and distributes it all over the body.

CLEAR

STEAMING
REABSORPTION

**Middle-Jiao
"Muddy Pool (*Ou*)"**

Ingested
Water

SPLEEN
STOMACH

DESCENDING
IMPURE

The Stomach receives water and directs the impure part downward to the Small Intestine.

TURBID

PURE

SMALL INTESTINE — PURE → KIDNEY

**Lower-Jiao
"Drainage Ditch (*Dou*)"**

The lighter impure part (urine) is stored and excreted by the Bladder. The heavier impure part (feces) is stored and excreted by the Large Intestine.

IMPURE

IMPURE

LARGE INTESTINE

BLADDER

Feces

Urine

Figure 8.5: Water metabolism and the three Jiao

Body Fluid Deficiency

Dryness is the primary clinical sign of Body Fluid Deficiency because Body Fluids are part of Yin in the body. Thus, Body Fluid Deficiency is also called Internal Dryness. Internal Dryness is part of Yin Deficiency. Body Fluid Deficiency may be considered a mild form of Yin Deficiency.

Etiology

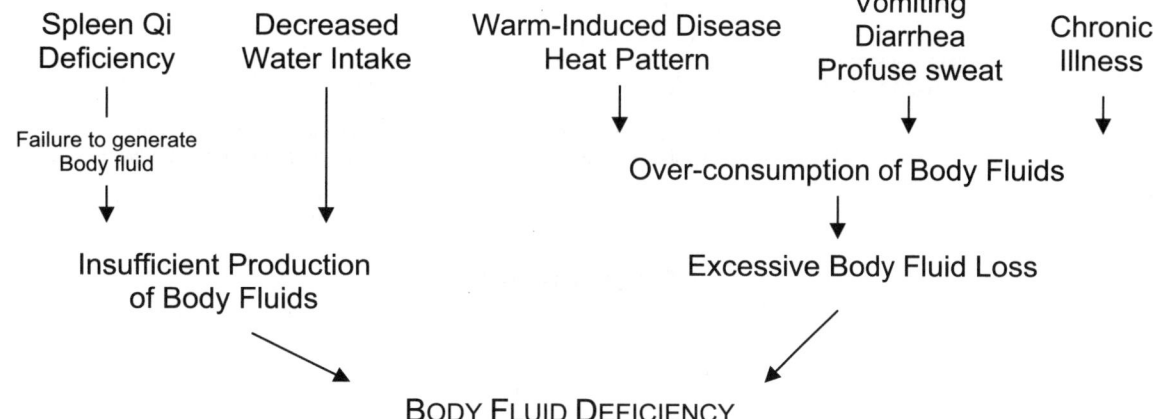

Clinical Signs

- Dryness of lips
- Dry skin

- Dry eyelids
- Joint stiffness
- Constipation

Acupoints

KID-3, BL-23, KID-10

Herbal Formula

Zeng Ye Tang

Retention of Water (Retained Liquid)

Water flows continuously in the San-jiao system. The clean part of the water is transformed and distributed to moisten the body. The impure and dirty part of the water is transported and excreted. If the water does not flow in this manner, it stagnates in the interior and causes pathology:

1. Retention of Water in the skin and muscle becomes edema

2. Retention of water in the Lung becomes Phlegm

3. Retention of water in the thoracic cavity becomes hydrothorax

4. Retention of water in the abdominal cavity becomes ascites

5. Retention of water in the Large Intestine becomes diarrhea

6. Retention of water in the joints becomes hydrarthrosis

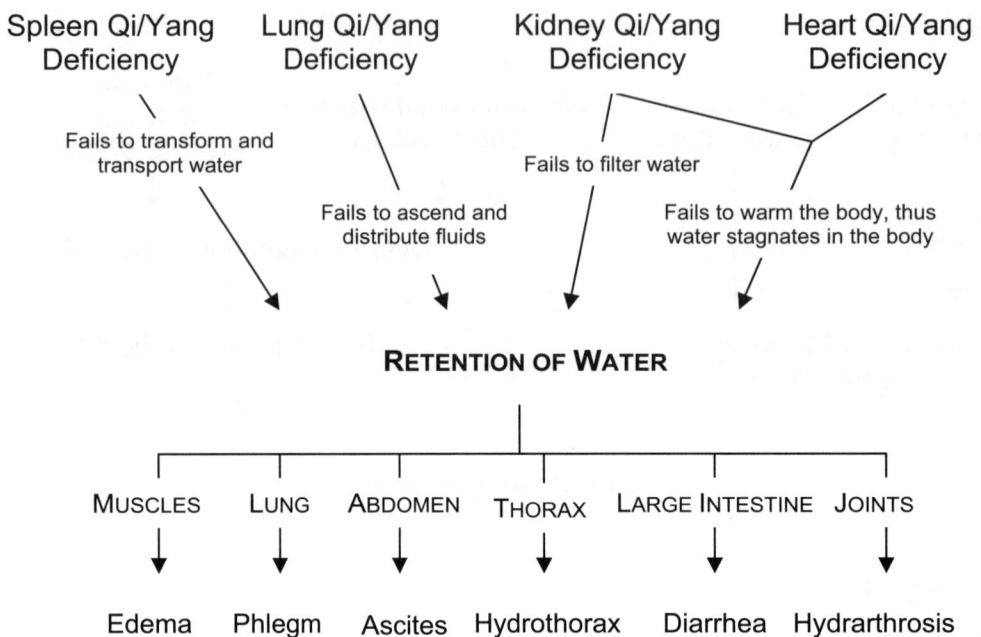

Edema

Edema arises from a Deficiency of Spleen, Lung, Kidney or a combination of these organs. There are four major patterns of edema: Spleen Qi Deficiency, Lung Qi Deficiency, Kidney Yang Deficiency, Spleen-Kidney Yang Deficiency, and Heart-Kidney Yang Deficiency.

Etiology

Same as the etiology of general water retention

Clinical Signs

- Edema
- Slow and weak pulse
- General weakness or exercise intolerance
- Wet, pale or pale purple tongue
- Greasy and white tongue coating

Edema Cause	Edema Characteristics
Lung Qi Deficiency:	Occurs in the top part of the body (Upper Jiao) including face, ears, eyes, lips, neck and front limbs (hands in humans). It is often triggered by invasion of Wind-Cold.
Spleen Qi Deficiency:	Tends to affect the middle part of the body (Middle Jiao) including the abdomen and flank areas
Kidney Yang Deficiency:	Occurs in the lower part of the body (Lower Jiao) including the pubis, tail and stifle areas
Spleen-Kidney Yang Deficiency:	Occurs in the lower abdomen, thighs, ankles and rear limbs
Heart-Kidney Yang Deficiency:	Occurs in the Lung and leads to cough

Acupoints and Herbal Formulas

Type of Edema	Signs	Acupoints	Herbal Formula
Lung Qi Deficiency	Dyspnea Cough Edema of face and front limbs	BL-13 CV-17 LU-9	*Bu Fei San*
Spleen Qi Deficiency	Anorexia Loose stool Edema in abdomen	ST-36 CV-6 SP-3	*Si Jun Zi Tang*
Kidney Yang Deficiency	Cold back and extremities Edema of scrotum, pubis, labia	GV-4 *Bai Hui* (Moxibustion)	*Jin Gui Shen Qi Tang*
Spleen + Kidney Yang Deficiency	Chronic diarrhea Coldness Edema in rear limbs	*Bai Hui* GV-1 (Moxibustion)	*Shi Pi Yin*
Heart + Kidney Yang Deficiency	Cough Dyspnea Coldness Fluid in the lungs	CV-22 GV-4 (Moxibustion)	*Zhen Wu Tang*

Phlegm

Phlegm is a secondary pathogen; it may result from the primary pathogens including Heat and Cold. However, Phlegm itself can lead to a disease. For instance, Phlegm can block the Heart Channel, mist the Heart and lead to Shen disturbance. Spleen Qi Deficiency is the primary cause of Phlegm formation. The Lung is the major system in which Phlegm dwells.

There are two types of Phlegm: Substantial Phlegm and Non-substantial Phlegm. The Substantial Phlegm may be defined as "thick, sticky, condensed fluid". It is also described as "the Phlegm having a form". This may be seen as sputum that is coughed up from the airways. Heat, Cold, Damp, Spleen Qi Deficiency, etc. may cause Substantial Phlegm.

The Non-substantial Phlegm is something that can cause a strange disease. Thus, it is said: "Where there is something strange, it must be Phlegm". It is the "Phlegm without form". This Phlegm may be retained subcutaneously or within the Channels. It obstructs the Channel that connects the Heart and its orifice, thus leading to manic or depression (misting in the Heart).

Heat and Damp Phlegm are the most common forms of Phlegm seen in practice.

Heat Phlegm:
- Fever
- Upper airway infection
- Cough
- Red tongue
- Fast and forceful pulse

Acupuncture points: LU-5, LU-9, *Xiong Tang*
Herbal formula: *Qing Qi Hua Tang*

Damp Phlegm:
- Wet Cough
- Pale tongue
- Slow and choppy pulse

Acupuncture points: ST-36, ST-40, SP-6
Herbal formula: *Er Chen Tang*

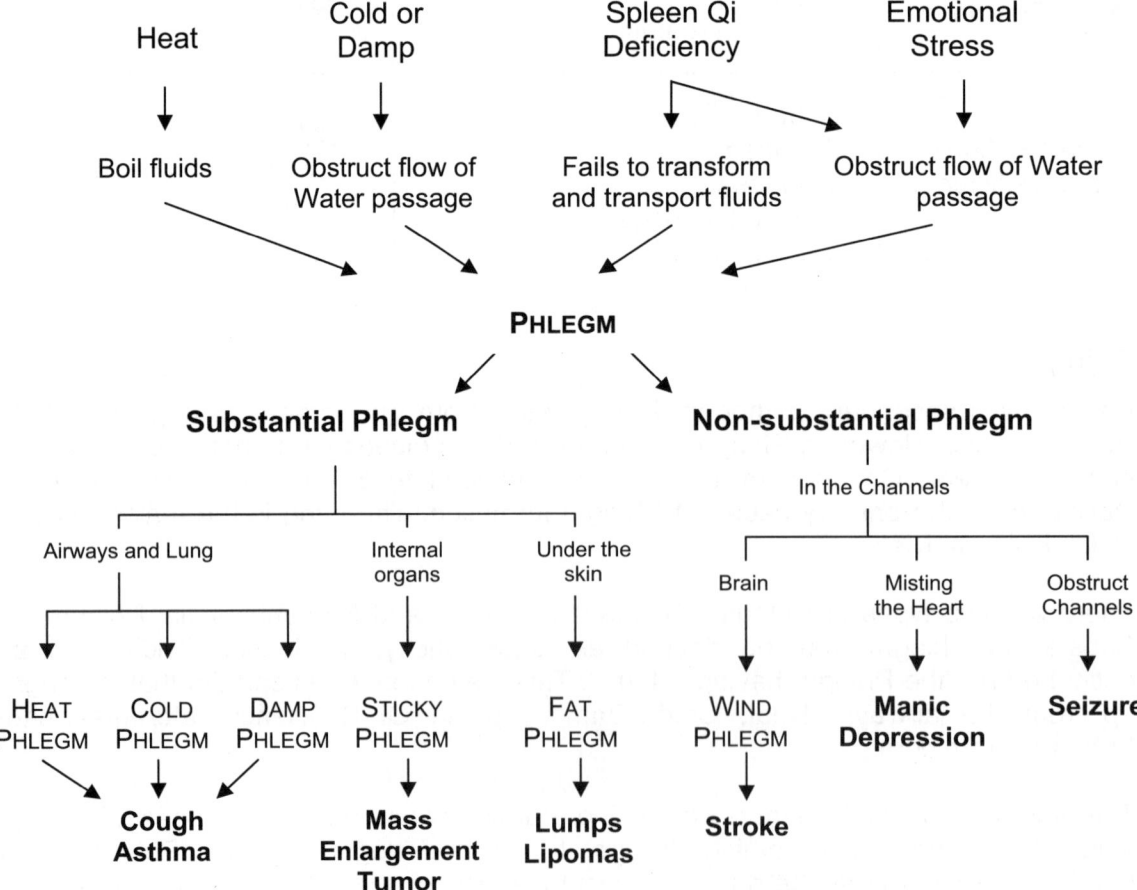

Figure 8.6: Identification and development of Phlegm types

Channel Patterns

Identification of Channel Patterns (Jing Luo Bian Zheng) is one of the oldest TCM diagnostic systems. It is based on the Jing Luo (Meridian) theories and Zang-Fu physiology and pathology.

The Channel Patterns include Twelve Regular Channel Patterns and Eight Extraordinary Channel Patterns.

Channel Patterns	Type of Patterns
Twelve Regular Channel Patterns	Lung Channel Pattern
	Large Intestine Channel Pattern
	Stomach Channel Pattern
	Spleen Channel Pattern
	Heart Channel Pattern
	Small Intestine Channel Pattern
	Bladder Channel Pattern
	Kidney Channel Pattern
	Pericardium Channel Pattern
	Triple Heater Channel Pattern
	Gall Bladder Channel Pattern
	Liver Channel Pattern
Eight Extraordinary Channel Patterns	Governing Vessel Channel Pattern
	Conception Vessel Channel Pattern
	Chong (Penetrating) Channel Pattern
	Dai (Girdle) Channel Pattern
	Yin-qiao Channel Pattern
	Yang-qiao Channel Pattern
	Yin-wei Channel Pattern
	Yang-wei Channel Pattern

LUNG CHANNEL PATTERN

Channel Pathway

	INTERNAL BRANCH	EXTERNAL BRANCH	EXTRA BRANCH
ORIGIN:	Middle Jiao (Stomach)	LU-1	LU-7
TERMINUS:	Zhong-Fu (LU-1)	LU-11	LI-1
CONNECTION:	Large Intestine	Enters the radial artery for pulse diagnosis	Large Intestine Channel

Clinical Signs

- Cough
- Dyspnea
- Shortness of breath, asthma
- Soreness of the forearm
- Sore throat
- Supraclavicular fossa pain

- Shoulder pain, coldness
- Chest fullness
- Problems with the throat, chest, lung, or front limbs
- Invasion of Wind Cold or Wind Heat
- Musculoskeletal conditions along the LU pathway
- Itching, pain, coldness or any other abnormal finding along the LU pathway

Acupoints

BL-13, LU-1, LU-11, LU-7, LU-1, *Fei Men* and *Fei Pan*
LU-5 and LI-4 for Excess; LU-9 and LI-11 for Deficiency

LARGE INTESTINE CHANNEL PATTERN

Channel Pathway

	INTERNAL BRANCH	SURFACE BRANCH	EXTRA BRANCH
ORIGIN:	Supraclavicular fossa	LI-1	Supraclavicular fossa
TERMINUS:	Large Intestine	Supraclavicular fossa	LI-20
CONNECTION:	Lung	Governing Vessel Channel	Stomach Channel

Clinical Signs

- Abdominal pain
- Diarrhea
- Constipation
- Sore throat
- Fever
- Toothache
- Nosebleed

- Musculoskeletal conditions along the LI pathway
- Laryngeal hemiplegia
- Soreness, coldness along shoulder, elbow, carpus
- Soreness of the first and second digits
- Nasal discharge or congestion
- Problems with the face, five sense organs, throat and larynx, pharynx

Acupoints

LI-1, LI-4, LI-10, BL-25, ST-25
LU-5 and LI-2 for Excess; LU-9 and LI-11 for Deficiency

STOMACH CHANNEL PATTERN

Channel Pathway

	LATERAL BRANCH	FACIAL BRANCH	SUPRACLAVICULAR BRANCH	STOMACH BRANCH	TIBIAL BRANCH
ORIGIN:	LI-20	ST-5	Supraclavicular fossa	Lower gate of the Stomach (pylorus)	ST-36
TERMINUS:	GV-24	Stomach	ST-30	ST-45	
CONNECTION:		Spleen		Supraclavicular Branch	

Clinical Signs

- Vomiting
- Abdominal pain
- Abdominal fullness
- Polydipsia
- Polyphagia
- High fever
- Sore throat
- Epistaxis
- Overexcited / frenzied
- Musculoskeletal conditions along the ST pathway
- Soreness, coldness along knees and chest
- Problems with gastrointestinal tract

Acupoints

ST-36, BL-20, BL-21, CV-12
ST-45 and ST-2 for Excess; ST-41 and LI-10 for Deficiency

SPLEEN CHANNEL PATTERN

Channel Pathway

	LATERAL BRANCH	INTERNAL BRANCH	EXTRA INTERNAL BRANCH
ORIGIN:	SP-1	Abdomen	Stomach
TERMINUS:	Chest (2nd intercostal space 6 cun lateral to ventral midline)	Root and lower surface of the tongue	Heart
CONNECTION:		Stomach	Heart Channel

Clinical Signs

- Gynecologic problems
- Infertility
- Epigastric pain
- Belching
- Abdominal fullness
- Loose stool
- Jaundice
- Fatigue

- Spleen and Stomach Patterns
- Gastrointestinal diseases
- Musculoskeletal conditions where SP influences
- Edema of the medial aspect of the rear limbs
- Stiffness and pain in the root of the tongue
- Vomiting immediately after eating
- Genital and uterine conditions
- Coldness of the rear limbs

Acupoints

BL-20, *Qi Hai Shu*, ST-36, LI-10, SP-6, SP-9 and SP-3

HEART CHANNEL PATTERN

Channel Pathway

	INTERNAL BRANCH	LATERAL BRANCH
ORIGIN:	Heart	Axilla
TERMINUS:	HT-1	HT-9
CONNECTION:	Small Intestine, Eyes	Small Intestine Channel

Clinical Signs

- Restlessness
- Palpitation
- Chest pain
- Dry throat
- Thirsty

- Pain in the medial aspect of the upper arm
- Hot paws/heels (hot palms in people)
- Musculoskeletal conditions along the HT Channel
- Shen (mind) or mental disorder
- Pain of the flank
- Yellow or red eyes

Acupoints

HT-7, PC-6, BL-14, BL-15, *An Shen*, *Shen Men*, PC-9 and SI-1

Small Intestine Channel Pattern

Channel Pathway

	LATERAL BRANCH	EXTRA LATERAL BRANCH	INTERNAL BRANCH
ORIGIN:	SI-1	Cheek	Supraclavicular fossa
TERMINUS:	SI-19	BL-1	Small Intestine
CONNECTION:	Governing Vessel (GV-14)	Bladder Channel	

Clinical Signs

- Lower abdominal pain
- Back pain
- Deafness
- Swelling of the cheek
- Sore throat
- Pain in the areas of the lateral shoulder
- Problems of the head, neck, ear, eye, throat
- Musculoskeletal conditions along the SI pathway
- Fever or febrile diseases
- Shen or mental disorders

Acupoints

SI-8, SI-3, SI-1, BL-27, ST-39 and SI-9

Bladder Channel Pattern

Channel Pathway

	LATERAL BRANCH	INTERNAL BRANCH	EXTRA INTERNAL BRANCH
ORIGIN:	BL-1 and BL-10 (inner and outer branch)	BL-23	Occipital area
TERMINUS:	BL-40 (Inner branch); BL-67 (outer branch)	Bladder	Brain
CONNECTION:	Brain, Kidney Channel	Kidney	

Clinical Signs

- Difficulty urinating
- Manic hyperactivity
- Malaria
- Nosebleed
- Headache
- Cervical pain
- Tears easily caused by exposure to wind
- Nasal discharge and congestion
- Internal organ disorders
- Urinary incontinence
- Musculoskeletal conditions along the BL Channel pathway
- Head, neck, eyes, back, lumbar-sacral, rear limbs
- Back pain

Acupoints

BL-39, TH-22, BL-28, BL-67, BL-40, BL-60 and KID-1

KIDNEY CHANNEL PATTERN

Channel Pathway

	LATERAL BRANCH	EXTRA LATERAL BRANCH	INTERNAL BRANCH	EXTRA INTERNAL BRANCH
ORIGIN:	Inferior aspect of small toe	Pubic bone (Internal Branch)	GV-1	Lungs
TERMINUS:	GV-1	KID-27	Root of the tongue	Chest
CONNECTION:	Inner Branch	Internal Branch	Bladder	Pericardium Channel

Clinical Signs

- Asthma, cough
- Dry tongue
- Edema
- Constipation
- Diarrhea
- Lumbar pain

- Musculoskeletal conditions along KID channel pathway
- Obstetrical and gynecological disorders
- Weakness and fatigue of rear limbs
- Hot rear paws or heels (hot soles of the feet)
- Sore and swollen throat
- Kidney, Lung and throat

Acupoints

KID-3, BL-23, *Shen Shu*, *Bai Hui*, *Wei Jian*, KID-7, KID-10, BL-20

PERICARDIUM CHANNEL PATTERN

Channel Pathway

	INTERNAL BRANCH	LATERAL BRANCH
ORIGIN:	Chest	PC-3
TERMINUS:	PC-3	PC-9, TH-1 (branch)
CONNECTION:	Upper, Middle, and Lower Jiao (San Jiao)	San Jiao Channel

Clinical Signs

- Chest pain
- Palpitation
- Shen disturbance
- Soreness

- Hot front paws/heels (hot sole of foot)
- Musculoskeletal conditions along the PC channel
- Soreness of the front paws/heals/soles
- Manic hyperactivity
- Elbow and forearm

Acupoints

PC-6, KID-3, BL-14, PC-9, PC-3, HT-7

TRIPLE HEATER CHANNEL PATTERN

Channel Pathway

	LATERAL BRANCH	INTERNAL BRANCH	EXTRA LATERAL BRANCH	AURICULAR BRANCH
ORIGIN:	TH-1	Supraclavicular fossa	Supraclavicular fossa	Retroauricular region
TERMINUS:	Supraclavicular fossa	San Jiao (Upper, Middle, Lower Jiao)	Infraorbital region	GB-1
CONNECTION:	Internal Branch	Pericardium Channel, San Jiao		Gall Bladder Channel

Clinical Signs

- Edema
- Sore throat
- Red eyes
- Fever
- Musculoskeletal conditions along the TH channel pathway
- Urinary incontinence
- Deafness or tinnitus
- Abdominal fullness

Acupoints

BL-22, TH-23, TH-1, TH-4, TH-5 and TH-10

GALL BLADDER CHANNEL PATTERN

Channel Pathway

	MAIN LATERAL BRANCH	AURICULAR BRANCH	EYE BRANCH	FOOT BRANCH	INTERNAL BRANCH
ORIGIN:	GB-1	Retroauricular area	Lateral eye canthus	GB-41	Supraclavicular fossa
TERMINUS:	GB-44	Lateral eye canthus	Supraclavicular fossa	LIV-1	GB-30
CONNECTION:			Main Lateral Branch	Liver Channel	Main Lateral Branch

Clinical Signs

- Headache
- Hypertension
- Tinnitus
- Fever
- Vomiting of bile
- Shen disturbance
- Eye problems
- Bitter mouth
- Musculoskeletal conditions along the GB channel pathway

Acupoints

GB-8, LIV-3, BL-18, BL-19, GB-34, GB-44, GB-20, *Yan Mai*

LIVER CHANNEL PATTERN

Channel Pathway

	LATERAL BRANCH	INTERNAL BRANCH
ORIGIN:	LIV-1	Lower abdomen
TERMINUS:	Hypochondriac Region	Apex of head
CONNECTION:		Gall Bladder, Lung Channel

Clinical Signs

- Hernia
- Lumbar soreness
- Genital diseases
- Eye problems

- Lower abdominal enlargement
- Chest fullness
- Nausea or vomiting
- Urinary incontinence
- Musculoskeletal conditions along the LIV channel path

Acupoints

BL-18, BL-19, SP-6, SP-3, SP-1, GB-34, GB-44, LIV-3

GOVERNING VESSEL CHANNEL

Channel Pathway

	LATERAL BRANCH	INTERNAL BRANCH
ORIGIN:	Lower abdomen (uterus and ovaries; prostate and testes)	Spinal Column of lower back
TERMINUS:	GV-28	Kidney
CONNECTION:	Brain	

Clinical Signs

- Fever
- Back pain
- Mental disorders
- Weak back or spine

- Musculoskeletal conditions along the GV channel path
- Degenerative Myelopathy
- Internal Wind syndromes
- Intervertebral disc disease
- Internal organs, brain (Mind), limbs, and spinal cord

Acupoints

GV-14, GV-1, *Da Feng Men, Bai Hui, Wei Jian, Hua Tuo Jia Ji*

CONCEPTION VESSEL CHANNEL

Channel Pathway

	LATERAL BRANCH	INTERNAL BRANCH
ORIGIN:	Lower abdomen (uterus and ovaries; prostate and testes)	Uterus or prostate
TERMINUS:	CV-24	Lower back
CONNECTION:	Infraorbital region	

Clinical Signs

- Back pain
- Hernia
- Genital discharge
- Infertility
- Musculoskeletal conditions along the CV channel path
- General mental conditions
- Abdominal enlargement
- Throat conditions

Acupoints

CV-4, CV-6, CV-24, CV-22 and CV-17

CHONG (PENETRATING) CHANNEL

Channel Pathway

	LATERAL BRANCH
ORIGIN:	Lower abdomen (uterus and ovaries; prostate and testes)
TERMINUS:	Lips
CONNECTION:	ST-30, CV and KID Channels

Clinical Signs

- Lower abdominal pain
- Chest pain
- Infertility
- Estrous disorders
- Musculoskeletal conditions along the Chong path
- Urinary or large intestinal incontinence
- Rebellious Qi
- Postpartum disorders

Acupoints

CV-1, CV-7, ST-30, KID-21, KID-13, KID-16

DAI (GIRDLE) CHANNEL

Channel Pathway

LATERAL BRANCH

ORIGIN: Below the hypochondriac region

TERMINUS: *Shen Jiao*, GV-3

CONNECTION: GB-26, GB-27, GB-28, *Yan Chi*

Clinical Signs

- Back pain
- Genital disorders
- Cycle disorders
- Musculoskeletal conditions along the Dai Channel path
- Weakness in the back
- Poor performance

Acupoints

GB-26, GB-27, GB-28, *Yan Chi*, GV-3

YIN-QIAO CHANNEL

Channel Pathway

LATERAL BRANCH

ORIGIN: KID-6

TERMINUS: Medial canthus of the eye

CONNECTION: Kidney Channel, Yang-Qiao Channel

Functions

Dominates activity and sleeping

Clinical Signs

- Hypersomnia
- Urinary incontinence

Acupoints

KID-6 and KID-8

YANG-QIAO CHANNEL

Channel Pathway

LATERAL BRANCH

ORIGIN: BL-62

TERMINUS: GB-20

CONNECTION: Yin-Qiao Channel and Bladder Channel

Clinical Signs

- Insomnia
- Soreness in the eyes
- Ataxia, imbalanced movement (Wobblers, EPM)

Acupoints

BL-62, BL-59, BL-1 and GB-20

YIN-WEI CHANNEL

Channel Pathway

LATERAL BRANCH

ORIGIN: KID-9

TERMINUS: CV-23

CONNECTION: Conception Vessel

Functions

Connects with all the Yin Channels

Clinical Signs

- Depression
- Chest pain
- Heart, kidney or liver failure

Acupoints

KID-9, CV-22 and CV-23

YANG-WEI CHANNEL

Channel Pathway

LATERAL BRANCH

ORIGIN: GB-63

TERMINUS: GV-15

CONNECTION: BL, GV, SI, TH and GB Channels

Clinical Signs

- Fever
- Chill
- Lumbar pain
- Bi syndrome
- Influenza
- Common cold
- Exterior Pattern
- IVDD

Acupoints

BL-63, GB-20, GV-15, SI-10, TH-15

Self Test

Questions 1-3 are based on the following case.

Cinnamon is an eleven-year old spayed female German shepherd who presents with severe chronic progressive hip dysplasia. When she stands on her hind limbs she will whine or moan because of the pain. Her hips are painful upon 45 degree extension or deep palpation. She is very stiff and painful in her lumbar area. Her tongue is purple with a red tip and has average moisture. Her pulses are deep, fast, wiry and forceful. She displays no temperature preference. She is a happy, friendly dog. She wags her tail but cries at the same time when her hip or lumbar areas are palpated.

Question 8.1: According to the Five Element/Five Constitutional Types, Cinnamon is considered to be which of the following types?

    a. Wood
    b. Fire
    c. Earth
    d. Metal
    e. Water

Question 8.2: Based on the Eight Principles, which is Cinnamon's diagnosis?

    a. Exterior Excess Pattern
    b. Exterior Deficiency Pattern
    c. Exterior Cold Pattern
    d. Interior Deficiency Pattern
    e. Interior Excess Pattern

Question 8.3: If she has an Interior Excess Pattern, Cinnamon can be further diagnosed with which of the following?

    a. Qi/Blood Stagnation
    b. Dryness
    c. Phlegm
    d. Damp-Heat
    e. Cold-Damp

Questions 4 and 5 are based on the following case.

Lady Red is a ten-year old female spayed Golden Retriever who presented with a two-year history of severe degenerative joint disease of the left carpus. The referring veterinarian suspected osteosarcoma due to the severe osteopenia. She has been given prednisone for the past two years. The owner describes Lady Red as easy-going, laid-back dog. Recently Lady Red has had great difficulty getting up, and she walks for less than one minute before she collapses. She prefers stay in cool places.

The physical exam reveals general weakness, hind limb paresis, generalized muscle atrophy, bilateral immature cataracts, a small right prescapular mass and reduced flexion of the left carpus. Her tongue was red and slightly dry. Her pulse was deficient on the left at the proximal, middle and distal positions.

Question 8.4: What is Lady Red's diagnosis based on the Eight Principles.

    a. Exterior Excess Pattern
    b. Interior Excess Pattern
    c. Interior Deficiency Pattern
    d. Interior Cold Pattern
    e. Exterior Cold Pattern

Question 8.5: What is Lady Red's diagnosis based on the Zang-Fu Patterns?

    a. Spleen Qi Deficiency
    b. Kidney Yin Deficiency
    c. Kidney Qi Deficiency with Kidney Yin Deficiency
    d. Spleen Qi Deficiency with Kidney Yin Deficiency
    e. Kidney Qi Deficiency with Spleen Qi Deficiency

Questions 6 and 7 are based on the following case.

Zack is a ten year old neutral male cross breed of Pit Bull and Catahoula Leopard Hound. He presents with a moderately differentiated mast cell tumor on his left lateral thorax. He had a history of unilateral chronic-progressive inflammatory intraocular disease which resulted in glaucoma. He has an ulcerated 2 x 3 centimeter ovoid mass on his left lateral thorax as well as increased respiratory strider with harsh large airway sounds. He has an occasional dry cough. His haircoat is dry. He also shows exercise intolerance and occasionally has loose stool. His tongue is slightly red and dry. His pulse was weak, deep and thready, especially at the right proximal position.

Question 8.6: Based on the Eight Principles, which of the following is Zack's diagnosis?

    a. Exterior Excess Pattern
    b. Interior Excess Pattern
    c. Interior Deficiency Pattern
    d. Interior Cold Pattern
    e. Exterior Cold Pattern

Question 8.7: Based on the Zang-Fu Patterns, which is Zack's diagnosis?

    a. Spleen Qi Deficiency
    b. Lung Yin Deficiency
    c. Kidney Yin Deficiency
    d. Lung Yin Deficiency with Lung Qi Deficiency
    e. Lung Yin Deficiency with Spleen Qi Deficiency

Lady is a six year old spayed female mixed breed hybrid who presented with a several-month history of "allergic skin disease". Her veterinarian prescribed Cephalexin (500 mg PO BID) and Thyroxine (0.5 mg, ½ tablet PO BID) but she showed little improvement. Recently her patchy alopecia and skin flaking were even worse. She has moderate dental calculus and dry flaky skin with hair loss. Her tongue was pale and dry. Her pulse was weak and thready on the left. After she received one acupuncture treatment and a month of daily Chinese herbal medications, her overall skin and haircoat became much better. She began to have hair regrowth. Her Thyroxine dose was reduced in half.

Question 8.8: Can you predict what type of TCVM treatment has been given for Lady?

    a. Nourish Yin
    b. Nourish Blood
    c. Tonify Yin
    d. Tonify Yang
    e. Calm the Shen

Mac B is a ten year old neutered male Dalmatian who presented with a history of severe chronic progressive hepatic cirrhosis. He has severe muscle wasting and a pendulous abdomen. Histopathology of the liver revealed degeneration and inflammation of hepatic tissue. Ten kilograms of ascitic fluid drained in the prior week. He tires very easily. His tongue is pale and wet, and his pulse is deep and weak. He is currently on five medications from his veterinarian.

Question 8.9: Based on Qi Blood and Body Fluid Patterns, what is Mac B's diagnosis?

    a. Retained Fluids (Retention of Water)
    b. Qi Stagnation
    c. Qi Deficiency
    d. Retained Fluids with Qi Stagnation
    e. Qi Deficiency with Retained Fluids

A five year old toy poodle, Mizie, has a nice personality and seems pretty calm except when her owner boards her for a few days. Recently she developed a bad case of bloody diarrhea when she was boarded. She remained active, and all of her blood work was normal the whole time. Her treatment included antibiotics, a low dose of prednisone and a highly digestible canned dog food. Her diarrhea and hematochezia stopped after a few days of this therapy. As she was finishing up her treatment, she developed a "hot spot" on the ventral aspect of her chin and neck. Her owner claims that she has always been prone to these skin lesions in exactly the same spot. They occur more often during the winter months. The rest of her skin appears normal. On physical exam she appears healthy and active. Her tongue is a red color with a yellow coating in the center, and there are no teeth marks or swelling. Her pulse is a little rapid and forceful.

Question 8.10: What is your TCVM diagnosis for Mizie based on Pathogen Patterns?

   a. Wind-Heat
   b. Damp-Cold
   c. Damp-Heat
   d. Wind-Dryness
   e. Summer Heat

A sixteen year old spayed female cat named Kittie has a history of life-long dermatitis. She was obtained from the shelter as a kitten, and she had a persistent upper respiratory infection. After several weeks of antibiotic treatment, the respiratory infection resolved. As a young cat, she had several dry coughing episodes that were worse in the summer. This resolved following treatment with prednisone and a homeopathic remedy. Kittie has always been a finicky eater, and every three weeks of her life she vomits bile. She has been quite an independent cat, but recently she is more clingy. Kitty has always sought warm places to sleep. For the past year, her kidney biochemical values have been elevated (BUN = 41, Creatinine = 2.7), and she has been treated with homeopathic remedies. Her owner also elected to treat her conjunctival erythema and edema homeopathically. She has had a moist dermatitis that started around her ears and eyes and now is spreading to the underside of her neck, belly and inner thighs. The owner is asking you to give her cat a TCVM evaluation and treatment. You find that Kittie's tongue is red with too much saliva and that her pulse deficient, deep, thin and easy to compress. She is sensitive upon palpation of BL-20 and CV-12. Also, her ears have been filled with a stinky waxy material for months now.

Question 8.11: After you have done the physical examination, what do you tell the owner about Kittie's TCVM diagnosis?

   a. Lung Heat with Gall Bladder Heat
   b. Lung Heat with Kidney Yang Deficiency
   c. Kidney Yang Deficiency with Gall Bladder Heat
   d. Heat in the Upper Jiao, Damp in the Middle Jiao, and Cold in the Lower Jiao
   e. Spleen Damp-Cold with Kidney Yang Deficiency

An eight year old Quarter Horse gelding named Firework presents with a sore back. He is used for barrel racing. About two weeks ago, he began to show signs of back pain, and it seems worse recently. For the past three days, he has thrown off his rider several times. Normally, he is a nice, easy-going, mellow horse. His Shen (mind) is alert. He is very sensitive on the left side from BL-17 to BL-22 upon palpation. His tongue is purple, and his pulse is forceful and wiry. An examination of the saddle revealed that the tree of the left side is broken.

Question 8.12: What is your TCVM diagnosis?

    a. Qi Stagnation
    b. Blood Stagnation
    c. Heat Pattern
    d. Cold Pattern
    e. Summer Heat Pattern

A seventeen year old Trakehner mare presents with a history of infertility. She was bred the last two years and as well as April and May of this year. In June, she was still open in June. She has normal cycles with normal follicles. She has multiple melanomas around her anus and tail and has an apple-sized mass caudal to her left eye. Her tongue is pale, swollen and wet. Her pulse is deep and weak.

Question 8.13: What is your TCVM diagnosis?

    a. Spleen Qi Deficiency
    b. Kidney Qi Deficiency
    c. Kidney Yin Deficiency
    d. Spleen Yin Deficiency
    e. Spleen Qi Deficiency with Kidney Yin Deficiency

CHAPTER NINE

PREVENTION AND TREATMENT STRATEGIES

> The aim of medicine is to prevent disease and prolong life; the ideal of medicine is to eliminate the need of a physician.
>
> – William J. Mayo

The ultimate goal of Traditional Chinese Veterinary Medicine (TCVM), according to *Su Wen* (*Plain Questions*), is to create a state in which "no illness occurs and long life is experienced". How does one achieve this goal? This chapter will address this question by focusing on disease treatment and prevention strategies.

Four Principles of Life

1. Harmony between Nature and the Body

To maintain health, creatures must keep a balanced state between the universe and the body. This harmony includes going to sleep when it becomes dark and waking up when the sun rises. Similarly, the body must stay warm during the cold winter, and it should remain cool during the hot summer weather.

2. Unification of a Quiet Mind and an Active Body

In TCVM, the Mind (Shen) and Body are unified. The Mind should remain in internal peace. The physical body should be moving and athletic. The health of the whole organism depends on both a quiet, peaceful Mind and an active body.

Su Wen said, "If the Mind (Shen) stays internally in peace, there are no causes of illness". People commonly use meditation, Qi-gong, and Tai-ji-quan to keep the Mind healthy. These exercises are not as practical in veterinary medicine; however, encouragement, positive influence, and minimizing stressful environments can help keep animals in good mental health.

Lu's Spring and Autumn states that an "inactive body leads to no flow of Jing (Essence). No flow of Jing leads to Qi Stagnation". Thus, physical exercise is very important to promote the free flow of Qi and Blood and to prevent illness. It is important to follow three rules when engaging in physical exercise:

1. Moderation: Do not over-do it. "The body is moving but not exhausted" (*Su Wen*).

2. Consistency: Practice every day. Only with consistent, regular physical exercise may one achieve fitness and health.

3. Versatility: Different species and different individuals should practice different forms of exercises depending upon their personal requirements. Old or weak animals should do mild exercises; however, young and strong animals can do more strenuous types of exercises. For example, a two-year-old German Shepherd can run for thirty minutes to one hour twice daily, but a fifteen-year-old toy poodle can only walk five to ten minutes twice daily.

3. Moderate Daily Life

In *Qian Jin Yao Fang* (*Thousand Ducat Prescriptions*), Dr. Sun Simiao of the Tang Dynasty (652 AD) described this principle well:

> To keep healthy, everyone has to keep everything from sleep to food in moderation. …Do not eat too much, do not drink too much, avoid overwork, avoid melancholy, avoid anger, not be frightened, not be hyperactive, do not talk too much, do not laugh too much…

Clearly, too much of anything can impair health. Too much rest is as deleterious as too much work. Gluttony can be as harmful as starvation. Even too much of any emotion may result in illness. The key to maintaining balance when confronted with the feast of life is to sample a little of everything at the buffet rather than serving up a heaping plateful of one item only.

4. Dietary Therapy

"Dietary therapy exceeds medicines" (Dr. Zhang Congzheng, Jin Dynasty).

Give cool foods such as fish, celery, or banana if the disease (skin itching) has a Heat Pattern. Use warmer foods such as mutton, fennel and ginger for Cold Pattern diseases (degenerative joint disease).

Dietary therapy is especially useful for geriatric patients or those with a chronic illness. Generally speaking, "the seniors should have meals which are warm, hot, well-cooked and soft. Sticky, hard, raw and cold meals are contraindicated for the seniors" (Dr. Chen Zhizeng, Song Dynasty).

Prevention Strategies

> The Best doctor does not treat the existing disease but engages in preventive medicine, does not treat the existing disorder but prevents the possible disorders… Giving a medicine for a disease that has already occurred or a treatment for a disorder that has occurred is like digging the well when thirsty and building up the army when the war occurs. It is just too late!
>
> *– Su Wen*

PREVENTING THE OCCURRENCE OF ILLNESS

The following prevention procedures are recommended for maintaining healthy animals:

Strengthen Zheng Qi

Zheng Qi refers to the general ability to resist any pathogens and pathological changes. According to *Su Wen*, "Pathogens have no effect if Zheng Qi is strong". Thus, strengthening Zheng Qi is the key to prevention. Regular, moderate physical exercise and a balanced diet are the most important tools to strengthen the Zheng Qi.

Regulate the Constitutional Weakness

Animals that easily feel cold (cold intolerance) tend to have a Kidney Yang Deficiency, which may be seen in the course of degenerative joint disease, intervertebral disc disease, or renal failure. The acupuncture points GV-3, *Bai Hui*, and *Shen Shu* along with the herbal medicine *Shen Qi Wan* are recommended for animals that tend to feel cold.

The animals that tend to be hot are likely to have a Yin Deficiency, which may be seen during the course of dermatological conditions and behavioral problems. The acupuncture points KID-3 and HT-7 and the herbal medicine *Liu Wei Di Huang Wan* may be used for prevention.

Irritable, hyperactive animals tend to have eye problems, liver problems, and Liver Qi Stagnation with Liver Yang Rising. For prevention, the acupoint LIV-3 and the herbal medicine *Xiao Yao San* are recommended.

Sickly animals and those that are born weak often have a Kidney Jing Deficiency. In this case, the acupuncture points KID-7, CV-4, CV-6 and the herbal medicine *Sheng Jing San* (Epimedium Powder) are recommended.

Avoid Exposure to Toxins or Pathogens

Toxins can be from food or water sources. Pathogens can be caused by a seasonal change or sudden weather change. Animals depend on the owner to provide the proper care to avoid these etiological sources.

Herbal Prevention

Herbal medications may be given to healthy animals that are at risk for certain health problems. In this way, the herbal medicine may help prevent illness from ever occurring. For example, Dryopteris root *Guan Zhong*, Isatis leaf *Da Qing Ye* and Isatis root *Ban Lan Gen* have been reported as effective herbal medicines for preventing the flu and upper airway infections. Garlic *Da Shuan* seems very useful as general preventive medication for gastrointestinal disorders.

Fan Mu Cuan Yan Fang (*Collection of Effective Prescriptions for Equine Diseases*), one of the early classical equine herbal medicine texts, was written by Dr. Wang Yu and published around 1086-1100 AD. Dr. Wang suggested that the herbal prevention be based on different seasons: *Yin Chen San* for the spring, *Xiao Huang San* for the summer, *Li Fei San* for the fall and *Hui Xiang San* for the winter.

Acupuncture Prevention

Healthy animals may receive acupuncture treatments that tonify the body's defenses and forestall some anticipated disorders. For example, stimulation of the acupuncture points ST-36, GV-14 and LI-10 will increase immune response and may be used for general prevention.

Since the horse is considered a Fire Animal and has sufficient Qi and Blood, the horse tends to develop a Heat Pattern. As a preventive measure, hemoacupuncture at *Xiong Tang* in the spring may prevent a Heat Pattern in the summertime.

PREVENTING AGGRAVATION OF THE DISEASE PROGRESS

The ideal situation is to prevent illness. However, when an illness has already occurred, the next best strategy is to prevent the disease from becoming worse. There are several procedures that may promote this goal.

Early Diagnosis

Early diagnosis and treatment for any disease usually achieves the best clinical results. To better reach this objective, the classical pulse and tongue diagnosis may be integrated with modern diagnostic techniques.

Stop the Shifting Pathway of a Disease

The transmission pathway of a pathogen is from body surface and Channels to the Zang and Fu organs. For example, a Warm Heat disease (*Wen Ren Bing*) starts with the Wei Stage. If not resolved in Wei Stage, the pathogens are transmitted into the Qi Stage. If still unresolved, the pathogens proceed into the Ying Stage. With continued illness, the pathogens shift into the final Xue stage.

Thus, the treatments should attempt to prevent the progressive pathogen invasion of deeper levels. Diaphoresis can treat illness in the Wei stage by opening the body surface and dispelling the pathogens from the Wei Stage. This prevents the pathogens from invading further into the Qi Stage. Should illness occur at the Qi Stage, the treatment should clear the Heat, dispel Heat from the Qi Stage, and prevent pathogen movement into the Ying Stage. Treatment of the Ying Stage should clear Heat from the Ying Stage and bring Heat to the Qi Stage.

3. Strengthen the Territory Before it is Affected

Five Element Theory

An organ in Excess tends to Cheng (over-control) another organ. Thus, strengthening the "grandchild" organ provides protection for that organ. For example, treatment of a Liver problem (Wood) should also include fortification of the Spleen (Earth). Even though there is no Spleen problem, it is beneficial to strengthen the Spleen because the Liver (Wood) tends to Cheng (over-control) the Spleen (Earth).

Yin Yang Theory

Yang Excess (Heat) pathology tends to damage Yin (Body Fluid). The major treatment plan for Excess Heat is to clear Heat. In addition to treating the Yang Excess, nourishment of Yin may help prevent damage to the Body Fluids.

Zang-Fu Theory

According to Zang-Fu pathology, any chronic illness will eventually be transmitted into the Kidney. Thus, when approaching a chronic disease condition, it is beneficial to tonify the Kidney even though there may be no clinical Kidney signs.

Treatment Strategies

TREATING THE ROOT AND TREATING THE MANIFESTATION

The Root (*Ben*) and the Manifestation (*Biao*) represent the two aspects of one entity. In Traditional Chinese Veterinary Medicine, the following are used to differentiate the Root and the Manifestation:

- When considering the body and the pathogenic factors, the Zheng Qi of the body is the Root and the Xie Qi is the manifestation.

- Regarding the Xie Qi and symptoms, the Xie Qi is the Root, and the symptoms are the Manifestation.

- During the clinical course of a disease, the original or the primary condition is the Root while the complication or secondary condition is the Manifestation.

- Regarding the location of a lesion, the internal organ is the Root, and the external surface is the Manifestation.

In general, the Root is the primary aspect of a disease, which should be treated first. Under certain circumstances, however, the Manifestation is critical and requires immediate treatment. The decision whether to treat the Root or the Manifestation depends on the severity and urgency of the disease. There are three possible treatment methods: treating the Root only, treating both the Root and the Manifestation, and treating the Manifestation first and the Root later.

Treating the Root Only

Generally, focusing on the Root alone can effectively treat many animal diseases. For instance, when encountering a case of diarrhea (the Manifestation) due to Spleen Qi Deficiency (the Root), the correct method of treatment is merely to tonify the Spleen Qi. Similarly, when the patient suffers from a common cold due to Wind-Cold, treating the Root only by eliminating Wind and Cold is enough to clear all clinical manifestations.

Treating Both the Root and the Manifestation

This method is widely used in clinical practice. In chronic cases when the clinical manifestations are severe, it is necessary to treat both the Root and the Manifestation. For example, when a patient has food retention (the Manifestation) due to a Spleen Qi Deficiency, the correct therapeutic method involves both tonifying Spleen Qi (treating the Root) and resolving the stagnated food (treating the Manifestation). However, during treatment, the Root should remain the focus and the Manifestation should provide an adjunct approach.

Treating the Manifestation First and the Root Later

Occasionally there are circumstances in which the clinical manifestations are very severe or life threatening. At these times, the Root becomes secondary, and the Manifestation should be treated first. For instance, immediate resolution of the gas is critical in a case with secondary intestinal gaseous colic (the Manifestation) due to impaction (the Root). Having relieved the intestinal distention, one may address the Root by purging the impaction (stagnated feces) from the intestines.

TONIFYING THE ZHENG QI AND ELIMINATING THE XIE QI

Combat between the Zheng Qi and the Xie Qi exists during all pathological conditions. Thus, the treatment principle is either to tonify the Zheng Qi or to eliminate the Xie Qi. There are three possible methods: 1) tonifying the Zheng Qi, 2) eliminating the Xie Qi, and 3) simultaneously tonifying the Zheng Qi and eliminating the Xie Qi.

Tonifying the Zheng Qi

Tonifying the Zheng Qi refers to any method that strengthens the body and increases its resistance. In this way, it is possible to eliminate the Xie Qi and cure the disease. The methods may include tonifying Qi, Blood, Yin or Yang. This approach is used to treat various Deficiency Patterns.

Eliminating the Xie Qi

Eliminating the Xie Qi refers to any method that eliminates the pathogenic factors. This includes procedures such as diaphoresis, purging, and eliminating Heat. It is mainly used to treat Excess Patterns.

Simultaneously Tonifying the Zheng Qi and Eliminating the Xie Qi

This method is commonly used in practice when the Zheng Qi is weak in the presence of a pathogenic factor. For example, if there is a Spleen Qi Deficiency that leads to the formation of Damp, the treatment method should tonify the Spleen Qi (Zheng Qi) and eliminate the Damp (Xie Qi).

STRAIGHT TREATMENT AND PARADOXICAL TREATMENT

Straight Treatment

Zheng Zhi, also known as Straight Treatment or Contrary Treatment, refers to the use of treatment methods and herbal medications whose nature is opposite to that of the disease. This is a common therapeutic approach.

When using this treatment principle, herbs with a Cold nature are used for Heat Patterns. Similarly, herbs with a hot nature are used for Cold Patterns. Tonifying herbs are used for Deficiency Patterns, and herbs with purging effects are beneficial for Excess Patterns.

Paradoxical Treatment

Fan Zhi, Paradoxical Treatment or Obedient Treatment, refers to treatment methods and herbs whose nature is similar to the nature of the disease. This method is used to treat the false symptoms of a disease.

This method of treatment includes four different approaches: 1) Treating Heat with Heat, 2) Treating Cold with Cold, 3) Treating Obstruction with Tonification, 4) Treating Diarrhea with Purgation.

- Treating Heat with Heat: Herbs with a hot or warm nature can treat Heat manifestations. This is beneficial for True Cold Patterns with pseudo-Heat symptoms.

- Treating Cold with Cold: Herbs with a cool or cold nature can treat Cold manifestations. It is used for a true Heat Pattern with pseudo-Cold symptoms. For example, a Heat Jue Pattern produces cold limbs, but this cold sign is a false or contrary manifestation. Gypsum *Shi Gao*, a very cold herbal medicine, is used even though limbs are cold. A detailed examination of the patient usually reveals signs such as a red tongue, fast pulse, high body temperature, and short, dark urination which indicate the presence of True Heat.

- Treating Obstruction with Tonification: Tonification methods can treat diseases due to obstruction. For instance, the appropriate treatment strategy for a patient with abdominal fullness due to Spleen Qi Deficiency is to tonify the Spleen Qi.

- Treating Diarrhea with Purgation: A purgative can treat diarrhea and dysentery due to food stasis.

COMPARATIVE TREATMENTS FOR THE SAME AND DIFFERENT DISEASES

Different Treatments for the Same Disease

The same disease may require different treatments. The common cold may result from either Wind-Cold or Wind-Heat. Therefore, the treatment varies depending upon the cause. A Pungent-Warm Diaphoretic is used for influenza due to Wind-Cold, and a Pungent-Cool Diaphoretic is for influenza due to Wind-Heat.

Same Treatment for Different Diseases

The same treatment may be used to treat several different diseases. Because an anal/rectal prolapse and a vaginal/uterine prolapse both result from a Spleen Deficiency, tonifying the Spleen and raising the Yang Qi are used in both situations despite the anatomical differences in the diseases.

Eight Treatment Methods

There are eight methods that form the basis of treatment in Traditional Chinese Veterinary Medicine: diaphoresis, emesis, purgation, harmonizing, warming, clearing, tonification, and dissipation.

DIAPHORESIS

Diaphoresis is artificially induced perspiration. Diaphoretic medicines cause sweating, which opens the skin and muscles via the sweat glands, in order to dispel the Xie Qi and to relieve the Exterior. Diaphoresis is divided into Pungent-Warm Diaphoresis and Pungent-Cool Diaphoresis.

Pungent-Warm Diaphoresis uses herbs with a pungent taste and warm nature to treat Exterior Cold Patterns. For example, the acupuncture point BL-10 and the herbal medicine *Ma Huang Tang* (Ephedra Decoction) may treat Cold Excess conditions.

Pungent-Cool Diaphoresis uses herbs with a pungent taste and cool nature to treat Exterior Heat Patterns. *Yin Qiao San* (Lonicera-Forsythia Powder) is one such formula.

Indications

- Exterior Pattern
- Common cold
- Influenza
- Initial stage of various infectious diseases
- Rheumatism
- Initial stage of wound healing
- Swelling
- Boils

Pharmacological Effect

The results of recent scientific experiments indicate that diaphoretic herbs can enhance the secretion of sweat glands, dissipate the body's Heat, and promote Blood circulation both locally and systemically.

Contraindications

Diaphoresis, by inducing perspiration, leads to consumption of Yin (Body Fluid). Diaphoretic medications are contraindicated in the following situations:

- The disease condition is not located in the Exterior.

- The patient suffers from weakness, dysentery, or loss of Blood. If diaphoresis must be used, combine its use with methods that tonify Qi or nourish Yin.

- The patient has already received abundant diaphoretic medications. Excessive sweating will impair Yin and Body Fluid.

- The patient has a weak constitution and is prone to sweating in the summer. Use diaphoresis with caution during the summer as Yin tends to be deficient at this time.

EMESIS

Some treatment methods are intended to induce vomiting. Emetic methods can help to dispel pathogenic factors or poisonous matter from the Stomach. It is a method that is used in emergencies. For example, the herb Dichroa root *Chang Shan* can induce vomiting in order to expel poisonous matter and food stasis from the stomach.

This method is used primarily in small animal medicine. With large animals such as horses and cattle, placement of a nasogastric tube and evacuation of stomach contents can achieve the same goal. Caution is required when a practitioner utilizes emesis as it is possible to impair the Kidney Qi and the Stomach with this method.

Indications

- Food retention
- Poisonous food in the Stomach

Contraindications

- Do not use in weak animals.

- Do not use in pregnant females.

- Do not use following parturition or Blood loss.

PURGATION

Purgation is the act of purging. It eliminates what is undesirable by evacuating the bowels. This method uses cathartics to keep the bowels open, relieve Stagnation, eliminate Excess Heat and excrete accumulated water. Purgation is divided into Drastic Purgation, Mild Purgation and Elimination of water.

Drastic Purgation: The therapeutic methods that purge the accumulation or Stagnation and Excess Heat from the intestines with strong cathartics.

Example: *Da Cheng Qi Tang* (Drastic Purgative Decoction)

Mild Purgation: Treatment methods that nourish Yin and Body Fluid and lubricate the feces. An appropriate treatment of deficient constipation in old, weak, or pregnant animals.

Example: Treat megacolon with *Ma Zi Ren Wan*

Eliminating Water: The methods that eliminate Water-Damp to treat the accumulation of Water-Damp in the body.

Example: Treat ascites with *Shi Zao Tang* (Ten-Dates Decoction).

Indications

- Constipation
- Excess Heat Pattern
- Food retention
- Stagnated Blood
- Accumulation of water

Pharmacological Effects

The results of recent scientific studies indicate that purgative herbs can increase the intestinal peristalsis and promote the blood circulation.

Contraindications

- Do not use if there is only an Exterior Pattern

- Do not use if there are no clinical signs indicating a disorder of the Interior.

- Do not use in vomiting patients.

- Drastic Purgation should not be used in weak, Yin-deficient or pregnant animals nor should it be used post-parturition or post-surgery.

HARMONIZING METHOD

The Harmonizing Method uses the regulating or mediating effects of herbs or acupuncture to eliminate the pathogenic factors, Xie Qi. One example of this method would be harmonizing the Liver and Spleen by using the acupoints GB-34, LIV-13, and LIV-3 with the herbal medicine *Xiao Yao San* to correct the disharmony between the Liver and Spleen.

Indications

- Shao-yang Pattern or Half Exterior and Half Interior Pattern
- Disharmony of the Liver and Spleen or Stomach

Contraindications

- Do not use for an Exterior Pattern without a Shao-yang Pattern.

- Do not use for an Interior Excess Pattern.

- Do not use for an Interior Cold Pattern.

WARMING METHOD

Warming Methods use herbs with a warm or hot nature to treat Cold Patterns by eliminating Cold and tonifying Yang Qi. The warming methods include: 1) Warming the Interior and Eliminating the Cold, 2) Reviving the Yang for Resuscitation, and 3) Dispersing Cold by Warming the Channels.

Warming the Interior and eliminating the Cold is the method that warms the Spleen Yang to treat a Cold Pattern due to Spleen Yang Deficiency. For example, moxibustion at the acupoints GV-4 and *Bai Hui* along with the herbal formula *Li Zhong Tang* can treat a Spleen Yang Deficiency.

Reviving the Yang for resuscitation is a method that treats Extreme Cold Patterns due to Kidney Yang Deficiency or collapse of Deficient Yang through tonification and warming of Kidney Yang. Use the acupoints GV-3 and GV-26 and the herbal formula *Si Ni Tang*.

Dispersing Cold by warming the Channels treats musculoskeletal soreness due to Wind-Cold or stagnated Qi and Blood. Use local acupuncture points and the herbal formula *Dang Gui Si Ni Tang*.

Indications

- Cold Pattern
- Collapse of Deficient Yang
- Yang Deficiency
- Rheumatism (musculoskeletal soreness)

Pharmacological Effects

It has been reported that warming herbs can enhance the function of the Heart, increase Blood pressure, and promote blood circulation.

Contraindications

- Do not use when there is Yin Collapse, coma, or dysentery with Heat.

- Do not use in animals with a Deficient Yin constitution or an Excess Heat Pattern.

- Do not use for a True Heat Pattern with Pseudo-Cold.

CLEARING METHOD

The clearing method uses herbs with a cool or cold nature and is used to treat Heat Patterns. The method includes: 1) Eliminating Heat and Fire, 2) Eliminating Heat and Toxin, 3) Eliminating Heat and Cooling Blood and 4) Eliminating Heat and Damp.

Eliminate Heat and Fire:	The methods used to treat Qi Stage Heat or an Interior Heat Pattern. For example, one may use the acupoints GV-14 and *Wei Jian* (tail tip) with *Bai Hu Tang* (White-Tiger Decoction).
Eliminate Heat and Toxin:	The methods that treat a Heat Toxin Pattern. Example: *Wei Jian* (tail tip) and *Huang Lian Jie Du Tang*
Eliminate Heat; Cool Blood:	Use treatment methods for Blood Stage Heat and Ying Stage Heat. Example: *Xiong Tang* and *Qing Ying Tang*
Eliminate Summer Heat:	This is the treatment method for sunstroke or heatstroke. Example herbal formula: *Xiang Ru San*
Eliminate Heat and Damp:	This method treats the Damp-Heat Patterns. Example herbal formula: *Zhi Li Tang* (Stopping-Dysentery Decoction) is designed to treat canine gastrointestinal Damp-Heat (parvovirus diarrhea).

Contraindications

- Do not use if there is fever due to an Exterior Pattern.
- Avoid in patients with a weak constitution, deficient Stomach Fire or loose feces.
- Do not use with a Deficient Heat Pattern due to Blood Deficiency or overwork.
- Do not use for a True Cold Pattern with Pseudo-Heat.

TONIFICATION

Tonfication is a method that enhances body condition and increases resistance to disease in order to treat various Deficiency Patterns. This method includes the Tonification of Qi, Blood or Yang and the Nourishment of Yin.

Tonifying Qi:	Used for Spleen Qi Deficiency, Lung Qi Deficiency, and Deficient Spleen Qi Sinking. Example: The acupoints CV-4 and ST-36 plus the herbal medicine *Shen Ling Bai Zhu San* are used to treat Spleen Qi Deficiency.
Tonifying Blood:	Used for Blood Deficiency. Example: BL-17, SP-10, and *Si Wu Tang* (Four Substance Powder)

Nourishing Yin: Used for Yin Deficiency Pattern or Deficient Heat Pattern.
Example: KID-3, SP-6, and *Liu Wei Di Huang Wan*

Tonifying Yang: Used for various Yang Deficiency Patterns.
Example: GV-3, *Bai Hui*, and *Shen Qi Wan*

Contraindications

- Pure tonification is not recommended. The herbal formulas for tonification should include a small amount of herbs that promote Qi and strengthen the Stomach.

- Do not use for an Excess Pattern. If the condition is a combination of an Excess Pattern and a Deficiency Pattern, combine tonification with purgation.

DISSIPATION

Dissipation uses stagnation-relieving and stasis-breaking herbs to relieve Qi Stagnation, Stagnated Blood, and food stasis. Because of its mild effects on the body, dissipation is widely used in veterinary practice.

The acupoints ST-37 and CV-12 and the herbal medicine *Qu Mai San* (Leaven-Barley Powder) may be used to relieve stasis or Stagnation.

External Therapy with Herbal Medicines

In some instances, the treatment may require direct application of herbs to an affected body surface such as the ears, nose, eyes, mouth, skin or anus. This method is widely used for surgical and traumatic diseases. There are several different methods of applying herbs externally: Smearing Application, Sprinkling Application, Dropping-into-the-Eyes, Blowing-into-the-Nose, Hot Packing and Cleaning Application.

Topical Application of Herbal Salve

Crush fresh herbs or grind dry herbs into a powder and mix with wine, vinegar, or vegetable oil to create a paste. The paste is smeared on the affected body surface. The mixture should be reapplied periodically to maintain the effectiveness of the salve. Normally, this will be used with a bandage.

This method is widely used for soreness, wounds, boils, acute superficial swellings with redness, fever and pain. *Ru Yi Jin Huang San* (Golden Yellow Salve) is an example of a topical herbal formula used for cuts, sores and acute injuries.

Topical Application of Herbal Tincture

This method is typically used for swelling and pain. Treat the affected location by massaging or gently rubbing the local areas with the tincture.

Eye or Ear Drops

Some herbal liquid extracts may be applied directly into the eyes or ears. The herbal extract, Ear Drop (*Di Er You*), may be used topically for the treatment of otitis.

Blowing Nose

This technique involves blowing or applying small amounts of finely powdered herbs into the nasal cavity. It is intended to open the orifice and to cause the patient to sneeze.

Commonly used for colic and Internal Wind syndrome (seizure), it may temporarily relieve the clinical signs. *Chui Bi San* (Blowing-Nose Powder) is one such powder that relieves colic pain when blown into the nasal cavity of horses. The major ingredients of *Chui-Bi-San* include Pepper *Hua Jiao*, Veratrum *Li Lu*, Dahurian Angelica *Bai Zhi*, Pinellia *Ban Xia*, Gleditsia *Zao Jiao*.

Hot Packing

Hot Packing can dispel Cold and warm the Channel to relieve Stagnation, and can be used for the treatment of Cold-Bi syndrome (arthritis), local muscle soreness.

Cleaning Application

This method uses a decoction of an herbal formula to clean the affected area. The herbal medicine liquid may be used to treat anal prolapse, mange, contusions and sprains.

Self Test

Nina is a fifteen-year-old spayed female mixed breed dog who presented with a history of chronic urinary incontinence and rear weakness. Recently, she has found walking to be difficult and painful. Her left carpus will only flex about 30 degrees. Radiographs indicate that she has extensive bridging spondylosis of the thoracic and lumbar vertebrae and has degenerative joint disease of the elbow and carpus. Upon palpation, her elbows and back were painful. Her tongue is purple with no coat. Her pulse is weak and deep. Based on the chronic urinary incontinence, the rear weakness, the deep and weak pulse and her old age, she is diagnosed with Kidney Qi Deficiency. In addition, she has Blood Stagnation evidenced by the painful walking, painful responses to palpation and purple tongue. The Kidney Qi Deficiency leads to bone weakness, degenerative joint disease and spondylosis, and it further results in Blood Stagnation (pain). Thus, the Kidney Qi Deficiency is the Root and Blood Stagnation is the Manifestation.

Question 9.1: What is your TCVM treatment strategy for Nina?

a. Treating the Root only
b. Treating the Manifestation only
c. Treating both the Root and the Manifestation
d. Not treating either the Root or the Manifestation
e. Strengthening Zheng Qi

Questions 2 and 3 are based on the following case.

A fourteen year old spayed female mixed breed dog named Sugar presented with a history of stiffness and pain of the back and rear limbs. She has received Rimadyl® (carprofen) for 2½ years. Her physical exam findings included bilateral nuclear sclerosis, painful hips upon extension (80 degrees), overall muscle atrophy, and stiffness and pain of the lumbar area. She has had occasional bouts of vertigo and geriatric disorientation. Her tongue is pale and lavender. Her pulse is deficient on the right side.

Question 9.2: What is your TCVM diagnosis for Sugar?

a. Qi Deficiency and Qi Stagnation Pattern
b. Qi and Blood Stagnation
c. Spleen Qi Deficiency and Heart Yin Deficiency
d. Kidney Yin Deficiency and Kidney Qi Deficiency
e. Spleen Qi Deficiency with Kidney Yin Deficiency

Question 9.3: What is your TCVM treatment strategy if Sugar is diagnosed with a combination of Deficiency and Excess (Stagnation)?

    a. Tonify the Deficiency only

    b. Eliminate the Pathogen (Stagnation) only

    c. Tonify the Deficiency and Tonify the Pathogen (Stagnation) at the same time

    d. Tonify the Deficiency and Eliminate the Pathogen (Stagnation) at the same time

    e. None of the above

Questions 4 and 5 are based on the following case.

Trickline is a two-year-old Thoroughbred colt who presented with a high fever and nasal discharge. He began showing the nasal discharge three days ago. His nasal discharge is thick and yellow. His body temperature is 104° F. His appetite and water intake are normal. He has a mild cough. His tongue is red, and his pulse is superficial, forceful and rapid. Three other horses also show similar clinical signs at the same barn.

Question 9.4: What is your TCVM diagnosis for Trickline?

    a. Wind-Cold Pattern

    b. Wind-Heat Pattern

    c. Lung Heat Pattern

    d. Exterior Deficiency Pattern

    e. Lung Yin Deficiency

Question 9.5: Which of the following treatment methods do you select for Trickline?

    a. Nourishing Yin

    b. Warming the Interior

    c. Pungent-Warm Diaphoresis

    d. Pungent-Cool Diaphoresis

    e. Eliminate Heat and Fire

Question 9.6: What is the goal of traditional Chinese veterinary medicine?

    a. The balance/harmony between the universe and the body

    b. The balance /harmony between individuals

    c. The balance/harmony between the mind and body

    d. A balanced/harmonious daily life and diet

    e. All of the above

CHAPTER TEN

CLINICAL CASE ANALYSIS

> If I have ever made any valuable discoveries, it has
> been owing more to patient attention than to any
> other talent.
>
> – Isaac Newton

Dealing with real clinical cases using a Traditional Chinese Veterinary Medical approach can be challenging. It requires an ability to integrate all of the aspects of TCVM diagnosis and treatment. Proficiency with clinical data collection, TCVM pattern differentiation, and treatment protocol selection are the keys to successful patient care.

This chapter contains real case examples. These are intended to illustrate the principles discussed in previous chapters and to provide some insight into a TCVM practitioner's clinical interpretation skills.

Case One: Jet the Quarter Horse Gelding

INTRODUCTION

Jet is a twenty-year-old Quarter Horse gelding that has been with his present owner since he was a yearling. He first visited a TCVM practitioner in April, 2000. At this time, the owner indicated that Jet suffered from chronic back pain and that he would swing out his right rear leg and kick out during horseback rides. He started to do this side-kicking during rides in June 1999.

Jet had a history of right hock osteoarthritis. Steroid Injections into the hocks did not appear to help the condition. The referring veterinarian had also diagnosed Equine Protozoal Myeloencephalitis (EPM) based upon CSF analysis. After three months of EPM medication, Jet seemed more alert, but he would still side-kick during rides. Jet would, however, walk and run normally without a saddle and rider on his back. Extensive massage (each session lasting a couple of hours) of his back and hip provided mild relief.

Generally, Jet is a very friendly horse who tolerates any type of treatment (e.g. dental work, injections, shoeing, acupuncture needling). He has remained pretty healthy for his entire life except for this side-kicking problem. As a pleasure riding horse (jumping and trotting), he is ridden about three times a week for about 60 minutes.

APRIL 21, 2000 (INITIAL VISIT)

Examination

- Overall, Jet appears alert with good Shen.

- Tongue Appearance: Blue-red, Purple

- Pulse Quality: Deep, fast

- Palpation: Jet was very sensitive to touch at the points BL-13 through BL-21, BL-54, the Coxa Hip point, BL-39 and BL-38.

Point Sensitivities upon Palpation:

	BL-13 to BL-21	BL-54, Coxa Hip	BL-38	BL-39
Left side	++++	+++	++	++
Right side	++++	+++	++	++

Initial Problem List

- Chronic sore back
- Side-kicking of the right rear leg during rides
- A purple tongue
- A deep, fast pulse
- Point sensitivities as listed above

TCVM Analysis

For the past fifteen years, Jet has been ridden three times weekly for an hour by an owner who weighs over 250 pounds. The chronic pressure of the rider's heavy weight on his back has gradually blocked the Qi in his back. This then leads to Qi stagnation in the back along BL-13 to BL-21 (the saddle areas). Consequently, a sore back occurs. Qi blockage of the back affects the Qi flow of the Bladder Channel, which leads to sensitivity of BL-54, BL-38 and BL-39 (possibly indicating soreness of the hip, stifle and hock).

He is an Earth type of animal who always tries his best to please his owner. As an Earth horse, Jet only side-kicks to show his discomfort during rides. A blue-purple indicates Qi Stagnation. A red tongue and fast pulse indicates Heat, which is secondary to Qi Stagnation. (Extended periods of Stagnation of any pathogen can lead to Heat.)

TCVM Diagnosis

Qi Stagnation of the back and rear limbs with Internal Heat

Treatment

The primary treatment strategy is to move Qi in order to relieve pain and Stagnation because the major issue is Qi Stagnation. The Heat that is present is a secondary finding. It results from the transformation of long-standing Qi Stagnation. When the Qi Stagnation is resolved, the Heat will disappear by itself.

The treatment includes acupuncture and herbal medicine. Dry needle acupuncture, electroacupuncture and aquapuncture are combined with a Chinese herbal formula. Fifteen grams of Body Sore should be given orally twice daily for 45 days. This herbal medication is a modification of the classical formula *Sheng Tong Zhu Yu Tang*, which moves Qi and Blood in order to relieve Pain and to resolve Stagnation.

The dry needle acupuncture is performed with the needles alone. The electroacupuncture is performed at bilaterally paired points for twenty minutes at 20 Hz. The aquapuncture involves injection of 5 ml of dilute Vitamin B_{12} into the acupoints. Together these help to extend the effects of the acupuncture point stimulation. Three acupuncture treatments should be planned for every three to five weeks.

Dry Needle Acupuncture: *Bai Hui*, BL-67, GB-44, BL-60

Electroacupuncture: *Shen Shu*, BL-15, BL-18, BL-21, BL-54, BL-40

Aquapuncture: *Hua Tuo Jia Ji* along BL-17 to BL-21

Bai Hui is used to relax the horse and to strengthen the back. BL-67 and GB-44 are the Jing-well points to open the Channel and to draw Qi flow from the head towards the foot. BL-60 helps resolve Qi Stagnation and clear Heat. BL-15, BL-18 and BL-21 are local points for back pain (Qi Stagnation of the back). *Shen Shu* helps to move Qi in the back and to strengthen the Kidney and bones. BL-54 is a local point for Qi Stagnation in the hip areas. BL-40 is an Earth point and a major point for resolving back and hip pain. The *Hua Tuo Jia Ji* points along BL-17 to BL-21 are local points for back pain.

Home Care Recommendations

- Turn Jet out into the pasture for rest.
- Do not ride Jet.
- Massage his back for ten minutes twice a day.
- Have a professional massage performed once every two weeks.

MAY 15, 2000 (SECOND VISIT)

Since the last visit, no improvement in the side-kicking (the side-kicking occurs only when somebody rides him) was noted. He does, however, seem more active after the initial acupuncture treatment and herbal medication.

Examination

- Tongue Appearance: Purple
- Pulse Quality: Weak and deep
- Shen Quality: Normal
- Skin Appearance: Normal

Point Sensitivities upon Palpation:

	BL-13 to BL-15	BL-17 to BL-18	BL-19 to BL-22	BL-23 to BL-25 *Shen Shu*	Coxa Hip
Left side	−	+++	−	++	+++
Right side	−	−	−	++++	+++

TCVM Analysis

Even though the side-kicking behavior has not changed since the previous acupuncture treatment, Jet has less sensitivity of the back and rear limbs upon palpation. This indicates improvement. The disappearance of the red tongue and the fast pulse indicates that the Heat has cleared. Currently, the major problem is the increase in sensitivity of the right coxofemoral areas (BL 23-25, *Shen Shu* and Coxa-hip point).

TCVM Diagnosis

Qi Stagnation in the back and coxofemoral areas (worse on the right side)

Treatment

The current treatment strategy is to move Qi to relieve pain. Once again a combination of dry needle acupuncture, electroacupuncture (20 Hz for twenty minutes at paired points) and aquapuncture (5 cc of vitamin B_{12}) are used. The herbal medicine is continued as previously prescribed.

Dry Needle Acupuncture: *Bai Hui*, BL-67, GB-44, ST-45

Electroacupuncture: BL-40, BL-54, *Shen Shu*, *Lu Gu*, *Da Kua* (right) with *Xiao Kua*

Aquapuncture: BL-15, BL-17, BL-18, BL-23, *Shen Shu*, BL-54

Lu Gu is the most important point for local coxofemoral Stagnation. As the Qi Stagnation is greater in right coxofemoral areas, the local points *Da Kua* and *Xiao Kua* are chosen. BL-17 is the local point for back pain. BL-23 is used to nourish the Kidney and to strengthen the back. ST-45, the Jing-well acupoint, opens the Channel to move Qi.

Home Care Recommendations

* Daily massage of the back
* Professional massage in two weeks
* Allow Jet to rest for three weeks, and then the light rider should ride Jet twenty minutes once a week.

JUNE 23, 2000 (THIRD VISIT)

The owner's friend, who weighs about 80 pounds, rode Jet twice during the past two weeks (20 minutes per ride). While horseback riding, Jet did not kick his right rear limb as much as before. This is his best behavior since he began side-kicking last year.

Examination

- Tongue Appearance: Pale
- Pulse Quality: Deep and weak

	LI-15 to LI-16	BL-13 to BL-23	Coxa hip, BL-54	BL-39
Left side	−	−	−	++
Right side	++	−	++	−

TCVM Analysis

When the branch manifestation (pain) improves, the underlying root Deficiency signs such as a pale tongue and deep, weak pulse become evident. Because the back is the house of the Kidney, the Kidney rules the back and the rear limbs. Based upon these signs, one may diagnose Kidney Qi Deficiency.

The normal reaction to palpation of the back indicates that there is no Qi blockage there. Slight sensitivity at the right LI-15 and LI-16 points indicate a slight Qi blockage of the right shoulder which may be secondary to the sore back and rear limbs. The other sensitivities indicate mild Qi blockage in the right hip and left hock.

The combination of rest, a light rider, acupuncture and herbal medicine seems to have improved the Qi Stagnation. Since the Excess Pattern (Qi Stagnation) is better, his underlying Deficiency shows up (pale tongue, deep/weak pulse) and becomes the focus of treatment. At twenty years of age, his Kidney Qi is in decline, leading to Kidney Qi Deficiency.

TCVM Diagnosis

Kidney Qi Deficiency with Qi Stagnation.

Treatment

The current treatment strategy is to Tonify Kidney Qi and to promote Qi Flow. Once again a combination of dry needle acupuncture, electroacupuncture (20 Hz for twenty minutes at bilaterally paired points) and aquapuncture (5 cc of vitamin B_{12}) are used. The herbal medicine, however, is discontinued.

Dry Needle Acupuncture: KID-1

Electroacupuncture: BL-23, *Shen Shu*, BL-54, *Ba Jiao*, and BL-40 with KID-3

Aquapuncture: BL-23, *Shen Peng*, *Shen Jiao*, *Lu Gu*, *Bai Hui*, GV-4

KID-1, KID-3, BL-23, *Shen Shu*, *Shen Peng*, *Shen Jiao*, *Bai Hui* and GV-4 are used to tonify Qi and to strengthen the Kidney. BL-54, BL-40, *Ba Jiao* and *Lu Gu* are used to clear the residue of Qi Stagnation.

Home Care Recommendations

- Add glucosamine in the feed.
- For the riding program, start with twenty minutes of light riding once weekly for a month. Progress to thirty minutes of light riding once weekly for the second month. Subsequently, Jet can move up to thirty to forty minutes of light riding twice weekly.

APRIL 16, 2001 (FOURTH VISIT)

During the past ten months since the last acupuncture treatment, Jet has been ridden once or twice a week (20 to 40 minutes) by a light rider. Occasionally his stool has been loose. He still side-kicks his right rear leg during riding, but the behavior is less severe. Also, he no longer side-kicks when returning to the barn (he used to do so) after riding.

Examination

- He looks depressed
- There is muscle atrophy of his right gluteal area (a 2 x 3 cm depression).
- Tongue Appearance: Pale
- Pulse Quality: Deep

	Qi Hai Shu BL-20 to BL-21	BL-22	Shen shu BL-23 to BL-25	BL-54, Lu gu, Coxa hip
Left side	++	−	++	++++
Right side	++	−	++	++

TCVM Analysis

A Kidney Qi Deficiency will cause a Spleen Qi Deficiency, which leads to loose stool, muscle atrophy and depression. The sensitivities indicate the presence of coxofemoral Qi Stagnation that is worse on the left side.

It is a good sign when the sensitivity switches from one side to another. The Qi flow of each Channel is bilateral. After acupuncture treatment, the Qi blockage moves from one side to another on the same Channel. It can continue to switch from one side to another until the Stagnation eventually resolves.

TCVM Diagnosis

Kidney and Spleen Qi Deficiency with Qi Stagnation

Treatment

The current treatment strategy is to Tonify Kidney and Spleen Qi and to move Qi for pain relief. Once again a combination of dry needle acupuncture, electroacupuncture (20 Hz for twenty minutes at bilaterally paired points) and aquapuncture (5 cc of vitamin B_{12}) are used. Two herbal medications are added to the treatment. Thirty grams of Equine *Du Huo* should be given once daily for the first two weeks, then fifteen grams can be given once daily for the following four weeks. In addition, thirty grams of Body Sore should be given daily for the first two weeks, followed by fifteen grams once daily for four weeks.

Dry Needle Acupuncture: BL-67, Bai-Hui

Electroacupuncture: *Shen Jiao, Shen Shu*, BL-54, BL-21, BL-40 with *Lu Gu*, and *Da Kua* with *Xiao Kua* (left)

Aquapuncture: BL-20, BL-21, *Qi Hai Shu*

Since Jet shows a Spleen Qi Deficiency, BL-20, BL-21 and *Qi Hai Shu* are added to tonify Spleen Qi. Equine *Du Huo, as a* modification of the herbal formula *Du Huo Ji Sheng Tang*, is intended to treat Bi syndrome due to Qi and Blood Deficiency.

Home Care Recommendations

The riding program should include complete rest for one month followed by one day of light riding for ten minutes during the first week. The second week after the rest period should include one twenty minute ride, and the third week should include one thirty-minute light ride.

JULY 25, 2001 (FIFTH VISIT)

Jet is doing great. He had only side-kicked two to three times for the past three months. His appetite, thirst and stool are normal.

Examination

- Tongue Appearance: Pale pink

- Pulse Quality: Normal

- Shen: Great

- Attitude: Great

	LI-18 to LI-15	BL-13 to BL-28	*Lu Gu*, BL-54	BL-39, Coxa hip
Left side	—	—	—	—
Right side	—	—	++	++

TCVM Analysis

Jet's physiological status is basically normal; there is balance of Yin-Yang and normal Qi flow. The normal appetite, thirst, stool, pulse, attitude and Shen indicate that the Spleen Qi has returned to normal and the Kidney Qi has greatly improved. However, there is still some Qi Stagnation of the right rear limb. The pale pink tongue, age and chronic rear limb soreness indicate a mild Kidney Qi Deficiency.

TCVM Diagnosis

Qi Stagnation and Kidney Qi Deficiency

Treatment

The current treatment strategy is to move Qi for pain relief and to tonify Kidney Qi. Again, a combination of dry needle acupuncture, electroacupuncture and aquapuncture (5 cc of vitamin B_{12}) are used. Fifteen grams of the *Ba Ji Tian San* should be given by mouth once daily for three months.

Dry Needle Acupuncture: BL-67, GB-44 (right)

Electroacupuncture: *Shen Jiao* with *Lu Gu*, *Shen Shu*, BL-54, and *Da Kua* with *Xiao Kua* (right)

Aquapuncture: BL-20, BL-23, ST-36

Since the problem is basically under the control, fewer acupuncture points are used. ST-36 is for general tonification. *Ba Ji Tian San* is the classical equine herbal formula for Kidney Qi Deficiency with back and rear limb soreness.

Home Care Recommendations

Allow Jet to rest for two weeks then gradually increase to normal riding schedule.
If needed, give an acupuncture treatment and a TCVM evaluation in six months.

Case Two: Markie the Warm Blood Gelding

INTRODUCTION

Markie is an eleven-year-old Dutch Warm Blood gelding. He is a successful jumper and dressage horse (4th class level) according to the owner. Markie is a dominant horse when in the pasture with other horses; he is aggressive towards other barn mates and charges them. He loves to run and compete. He is irritable, alert, nimble, impatient, and a good athlete.

Unfortunately, Markie ran into a tree and injured his right rear limb last September. After resting for four months, he seemed to be doing well. The owner started to train him at the end of January 2001. He showed a little lameness of the right rear limb, which responded well to oral phenylbutazone.

About six days prior to his initial TCVM visit, Markie showed significant lameness. The referring veterinarian performed a nerve block and hock injection, but the lameness remained unchanged. Subsequently, Markie was presented to the referral veterinary hospital for a lameness examination and treatment. Nerve blocks, stifle and hock flexion tests, radiographs and Magnetic Resonance Imaging (MRI) did not reveal any abnormal findings. Gait analysis indicated a 3 of 5 grade right rear limb lameness. At this time he was referred to the acupuncture service.

APRIL 2, 2001 (INITIAL VISIT)

Examination

- Tongue Appearance: Purple
- Pulse Quality: Wiry
- Shen: OK
- Personality Type: Wood
- Skin: Good

	LI-18 to LI-15	BL-13 to BL-21	Lu Gu BL-54	BL-37 to BL-38	BL-39 Coxa hock
Left side	+++	++	++	—	—
Right side	—	++	++++	—	++

Initial Problem List

- Right rear limb lameness (grade 3/5)
- A purple tongue
- A wiry pulse
- Point sensitivities as listed above

TCVM Analysis

The injuries had caused Qi and Blood Stagnation of the right coxofemoral area. Thus, BL-54 and *Lu Gu* are very sensitive to palpation. Sensitivity at BL-39 and the Coxa Hock point indicate hock soreness (Qi Stagnation), which is secondary to the coxofemoral Qi Stagnation. The sensitivity of the left LI-18 and LI-15 indicate left front foot Qi Stagnation, which is also secondary to right coxofemoral Qi Stagnation. Sensitivity at BL-13 to BL-21 indicates Qi Stagnation of the back which can be caused by excessive or improper jumping and dressage work. A purple tongue and wiry pulse indicate Stagnation.

TCVM Diagnosis

Qi Stagnation at right coxofemoral areas and back

Treatment

The treatment strategy is to move Qi for pain relief and to move Blood for resolution of the Stagnation. Dry needle acupuncture, electroacupuncture (pairs of points stimulated at 20 Hz for twenty minutes), and aquapuncture with 5 cc of diluted Vitamin B_{12} are used in addition to the herbal formula "Body Sore". For two weeks, thirty grams of the herbal medicine should be given by mouth twice daily, and then it can be decreased to fifteen grams twice daily. Three acupuncture treatments one to three months apart are recommended.

Dry Needle Acupuncture:	BL-67, GB-44, LI-1 (left), LU-11 (left)
Electroacupuncture:	*Shen Shu*, BL-54, *Shen Jiao* with *Lu Gu*, *Da Kua* with *Xiao Kua* (right), BL-35 with Coxa Hip point (right)
Aquapuncture:	BL-18, BL-19, BL-40, Coxa Hip point, *Lu Gu*

The points BL-67 and GB-44 are Jing-well points which open the Channel and draw Qi flow from the head toward the foot. *Shen Shu* and *Shen Jiao* are used to move Qi in the back and to strengthen the Kidney and bones. BL-54 is a local point for Qi Stagnation in the hip areas. BL-40 is an Earth point and a master point for resolving back and hip pain. BL-35, *Lu Gu*, Coxa Hip point, *Da Kua* and *Xiao Kua* are the local points for coxofemoral Qi Stagnation. LI-1 and LU-11 are Jing-well points that open the Channel and draw Qi Flow from the chest to the foot. BL-18 and BL-19 are the association points of the Liver and Gallbladder, which act to relieve local back pain and to soothe the Liver Qi of a Wood-type horse.

Home Care Recommendations

- Turn Markie out and allow him to rest for one month, and then gradually ease back into the training program.

- Massage the right hip for ten minutes once daily for one month.

MAY 18, 2001 (SECOND VISIT)

By Markie's second presentation for acupuncture treatment, the owners had begun to ride him about one month ago. He had been doing well. According to the owner and trainer, his lameness had improved by 90 percent. The trainer felt only slight stiffness of his right rear limb.

About one week ago, Markie began to stop sweating. Also, during the four hour drive to the hospital the previous evening, Markie experienced some mild colic. His appetite and thirst were depressed. In a day, he took in ¼ bucket of water, 1/3 scoop bran mash, ¼ scoop oats mixed with water, and ¼ flake of timothy hay. He had a decrease in gut sounds and has produces no stool since his arrival.

Examination

He looks depressed. His body surface feels hot, and his whole body surface is dry. Within the same barn, the other horses are sweating because of the hot environment. He shows no desire to drink water and is demonstrating mild colic signs. The rectal exploration indicates impaction in the colon.

- Shen: Low

- Tongue Appearance: Red and dry with yellow coating

- Pulse Quality: Fast

	LI-18 to LI-15	BL-13 to BL-18	Lu Gu BL-54	BL-19 to BL-21	BL-39 Coxa hock
Left side	–	–	–	+++	–
Right side	–	–	+++	+++	–

Problem List

- Colic
- Anhidrosis
- Depression
- Red, dry tongue with yellow coating
- Fast pulse

TCVM Analysis

The right coxofemoral Qi Stagnation has greatly improved; however, Summer Heat has invaded the body and shut down the sweating ability. Summer Heat is very hot and also tends to consume Large Intestine body fluids. Food impaction (Food Stasis at Large Intestine) occurs as a consequence. The colic signs, the red and dry tongue, the yellow coating and fast pulse indicate Food Stasis and Heat. Lack of thirst and non-sweating indicates the presence of Summer Heat. Summer Heat is almost always combined with Damp. Damp makes a horse lose the desire to drink and the ability to sweat.

TCVM Diagnosis

Food Stasis of the Large Intestine and Summer Heat

Treatment

The treatment strategy is to purge the Large Intestines to resolve impaction and clear Heat. Even though the pathogen Summer Heat is the underlying cause of Food impaction and anhidrosis, the colic (Large Intestine Food stasis) is a most urgent clinical sign to eliminate. Thus purging the Large Intestine to resolve impaction is the primary issue. At this time, hemoacupuncture will also be performed to clear Heat. Electroacupuncture is performed at paired points at 20 Hz for ten minutes followed by 80-120 Hz for another ten minutes.

Hemoacupuncture:	*Tai Yang*, *Wei Jian* (tail tip), *San Jiang* (ST-2), TH-1
Electroacupuncture:	BL-20, BL-21, *Qi Hai Shu*, *Mi Jiao Gan*, BL-22, BL-13, GV-14 with LI-11 (right)
Aquapuncture:	KID-7, LI-10

Hemoacupuncture at *Tai Yang*, Tip of the Tail, ST-2 and TH-1 is to clear Heat, detoxify, and resolve Stagnation. GV-14 and LI-11 also clear Heat. BL-20, BL-21 *Qi Hai Shu*, *Mi Jiao Gan* and LI-10 strengthen Spleen and Stomach, promote appetite, and promote gastrointestinal motility. BL-22 and BL-13 help to open and distribute fluids including sweat. KID-7 nourishes Yin and body fluids. During the acupuncture treatment, Markie excreted a clear serous nasal discharge. This is one of De-Qi (arrival of Qi) responses.

In addition, the 200 grams of the Chinese Herbal medicine *Da Cheng Qi Tang* should be given once daily by nasogastric tube for two days. *Da Cheng Qi Tang* is the classical herbal formula used to purge the Large Intestine and to resolve impaction. Because it is very potent, it should only be used for a short period of time.

Continued Care Recommendations

- Stop feeding grains.
- Allow free access to water
- Feed timothy hay three times a day
- Monitor gut sounds and bowel movements. If the colic is severe, surgical removal of impaction might be an option.

JUNE 20, 2001 (THIRD VISIT)

Markie has had soft-formed, almost-normal feces. He has eaten two flakes of timothy hay three times a day, however, he only drank ½ bucket of water each day. His gut sounds are almost normal. He was allowed to graze on pasture for ten minutes twice a day (during which time he wants to run). His body surface is still always dry (non-sweating).

Examination

- His body surface feels hot
- He is restless and irritable.
- Tongue Appearance: Red and dry
- Pulse Quality: Thready

	LI-18 to LI-15	BL-42 to BL-44	*Lu Gu*, BL-54	BL-39, Coxa hock
Left side	–	++	++	++
Right side	–	++	++++	++

TCVM Analysis

The food impaction has resolved, however, Markie still has a hot body surface, red tongue, anhidrosis, and a decrease in water intake, which indicate Summer Heat. A dry tongue and thready pulse indicate Yin Deficiency, which can be secondarily caused by Summer Heat. When the critical signs (colic) are cleared, the chronic signs (right hip soreness) become more active (greater sensitivity is found on the right side of BL-54 and *Lu Gu*). Sensitivity at BL-39 and the Coxa Hock point indicates hock Qi Stagnation, which may result from the primary hip soreness.

Markie is a Wood horse and loves to run. However, the constraints in the hospital barn can lead to emotional stress, which can turn on sensitivity at BL-42 to 44 (as Heat tends to flare up and affect the upper jiao including the Lung, Pericardium and Heart organs).

TCVM Diagnosis

Summer Heat, Yin Deficiency, Qi Stagnation of the right coxofemoral areas

Treatment

The treatment strategies are to clear Summer Heat, to nourish Yin, and to move Qi for pain relief. Dry needle acupuncture, electroacupuncture (paired points, 20 Hz for twenty minutes), and aquapuncture are combined.

Dry Needle Acupuncture:	*Bai Hui*, BL-67, GB-44
Electroacupuncture:	*Shen Shu*, BL-42, BL-44, BL-17, BL-22, BL-54, *Lu Gu* (right) with *Da Kua*
Aquapuncture:	*An Shen*, LI-11, GV-14, KID-7

BL-67 and GB-44 are Jing-well points that open the Channel and draw Qi flow from the head toward the foot. *Shen Shu* is used to nourish the Kidney. BL-42 can open the Lung and body surface. BL-44 and *An Shen* calm the Shen and strengthen the Heart. BL-17 nourishes the Blood, and BL-22 helps distribute body fluids. BL-54 is a local point for Qi Stagnation in the hip area. *Lu Gu* and *Da Kua* are local points for coxofemoral Qi Stagnation. LI-11 and GV-14 clear Heat, and KID-7 nourishes Yin and body fluids.

Markie became more relaxed and stood more quietly after the needles were inserted into *Bai Hui* and *An Shen*.

JUNE 22, 2001 (FOURTH VISIT)

Markie has been eating well, and his gut sounds have been within normal limits since June 20. He still seems to not be drinking as much as he should, and he still does not sweat. His body surface still feels hot.

Examination

- Tongue Appearance: Red and dry
- Pulse Quality: Weak

	BL-13 to BL-21	BL-42 to BL-44	*Lu Gu*, BL-54	BL-39, Coxa hock
Left side	—	++	+	++
Right side	—	+	+	—

TCVM Analysis

Qi Stagnation of the coxofemoral areas seemed to have cleared, but anhidrosis is still a major concern. Because of the inability to sweat, Heat accumulates in the Interior. He has no thirst due to the Summer Heat. The red, dry tongue indicates Heat and Yin Deficiency. The weak pulse indicates a Yin Deficiency that fails to support Qi.

TCVM Diagnosis

Interior Heat due to Summer Heat, Yin Deficiency

Treatment

The treatment strategies are to clear Summer Heat and to nourish Yin. Dry needle acupuncture, Hemoacupuncture, electroacupuncture (paired points, 20 Hz for twenty minutes), and aquapuncture are combined at this visit. In addition, fifty grams of the Chinese herbal medicine *Xin Xiang Ru San* should be given twice daily for two weeks. *Xin Xiang Ru San* is the classical herbal formula *Xiang Ru San* modification for anhidrosis due to Summer Heat.

Dry Needle Acupuncture: LI-4

Hemoacupuncture: *Xiong Tang, Yan Mai, Da Mai*

Electroacupuncture: *Shen Shu, Tai Yang*, BL-13, BL-22, *Ding Chuan*, KID-7

Aquapuncture: SP-6, BL-42 and BL-44

The points LI-4, Ding-chuan, and *Tai Yang* open the body surface to clear Heat. *Xiong Tang, Yan Mai* and *Da Mai* are also used to clear Heat. BL-13 and BL-22 help to distribute Body Fluids normally, while KID-7 and SP-6 help to nourish Yin.

JUNE 25, 2001 (FIFTH VISIT)

Since June 25th Markie has begun to sweat normally. He also drinks a normal amount of water and eats normally. His Shen is great and both the tongue and pulse are normal.

Today Markie will be discharged from the hospital today. He should be allowed to rest for two weeks, and then he may gradually be brought back into normal training.

FEBRUARY 27, 2002 (FOLLOW-UP VIA TELEPHONE)

Markie has returned to normal training and is doing very well. He loves to run and compete, and he is full of energy and has a good attitude. There is no longer any lameness. He eats, drinks, and sweats normally.

Case Three: Mr. Flopp the Lop Eared Rabbit

INTRODUCTION

Mr. Flopp is a picky 1½ year old Lop Eared Rabbit. The owner indicated that he is the first and only pet she has ever had. Mr. Flopp lives in a town house. The owner tries very hard to please the rabbit by giving him different types of hay (timothy, oat, etc.), pellets, fruits, curly kale, alfalfa sprouts, oats, wheat crackers, all kinds of rabbit drinking bowls, and freedom to run and play in the living room and bedroom.

During the last week of November, 2000, the rabbit started refusing water and hay. At this time, the referring veterinarian diagnosed an impaction and an ear infection. The veterinarian treated the rabbit with ear drops, a two-week course of antibiotics, and subcutaneous fluids.

Mr. Flopp did not improve to the owner's satisfaction, so she brought Mr. Flopp to the referral hospital on December 1, 2000. He presented with a poor appetite, dry fecal balls, dark orange urine, and depression. Skull radiographs and abdominal ultrasound showed no abnormalities. The complete blood count was within normal limits, but the biochemistry panel revealed a low BUN (10 mg/dL). He was diagnosed with anorexia and delayed gastric emptying. He was hospitalized for four days, treated with IV fluids, and force fed three times daily via a syringe with Oxbow mixed with baby food, greens, veggies, fruit, hay and water.

DECEMBER 4, 2000 (INITIAL VISIT)

Examination

Mr. Flopp looks fatigued and emaciated. He refuses to eat and drink. The feces appear normal, but he has decreased gastrointestinal (GI) motility and is dehydrated.

- Shen: Low (depression)
- Personality: As a friendly, laid-back rabbit who is very cooperative during the TCVM exam, Mr. Flopp is an Earth type of rabbit.
- Tongue Appearance: Red, dry
- Pulse Quality: Deep and weak

TCVM Analysis

Earth type animals tend to develop gastrointestinal disorders and Spleen Qi Deficiency. The deep and weak pulse, decreased GI sounds, weariness, emaciation, anorexia and lack of thirst all indicate a Spleen Qi Deficiency. As Spleen Qi Deficiency can lead to a Heart Deficiency ("The Child's illness affects the Mother"), Mr. Flopp thus shows weariness and low Shen. The rabbit's Spleen Qi Deficiency leaves him with no energy to eat and drink, and the secondary Heart Deficiency decreases his desire to drink and eat. Insufficient water intake gradually leads to Yin Deficiency, thus causing a red, dry tongue and dehydration.

TCVM Diagnosis

Spleen Qi Deficiency with Yin Deficiency

Treatment

The treatment strategy is to tonify the Spleen Qi. Because the signs of Heart Deficiency and Yin Deficiency are very mild and secondary to the Spleen Qi Deficiency, tonification of the Spleen Qi remains the focus of treatment.

Dry Needle Acupuncture: BL-20, BL-21, GV-20, ST-36

Aquapuncture: GV-1, GB-34, *Shan Gen*
(0.3 cc of vitamin B_{12})

BL-20 and BL-21 tonify the Spleen Qi and strengthen the Stomach. GV-20 is used for general relaxation. ST-36 is beneficial for general Qi tonification. GB-34 harmonizes the Liver and Spleen and promotes good Qi flow of the middle jiao. GV-1 and *Shan Gen* promote appetite and thirst.

Recommended Care

- Discharge from the hospital
- Give Mr. Flopp subcutaneous fluid injections twice a day if he still does not drink water by himself.

DECEMBER 12, 2000 (SECOND VISIT)

Since December 9th Mr. Flopp has had a good appetite. He was offered a variety of items including oat and timothy hay, Oxbow pellets, oats, fruit, vegetables, sunflower seeds and kale. He still does not drink, and the owner has given him subcutaneous fluids twice daily. Some wounds or scar tissues were noted on his cranial ventral abdomen.

Examination

- Overall: Mr. Flopp appears happier and more active.
- Tongue Appearance: Pale
- Pulse Quality: Weaker on right side
- Shen: Normal

TCVM Analysis

A good appetite, greater activity and a more cheerful attitude indicate improvement. However, the pale tongue, right-sided weak pulse, and lack of thirst indicate that Mr. Flopp still has some degree of Spleen Qi Deficiency. The wound or scar tissue on his cranioventral abdomen indicates Blood Stagnation.

TCVM Diagnosis

Spleen Qi Deficiency with Blood Stagnation of the local abdomen

Treatment

The strategies are to tonify the Spleen Qi and to move Blood to resolve Stagnation.

Dry Needle Acupuncture: Circle the dragon around the cranial abdominal wound

Electroacupuncture: BL-20, *Jian Wei*, and ST-36 bilaterally
(20 Hz for twenty minutes)

Aquapuncture: BL-21, ST-36, LI-10 and *Shan Gen*
(0.3 cc of vitamin B$_{12}$)

Jian Wei is an extra point that promotes appetite and thirst. LI-10 can tonify Spleen Qi. "Circling the dragon" with the acupuncture needles promotes Qi and Blood circulation and hastens the healing process.

Home Care Recommendations

- For the next two weeks, massage BL-20, BL-21, and CV-12 for five minutes daily.
- Moxibustion at BL-20 and BL-21 for five minutes daily during the next two weeks.
- Repeat acupuncture treatment in one month if his appetite is not 100% normal.

FEBRUARY 6, 2001 (THIRD VISIT)

Mr. Flopp has been eating well; however, he recently began eating only about one cup of hay at night (he only eats at night). He still does not drink much water and receives a subcutaneous fluid injection every other day. His stool seems a little dry, and his urine is dark and orange.

Examination

His Shen looks good. He is active (maybe a little hyperactive). His eyes are red and dry. The abdominal wound has completely healed. He dislikes needling this time.

- Tongue Appearance: Red
- Pulse: Deep and weak

TCVM Analysis

The red tongue, red and dry eyes, hyperactivity, dry stool, and dark urine all indicate Yin Deficiency. The lack of thirst and poor appetite during the daytime as well as the weak, deep pulse indicate a Spleen Qi Deficiency. The Yin Deficiency is secondary to the decreased thirst (a decrease in water intake).

TCVM Diagnosis

Spleen Qi Deficiency with Yin Deficiency

Treatment

The treatment strategies are to tonify Spleen Qi and to nourish Yin. In addition to the acupuncture, the Chinese herbal medicine *Si Jun Zi Tang* is recommended for one to two months. One pill should be given daily in the morning. (The owner loves the rabbit very much and spoils him. She cannot do anything he dislikes. Thus, the herbal medication was discontinued on February 25th because Mr. Flopp refused the pill.)

Dry Needle Acupuncture: *An Shen*, BL-20 BL-21, *Bai Hui*

Aquapuncture: CV-4, CV-6, ST-36, KID-3
(0.3 cc of vitamin B_{12})

An Shen and *Bai Hui* are used to calm him down. CV-4 and CV-6 are for general tonics. KID-3 is a Yin tonic. *Si Jun Zi Tang* is a classical herbal formula for Spleen Qi Deficiency.

Recommendation

- Stop the subcutaneous fluids therapy
- Come for another acupuncture treatment in four months

JUNE 5, 2001 (FOURTH VISIT)

Mr. Flopp will drink now, but he recently has become lethargic. He is occasionally constipated, and he scratches his ears (chronic and intermittent). He will not eat hay (Timothy, oat, costal), but he will eat parsley, carrot tops, kale, pellets, rabbit seed mixture. He runs free in the house and eats a lot of inappropriate items such as wood, paint, and carpet.

Examination

He is nice and quiet in the exam room (even though the owner claims that he is very dominant at home). He has gained one pound since February. There is alopecia on his ears, but there is no discharge inside the ears. No sensitivity was found of his back-shu points upon palpation.

- Tongue Appearance. Deep red
- Pulse Quality: Thready
- Shen: Good

TCVM Analysis

His ear-scratching, constipation, and strange eating habits (avoiding dry hay and eating inappropriate items) indicate a Yin Deficiency. The deep red tongue and thready pulse also indicate Yin Deficiency.

TCVM Diagnosis

Yin Deficiency

Treatment

The treatment strategy is to nourish Yin. BL-23, KID-3 and KID-10 can help to nourish Kidney Yin. HT-7 and LIV-3 tonify the Heart and Liver Yin. In addition, the herbal medicine *Liu Wei Di Huang Wan* should be given to nourish Yin. One pill of the herbal medication is given in the evening for two months.

Dry Needle Acupuncture: *An Shen*, BL-23, KID-3, KID-10

Aquapuncture: CV-4, CV-6, HT-7, LIV-3
(0.3 cc of vitamin B_{12})

Recommendation

Provide free access to water and different kinds of vegetable leaves, grasses, and hay.

AUGUST 7, 2001 (FIFTH VISIT)

Mr. Flopp now eats and drinks very well. He still scratches his ears sometimes, but no alopecia or discharge is visible.

Examination

- Tongue Appearance: Pink
- Pulse Quality: Normal
- Shen: Great

TCVM Diagnosis

Yin-Yang Equilibrium (Overall, Mr. Flopp's health status is good)

Treatment

Dry Needle Acupuncture: SI-19, BL-21, BL-23

Aquapuncture: ST-36, *An Shen*
(0.3 cc of vitamin B_{12})

The points SI-19 and *An Shen* are local points which help stop ear itching.

Recommendation

Monitor the ear scratching. If he becomes worse, either take him to the dermatologist or try topical application of the herbal ointment Ear Drop (*Di Er You*).

Case Four: Galahad the Doberman Pinscher

INTRODUCTION

Galahad is a four year old intact male Doberman Pinscher. He was diagnosed with lymphocytic-plasmacytic dermatitis in January 2000. The owner was given the options of alternative medicine or chemotherapy; she chose alternative medicine.

Galahad had a history of various skin problems over the past four years. He had white, thick skin lesions that were about 3 cm x 3 cm in size. The skin lesions started on the right side of the trunk, spread to the dorsal back, and extended to the left trunk.

The owner has owned Galahad since he was born. Galahad is a performance dog. The owner believes in a holistic approach and she is willing to try everything possible to resolve the dog's skin problem. Except for the skin conditions, the dog has been very healthy all his life.

JULY 11, 2000 (INITIAL VISIT)

Examination

The skin lesions were found on about twenty-five locations around flank areas. It was worse on the right side and dorsum. Each lesion looks like a Quarter, as they are silver in color and about 3 x 3 cm in size. These areas feel thickened, appear raised above the normal skin area, and exhibit some hair loss. Galahad's nose and hair coat are dry; his eyes are red.

- Personality: As he is very competitive and aggressive, he has a Wood personality.
- Tongue Appearance: Purple
- Pulse Quality: Wiry

TCVM Analysis

Wood type dogs tend to have Liver Qi Stagnation which is evidenced by the purple tongue and wiry pulse. Liver Qi Stagnation (Excess) can insult (counter-control) the Lung (Excessive Wood insults Metal). Liver is a Yang organ; and when Liver Qi is stagnant, the Liver Yang rises up, leading to Liver fire (red eyes). Liver Fire insults and consumes the Lung Yin, gradually resulting in a Lung Yin Deficiency. The dry nose and dry hair reflect the Lung Yin Deficiency.

The skin lesions are found mostly in Liver territories (sides of flank areas), indicating a disharmony between the Lung and Liver. When the Lung Yin is deficient and fails to nourish the body surface, the skin lacks nourishment and shrinks which leads to depigmentation (silver color), thickness, and hair loss.

TCVM Diagnosis

Liver Qi Stagnation, Disharmony between Lung and Liver, and Lung Yin Deficiency

Treatment

The treatment strategies include soothing the Liver Qi, moving Blood, and nourishing Yin. In addition to acupuncture, two herbal formulas are recommended. Three teaspoons each of *Mu Dan Pi San* and Damp Heat Skin Powder should be given by mouth twice daily for two months.

Dry Needle Acupuncture: BL-13, BL-18, LU-5, KID-3 and SP-10

Aquapuncture: BL-17 and LIV-3
(0.5 cc of vitamin B_{12})

BL-13 and LU-5 open the Lung and nourish the Lung Yin. LIV-3 and BL-18 soothe the Liver Qi. KID-3, SP-10 and BL-17 nourish Yin and Blood. The herbal formula *Mu Dan Pi San* is designed to soothe Liver Qi, to move blood and resolve Stagnation, and to harmonize the Liver and Lung. The Damp-Heat Skin Formula is designed to clear Heat and to open the body surface. *Mu Dan Pi San* is the modified *Chai Hu Shu Gan Wan*. Damp-Heat Skin Formula is the classical formula *Bi Xie Sheng Shi Tang* modification.

Recommendations

- Supplement Galahad's food with one teaspoon each of Flax oil and Barley Green
- Give Galahad 200 IU of Vitamin E, 80 mcg of Selenium, and 1000 g of Vitamin C
- Fast him one day per week.

Fasting is a special form of the TCVM purgation method. It allows the bowels to maximally evacuate the undesirable contents and leads to the greatest descending flow of Stomach Qi. When the Stomach Qi descends normally, it promotes better flow of Qi in the whole body.

AUGUST 8, 2000 (SECOND VISIT)

Examination

The skin lesion seems a little flatter. The color of lesion appears grayer. The body surface feels hot. The rest of his signs had not changed.

- Tongue Appearance: Purple
- Pulse Quality: Deep, thready

Treatment

The TCVM diagnosis is the same as at the previous visit. The herbal medication will remain the same as previously prescribed. In addition to some of the acupuncture points used previously, GV-14 and LI-11 are added to clear Heat because the body surface feels hot.

Dry Needle Acupuncture: BL-13, BL-18, LI-11, KID-3, LIV-3, GV-14

Aquapuncture: BL-17 and LIV-3
(0.5 cc of vitamin B_{12})

Recommendations

- Fast one day for every five days.
- Keep the food supplements the same.

SEPTEMBER 5, 2000 (THIRD VISIT)

Examination

The skin lesions are more flat (almost at the same level of the normal skin) but are much wider. Galahad prefers warmth and dislikes air-conditioning. He was barking during the exam, but was very quiet after needling.

- Tongue Appearance: Purple
- Pulse Quality: Thready

Treatment

The TCVM Diagnosis is Liver Qi Stagnation and Yin Deficiency. The herbal medication and dietary supplements were continued as previously prescribed. This acupuncture treatment consisted of dry needling at *Bai Hui*, GV-20, KID-3, BL-23, and BL-18

OCTOBER 3, 2000 (FOURTH VISIT)

Examination

Some small, lump-like, grey lesions were seen on dorsum. These areas appear raised on some days and flat on other days. In the past six months, he lost about six pounds.

Galahad refused to be needled. He became more irritable and aggressive, and he tried to snap at the veterinarian who performed the examination. He had red eyes.

- Tongue Appearance: Pale purple
- Pulse Quality: Fast and forceful

TCVM Analysis

An extended period of Liver Qi Stagnation can lead to Liver Yang Rising. This generates Liver Fire which is reflected in the red eyes, the fast, forceful pulse, and the irritable, aggressive attitude. The non-painful lumps on the skin indicate phlegm accumulation. Also, the onset of additional lumps and the pale tongue indicate a Qi Deficiency.

TCVM Diagnosis

Liver Yang Rising with Fire, Phlegm accumulation, and Qi Deficiency

Treatment

The treatment strategies are to soothe the Liver Qi, move Blood to resolve lumps, and tonify Qi to prevent Phlegm. There was no way to perform the acupuncture procedures at this visit. Three herbal medications were prescribed at this time, *Long Dan Xie Gan Tang* Pills, Wei Qi Booster (Modified *Si Jun Zi Tang*), and Max Formula (*Nei Xiao San*).

Long Dan Xie Gan Tang Pills:	Give six pills twice daily for six weeks
Wei Qi Booster	Give three teaspoons twice daily for six weeks
Max Formula:	Give three teaspoons twice daily for six weeks

Long Dan Xie Gan Tang is a classical herbal formula used to clear the Liver and drain Fire/Heat. Wei Qi Booster is designed to tonify Wei Qi and to prevent the accumulation of Phlegm (neoplastic masses). Max Formula is designed to move Blood for resolution of lumps and Stagnation.

NOVEMBER 7, 2000 (FIFTH VISIT)

Examination

The skin lesions are much more flat and less gray. Galahad is still irritable and aggressive in the exam room. His nose seems a little dry. His tongue is pale purple and his pulse is weaker on the left side.

Treatment

The TCVM diagnosis is Liver Yang Rising with Fire and Yin Deficiency. Since the lumps have become flat, the Max Formula is discontinued. The left-sided weak pulse and the dry nose indicate Yin Deficiency, which may be a secondary result of the Liver Fire. Thus, *Liu Wei Di Huang Wan* is also added to nourish Yin.

Long Dan Xie Gan Wan:	Give six pills twice daily for six weeks
Wei Qi Booster:	Give three teaspoons twice daily for six weeks
Liu Wei Di Huang Wan:	Give six pills twice daily for six weeks

DECEMBER 12, 2000 (SIXTH VISIT)

Galahad has been doing well physically and during competitive events. According to the owner, the thick skin lumps returned after discontinuing Max's Formula.

Examination

The skin lumps still look grayish and feel elevated. Galahad is still aggressive and nasty towards the examiner.

- Tongue Appearance: Red-purple
- Pulse Quality: Wiry and fast

Treatment

The Liver Qi is still deeply stagnant. The Fire generated from Stagnation boils the body fluid and produces phlegm. The TCVM diagnosis is Liver Qi Stagnation, Liver Fire, and Phlegm Accumulation. A combination of *Long Dan Xie Gan Tang* and *Xiao Yao San* may be used to soothe Liver Qi and clear Liver Fire simultaneously. Give six pills of *Long Dan Xie Gan Tang* and *Xiao Yao San* twice daily for six weeks. Also give three teaspoons of Max Formula twice daily for six weeks

JULY 3, 2001 (SEVENTH VISIT)

Examination

The skin lesions are almost completely healed and the hair has regrown. Galahad looks much calmer. He still growls, but he stays still during the examination. His nose is a little dry and there is dry, thick, yellow discharge from his eyes.

- Tongue Appearance: Red
- Pulse Quality: Soft and thready at the Liver position

Treatment

The TCVM diagnosis is Liver Yin Deficiency. Chronic Liver Fire leads to Liver Yin Deficiency which causes a dry nose, dry and thick ocular discharge, a red tongue and a soft, thready pulse.

The herbal medications are changed to *Yi Guan Jian* and *Xiao Yao San*. Use one tablespoon of *Yi Guan Jian* twice daily for two months, and then give six pills *Xiao Yao San* daily for four months. The condition is under control. Only use a low dosage of the Liver Yin Tonic, *Yi Guan Jian,* for two months. His Liver Yin should be balanced by this time, so follow up by using *Xiao Yao San* to maintain the normal flow of Liver Qi.

FEBRUARY 25, 2002 (TELEPHONE FOLLOW-UP)

Galahad is still doing well. The skin lesions are completely healed. He won the state dog field trials championship.

Case Five: Lady Bird the Greyhound

INTRODUCTION

Lady Bird is a thirteen year old spayed female Greyhound. She presented to the emergency service the evening of April 3, 2001 because she had a great deal of pain, vomiting, and mild to moderate bloating. She was diagnosed with gastric dilation and volvulus. An incisional gastropexy was performed the next day.

On April 27, the neurology service reported a left-sided Horner's syndrome due to otitis media/interna of both ears. In addition, there was left-sided trigeminal nerve dysfunction causing temporalis and masseter muscle atrophy as well as ankylosing spondylosis (involving the entire T-L spine) causing hind limb weakness.

JUNE 12, 2001 (INITIAL VISIT)

According to the owner, Lady Bird began to show hind limb weakness and stiffness several months ago. The stiffness and weakness has become worse recently. There has been no change in her appetite, urine or stool. Recently she shows a preference for lying on the carpet and warm-seeking behavior. Lady Bird is a nice, laid-back dog who has been with her owner for the past year and a half.

Examination

Lady Bird is slightly lethargic. Her confirmation and hair coat appear normal. Her nose is of normal moisture to slightly wet. Her right metatarsal joint is moderately dropped compared to left. Lady Bird's extremities, nose, and lumbosacral area feel cold.

- Point Sensitivities: BL-20, BL-21, BL-23 and thoracolumbar area
- Tongue Appearance: Pale purple
- Pulse Quality: Deep and weaker on the right side
- Shen: Good
- Personality Type: Earth

TCVM Analysis

Lady Bird is a thirteen year old dog. With age, Lady Bird's Kidney Jing has begun to decrease. The Kidney Jing comprises both Yin and Yang. Her moisture status (Yin) seems normal. However, the pale purple tongue, the weak right-sided pulse and the coldness of the extremities and lumbosacral area indicate a Yang Deficiency. The lumbosacral area (lower back) is the house of Kidney. The Kidney rules the knees and rear limbs. Thus, a Kidney Yang Deficiency leads to weakness and stiffness of the rear limbs and to warm-seeking behavior.

Spleen Qi requires Kidney Yang for support; thus, deficient Kidney Yang may lead to Spleen Qi Deficiency. This results in muscle atrophy and lethargy. The spondylosis can be considered Blood Stagnation which causes thoracolumbar sensitivity upon palpation.

TCVM Diagnosis

Kidney Yang Deficiency and Blood Stagnation of the spine

Treatment

The treatment strategies are to warm the Kidney and tonify Kidney Yang, to move Qi for pain relief, and to move Blood to resolve the Stagnation. In addition to the acupuncture treatment, the herbal medicines *Xiao Huo Luo Dan* and Loranthus Powder (Modified *Ba Ji San*) are prescribed. Six pills or capsules of each of these should be given twice daily for one month.

Dry Needle Acupuncture:	KI-7
Electroacupuncture: (20 Hz for twenty minutes)	BL-23, *Shen Shu*, BL-11, BL-40. GV-3 with *Bai Hui*
Aquapuncture: (dilute vitamin B_{12})	1 ml at BL-40 0.5 cc at *Hua Tuo Jia Ji* points T_{11-12}, T_{12-13} and T_{13}-L_1

KID-7, *Shen Shu*, BL-23 are used to tonify the Kidney. GV-3 and *Bai Hui* are used to warm the Kidney Yang. BL-11 strengthens the bones. BL-40 moves Qi to resolve pain. *Hua Tuo Jia Ji* moves Qi and Blood to resolve Stagnation. *Xiao Huo Luo Dan* is a classical herbal formula that warms the Channel to dispel Cold and moves Qi and Blood to resolve Stagnation. Loranthus Powder is designed to tonify Kidney Yang and to move Qi to stop the pain.

Home Care Recommendations

- Allow Lady Bird 20 to 30 minutes of exercise (walking) twice daily.
- Massage along the spine twice daily.
- Change the diet to include ingredients such as lamb, chicken, black beans, kidney beans, carrots, broccoli and sweet potatoes. Avoid fish and other cooling meats.

JULY 3, 2001 (SECOND VISIT)

The owner reported that the hind limb weakness is much improved after the initial acupuncture treatment. She prefers to sleep on the cooler areas of the floor.

Examination

Lady Bird's extremities and *Bai Hui* areas feel almost normal (much warmer now than during the initial visit). There are no strong sensitive points found along the Bladder Channel shu points upon palpation.

- Shen: Great
- Tongue Appearance: Purple
- Pulse Quality: OK

Treatment

Lady Bird's Kidney Yang has increased greatly in response to herbal and dietary management. Her current TCVM diagnosis is Blood Stagnation of the spine. The herbal medication should be continued as previously prescribed.

Dry Needle Acupuncture:	LIV-3 (right) and KID-3 (right)
Electroacupuncture: (20 Hz for twenty minutes)	BL-20, BL-23, *Shen Shu*, BL-54, *Bai Hui* with GB-34 (left), ST-41 (left) with ST-36
Aquapuncture: (0.5 cc vitamin B$_{12}$)	BL-40, ST-36, ST-41 and LIV-3

LIV-3 moves Qi to relieve pain. KID-3 nourishes Yin and provides balance when tonifying Yang (herbal prescription). BL-20 is used to tonify the Spleen, and it is a local point for spondylosis. ST-36, ST-41, BL-54 and GB-34 are for general rear limb weakness.

AUGUST 6, 2001 (THIRD VISIT)

Lady Bird's hind limb weakness has completely resolved. There are no other health complaints except allergic signs including intermittent nasal discharge and red eyes for the past 1.5 years.

Examination

Her eyes are slightly red. Mild scratches are noted on the ear. There is a slightly clear nasal discharge.

- Tongue: Pink
- Pulse: Normal
- Shen: Great

TCVM Analysis

Skin allergy is often considered a Wind-Toxin or Wind-Heat problem. The Wind-Heat pathogen residing in the body surface leads to itchy ears, nasal discharge and red eyes.

TCVM Diagnosis

Wind-Toxin (Wind-Heat)

Treatment

Two herbal medications, Kidney Qi/Yin formula (*Shen Qi Yin Xu Fang*) and External Wind (*Wai Feng San*), are prescribed in addition to the acupuncture treatments. Lady Bird should receive three capsules of Kidney Qi/Yin formula twice daily for one month followed by two capsules twice daily for the second month, and then one capsule twice daily for the third month. She should also receive six capsules of External Wind twice daily for two months.

Electroacupuncture: (20 Hz for twenty minutes)	BL-23, *Shen Shu*, ST-36 with GB-34, BL-54
Aquapuncture: (0.5 cc vitamin B$_{12}$)	SP-10, ST-40, ST-36, KID-1, BL-20, SI-19, LI-10 and LI-11

BL-23, *Shen Shu*, KID-1 are used to maintain the normal Kidney physiological activities. ST-36, GB-34, BL-54 and BL-40 are general points for strengthening the rear limbs. The point SP-10 helps move Blood and clear Wind. BL-20 strengthens the Spleen to maintain the Earth Element. SI-19 is a local point for the ear itching. LI-10 and LI-11 are used to clear Wind-Heat. Kidney Qi/Yin Formula is designed as a general Kidney Qi/Yin tonic that strengthens the rear limbs. The formula External Wind can clear Wind-Heat and detoxify.

DECEMBER 21, 2001 (TELEPHONE FOLLOW-UP)

Lady Bird is still doing well. She walks and runs 30 minutes twice a day without problems. There are no abnormal findings of her nose, eyes, and ears.

Case Six: Roxa the Great Dane

INTRODUCTION

Roxa is a twelve year old Great Dane. She has had a history of weight loss, poor appetite, decreased thirst and lethargy (exercise intolerance) for several months. The owner did not report any vomiting, skin itching, lameness, or diarrhea. She has, however, had some hair loss over the past two months.

AUGUST 3, 1999 (INITIAL VISIT)

Examination

Overall, Roxa appears depressed and emaciated. She weighs only 80 pounds. She is anorexic and lethargic. Roxa's hair falls out very easily when brushed.

She is a laid back dog. She will bark in one tone to let the owner know when someone visits the house, and she will use a different tone to bark at another dog. She is friendly and has never bitten anyone.

- Point Sensitivities: BL-19, BL-21 and BL-23
- Shen: Low
- Tongue Appearance: Pale
- Pulse Quality: Deep and weak
- Personality Type: Earth

TCVM Analysis

The Earth type dogs tend to develop Spleen Qi Deficiency. Weight loss, lethargy, decreased thirst, poor appetite, pale tongue and a weak pulse are typical signs of Spleen Qi Deficiency. Due to this Deficiency, the Spleen Qi fails to hold the hair, thus contributing to hair loss.

TCVM Diagnosis

Spleen Qi Deficiency

Treatment

The treatment strategy is to strengthen the Spleen and to tonify Qi. Dry needle acupuncture and electroacupuncture will be used in addition to herbal therapy. Eight pills of *Si Jun Zi Tang* should be given by mouth twice daily for three to six months. *Si Jun Zi Tang* is a classical herbal formula to tonify Spleen Qi. It may be safely used on a long-term basis for Spleen Qi Deficiency.

Dry Needle Acupuncture: *Shan Gen*
(Twenty minutes)

Electroacupuncture: BL-20, BL-21, ST-36, LI-10
(20 Hz for twenty minutes)

Shan Gen is a transpositional point from cattle to stimulate appetite and thirst. BL-20 is the Spleen association point is to tonify Qi and to strengthen the Spleen. BL-21, the Stomach association point, is used to regulate Stomach Qi and to strengthen the Spleen. The point ST-36, which is called "rear three miles", is a Qi general tonic point. LI-10, known as "front three miles", may be used as a substitute for ST-36. LI-10 and ST-36 can be also used together to reinforce Qi tonic effect.

FEBRUARY 1, 2000 (SECOND VISIT)

The dog had shown great improvement within four to five weeks following the initial acupuncture treatment. According to the owner, she has had a good appetite and thirst, more energy, an increase in muscle tone.

About three days ago her appetite decreased again. She has developed watery and brown diarrhea (especially in the early morning). Three or four days ago, she vomited once a small amount of yellow, mucoid fluid. She has been slightly more lethargic in the morning and has been weak in the hind end. There were no signs of itching, coughing, sneezing or lameness noted.

Examination

She weighed 92 pounds, having gained 12 pounds since the last visit. Her hair coat had improved greatly. Palpation revealed sensitivity at BL-23 and coldness of *Bai Hui*.

- Shen: Normal
- Tongue Appearance: Pale and purple
- Pulse Quality: Weak on the right side

TCVM Analysis

The Spleen is the post-natal root while the Kidney is the pre-natal root. The poor appetite and watery diarrhea indicate a Spleen Qi Deficiency. Chronic or recurrent Spleen Qi Deficiency can lead to Kidney Yang Deficiency. In addition, Roxa is twelve years old and with age her Kidney Yang will gradually decrease. Weakness of the hind end and coldness at *Bai Hui* indicate Kidney Deficiency. In addition, the pale purple tongue and the deep, weak pulse also indicate Qi and Yang Deficiency.

Stomach and Spleen dominate the time frame in the morning (7 to 11 am), thus signs of a Spleen Qi Deficiency (diarrhea and lethargy) are worse in the morning. According to the Eight Diagrams (*ba-gua*) and Yin-Yang theory, the early morning is the first rising of Yang. Yang is very fragile during this time. When Kidney Yang is deficient, the diarrhea is worse in the early morning.

TCVM Diagnosis

Spleen Qi and Kidney Yang Deficiency

Treatment

The treatment strategy is to tonify Spleen Qi and to warm Kidney Yang. In addition to twenty minutes of electroacupuncture (20 Hz) and aquapuncture, five grams of the herbal medicine *Si Shen Wan* (Four Immortals) is recommended twice daily for one month.

Electroacupuncture: GV-4 with *Bai Hui*, BL-20, BL-21, *Shen Shu*, ST-36 with GB-34

Aquapuncture: BL-21, BL-23 and GV-1, GV-3

GV-3, GV-4, *Bai Hui*, BL-23, and *Shen Shu* are used to warm the Yang and to tonify the Kidney. GV-1 is a special point used to stop diarrhea. GB-34 is an Earth point and can regulate the Stomach and Spleen to stop diarrhea and vomiting. *Si Shen Wan* is a classical formula for diarrhea due to Spleen Qi and Kidney Yang Deficiency.

MAY 15, 2001 (THIRD VISIT)

The owner reports that Roxa had reduced diarrhea and a better appetite the day after the second acupuncture treatment. Her gastrointestinal complaints (poor appetite and loose stool) were completely resolved by the end of February. She had gained fourteen pounds since February 1, 2000 (now she weighs 116 lb) and has had a good appetite and normal stool.

About two months ago she had one or two episodes of falling down during which times she had an irregular pulse and appeared unaware of her surroundings, but did not totally lose consciousness. Last month, she had about four episodes of falling down. This month, only two episodes were noted during which she had urinary incontinence. Her stool is normal, but sometimes she can not hold her bowels long enough to defecate outdoors.

Examination

When she stands, she loves to lean on somebody to help support her rear limbs. She is lethargic and has bilateral hind leg muscle atrophy, hind limb weakness, and severe gingivitis. Sensitivity was found at BL-13, BL-20 and BL-23 upon palpation.

- Shen: Normal

- Skin: Scaly and malodorous

- Tongue Appearance: Pale

- Pulse Quality: Deep and feeble

TCVM Analysis

Muscle atrophy and lethargy still indicate Spleen Qi Deficiency. Chronic Spleen Qi Deficiency can lead to Heart Qi Deficiency (a child's illness affects the mother). Deficient Heart Qi fails to host the Shen/Mind, leading to disconnection between the physical body and spiritual Mind. As a consequence, falling down and disorientation (unawareness of the surroundings) occurs. Weakness of rear limbs, urinary incontinence and fecal incontinence indicate a Kidney Qi Deficiency. Kidney Qi Deficiency can be caused by chronic illness and old age.

TCVM Diagnosis

Spleen-Heart-Kidney Qi Deficiency

Treatment

The treatment strategy is to tonify the Qi of the Spleen, Heart and Kidney. The herbal medications *Bu Yang Huan Wu* Powder and *Si Ni Tang* are prescribed in addition to the dry needle acupuncture (20 minutes) and aquapuncture (0.5cc Vitamin B_{12} per point). Five grams *Bu Yang Huan Wu* Powder should be given twice daily for three to six months and two grams of *Si Ni Tang* should be given twice daily for only one month.

Dry Needle Acupuncture: HT-7, BL-15, BL-20, GV-4, *Bai Hui*, KID-7, KID-10

Aquapuncture: CV-17, CV-4, CV-6, BL-21, ST-36

HT-7 and BL-15 tonify Heart Qi. BL-20 and BL-21 tonify Spleen Qi. GV-4, *Bai Hui*, KID-10, KID-7 tonify Kidney Qi. ST-36, CV-17, CV-4 and CV-6 are general tonic for Qi of the whole body. *Bu Yang Huan Wu Tang* is a classical herbal formula used to tonify Spleen and Kidney Qi Deficiency. *Si Ni Tang* is a classical formula used to tonify Heart and Kidney Qi. Since this formula is potent and very hot, it should not be over-dosed or used for a long time.

Recommendations

- If the episodes of collapse and disorientation persist or worsen over the next month, she should be examined by the neurological service.

JUNE 12, 2001 (FOURTH VISIT)

Roxa has been more alert and energetic. Her appetite and thirst are fine. She had only one episode of falling down during past month. Her hindquarters appear stronger. However, her urinary and large intestine incontinence have not improved significantly.

Examination

- Shen: Normal
- Tongue Appearance: Pale pink
- Pulse Quality: Weak on the right side

TCVM Diagnosis

Kidney Qi Deficiency

Treatment

The treatment strategy is to tonify Qi and to warm Yang. Electroacupuncture (80-120 Hz for 20 minutes), aquapuncture (0.5 cc Vitamin B_{12}), moxibustion, and herbal therapy are used. Moxibustion should be performed for ten minutes each day for thirty days. Five grams each of the herbal formulas *Suo Quan Wan* and *Bu Yang Huan Wu Tang* are recommended twice daily for three months.

Electroacupuncture:	*Shen Shu*, BL-23, BL-39 with ST-36, GV-1 with *Bai Hui*, *Er Yan*
Aquapuncture:	BL-39, CV-4, CV-6
Moxibustion:	CV-8, *Bai Hui*

Shen Shu and BL-23 are used to tonify Kidney Qi. BL-39, the lower He-sea point for Triple Heater, holds the Bladder to resolve urinary incontinence. GV-1, *Bai Hui* and *Er Yan* tonify the Kidney to resolve incontinence of bladder and large intestines. CV-4, CV-6 and ST-36 are used as general tonics. *Suo Quan Wan* warms the Kidney to resolve incontinence.

JULY 10, 2001 (FIFTH VISIT)

Roxa eats, drinks and walks normally. Her urinary and fecal incontinence are almost resolved (only one occurrence in the past month).

- Shen: Normal

- Tongue Appearance: Pale pink

- Pulse Quality: Normal

Treatment

The TCVM diagnosis is Kidney Qi Deficiency. The treatment strategy is to tonify Qi and to warm Yang. The acupuncture and herbal treatments remain the same.

DECEMBER 18, 2001 (TELEPHONE FOLLOW-UP)

Roxa seems to be doing well. No accidental urination or defecation has occurred since the previous acupuncture treatments.

Case Seven: Doc the Labrador Retriever

INTRODUCTION

Doc is a nine year old male Labrador Retriever. On May 24, 2000 he presented to the neurology service with a history of intermittent pain and hind limb weakness of several years duration. The owner indicated that he falls down a lot when walking. He was able to get up without assistance. He was diagnosed with multifocal type II intervertebral disc disease (IVDD) with spondylosis at C7-T1, T13-L1, L1-L2, L2-L3, and L7-S1. At this time, he was referred for acupuncture because the option of surgery was considered to be the last resort.

MAY 1, 2000 (INITIAL VISIT)

Doc presented for his first acupuncture treatment for severe hind limb weakness. He fell down several times between the front desk and the exam room and was having a very hard time walking without assistance. He sought a cool place to rest and he was very sensitive along the entire spine upon palpation.

- Tongue Appearance: Purple

- Pulse Quality: Fast and thready

- Shen: Normal

- Constitution: Fire

TCVM Analysis

Doc is considered a Fire-type dog because of personality. He is a handsome dog who loves to be petted. He greets strangers warmly, wags his tail and tries to kiss everybody. He has never attacked any human beings or animals. He is an easily excitable dog who is difficult to keep quiet and still. As a very sensitive dog, he "talks" a lot during the acupuncture treatment.

A Fire-type of animal tends to have Excess Heat/Fire, which can easily consume body fluids and gradually lead to Yin Deficiency. When a Yin Deficient body is invaded by Wind-Cold-Damp, multiple IVDD lesions may occur. The signs of pain, weakness and stiffness of the body and limbs are considered Bi Syndrome. Bi Syndrome may be divided into five categories: Wind Bi, Cold Bi, Damp Bi, Heat Bi and Bony Bi. Bony Bi can be subgrouped into Yin Deficiency and Yang Deficiency. In this case, Doc has a typical Bony Bi due to Yin Deficiency, which is evidenced by the fast, thready pulse and the cool-seeking behavior. The pathogen Wind-Cold-Damp obstructs the Qi flow along the back. Where Qi does not flow freely, there must be pain. The sensitive back and the purple tongue are signs of the obstructed Qi.

TCVM Diagnosis

Bony Bi due to Yin Deficiency

Treatment

The treatment strategy is to Clear Wind-Damp, move Qi to relieve pain, nourish Yin and tonify Kidney. The treatment consisted of dry needle acupuncture, electroacupuncture for twenty minutes at 20 Hz, and aquapuncture using 0.5 cc vitamin B_{12} per point. In addition, the herbal formulas *Di Gu Pi* Powder (2 teaspoons) and *Sheng Tong Zhu Yu Tang* (6 pills) are prescribed for use twice daily for one month.

Dry Needle Acupuncture:	GV-20 and Bai-Hui
Electroacupuncture:	BL-23, KID-3 with BL-40, BL-21, *Shen Shu*, GB-21, *Wei Gen* with GV-14
Aquapuncture:	*Hua Tuo Jia Ji* points at C7-T1, T13-L1, L1-L2, L7-S1; LIV-3

GV-20 and *Bai Hui* calm the Shen and relax the animal. KID-3 and BL-23 tonify the Kidney and nourish Yin. *Bai Hui*, GB-21, BL-21, GV-14, and *Wei Gen* are local points used to move Qi for pain relief of IVDD conditions. BL-40 is used to open the back and to relieve pain of the back. *Hua Tuo Jia Ji* points are used to move Qi and to relieve the pain of IVDD. LIV-3 moves Qi and stops pain. *Di Gu Pi Powder* is designed for use in the Bony Bi syndrome due to Yin Deficiency. *Sheng Tong Zhu Yu Tang* is a classical formula used to move Blood and to resolve Stagnation for pain relief.

Recommendations

- Avoid hot and spicy foods such as lamb or deer meat, ginger, and garlic.
- Cool diet consisting of such foods as fish and tofu is encouraged.
- Massage his back for ten minutes once a day.

JUNE 12, 2000 (SECOND VISIT)

Doc has not been falling down since the initial acupuncture treatment. He can walk and even trot. He appears very happy. The owner is very pleased with the results.

A "hot spot" was noticed by the owner yesterday. A large area (about 8 cm x 10 cm) of moist dermatitis was found around the sacrum and the base of the tail. The lesion is red and bloody with hair loss. He is much less sensitive to palpation of his back.

- Shen: Very good
- Tongue Appearance: Red
- Pulse Quality: Thready and fast

TCVM Analysis

His Bony Bi syndrome due to Yin Deficiency is almost under control. When the body has Yin Deficiency, the cooling system is too weak to balance any random Heat factors. Thus, the pathogen Heat Toxin invades the body surface, leading to the acute onset of the "hot spot".

TCVM Diagnosis

Heat Toxin with Bony Bi syndrome due to Yin Deficiency

Treatment

The treatment strategies are to cool Blood and clear Heat, to nourish Yin, and to move Blood to resolve blockage. The treatment consisted of electroacupuncture for twenty minutes at 20 Hz, hemoacupuncture and aquapuncture using 0.5 cc vitamin B_{12} per point. The herbal treatment shall remain the same.

Electroacupuncture: GV-14 with Wei-Gen, BL-23, *Shen Shu*, KID-3 with BL-40, BL-11

Hemoacupuncture: *Wei Jian* and *Er Jian*

Aquapuncture: Injections located around the "hot spot" using the "circling-the-dragon" technique

Hemoacupuncture at *Wei Jian* and *Er Jian* is a fast and effective way to clear Heat and cool the blood. The circling-the-dragon aquapuncture technique can promote Blood flow and relieve toxins.

Recommendations

- Encourage exercise consisting of 20 to 30 minute walks twice daily.
- Massage the lower back, ten minutes once a day for one month.

JULY 10, 2000 (THIRD VISIT)

According to the owner, Doc is completely normal now. Doc walks and/or runs about thirty minutes twice a day. His "hot spot" disappeared completely three days after the second acupuncture treatment.

- Shen: Very good

- Tongue Appearance: Pink

- Pulse Quality: Normal

TCVM Diagnosis

Health check and Tune up for Fire Animal

Treatment

The treatment strategies are to nourish Yin, strengthen Heart and clear Heat. The treatment consisted of dry needle acupuncture and aquapuncture using 0.5 cc vitamin B_{12} per point. Two herbal formulas are prescribed. *Liu Wei Di Huang Wan* should be given in the evening for two months and *Sheng Tong Zhu Yu Tang* should be given in the morning for two months.

Dry Needle Acupuncture: HT-7, *An Shen*, BL-15, LI-11, KID-3

Aquapuncture: PC-8, KID-1 and LIV-3

HT-7, *An Shen*, BL-15 and PC-8 are used to strengthen the Heart and to calm the Shen (the Mind). LIV-3, KID-1, KID-3 and LI-11 nourish Yin and clear Heat. *Liu Wei Di Huang Wan* is the classical herbal formula used to nourish Yin.

JULY 10, 2001 (FOURTH VISIT)

Doc has been doing very well for past year. He has no medical complaints. He eats, drinks, walks and runs normally.

- Shen: Good

- Tongue Appearance: Pink

- Pulse Quality: Normal

Treatment

The plan for this visit is to perform an annual health check and tune-up. The strategies include strengthening the Kidney to prevent IVDD and nourishing the Yin to prevent Heat. The treatment consisted of electroacupuncture for twenty minutes at 20 Hz and aquapuncture using 0.5 cc vitamin B_{12} per point. No herbal therapy shall be prescribed. Another recheck and tune-up acupuncture treatment is recommended in one year.

Electroacupuncture: BL-23, *Shen Shu*, GV-14 with LI-11 (right), BL-11

Aquapuncture: BL-15 and HT-7

JULY 2, 2002 (FIFTH VISIT)

According to the owner, Doc has been doing very well. He eats, drinks, walks/runs about thirty minutes twice a day.

- Shen: Good

- Tongue Appearance: Pink

- Pulse Quality: Normal

Treatment

This visit is another annual health check and tune-up program. The strategies and treatments are similar to the previous visit (July 10, 2001).

Case Eight: Red the Quarter Horse Thoroughbred Mix

INTRODUCTION

Red is a seventeen year old gelding with a history of navicular disease of the left front limb. His condition was diagnosed with radiographs and nerve blocks in March 2000.

Red is a friendly, sensitive and smart horse. He loves to be petted and touched but he becomes irritable and restless as soon as he realizes that you will needle him. He is sensitive to acupuncture needling as well as the regular injections. He was submissive to the one other household gelding that shared the pasture until that old gelding died at twenty years of age. In other words, the old gelding was always his boss. One year later, a little pony was placed in the same pasture and Red started to boss him around. He kicked and controlled the little pony. When the little pony left, a mare of his same age shared the pasture, and he started to boss her around as well.

Red's owner has owned him since he was born and is very fond of him. She often gives him treats. She rides him for pleasure about once or twice a week. He loves to run and play, but he will let the mare in the same pasture go first if there is something that is unfamiliar (such as deer).

APRIL 12, 2000

Examination

Red presents with a grade 3 of 5 left front limb lameness. Red shows sensitivity to palpation at LI-18, LI-15, LI-16, BL-18, BL-19, PC-1, and BL-13. His personality type is Fire with Water.

- Tongue Appearance: Purple
- Pulse Quality: Fast

	LI-18	LI-16 LI-15	BL-13 PC-1	BL-18 to BL-21	Lu Gu BL-54	Hock / Stifle points
Left side	+++++	+++	+++	++	-	-
Right side	++	++	++	++	++	-

TCVM Analysis

The purple tongue, the fast pulse and the lameness indicate pain due to Qi Stagnation. Sensitivity at LI-18, LI-16, LI-15, BL-13 and PC-1 indicates front foot soreness. This is Qi Stagnation localized in the left front foot. Mild soreness of the right front foot and the coxofemoral areas (sensitivity at BL-54 and Lu Gu) may be secondary to the left front foot problem. Sensitivity at BL-18 to BL-21 may indicate local back pain.

TCVM Diagnosis

Qi and Blood Stagnation of the front foot (front foot lameness).

Treatment

The treatment principles include moving Qi to relieve pain and moving Blood to resolve Stagnation. The treatment includes dry needle acupuncture, electroacupuncture for twenty minutes at 20 Hz, aquapuncture and hemoacupuncture.

Dry Needle Acupuncture: BL-18, BL-19

Electroacupuncture: PC-9, *Qian Ti Men* (medial + lateral) of the same foot, *Shen Shu*, SI-3 (left) with LI-1

Hemoacupuncture: TH-1, SI-1

Aquapuncture: PC-9, SI-9

PC-9, *Qian Ti Men*, LI-1, TH-1 and SI-1 are the local points which move Qi to relieve pain. *Shen Shu* strengthens the Kidney and bones including the navicular bone. BL-18 and BL-19 regulate the Liver and Gallbladder and strengthen the hooves.

Recommendation

- Allow Red to rest.
- Turn him out in the pasture.

MAY 24, 2000 (SECOND VISIT)

The owner reported that Red walks more comfortably. However, after the initial acupuncture treatment, the owner did not notice any improvement when Red runs in the pasture. He is still lame.

Examination

Upon palpation, Red is sensitive at LI-18 / LI-15. There are no trigger points on the back or rear end.

- Lameness: Grade 2 of 5
- Tongue Appearance: Purple
- Pulse Quality: Normal

	LI-18	LI-16 LI-15	BL-13 PC-1	BL-18 to BL-21	*Lu Gu* BL-54	Hock / Stifle points
Left side	+++++	++	++	-	-	-
Right side	+	+	-	-	-	-

TCVM Analysis

Even though clinical signs (lameness) do NOT change significantly after initial treatment, the reduced sensitivity of the acupuncture points indicate that Qi flow is better.

TCVM Diagnosis

Qi Stagnation

Treatment

The strategy is to move Qi for pain relief. The treatment includes electroacupuncture for twenty minutes at 20 Hz and aquapuncture. In addition, the herbal medicine *Si Sheng Gao* (Four Herbs Salve) should be applied topically around the coronary band of left front foot and wrapped normally. Leave this on for twelve hours, off for twelve hours, and change every day. Use this for only 21 days.

Electroacupuncture: PC-9 (left) with SI-3, LU-11 (left) with *Qi Ti Men*,
                                HT-9 (left) with *Qi Ti Men*

Aquapuncture: TH-15, GB-21, SI-9, LI-15

PC-9, HT-9, LU-11 are all local points for foot pain. TH-15, GB-21, SI-9 and LI-15 can promote Qi flow in the front limb and help resolve Qi Stagnation in the foot. *Si Sheng Gao* is based on the *Xiao Huo Luo Dan* formula, which can move Qi to relieve pain and move Blood to resolve Stagnation.

JULY 19, 2000 (THIRD VISIT)

Red has significantly improved after the second acupuncture and herbal treatment.

Examination

He is only slightly lame. He tried to avoid needling. Red did not like a twitch on his nose, but he behaved well with an ear twitch.

- Lameness: Grade 0.5 of 5
- Tongue Appearance: Slightly purple
- Pulse Quality: Normal

	LI-18	LI-16 LI-15	BL-13 PC-1	BL-18 to BL-21	*Lu Gu* BL-54	Hock / Stifle points
Left side	++	+	+	-	+	-
Right cido					+	

TCVM Diagnosis

Qi Stagnation is almost resolved

Treatment

The treatment strategy is to move Qi, to tonify the Kidney and to strengthen bones. The treatment includes dry needle acupuncture, electroacupuncture for twenty minutes at 20 Hz, aquapuncture and hemoacupuncture. In addition, fifteen grams of the herbal medication Hot Hoof 2 should be used twice daily for thirty days.

Dry Needle Acupuncture: TH-1, LU-11 (left), LI-1

Electroacupuncture: *Shen Shu*, BL-54, PC-9 (left) with *Qian Ti Men*

Aquapuncture: SI-9, BL-11

BL-54 is a local point to relieve the secondarily Qi blockage of the coxofemoral areas. SI-9 is a strong point for promoting Qi flow in the front limb. BL-11 strengthens bones. Hot Hoof 2 is an herbal medication based on the classical equine herbal formula *Yin Chen San*, which is designed to clear Liver Heat, to move Qi for pain relief and to move Blood for resolution of Stagnation in the feet.

Recommendation

- Gradually start to work and then ride Red.

NOVEMBER 2, 2000 (FOURTH VISIT)

The owner reported that Red became completely sound about one week after the third acupuncture treatment. He has been ridden two to three times a week for about 60 minutes each time. About four days ago, he was slightly off on his left front limb when he was ridden and trotted, but he was fine when walking. He seems fine when he is running in the pasture.

Examination

- Tongue Appearance: Pale
- Pulse Quality: Deep and weak

	LI-18	LI-15	BL-13 PC-1	BL-18 to BL-21	*Lu Gu* BL-54	Hock / Stifle points
Left side	+++	++	-	-	-	-
Right side	-	-	-	-	-	-

TCVM Analysis

Aging and chronic recurrent bony conditions can gradually lead to Kidney Deficiency. The pale tongue and deep, weak pulse indicate a Kidney Qi Deficiency.

TCVM Diagnosis

Qi Stagnation of the left front limb with a Kidney Qi Deficiency

Treatment

The treatment strategies include moving Qi to relieve pain, tonifying Qi and strengthening bones. The treatment includes dry needle acupuncture, aquapuncture (5 cc of vitamin B_{12} per point) and *Tui-na* (stretching and manipulation) both front limbs. In addition, fifteen grams of the herbal medication Hot Hoof 2 should be used twice daily for the first month then fifteen grams of *Equine Du Huo* should be used twice daily for the second and third months.

Dry Needle Acupuncture: *Bai Hui*, *Shen Shu*, PC-9 (left), LI-1 (left), LU-11 (left), TH-1 (left), SI-9 (left), PC-9 (right), LU-11 (right)

Aquapuncture: *Bo Jian*, *Bo Zhong*, SI-9, BL-23, BL-11

BL 23, *Shen Shu* and *Bai Hui* can tonify Kidney Qi and strengthen bones. *Equine Du Huo* is based on the classical herbal formula *Du Huo Ji Sheng Tang*, which clears Wind-Cold-Damp and moves Qi and Blood to relieve joint pain.

JANUARY 26, 2001 (FIFTH VISIT)

Red seems to be doing great. When the owner rides him, she feels a slight unbalance in his left front limb, but there is no lameness when trotting or lunging him.

Examination

- Tongue Appearance: Pink
- Pulse Quality: Normal

	LI-18	LI-15	PC-1	BL-18 to BL-21	*Lu Gu* BL-54	Hock / Stifle points
Left side	++	++	+	-	-	-
Right side	-	-	-	-	-	-

TCVM Diagnosis

Qi Stagnation

Treatment

The treatment strategies are to move Qi and Blood and to strengthen the Kidney and bones. The treatment includes dry needle acupuncture and aquapuncture. In addition, fifteen grams of the herbal medication Hot Hoof 2 should be given once daily in the evening for sixty days and fifteen grams of *Sang Zhi San* should be given once daily in the morning for sixty days. The herbal formula *Sang Zhi San* is designed to clear Qi and Blood blockage of joints.

Dry Needle: *Bai Hui*, *Shen Shu*, TH 1, SI 9, *Bo Zhong*, *Bo Jian*, *Qian Ti Men*

Aquapuncture: BL-11, BL-23

MAY 2, 2001 (SIXTH VISIT)

Red had been sound until two weeks ago. He was ridden three times a week and was a pleasant to ride. He could trot and run without lameness. However, about two weeks ago, he began to show lameness of both front limbs.

Examination

Radiographs and nerve blocks confirmed navicular disease in both front feet.

- Lameness: Grade 2 of 5
- Tongue Appearance: Pale purple
- Pulse Quality: Deep and weak

	LI-18	LI-16, LI-15	BL-13, PC-1	BL-23 to Shen Shu	Lu Gu BL-54	Hock / Stifle points
Left side	++++	+++	++	+++	-	-
Right side	+++	++	++	++	-	-

TCVM Analysis

This may be caused by infrequent acupuncture and herbal treatment due to the owner's relocation. Aging and chronic illness leads to Kidney Qi Deficiency. Deficient Kidney fails to nourish and support bones and joints, leading to Bony Bi syndromes.

TCVM Diagnosis

Front leg lameness (worse on the left) and Bony Bi syndrome due to Kidney Qi Deficiency

Treatment

The treatment strategies include tonification of the Kidney Qi to strengthen bones and moving Qi and Blood to resolve Stagnation. The treatment includes dry needle acupuncture, electroacupuncture for twenty minutes at 20 Hz and aquapuncture (5 cc of diluted vitamin B$_{12}$). In addition, fifteen grams each of the herbal medication Equine *Du Huo* and *San Zhi San* should be used twice daily for one month.

Dry Needle Acupuncture:	LU-11, LI-1, SI-1, TH-1
Electroacupuncture:	*Shen Shu*, *Shen Peng*, *Shen Jiao*, BL-23, BL-11, *Qian Ti Men* (medial and lateral)
Aquapuncture:	*Bai Hui*, PC-9, SI-1, *Bo Jian*, *Bo Lan*

Recommendations

- Rest him for three weeks.
- Ride him ten to thirty minutes twice during the fourth week.

MAY 30, 2001 (SEVENTH VISIT)

Red was doing okay when the owner rode him Monday and today. He was a little stiff and slightly lame.

Examination

- Lameness: Grade 1 of 5
- Tongue Appearance: Pale pink
- Pulse Quality: Normal

	LI-18	LI-16, LI-15	BL-13, PC-1	BL-23, Shen Shu	*Lu Gu* BL-54	Hock / Stifle points
Left side	++	++	+	+	-	-
Right side	+	+	+	++	-	-

TCVM Diagnosis

Bony Bi syndrome due to Kidney Qi Deficiency

Treatment

The treatment strategies include tonification of Kidney Qi to strengthen bones and moving Qi and Blood to resolve Stagnation. The treatment includes dry needle acupuncture, electroacupuncture for twenty minutes at 20 Hz and aquapuncture (5 cc of diluted vitamin B$_{12}$). In addition, fifteen grams each of the herbal medication Hot Hoof 2 and *Ba Ji San* should be used twice daily for four months.

Dry Needle Acupuncture:	LU-11, LI-1, SI-1 and TH-1
Electroacupuncture:	*Shen Shu*, *Shen Peng*, *Shen Jiao*, BL-23, BL-11,
Aquapuncture:	*Bai Hui*, PC-9, SI-1, *Bo Jian*, *Bo Lan*

Comments

Bony Bi syndrome is too difficult to cure. In order to maintain his Kidney Qi, he has to be medicated alternately using a low dosage of Kidney Qi Tonic herbal formulas including *Ba Ji San*, *Sang Ji Sheng San* or *Du Huo Ji Sheng Tang* for the rest of his life.

MAY 22, 2002 (EIGHTH VISIT)

The owner reported that Red is still doing fine. He is ridden twice to three times a week. He is basically sound when he is ridden even though he walks and runs a little slower than he used to. He eats, drinks and defecates normally.

Examination

- Shen: Normal
- Tongue Appearance: Pale pink
- Pulse Quality: Normal

	LI-18	LI-16, LI-15	BL-13, PC-1	BL-23, Shen Shu	Lu Gu BL-54	Hock / Stifle points
Left side	+	+	-	-	-	-
Right side	-	-	-	-	-	-

Treatment

The plan for this visit is to perform an annual health check and tune-up. The strategies include strengthening the Kidney to prevent further bony change and moving Qi-Blood to prevent Stagnation. The treatment consisted of electroacupuncture for twenty minutes at 20 Hz and aquapuncture using 0.5 cc vitamin B_{12} per point.

Electroacupuncture: *Shen Shu*, PC-9, Qian Ti Men, TH-1, LI-4, BL-11

Aquapuncture: BL-23, SI-9, BL-21 and LI-10

No herbal therapy shall be prescribed. Another recheck and tune-up acupuncture treatment is recommended in one year.

Case Nine: Rosie the Quarter Horse

INTRODUCTION

Rosie is a Quarter Horse mare who has a history of a bad injury to her right hock in June 1997. Since that time, she has been never sound despite a variety of treatments including conventional drugs, chiropractic, massage, and acupuncture. In addition, Rosie has failed to conceive in the past two years.

Rosie has been with her current owner since 1996. The owner is a novice rider and Rosie is her first horse. Rosie is lame in both hocks, has hives occasionally and experiences female behavior problems when she is in heat. She is a nice, friendly horse. She enjoys relaxing, moves slowly and is mellow and eager to please; she tries very hard to please the rider (the owner).

SEPTEMBER 22, 2000 (INITIAL VISIT)

Rosie has bilateral hock lameness. She also shows behavior problems when she is in heat. Injections of her hock have not helped her lameness. She does not seem to be drinking as much water as the owner expects.

Examination

She has a grade 3 of 5 lameness of both rear limbs. Upon palpation of her hocks, she reacted by kicking (worse on the left side than right). Rosie appears overweight and has mild hives on her neck and trunk.

- Shen: Ok
- Tongue Appearance: Pale
- Pulse Quality: Deep and weak on the right side
- Personality: Earth

	LI-18, LI-16, LI-15	BL-13, PC-1	BL-14 to BL-21	BL-54, *Lu Gu*	Coxa Hock, BL-35	BL-39
Left side	-	-	-	-	++++	+++
Right side	-	-	-	-	++	+

TCVM Analysis

The lameness and the sensitivity at BL-35, BL-39 and coxa hock point indicate Blood Stagnation of the hock. Originally, injury of the right hock blocked Qi flow of the right hock and led to Blood Stagnation. The horse tried to compensate by using the left rear limb, thus resulting in greater sensitivity of the left hock.

Presentation with a pale tongue, deep and weak pulse, obesity, lack of thirst and infertility indicates Kidney and Spleen Qi Deficiency. When Wei Qi is deficient, the pathogen Wind-Heat can easily invade the body and Lung system, leading to hives. Hives are *Fei Feng Huang* or Lung Wind-Heat syndrome.

TCVM Diagnosis

Blood Stagnation of the hock, Kidney and Spleen Qi Deficiency, and Lung Wind-Heat

Treatment

The treatment plan includes moving Qi to relieve pain, moving Blood to resolve Stagnation, and tonifying Kidney to strengthen bones. This condition is a combination of Excess (Blood Stagnation and Lung Wind-Heat) and Deficiency (Kidney and Spleen Qi Deficiency). Since the lameness is the major concern and the most severe clinical sign, the Blood Stagnation should be the primary focus of treatment.

The treatment includes dry needle acupuncture, electroacupuncture for twenty minutes at 20 Hz and aquapuncture (5 cc of diluted vitamin B_{12}). In addition, fifteen grams of the herbal medication Body Sore should be used twice daily for two months. *Huo Xue Hua Yu Gao* (Relief Salve) should be topically applied and massaged into the hocks once daily for one month.

Dry Needle Acupuncture:	*Bai Hui*, BL-67
Electroacupuncture:	BL-23, *Shen Shu*, BL-54, *Yan Chi*, Coxa hock point, BL-39 with BL-60
Aquapuncture:	*An Shen*, BL-54, BL-39

Bai Hui, BL-23, Shen-shen, Yan-chi, and Coxa Hock point are to strengthen the back and rear limbs and to tonify the Kidney and bones. BL-39 and BL-60 are local points for hock soreness. BL-67 promotes Qi flow to relieve blockage of the Bladder Channel. Body Sore is based on the classical herbal formula *Sheng Tong Zhu Yu Tang*, which activates Blood to resolve Stagnation and moves Qi to relieve pain. Relief Salve is a topical herbal salve that is designed to resolve Blood Stagnation.

Recommendations

- Reduce sweet feed and supplement the food with one tablespoon flax seed daily.
- Rest for Rosie for week one.
- Ride her one time during week two. Ride her twice during week three, and then ride four times weekly until the recheck.

OCTOBER 30, 2000

According to the owner, Rosie's lameness is about 50% improved. She still has hind limb lameness, but the owner feels more comfortable riding her. She has been ridden for 30 minutes (walking and trotting) four times a week.

Examination

Her lameness is grade 2 of 5 for both rear limbs.

- Tongue Appearance: Pale purple
- Pulse Quality: Fast

	LI-18, LI-17, LI-15	BL-15 to BL-20	BL-23	Hip / Stifle	Hock point, BL-39
Left side	+++	-	-	-	++++
Right side	+	-	+++	-	++

TCVM Analysis

Sensitivity at LI-18, LI-17 and LI-15 indicate left front foot soreness, which is secondary to hock soreness.

TCVM Diagnosis

Blood Stagnation of the hock, Kidney and Spleen Qi Deficiency, and Lung Wind-Heat

Treatment

The treatment includes dry needle acupuncture, electroacupuncture for twenty minutes at 20 Hz and aquapuncture (5 cc of diluted vitamin B$_{12}$). In addition, fifteen grams each of the herbal medications Equine *Du Huo* and *Sang Zhi San* should be used twice daily for five weeks.

Dry Needle Acupuncture:	*Bai Hui*, BL-67, LI-1 (left), LU-11, PC-9
Electroacupuncture:	*Shen Shu*, *Shen Peng*, BL-54, BL-60 with BL-39, Coxa hock point
Aquapuncture:	BL-60, BL-39

LI-1, LU-11 and PC-9 are added for left front foot soreness. Equine *Du Huo* is based on the classical herbal formula *Du Huo Ji Sheng Tang*, which clears Wind-Cold-Damp and moves Qi and Blood to relieve joint pain. The herbal formula *Sang Zhi San* is designed to clear Qi and Blood blockage of joints.

Recommendations

- Rest her for at least one week, then progress to ten-minute rides once a week.
- Massage *Huo Xue Hua Yu Gao* (Relief Salve) for ten minutes once daily for a month.
- Walk her by hand for ten minutes twice a day.

DECEMBER 6, 2000 (THIRD VISIT)

The owner reported that Rosie is doing well despite a slight lameness. She has a good attitude and is pleasant to ride, but she resists when asked to go to the left lead.

Examination

- Lameness: Grade 1 of 5
- Tongue Appearance: Purple
- Pulse Quality: Normal
- Shen: Good

	LI-18, LI-16, LI-15	BL-13 to BL-20	Hip	Stifle	Hock point, BL-39
Left side	-	-	-	-	+++
Right side	-	-	-	-	+

TCVM Diagnosis

Hock Blood Stagnation

Treatment

The treatment includes dry needle acupuncture, electroacupuncture for twenty minutes at 20 Hz and aquapuncture (5 cc of diluted vitamin B_{12}). GB-32 and GB-44 are added for the local hock soreness. In addition, fifteen grams of the herbal medication *Sang Zhi San* should be used twice daily for thirty days.

Dry Needle Acupuncture:	BL-67 and GB-44
Electroacupuncture:	BL-39 (left) with Coxa Hock point, GB-32 with BL-60, BL-39 (right) with Coxa Hock point, *Shen Shu*
Aquapuncture:	BL-39, BL-60, Coxa Hock point

Recommendation

- Gradually increase the length of her rides.

JANUARY 17, 2001 (FOURTH VISIT)

The owner reported that Rosie is doing very well. She is willing to run and trot when she is ridden. The rider still feels some stiffness when she leads on the left, but she is basically sound. Now, the owner's major concern is to help her fertility and her hives.

Examination

Rosie has hives and lumps (about 2 x 2 cm) around the neck/chest/back are easily seen. The body feels warm.

- Tongue Appearance: Pale
- Pulse Quality: Deep and weak
- Shen: Good

	LI-18, PC-1	BL-13 to BL-20	Hip	Stifle	Hock point, BL-39
Left side	-	-	-	-	-
Right side	+++	-	-	-	-

TCVM Analysis

The pale tongue, the deep and weak pulse and the infertility indicate a Kidney Jing Deficiency. A Kidney Jing Deficiency can lead to a Wei Qi Deficiency. When the Wei Qi is deficient, the pathogen Wind-Heat can easily invade the body and Lung system, which leads to hives. In TCVM, hives are called *Fei Feng Huang* or Lung Wind-Heat syndrome. Sensitivity at LI-18 and PC-1 indicate right front foot soreness, which can be secondary to the rear limb lameness.

TCVM Diagnosis

Kidney Jing Deficiency with Lung Wind Heat Syndrome

Treatment

The treatment strategies include tonifying the Kidney Qi, nourishing Jing, and opening the body surface to clear the Wind-Heat. The treatment includes dry needle acupuncture, electroacupuncture for twenty minutes at 20 Hz and aquapuncture (5 cc of diluted vitamin B_{12}). In addition, fifteen grams of the herbal medication *Sheng Jing San* (Epimedium Powder) should be used twice daily for two months.

Dry Needle:	ST-45, LI-1, LI-4, LI-10, SP-6, TH-1 (right), PC-9
Electroacupuncture:	BL-21, BL-23, *Shen Shu*, *Shen Peng*, GV-3 with *Bai Hui*, *Yan Chi*
Aquapuncture:	LI-11, GV-14

ST-45, LI-1, LI-4, LI-11 and GV-14 clear the Pathogen Wind-Heat. BL-21, SP-6 and LI-10 tonify the Spleen to reinforce the Postnatal Jing. BL-23, *Shen Shu*, *Shen Peng*, *Bai Hui*, GV-3 and Yan-chi tonify the Kidney and reinforce the Prenatal Jing. TH-1 and PC-9 are the local points for foot soreness. *Sheng Jing San* is designed to tonify Kidney Qi, to warm Kidney Yang, to nourish Yin and Blood and to reinforce Jing.

JUNE 27, 2001 (FIFTH VISIT)

After two months of *Sheng Jing San*, Rosie had a normal follicle. She was bred once in March, and she conceived. Because her progesterone level was very low, she was given *Bai Zhu San* (Pregnancy Smoother) for three months. Her progesterone level gradually maintained a normal level.

Rosie is sound. There are no lameness problems. Her major complaint for this visit is severe hives. Rosie has a history of developing hives whenever she receives an inoculation. She is three months pregnant, and she had received a Pneumabort-K vaccine last Wednesday to protect against EHV-1 (Equine Herpes Virus 1). After the inoculation, she once again broke out with hives on her neck and lateral abdomen.

Examination

Rosie has severe hives on the left cervical area (where vaccine was injected) and the right lateral abdomen. She has moderate hives on the right cervical region and the left lateral abdomen.

- Tongue Appearance: Deep red
- Pulse Quality: Stronger on the right side
- Shen: Good

	LI-18, LI-15, PC-6	BL-13 to BL-20	Hip	Stifle	Hock point, BL-39
Left side	-	-	-	-	-
Right side	-	-	-	-	-

TCVM Analysis

When Wei Qi is challenged and overwhelmed by vaccines, it may become imbalanced. Subsequently, the pathogen Wind-Heat easily invades the body and Lung system leading to a Lung Wind-Heat syndrome.

TCVM Diagnosis

Lung Wind Heat (Lung Wind Huang Syndrome)

Treatment

The treatment includes dry needle acupuncture and aquapuncture (5 cc of diluted vitamin B$_{12}$). In addition, fifteen grams of the herbal medication Lung Wind Huang Powder should be used twice daily for three months.

Dry Needle: BL-13, LU-5, LI-11, LI-1, LU-1, GV-14

Aquapuncture: GV-14, LI-11, LU-5

LI-11, LI-1, GV-14 and LU-5 open the body surface and clear the Wind-Heat. LU-1 and BL-13 strengthen the Lung system. Lung Wing Huang Powder (*Xiao Huang San*) is a classical equine herbal formula that clears Wind-Heat and resolves the hives.

Recommendations

- Rest for two weeks and gradually go back to the normal riding schedule.
- Strong manipulation is contraindicated around lumbosacral and abdominal areas.

SEPTEMBER 21, 2001 (E-MAIL COMMUNICATION)

Rosie's hives disappeared gradually about ten days after the acupuncture therapy.

Rosie passed a big test last week when she was vaccinated against West Nile virus; she has not shown any sign of hives. Her pregnancy continues normally. She is ridden three to four times a week. The owner was instructed to discontinue the herbal medication Lung Wind Hung Formula.

FEBRUARY 27, 2002 (E-MAIL COMMUNICATION)

Rosie is doing well. She gave birth to a nice, handsome colt yesterday.

Self Test

Max is a seven year old male Basset Hound. He is a very friendly and happy dog who greets everybody and loves to be petted. Max has a history of chronic impacted anal glands and other illnesses. He was very sick when was born. When he was 1½ years old, he developed a temporary lameness of one hind limb (the owner believes he still has some residual lameness). When he was two years old, he developed a high fever, diarrhea and vomiting post-boarding.

For over a month, Max has shown lethargy, listlessness, and warm-seeking behavior. The owner spoon feeds him because it takes Max too much effort to eat otherwise. His condition has progressed in the past month. Recently, he has been very anorexic and lethargic. He has been drooling and has had some loose stool and vomiting. Max had not eaten at all for two days, but he ate a little with some assistance yesterday. He was diagnosed with dilated cardiomyopathy on July 8, 2001. The medications prescribed include Enalapril and Furosemide. His diet has consisted of brown rice, meat and vegetables.

Question 10.1: What is Max's personality type?

    a. Wood
    b. Fire
    c. Earth
    d. Metal
    e. Water

Question 10.2: Why does Max have so many illness at his young age?

    a. Spleen Qi Deficiency
    b. Spleen Jing Deficiency
    c. Kidney Qi Deficiency
    d. Kidney Jing Deficiency
    e. Heart Jing Deficiency

Question 10.3: Which Zang system (Element) is of major concern based on the information provided above?

    a. Liver
    b. Heart
    c. Spleen
    d. Lung
    e. Kidney

Physical examination on July 10, 2001, reveals that Max is very lethargic and depressed. His pulse is weaker on the right side. His tongue is pale purple with a white coating. His nose is dry. Upon palpation, BL-17 on the left side is very sensitive. Max is considered a Fire-type because he is a friendly dog that greets everyone warmly even when he is not feeling well. He comes to strangers when called. He is interested in what the other patients in the hallway outside the exam room are doing.

Question 10.4: What is Max's TCVM diagnosis?

    a. Kidney Jing Deficiency
    b. Heart Yang Deficiency
    c. Spleen Qi Deficiency
    d. All of the above
    e. None of the above

Question 10.5: Which of Max's signs correspond to a Kidney Jing Deficiency?

    a. History of serious disease at an early age
    b. Fire personality, dilated cardiomyopathy and pale purple tongue
    c. Anorexia
    d. Listlessness
    e. Dry nose

Question 10.6: Which of Max's signs correspond to a Heart Yang Deficiency?

    a. Listlessness
    b. Warm-seeking behavior
    c. Fire personality, dilated cardiomyopathy and pale purple tongue
    d. All of the above
    e. None of the above

Question 10.7: Which of Max's signs correspond to a Spleen Qi Deficiency?

    a. Anorexia
    b. Lethargy
    c. Vomiting and drooling
    d. Weak pulse on the right side
    e. All of the above

Question 10.8: Assuming that Max's TCVM diagnoses include Kidney Jing Deficiency, Heart Yang Deficiency and Spleen Qi Deficiency. What are your Treatment strategies?

    a. Nourish Kidney Jing Only
    b. Tonify Heart Yang Only
    c. Tonify Kidney Jing and Heart Yang
    d. Tonify Spleen Qi and Kidney Jing
    e. Tonify Spleen Qi and Heart Yang

Question 10.9: Which of the following acupoint formulas is best for Max today?

    a. *Shan Gen*, *Bai Hui*, BL-20, ST-36, LI-10, HT-7, BL-15
    b. *Shan Gen*, *Bai Hui*, BL-20, ST-36, GV-1, *Wei Jian* (tail tip)
    c. *Shan Gen*, *Bai Hui*, GV–3, GV-4, CV-4, BL-23, KID-3, KID-7
    d. KID-3, KID-10, KID-7, BL-23, *Shen Shu*, *Bai Hui*
    e. HT-7, HT-9, BL-14, BL-15, *Bai Hui*, CV-17

Question 10.10: Which of the following herbal formulas is best for Max today?

    a. *Jin Gui Shen Qi Wan*
    b. *Lie Wei Di Huang Wan*
    c. *Ginseng Jian Pi* and *Zhen Wu Tang*
    d. *Zhen Wu Tang*
    e. *Zhen Wu Tang* and *Jin Gui Shen Qi Wan*

SELF TEST ANSWER KEY

CHAPTER 1

Question 1.1: **A**
Question 1.2: **A**
Question 1.3: **B**
Question 1.4: **B**
Question 1.5: **A**
Question 1.6: **B**
Question 1.7: **B**
Question 1.8: **B**
Question 1.9: **A**
Question 1.10: **B**
Question 1.11: **A**
Question 1.12: **D**
Question 1.13: **B**
Question 1.14: **B**

CHAPTER 2

Question 2.1: **C**
Question 2.2: **D**
Question 2.3: **A**
Question 2.4: **B**
Question 2.5: **C**
Question 2.6: **D**
Question 2.7: **E**
Question 2.8: **E**
Question 2.9: **D**
Question 2.10: **B**
Question 2.11: **D**
Question 2.12: **D**
Question 2.13: **C**
Question 2.14: **C**
Question 2.15: **E**
Question 2.16: **A**
Question 2.17: **B**
Question 2.18: **B**

CHAPTER 3

Question 3.1: **A**
Question 3.2: **B**
Question 3.3: **C**
Question 3.4: **E**
Question 3.5: **A**
Question 3.6: **A**
Question 3.7: **B**
Question 3.8: **D**
Question 3.9: **C**
Question 3.10: **A**
Question 3.11: **D**
Question 3.12: **E**
Question 3.13: **D**

CHAPTER 4

Question 4.1: **A**
Question 4.2: **C**
Question 4.3: **E**
Question 4.4: **B**
Question 4.5: **A**
Question 4.6: **D**
Question 4.7: **A**
Question 4.8: **E**
Question 4.9: **B**
Question 4.10: **D**
Question 4.11: **E**
Question 4.12: **C**

CHAPTER 5

Question 5.1: **C**
Question 5.2: **B**
Question 5.3: **C**
Question 5.4: **D**
Question 5.5: **A**
Question 5.6: **C**
Question 5.7: **E**
Question 5.8: **C**
Question 5.9: **E**
Question 5.10: **C**
Question 5.11: **B**
Question 5.12: **B**
Question 5.13: **A**
Question 5.14: **A**

CHAPTER 6

Question 6.1: **B**
Question 6.2: **C**
Question 6.3: **E**
Question 6.4: **D**
Question 6.5: **E**
Question 6.6: **C**
Question 6.7: **C**
Question 6.8: **A**
Question 6.9: **A**
Question 6.10: **B**
Question 6.11: **D**
Question 6.12: **E**
Question 6.13: **A**
Question 6.14: **D**

CHAPTER 7

Question 7.1: **B**
Question 7.2: **D**
Question 7.3: **B**
Question 7.4: **C**
Question 7.5: **E**
Question 7.6: **A**
Question 7.7: **E**
Question 7.8: **C**

CHAPTER 8

Question 8.1: **B**
Question 8.2: **E**
Question 8.3: **A**
Question 8.4: **C**
Question 8.5: **D**
Question 8.6: **C**
Question 8.7: **E**
Question 8.8: **B**
Question 8.9: **E**
Question 8.10: **C**
Question 8.11: **D**
Question 8.12: **A**
Question 8.13: **B**

CHAPTER 9

Question 9.1: **C**
Question 9.2: **A**
Question 9.3: **D**
Question 9.4: **B**
Question 9.5: **D**
Question 9.6: **E**

CHAPTER 10

Question 10.1: **B**
Question 10.2: **D**
Question 10.3: **C**
Question 10.4: **D**
Question 10.5: **A**
Question 10.6: **D**
Question 10.7: **E**
Question 10.8: **E**
Question 10.9: **A**
Question 10.10: **C**

HISTORY OF TRADITIONAL CHINESE MEDICINE

Traditional Chinese Veterinary Medicine originated with China's primitive society. As the years passed, TCVM practitioners gained greater medical knowledge until they created an academic system with generally accepted core principles for diagnosis and treatment. These basic principles still remain the foundation of present day TCVM practice, even though new discoveries continuously enrich this developing field. Many of today's common treatment techniques such as acupuncture, herbal therapy and moxibustion have been used for disease prevention and treatment since the early years of this system. Except for a stagnant period during which China was ruled as a semi-feudal society, Traditional Chinese Veterinary Medicine has been constantly expanding. Since 1949, the Chinese government has paid close attention to traditional Chinese medicine and has made efforts to preserve and promote this system. Subsequently, TCVM enjoyed renewed growth and has spread across the world at a staggering rate.

Origin

The origin of Traditional Chinese Veterinary Medicine can be traced to ancient society when man began to domesticate animals. To protect the animals they raised, the primitive humans used various methods to treat or prevent animal diseases, subsequently developing the first seeds of veterinary knowledge. These people used the tools at their disposal including fire, stone, and bone to combat human and domestic animal diseases. This became the origin of heat therapy, acupuncture and moxibustion. The discovery of a stone knife ("*Bian Shi*") in Inner Mongolia is evidence that acupuncture originated in a primitive society. This knife is believed to have been used to cut boils and to stimulate acupuncture points.

The development of veterinary medicine originated with observation of animal selection and reaction to various stimuli and ingested matter. The majority of the early medicines were from plants, thus the formulas were called herbal medicines even though some of the ingredients may be of mineral or animal origin. These formulas were later gathered together and written into works known as the *Ben Cao* (materia medica).

Shang Dynasty (16th to 11th century B.C.)

- First development of veterinary knowledge in China

- People paid great attention to domestic animal breeding and health, especially horses due to their uses as beasts of burden and transportation and for war.

- Inscriptions on bone describe human and animal disease.

- Pictographic characters inscribed on bones indicate that a method of castration surgeries had been developed.

- Chinese medicines such as bunge, cherry seed and peach pit were excavated from the *Gaocheng* ruins of the *Hebei* Province.

- Bronze knives and needles were available for castration surgery and acupuncture.

- The pigsty, cowshed, stable and sheepfold came into use.

Western Zhou Dynasty to Spring and Autumn Period (11th century-476 B.C.)

- A large quantity of veterinary medical knowledge was documented during this period.

- *Zhou Li Tian Guan*, a history book of the Zhou Dynasty, records the existence of full-time veterinarians treating animal disease.

- *Zhou Li* (*The Rites of Zhou Dynasty*), *Shi Jing* (*The Book of Songs*) and *Shan Hai Jing* (*The Book of Mountains and Rivers*) described more than one hundred Chinese medicines.

- *Li Ji* (*The Book of Rites*) contains records of collecting medicinal herbs in summer and of some serious domestic animal diseases.

- Famous people involved with animal husbandry and veterinary medicine during this time included Zao Fu, Bo Le and Wang Liang.

Warring States Period (475 to 221 B.C.)

- Veterinarians specializing in equine diseases emerged.

- The books of this period contained records of a variety of domestic animal diseases including boils, weakness, wounds and sudden death in cattle and horses.

- *Huang Di Nei Jing* (*The Yellow Emperor's Classic of Internal Medicine*) collects the theories and experiences of the ancient Chinese people in struggle against disease, thereby documenting the basic theories of Traditional Chinese Medicine and Traditional Chinese Veterinary Medicine.

Qin Dynasty (221 B.C. to 209 B.C.)

- The government created the initial rules governing animal husbandry and veterinary medicine in China.

- These laws were written in the *Jiu Yuan Lu* (Animal Husbandry and Veterinary Medicine Laws).

Han Dynasty (206 B.C. to 220 A.D.)

- The animal husbandry laws became known as *Jiu Lu*.

- *Shen Nong Ben Cao Jing* (*The Shen Nong's Book of Medical Herbs*), a collection of information on 365 medicinal herbs, became the earliest Chinese materia medica.

- Veterinary prescriptions for oral medications were found to be written upon bamboo slips.

- Zhang Zongjing (150-219 A.D.) wrote *Shang Han Za Bing Lun* (*Treatise on Cold-Induced Disorders and Miscellaneous Diseases*) which further developed the process of treatment determination based upon pattern differentiation. This text has been used as a veterinary reference ever since.

- A set of nine different types of iron needles were developed, although needles made of gold or silver were also common.

- Some books record using a combination of acupuncture and herbal medicine to treat animal diseases.

- There was greater understanding of epidemic diseases during this time and some Chinese characters were even created to represent them.

- Leather horseshoes and hoof trimming were used to prevent hoof diseases.

- Veterinarians specializing in cattle diseases emerged.

- Hua Tuo invented a general anesthetic formula named *Ma Fei San*, which promoted the progress of surgical knowledge.

Jin Dynasty to South-North Period (265 to 581 A.D.)

- Ge Hong (281-340 A.D.) wrote *Zhou Hou Bei Ji Fang* (*Pocket Book for Emergency Therapies*) which included descriptions of disease treatment and of rectal palpation methods.

- Around 533 to 544 A.D., Jia Sixie wrote *Qi Min Yao Shu* (*Basic Techniques for Farmers*), which contains information about more advanced animal husbandry and veterinary medical techniques.

- *Bo Le Liao Ma Jing* (*Bole's Classics on Treatment of Equine Diseases*) was published during the Liang stage (502 - 557 A.D.).

Sui Dynasty (581 to 618 A.D.)

- Veterinary medicine began to branch out as more specific books on diagnosis, treatment, medicinal herbs, acupuncture and moxibustion were published.

- *Tai Pu Si*, a branch of government in charge of animal husbandry and veterinary medicine, was established with 120 veterinarians in the country.

- *Sui Shu Jing Ji Zhi* cataloged the books published in Sui Dynasty including the following veterinary medical books:

  o *Liao Ma Fang* (*Prescriptions for Horse*), one volume

  o *Bo Le Zhi Ma Za Bing Jing* (*Treatise on Treatment for Sick Horses by Bo Le*), one volume

  o *Yu Ji Liao Ma Jing* (*Classic on Treatment of Equine Diseases by Yu Ji*), three volumes

  o *Liao Ma Jing* (*Classics on Treatment of Equine Diseases*), four volumes

  o *Zhi Ma Jing Tu* (*Classics on Treatment of Equine Diseases with Pictures*), two volumes

- *Ma Jing Kong Xue Tu* (*Atlas of Equine Meridians and Acupuncture Points*), one volume
- *Zhi Ma Niu Tuo Luo Deng Jing* (*The Classics on Treatment of Diseases in Horses, Cattle, Camel and Mule*), three volumes.

Tang Dynasty (618 to 907 A.D.)

- A comprehensive veterinary education system was established.

- From 705 to 707 A.D., there were 600 veterinarians, 4 veterinary teachers and 100 veterinary students in *Tai Pu Si* (a government-funded educational institution).

- The earliest veterinary medical textbook in China, *Si Mu An Ji Ji* (*A Collection of Ways to Care for and Treat Horses*), systematically narrated the basic theories, diagnostics and treatment techniques of Traditional Chinese Veterinary Medicine. This book was written by Li Shi who was once a government official.

- The government created animal husbandry and veterinary medical laws in order to guarantee animal husbandry development.

- Veterinary medicine developed greatly in the nations surrounding China, and these nations published some veterinary medical books.

- In 659 AD, the government published *Xin Xiu Ben Cao* (*Newly Revised Materia Medica*), which described 844 Chinese herbal medicines and was China's earliest pharmacopeia for human and veterinary medicine.

Song Dynasty (960 to 1279 A.D.)

- In 1007, the government established "*Bing Ma Jian*" (Hospital of Sick Horses) to treat sick horses near the capital. *Bing Ma Jian* was the first animal hospital in China.

- In 1036, the government pronounced that horses with mild illness should be sent to a different hospital.

- An organization known as "*Pi Bao Suo*" (Institute of Pathological Autopsy) was established to perform animal postmortem examinations in China.

- The government also established the "*Yao Mi Ku*" (Storage of Honey and Medicine), which was the first veterinary dispensary in China.

- Papermaking tools and printing technique promoted the spread of veterinary medical works.

- A famous veterinarian named Chang Shun lived during this time in Yang Cheng of the *Shanxi* Province.

Yuan Dynasty (1206 to 1368 A.D.)

- Bian Bao or Bian Guangou wrote *Quan Ji Tong Xuan Lun* (*Treatment of Sick Horses*) which described the pathology of the visceral organs and the treatment of common animal diseases.

Ming Dynasty (1368 to 1644 A.D.)

- The government made veterinary training a law. Every head caretaker of at least 25 horses (later 50 horses) should select 2 or 3 clever young men to study veterinary medicine and treat horse diseases.

- The widespread book *Yuan Heng Liao Ma Ji Fu Niu Tuo Jing* (*Yuan-Heng's Therapeutic Treatise of Horses*) was written in 1608 A.D. by two famous veterinarians, Yu Benyuan and Yu Benheng, with a preface by Ding Bin. It was a representative work of traditional Chinese veterinary medicine and was widely spread in China.

- *Ma Shu* (*The Book of Horses*), edited and published by Yang Shiqiao in 1594 AD, contained substantial quantities of information about treatment of equine diseases.

- In 1633 AD, two Korean authors Zhao Jun and Jin Shiheng wrote the book *Xin Bian Ji Cheng Ma Yi Fang Niu Yi Fang* (*New Collection of Prescriptions for Horses and Cattle*) in the Chinese language.

- After 30 years experience and consultation of more than 800 books including veterinary medical texts, Li Shizhen (1518-1593) wrote *Ben Cao Gang Mu* (*Compendium of Materia Medica*) which described 1,892 Chinese herbs and 11,096 Chinese herbal formulas. Not long after this book was published in 1596, it spread overseas greatly contributed to development of both the Chinese and foreign materia medica.

- In many books published during this time contained records of castration in horses, cattle, sheep, pigs, dogs and chickens.

Qing Dynasty to the Opium War (1644 to 1840 A.D.)

- Traditional Chinese veterinary medicine developed slowly during this period.

- In 1736 AD, Li Yushu wrote an adaptation of *Yuan Heng Liao Ma Ji* with a preface by Xu Keng. This text became the most popular one in use today.

- In 1785 AD, Guo Huaixi annotated *Yuan Heng Liao Ma Ji* and gave it the title *Ma Niu Tuo Jing Da Quan* (*The Complete Collection of Diseases of Horses, Cattle and Camels*).

- In 1800, Fu Shufeng wrote *Yang Geng Ji* (*A Collection on Management of Draught Cattle*) which consisted of the diagnosis, treatment and prescriptions of cattle diseases, as well as acupuncture and moxibustion techniques.

- *Niu Yi Jin Jian* (*Golden Guide for Bovine Veterinarians*) and *Bao Du Ji* (*Treatise On Calf Diseases*) were published during this period.

Modern Times (1840 to 1949 A.D.)

- China was a semi-colonial, semi-feudal society.

- Development of Traditional Chinese Veterinary Medicine suffered during this period.

- Traditional Chinese Veterinary Medicine nearly perished due to a general lack of interest and attention.

- Folk veterinarians kept the traditions alive by collecting and practicing the techniques of Traditional Chinese Veterinary Medicine.

- Li Nanhui wrote the book *Hou Shou Ci Zhou* (*Human Care of Animals*) which provided detailed explanations of disease patterns in a variety of species including yellow cattle, buffaloes, pigs, horses, sheep, dogs and cats.

- *Zhu Jin Da Quan* (*Complete Collection of Swine Diseases*) was a unique book about swine medicine that described therapeutics for 48 kinds of pig diseases.

- Western veterinary medical school of thought was imported into China at the beginning of the 20th century.

Recent Developments (1949 to Present)

- With the establishment of the People's Republic of China in 1949, great importance was attached to revival and development of Traditional Chinese Veterinary Medicine.

- The government issued a policy in 1956 that required unity, use, teaching and improvement of Traditional Chinese Veterinary Medicine.

- The first National Congress of Folk Veterinary Medicine was held in Beijing in September, 1956. It proposed combining Traditional Chinese Veterinary Medicine with Western veterinary medicine, thereby resulting in quick advancement of traditional Chinese veterinary medicine.

- Institutes of TCVM education and research were founded.

- A series of TCVM books published during this period were based on clinical experiences with disease prevention and treatment, Chinese herbal medicines, acupuncture and castration.

- Chinese and Western experts noticed the success of acupuncture analgesia in animals.

- Effective diagnostic and treatment methods were developed for constipation, gastric distension, fractures, diarrhea, back and limb problems, obstetrical disorders and encephalitis.

- New acupuncture techniques and herbal formulas were invented.

- Since 1978, much attention has been directed towards research and education in TCVM, and modern, advanced technologies have been applied to the field.

- Laser-acupuncture, microwave acupuncture, magnetic acupuncture and auriculotherapy were applied to treatment of animal disease.

- Computers were applied to identification of Patterns and selection of acupuncture points and herbal additives.

- Microscopes were used to examine the histologic structure of acupuncture points.

Propagation of Traditional Chinese Veterinary Medicine

Today, Traditional Chinese Veterinary Medicine has spread worldwide. The success of acupuncture analgesia especially has had great influence on the veterinary field. Although Traditional Chinese Veterinary Medicine seems new to people in the United States, it has been well known in many countries for a long time.

Traditional Chinese veterinary medical techniques were exported to Korea and Japan as early as 1,500 years ago. In 595 A.D., a Korean monk commented on the treatment of equine diseases in Japan, "There are doctors who are experts in equine diseases in China." Possibly following this sage advice, Naka Kuni Taira, a Japanese native, visited China to learn veterinary medicine in 804 A.D. After returning home, he trained numerous veterinary workers and established a branch of veterinary study known as the "Kuni Sect".

The proliferation of written works by authors outside of China is some evidence of TCVM expansion throughout the Asian world and beyond:

- Both the early Japanese book *Jia Ming An Ji Ji* (*A Collection of Ways to Care and Treat Horses in Japanese*) and the Korean book *Xin Bian Ji Cheng Ma Yi Fang Niu Yi Fang* (*New Integrated Prescriptions for Equine and Bovine Diseases*) were based on ancient Chinese veterinary literature.

- An important ancient Chinese veterinary work, *Yuan Heng Liao Ma Ji* (*Yuan-Heng's Therapeutic Treatise of Horses*), was disseminated to Japan, Korea, Vietnam, Europe and the United States throughout the years. Since the 18th century, a number of articles have been published on the application of traditional Chinese veterinary therapeutics including acupuncture and herbal medicine.

- The book *Chinese Veterinary Medicine and Animal Acupuncture*, which was published in Japan in 1987 contained detailed information about TCM principles, theories, formulas, herbs and acupuncture techniques.

The Future of TCVM

Since the People's Republic of China was founded in 1949, integration of Traditional Chinese Veterinary Medicine (TCVM) and Western veterinary medicine (WVM) has been a guiding principle for development of Chinese veterinary medicine. A new, effective veterinary medical science emerges as it absorbs the advantages of both TCVM and modern Western veterinary medicine.

Three kinds of veterinary study may be found today. These include Traditional Chinese Veterinary Medicine, Western veterinary medicine and integrated traditional Chinese and Western medicine. Clinically, both TCVM and WVM both attempt to prevent and treat animal diseases, but each has its own strengths and weakness. TCVM uses therapeutic methods such as Chinese herbs, acupuncture and moxibustion to treat animal diseases and to improve resistance to disease. On the other hand, WVM has advanced diagnostic techniques which directly contend with disease etiologies and pathogens (microorganisms, parasites and mechanical lesions). Integrative medicine is formed when TCVM and WVM supplement each other, thereby forming a stronger and more versatile system.

From an academic perspective, integrated traditional Chinese and Western veterinary medicine consists of three areas: theory, pharmacology and disease identification. The principles of TCVM stress whole-body homeostasis and resistance for disease prevention and treatment. On the other hand, WVM principles emphasize experimental research and disease prevention and treatment through identification and therapy directed at specific etiologic agents. By combining TCVM's dynamic, whole-body views of health with the more mechanistic, pathologic views of Western veterinary medicine, an integrative theory emerges and provides better results than either system alone.

From a pharmacological perspective, the traditional Chinese medicines are natural substances including plants, animal parts or minerals. They are intended to exert effects along the Meridians and to regulate the balance within the body. Generally, they produce few to no side-effects or drug residues. Most western medicines are chemical and biological drugs, which are directed toward a specific disease process or etiologic agent. Typically, they exert their effects faster than Chinese herbs, but may have more side effects. Combinations of Chinese herbs with Western drugs can produce beneficial synergistic effects.

TCVM uses Pattern Identification to recognize and diagnose diseases. By analyzing a patient's clinical signs, a TCVM practitioner can identify the etiology and location of lesions as well as the associated pathologic changes. Conversely, WVM diagnoses disease by identifying an etiological agent. This is accomplished by interpreting clinical signs and diagnostic test results. In general, the TCVM Pattern is related to but different from the WVM disease. A disease may include several Patterns. For instance, gastroenteritis includes the Damp-Heat Pattern, Cold-Damp Pattern, Spleen Qi Deficiency Pattern and Overfeeding Pattern. On the other hand, a Pattern may appear in several diseases. For example, a Heat Pattern may be exhibited in infectious diseases, parasitic diseases and internal medical diseases. Thus, when evaluating patients, both a TCVM Pattern and a Western disease diagnosis may be applied. Subsequent treatment with both appropriate Western and Chinese medicines will provide superior therapeutic results.

DIAGRAMS

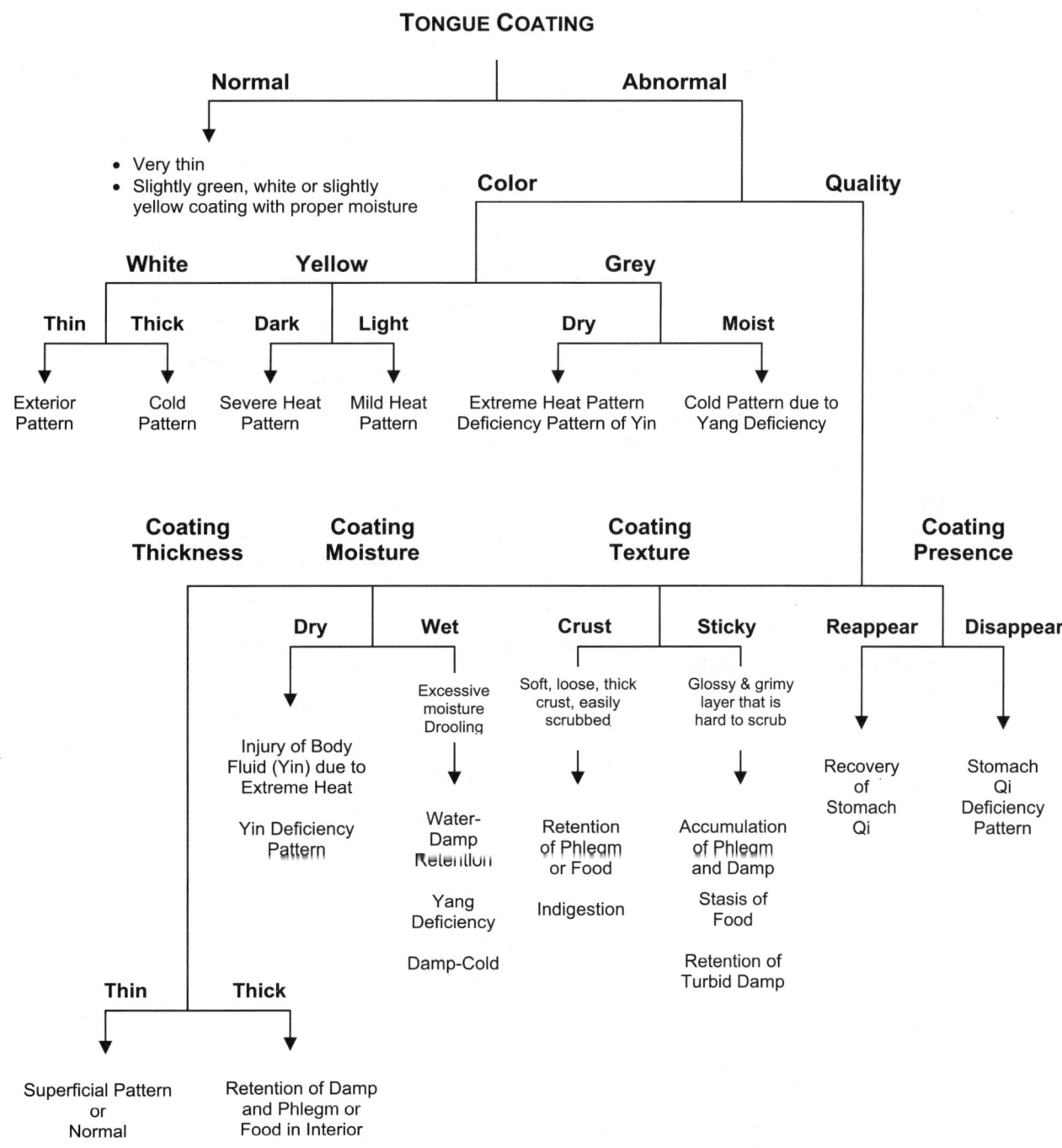

TONGUE COATING

Normal

- Very thin
- Slightly green, white or slightly yellow coating with proper moisture

Abnormal

Color

Quality

White

Thin → Exterior Pattern

Thick → Cold Pattern

Yellow

Dark → Severe Heat Pattern

Light → Mild Heat Pattern

Grey

Dry → Extreme Heat Pattern Deficiency Pattern of Yin

Moist → Cold Pattern due to Yang Deficiency

Coating Thickness

Coating Moisture

Coating Texture

Coating Presence

Dry → Injury of Body Fluid (Yin) due to Extreme Heat

Yin Deficiency Pattern

Wet → Excessive moisture Drooling → Water-Damp Retention

Yang Deficiency

Damp-Cold

Crust → Soft, loose, thick crust, easily scrubbed → Retention of Phlegm or Food

Indigestion

Sticky → Glossy & grimy layer that is hard to scrub → Accumulation of Phlegm and Damp

Stasis of Food

Retention of Turbid Damp

Reappear → Recovery of Stomach Qi

Disappear → Stomach Qi Deficiency Pattern

Thin → Superficial Pattern or Normal

Thick → Retention of Damp and Phlegm or Food in Interior

TONGUE COLOR

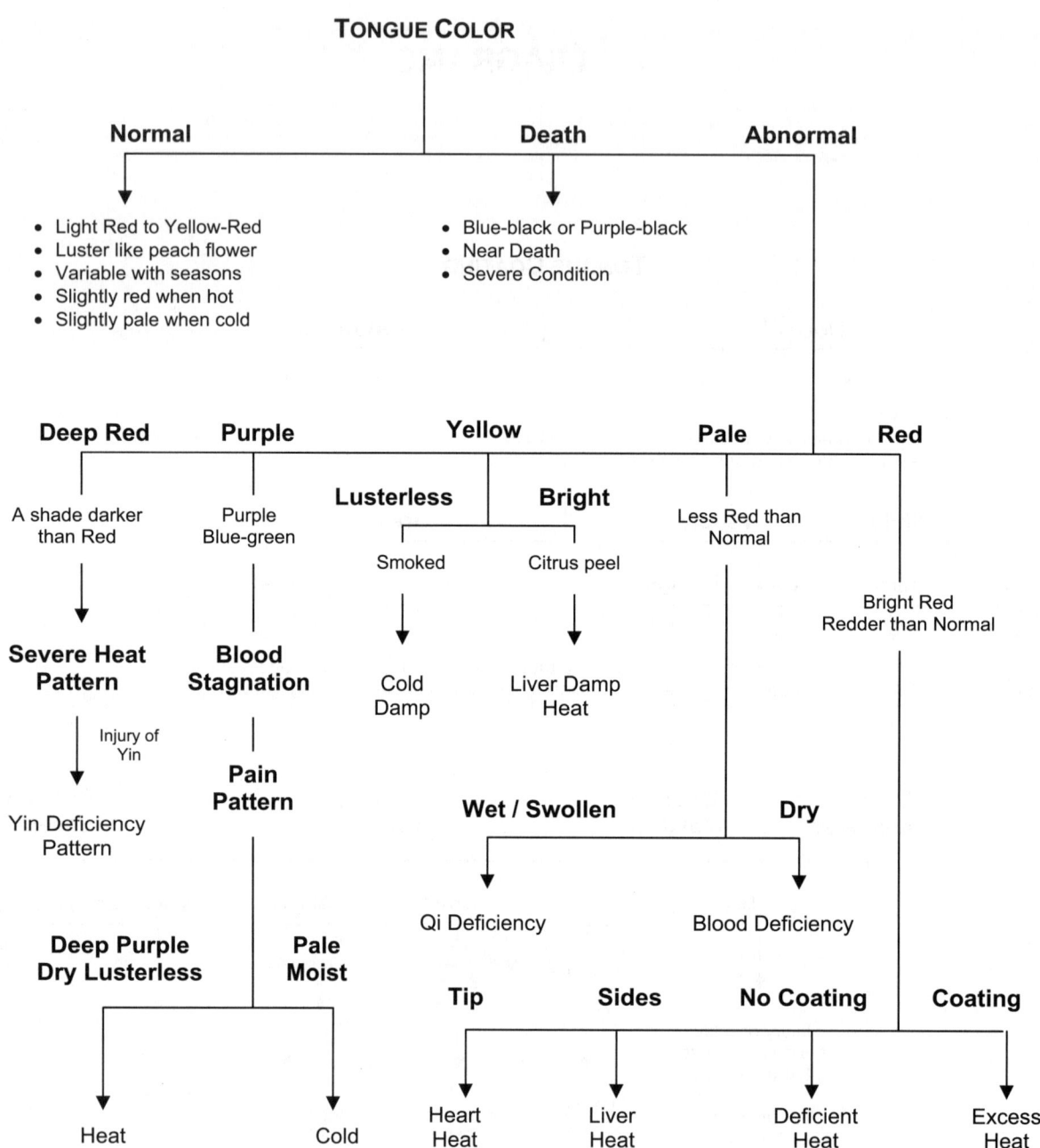

Normal
- Light Red to Yellow-Red
- Luster like peach flower
- Variable with seasons
- Slightly red when hot
- Slightly pale when cold

Death
- Blue-black or Purple-black
- Near Death
- Severe Condition

Abnormal

Deep Red

A shade darker than Red

↓

Severe Heat Pattern

↓ Injury of Yin

Yin Deficiency Pattern

Purple

Purple Blue-green

Blood Stagnation

Pain Pattern

Deep Purple Dry Lusterless → Heat

Pale Moist → Cold

Yellow

Lusterless

Smoked

↓

Cold Damp

Bright

Citrus peel

↓

Liver Damp Heat

Pale

Less Red than Normal

Wet / Swollen

↓

Qi Deficiency

Tip → Heart Heat

Sides → Liver Heat

Dry

↓

Blood Deficiency

No Coating → Deficient Heat

Coating → Excess Heat

Red

Bright Red Redder than Normal

TONGUE SHAPE

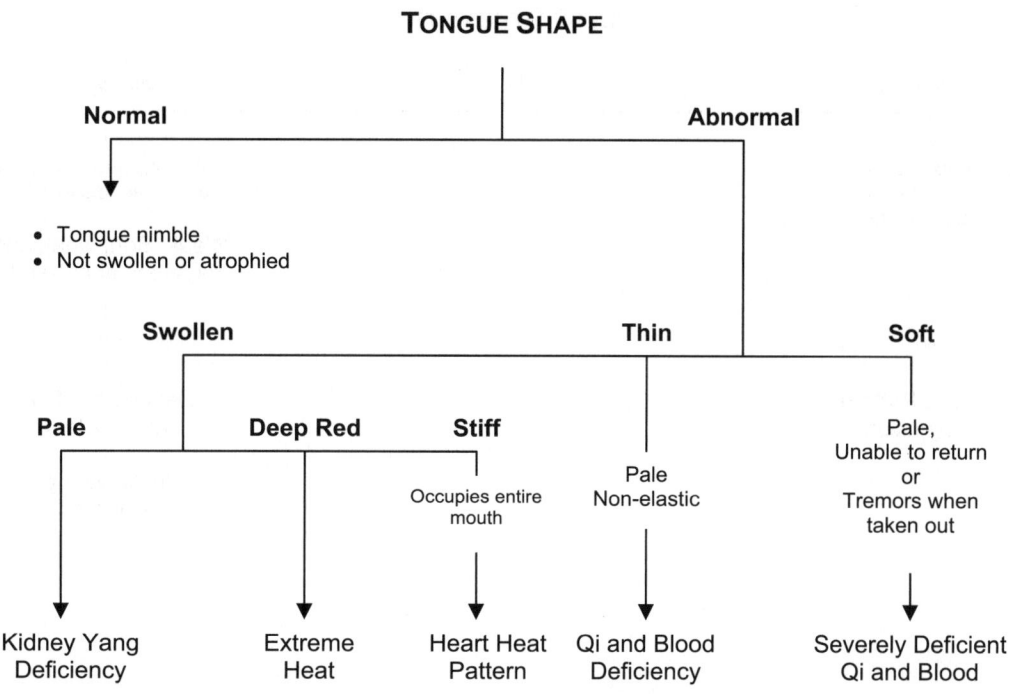

PULSE DEPTH

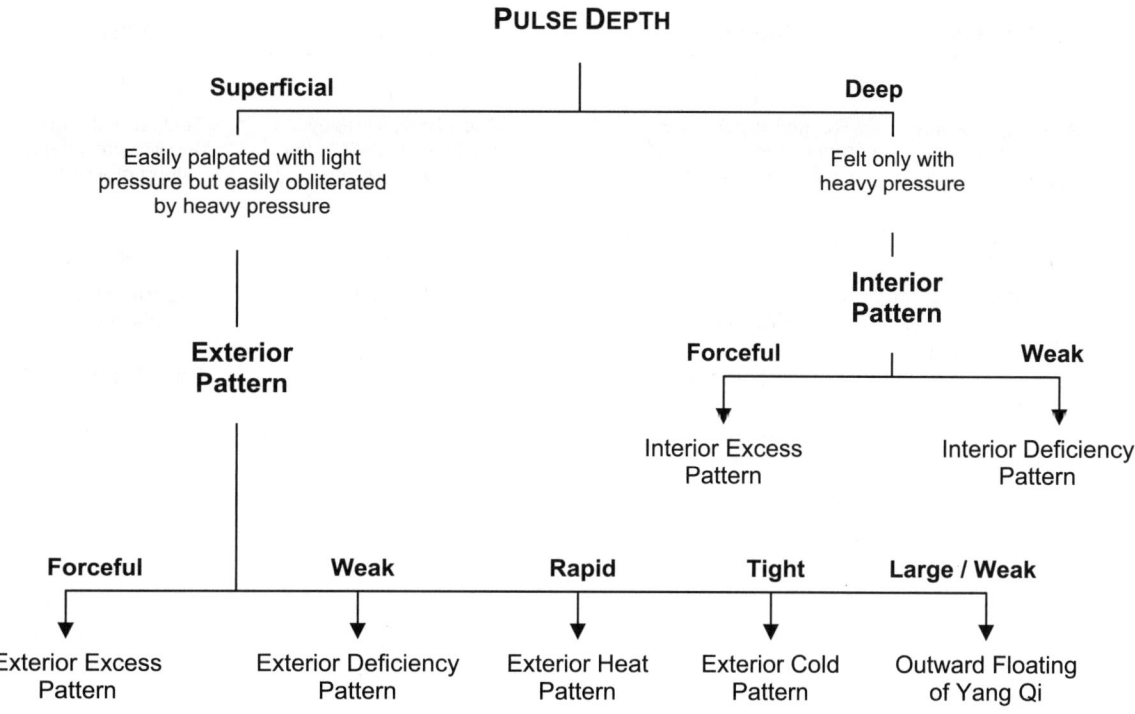

PULSE STRENGTH

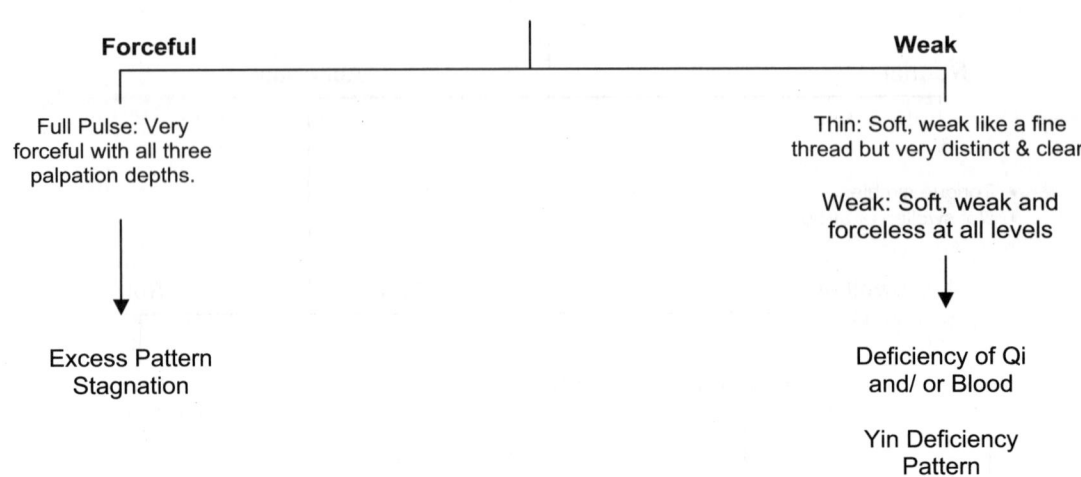

Forceful

Full Pulse: Very forceful with all three palpation depths.

↓

Excess Pattern Stagnation

Weak

Thin: Soft, weak like a fine thread but very distinct & clear.

Weak: Soft, weak and forceless at all levels

↓

Deficiency of Qi and/ or Blood

Yin Deficiency Pattern

PULSE QUALITY

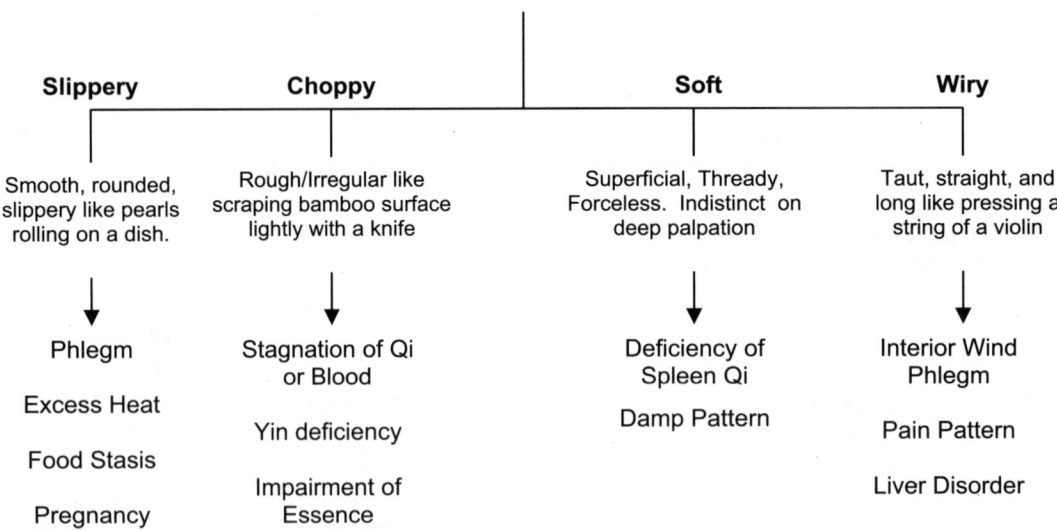

Slippery

Smooth, rounded, slippery like pearls rolling on a dish.

↓

Phlegm

Excess Heat

Food Stasis

Pregnancy

Choppy

Rough/Irregular like scraping bamboo surface lightly with a knife

↓

Stagnation of Qi or Blood

Yin deficiency

Impairment of Essence

Soft

Superficial, Thready, Forceless. Indistinct on deep palpation

↓

Deficiency of Spleen Qi

Damp Pattern

Wiry

Taut, straight, and long like pressing a string of a violin

↓

Interior Wind Phlegm

Pain Pattern

Liver Disorder

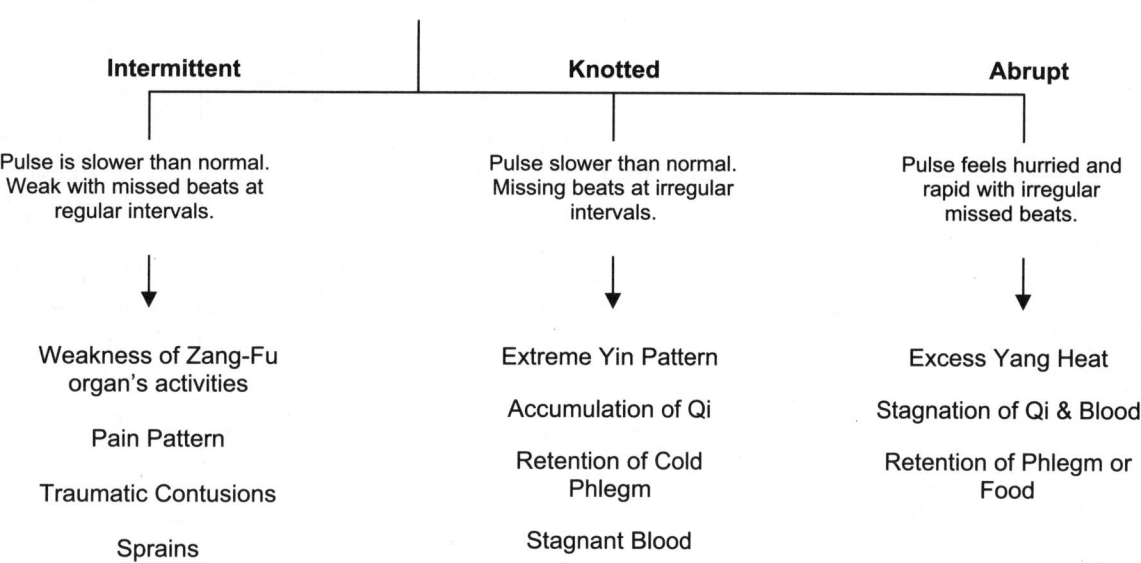

PULSE RHYTHM

Intermittent	Knotted	Abrupt
Pulse is slower than normal. Weak with missed beats at regular intervals.	Pulse slower than normal. Missing beats at irregular intervals.	Pulse feels hurried and rapid with irregular missed beats.
Weakness of Zang-Fu organ's activities	Extreme Yin Pattern	Excess Yang Heat
Pain Pattern	Accumulation of Qi	Stagnation of Qi & Blood
Traumatic Contusions	Retention of Cold Phlegm	Retention of Phlegm or Food
Sprains	Stagnant Blood	

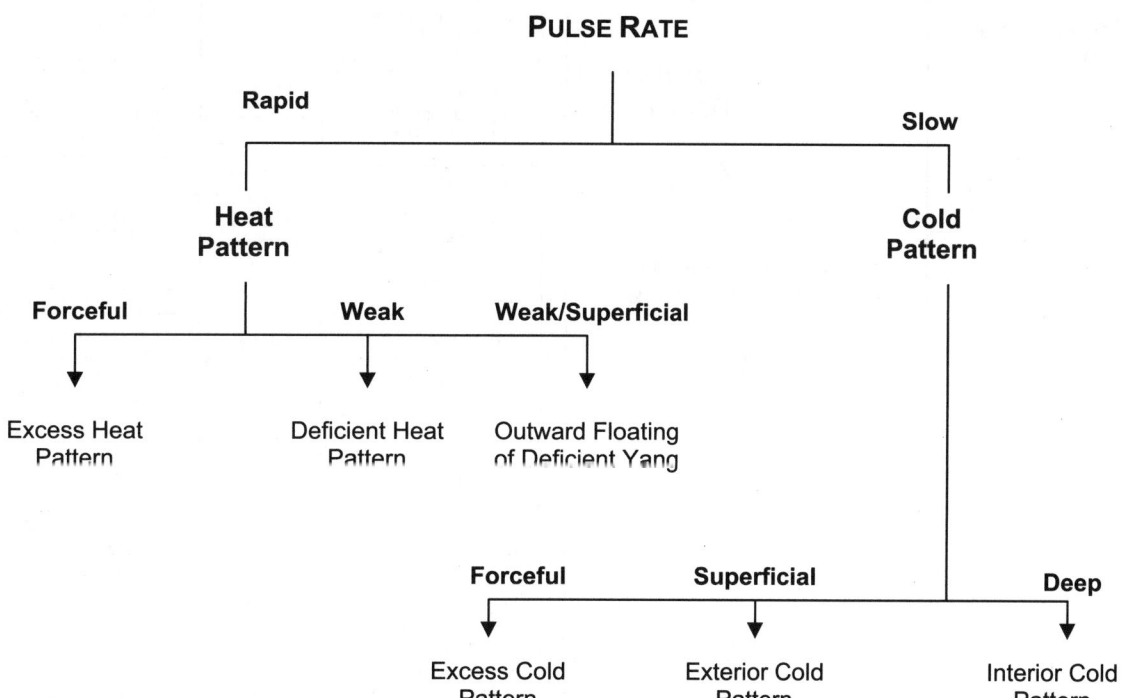

PULSE RATE

Rapid

Slow

Heat Pattern

Cold Pattern

Forceful — Excess Heat Pattern

Weak — Deficient Heat Pattern

Weak/Superficial — Outward Floating of Deficient Yang

Forceful — Excess Cold Pattern

Superficial — Exterior Cold Pattern

Deep — Interior Cold Pattern

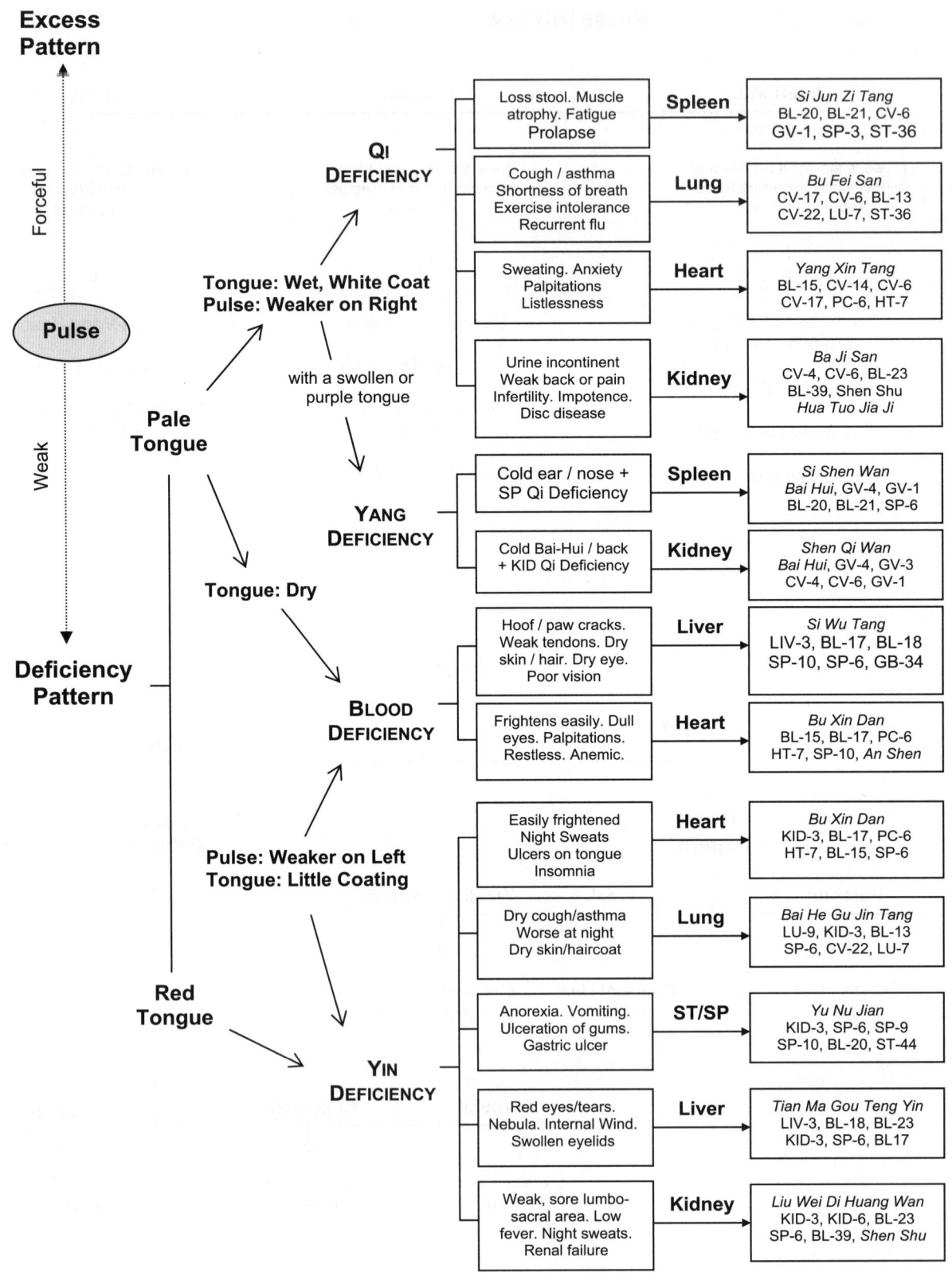

Excess Pattern

Forceful

Weak

Pulse

Deficiency Pattern

Pale Tongue

Red Tongue

Tongue: Wet, White Coat
Pulse: Weaker on Right

with a swollen or purple tongue

Tongue: Dry

Pulse: Weaker on Left
Tongue: Little Coating

QI DEFICIENCY

Loss stool. Muscle atrophy. Fatigue Prolapse	**Spleen**	*Si Jun Zi Tang* BL-20, BL-21, CV-6 GV-1, SP-3, ST-36
Cough / asthma Shortness of breath Exercise intolerance Recurrent flu	**Lung**	*Bu Fei San* CV-17, CV-6, BL-13 CV-22, LU-7, ST-36
Sweating. Anxiety Palpitations Listlessness	**Heart**	*Yang Xin Tang* BL-15, CV-14, CV-6 CV-17, PC-6, HT-7
Urine incontinent Weak back or pain Infertility. Impotence. Disc disease	**Kidney**	*Ba Ji San* CV-4, CV-6, BL-23 BL-39, Shen Shu *Hua Tuo Jia Ji*

YANG DEFICIENCY

Cold ear / nose + SP Qi Deficiency	**Spleen**	*Si Shen Wan* *Bai Hui*, GV-4, GV-1 BL-20, BL-21, SP-6
Cold Bai-Hui / back + KID Qi Deficiency	**Kidney**	*Shen Qi Wan* *Bai Hui*, GV-4, GV-3 CV-4, CV-6, GV-1

BLOOD DEFICIENCY

Hoof / paw cracks. Weak tendons. Dry skin / hair. Dry eye. Poor vision	**Liver**	*Si Wu Tang* LIV-3, BL-17, BL-18 SP-10, SP-6, GB-34
Frightens easily. Dull eyes. Palpitations. Restless. Anemic.	**Heart**	*Bu Xin Dan* BL-15, BL-17, PC-6 HT-7, SP-10, *An Shen*

YIN DEFICIENCY

Easily frightened Night Sweats Ulcers on tongue Insomnia	**Heart**	*Bu Xin Dan* KID-3, BL-17, PC-6 HT-7, BL-15, SP-6
Dry cough/asthma Worse at night Dry skin/haircoat	**Lung**	*Bai He Gu Jin Tang* LU-9, KID-3, BL-13 SP-6, CV-22, LU-7
Anorexia. Vomiting. Ulceration of gums. Gastric ulcer	**ST/SP**	*Yu Nu Jian* KID-3, SP-6, SP-9 SP-10, BL-20, ST-44
Red eyes/tears. Nebula. Internal Wind. Swollen eyelids	**Liver**	*Tian Ma Gou Teng Yin* LIV-3, BL-18, BL-23 KID-3, SP-6, BL17
Weak, sore lumbo-sacral area. Low fever. Night sweats. Renal failure	**Kidney**	*Liu Wei Di Huang Wan* KID-3, KID-6, BL-23 SP-6, BL-39, *Shen Shu*

Differentiation of Excess Patterns (Shi Patterns)

Parameter	Wind-Cold	Wind-Heat	Damp-Heat	Cold-Damp	Wind-Cold-Damp	Phlegm	Blood Stagnation	Qi Stagnation
Course of Illness	< 3 days	< 7 days	< 5 days	< 10 days	Acute or Chronic	Sub-acute	Acute or Chronic	Acute or Chronic
Nasal Discharge	Clear	Thick	±	±	±	±	±	±
Cough	No	Yes	±	±	±	Yes	±	±
Preference of Massage	±	±	No	Yes	Yes	±	No	No
Stool	Normal	Normal	Bloody	Loose	Normal	Loose	Normal	Normal
Temperature Preference	Warm	Cool	Cold	Warm	Warm	±	±	±
Fever	Yes	Yes	Yes	No	No	No	No	No
Cold Shivers	Yes	No	No	±	-	-	-	-
Tongue Color	Purple Pale	Red	Red Yellow	Purple Pale	Purple	Red or Pale	Purple	Purple
Tongue Coating	Thin White	Thin Yellow	Thick Yellow	Thick White	Thin	Thick Greasy	Thin	Thin
Pulse	Floating	Floating Fast	Forceful	Slow	Tight	Choppy	Tight	Tight
Acupoints	BL-10, GB-20, LI-4	LI-4, LI-11, GV-14	LI-10, LI-11, Wei Jian	SP-9, SP-6, ST-40	LIV-3, Bai Hui, Local points	ST-36, LU-9, SP-6	BL-17, LIV-3, Local points	LIV-3, ST-36, Local points
Classical Formula	Ma Huang Tang	Yin Qiao San	Long Dan Xie Gan Tang	Wei Ling San	Du Huo Ji Sheng Tang	Er Chen Tang	Sheng Tong Zhu Yu Tang	Xiao Yao San

ACUPUNCTURE POINT LOCATIONS

Lung Meridian (LU): Taiyin; 3 am - 5 am; Thoracic limb (begins on chest; ends on distal leg)

Name	Location	Indications
LU-1 *Zhong Fu* Central Storage	• Canine: In the space medial to the greater tubercle of the humerus in the Superficial Pectoral muscle at the level of the 1st intercostal space • Equine: A depression in the middle of the transverse pectoral muscle (1.5 cm lateral to ventral end of the medial pectoral sulcus)	Front-Mu (Alarm) point for Lung Immune Regulation
LU-5 *Chi Ze* Cubit Marsh	• On the cubital crease, just lateral to the tendon of the biceps brachii muscle with the elbow flexed. • Equine: At the elbow, lateral to the biceps tendon	He-sea point (water) Water point (sedate) for Lung, Lung Heat, fever, cough, asthma
LU-7 *Lie Que* Broken Sequence	• Canine: Proximal to the styloid process of the radius, 1.5 cun above the radiocarpal joint. • Equine: Craniomedial edge of radius, 0.5 cun (1 finger) in front of cephalic vein at level of distal border of chestnut (just proximal to the medial styloid process of the radius).	Luo-connecting point to Large Intestine Meridian (LI-6) Confluent point of CV Meridian Master point for head and neck
LU-9 *Tai Yuan* Great Abyss	• Canine: On the medial end of the radiocarpal joint, medial to the radial artery.	Shu-stream (earth) point Yuan (Source) point Influential point of blood vessels
LU-11 *Shao Shang* Minor Trade	• Equine: Caudomedial; Jing-well point (0.5 cun proximal to coronary band, just cranial to medial collateral cartilage) of forelimb	Jing-well point (wood). Use for asthma, bleeding, cough, allergy (dust, mold, pollen), nasal discharge, lung problems, fatigue, sole bruising

Large Intestine Meridian (LI): Yangming; 5 am - 7 am; Thoracic limb (begins distal leg, ends on head)

Name	Location	Indications
LI-1 *Shang Yang* Trade Yang	• Equine: Craniomedial: 0.5 cun proximal to the coronary band, halfway between the cranial midline and LU-11	Jing-well point (metal) for nasal discharge, reluctance to lead in a race, lame in forelimb or shoulder
LI-4 *He Gu* Union Valley	• Canine: Between the 2nd and 3rd metacarpal bones approximately in the middle of the 3rd metacarpal bone on the radial side. • Canine Alternative: Between the 1st and 2nd metacarpal bones, approximately in the middle of the 2nd metacarpal bone on the radial side. • Equine: Proximal 1/3 between the cannon bone and base of the medial splint bone.	Yuan (Source) point Master point for face and mouth
LI-5 *Yang Xi* Yang Ravine	• Equine: Depression between 2nd and 3rd carpal bones on the craniomedial aspect of carpus	Jing-river point (fire)
LI-6 *Pian Li* Veering Passageway	• Equine: 3 cun (6 fingers) above LI-5 in the most cranial muscle groove on the lateral surface (between extensor carpi radialis and common digital extensor)	Luo connecting point with LU-7
LI-7 *Wen Liu* Warming Dwelling	• Equine: 2 cun (4 fingers) above LI-6 in the same muscle groove	Xi cleft point for acute borborygmi or acute abdominal pain
LI-10 *Qian San Li* Front 3 Mile	• Canine: 2 cun distal to LI 11 (1/6 of the way below the elbow) between the extensor carpi radialis and the common digital extensor muscle. • Equine: 2 cun (4 fingers) below LI-11 in same muscle groove as LI-6	
LI-11 *Qu Chi* Pool on the Bend	• Canine: At the end of the lateral cubital crease, halfway between the biceps tendon and the lateral epicondyle of the humerus with the elbow flexed. • Equine: In the transverse cubital crease (formed when carpus flexed) in a depression cranial to the elbow	He-sea point (earth) Mother point for Deficiency
LI-15 *Jian Yu* (Jian Jing) Shoulder Bone	• Canine: Cranial and distal to the acromion on the cranial margin of the acromial head of the deltoideus muscle. • Equine: Cranial to acromion at the point of shoulder	Treatment and diagnostic point for the shoulder

LI-16 *Ju Gu* Giant Bone	• Equine: Along cranial border of scapula, in a depression 2/3 of distance from TH-15 to point of shoulder.	Fetlock and shoulder diagnostic and treatment points
LI-17 *Tian Ding* Celestial Tripod	• Equine: 2 cun craniodorsal to L-16 on the sternocleidomastoid muscle at the level of C-6	Carpal diagnostic and treatment point
LI-18 *Fu Tu* Protuberance Assistance	• Equine: With head extended, follow the ventral mandible to the depression just above jugular groove	Diagnostic point for a hoof problem
LI-20 *Ying Xiang* Welcome Aroma	• Canine: In the nasal labial groove, at the level of the widest part of the nostril approximately 0.1 cun outside the haired-nonhaired border. • Equine: 2/3 of way upward along lateral edge of nares (from ventral edge), 1 cun caudal to nares	Use for sinusitis or nasal discharge

Stomach Meridian (ST): Yangming; 7 am – 9 am; Pelvic limb (begins on face, ends on distal leg)

Name	Location	Indications
ST-1 *Cheng Qi* Receiving Tears	• Canine: Directly below the center of the pupil just inside the infraorbital ridge. Penetrate the point by retropulsing the eyeball dorsally and directing the needle over the infraorbital ridge through the skin and under the eye. • Equine: Lower eye lid, 1/3 of way from medial canthus	Use for uveitis, Liver Heat
ST-2 *Si Bai* Four Whites	• Canine: In the depression at the center of the infraorbital foramen • Equine: Ventral to medial canthus at bifurcation of angular vein	Uveitis, colic
ST-4 *Di Cang* Earth Granary	• Canine. At the lateral corner of the mouth 0.1 cun outside the mucocutaneous border.	
ST-6 *Jia Che* Jawbone	• Canine: In the depression in the middle of the masseter muscle just rostral to the angle of the mandible.	
ST-10 *Shui Tu* Water Prominence	• Equine: Put heel of hand on the point of the shoulder (right hand on right shoulder, left on left). Grab the muscle above jugular groove with thumb and index finger. The index finger marks ST-10	Diagnostic point for ipsilateral stifle

ST-25 *Tian Shu* Celestial Center	• Canine: 2 cun lateral to the center of the umbilicus. • Equine: 1.5 cun lateral to umbilicus	Front-Mu (Alarm) point for LI Release Heat and relieve constipation
ST-35 *Du Bi* Calf's Nose	• Canine: In the depression below the patella and lateral to the patellar ligament. Also referred to as "lateral eye of the knee" or *Wei Xi Yan*. • Equine: Between lateral and middle patellar ligaments.	Lateral eye of knee Stifle problems, rear limb weakness
ST-35b *Xi Ao* Knee Curve	• Canine: In the depression below the patella and medial to the patellar ligament is a point also referred to as "the medial eye of the knee" or *Nei Xi Yan*. Together with ST-35, the two points are referred to as *Xi Yan*.	Medial Eye of Knee Stifle problems, rear limb weakness
ST-36 *Hou San Li* Rear 3 Miles	• Canine: 3 cun below ST-35, one finger-width from the cranial crest of the tibia in the belly of the cranial tibial muscle. This is a long linear point. • Equine: 0.5 cun lateral to and 1.5 cun below distal aspect of tibial crest over the cranial tibialis muscle	He-sea (earth) point Master point for gastrointestinal tract and abdomen Use for nausea, vomiting, gastric pain, gastric ulcer, food stasis
ST-40 *Feng Long* Bountiful Bulge	• Canine: One half of the distance between the lateral malleolus and the tibial plateau (top of the tibia), 2 cun lateral to the anterior tibial midline in the groove (the second muscle groove) between the cranial tibial and long digital extensor muscles.	Luo-connecting point to Spleen Influential point for Phlegm
ST-41 Jie Xi Ravine Divide	• Canine: On the dorsum of the rear foot at the level of the hock in the depression directly on the midline. The point lies at the level of the malleolus between the ligaments of the long digital extensor and the cranial tibial muscles.	Jing-river point (fire)
ST-44 *Nei Ting* Inner Court	• Canine: Proximal to the web margin between the 2nd and 3rd toes in the depression distal and lateral to the 2nd metatarsophalangeal joint. • Canine Alternative: Proximal to the web margin between the 3rd and 4th toes in the depression distal and lateral to the 3rd metatarsophalangeal joint. • Equine: At the level of the ergot, 0.5 cun lateral to the midline.	Ying-spring point (water) Use for Stomach Heat and gastric ulcers
ST-45 *Li Dui* Severe Mouth	• Canine: On the lateral side of the 2nd digit nail base • Canine Alternative: On the lateral side of the 3rd digit at the nail base • Equine: cranial midline 0.5 cun proximal to coronary band of hind limb	Jing-well (metal) point Son point for Excess Diagnostic and treatment points for appetite

Spleen Meridian (SP): Taiyin; 9 am – 11 am; Pelvic limb (begins on distal leg, ends on chest)

Name	Location	Indications
SP-1 *Yin Bai* Hidden White	• Equine: Caudomedial 0.5 cun proximal to coronary band of hind limb, just cranial to medial collateral cartilage	Jing well point (wood)
SP-4 *Gong Sun* Yellow Emperor	• Canine: In the depression distal to the base (proximal end) of the 1st metatarsal bone on the most medial aspect of the rear foot. • Canine Alternative: In the depression just distal to the base (proximal end) of the 2nd metatarsal bone on the most medial aspect of the rear foot.	Luo-connecting point to Stomach Confluent point to Chong Meridian
SP-6 *San Yin Jiao* 3 Yin Crossing	• Canine: 3 cun above the tip of the medial malleolus on the posterior border of the tibia in the small depression trailing the tibia. The point is directly opposite GB-39 which is on the lateral side. • Equine: Caudal to tibia, 3 cun proximal to medial malleolus	Master point for the caudal abdomen and urogenital system Yin/Blood tonic Clears Damp
SP-9 *Yin Ling Quan* Yin Mound Spring	• Canine: On the lower border of the medial condyle of the tibia in the depression between the posterior border of the tibia and the gastrocnemius muscle. The point is found by following the back of the tibia cranially until it bends caudally just below the medial tibial condyle. It is opposite GB-34 on the lateral side of the fibula. • Equine: Distal border of medial condyle of tibia (opposite to GB-34)	He-sea point (water) Yin tonic Clears Damp
SP-10 *Xue Hai* Sea of Blood	• Canine: When stifle is flexed, the point 2 cun above and medial to the patella (diagonally) in a depression just anterior to the sartorius muscle. The point is just proximal and medial to the top of the medial patellar groove on the femur. • Equine: 2 cun proximal to the patella, in the belly of the vastus medialis m.	Sea of Blood Cools Blood Nourishes Blood Invigorates Blood
SP-21 *Da Bao* Great Embracement	• Equine: 10th intercostal space, at the same level as point of shoulder	Spleen major Lou

Heart Meridian (HT): Shaoyin; 11 am – 1 pm; Thoracic limb (begins on chest, ends on distal leg)

Name	Location	Indications
HT-1 *Ji Quan* Highest Spring	• Canine: In the center of the axillary space (between the trunk and the foreleg) over the superficial pectoral muscle	
HT-3 *Shao Hai* Minor Sea	• Canine: On the medial side of the elbow just lateral to the medial epicondyle. The point is between the end of the cubital crease and the medial epicondyle of the humerus.	He-sea point (water)
HT-7 *Shen Men* Spirit Gate	• Canine: On the transverse crease of the carpal joint in the depression lateral to the tendon of the flexor carpi ulnaris muscle. • Equine: On the caudolateral aspect of the radius, just proximal to the accessory carpal bone	Shu-stream point (earth) Yuan (Source) point Son point for Excess
HT-8 *Shao Fu* Lesser Mansion	• Canine: On the palmar surface of the paw between the 4th and 5th metacarpal bones, proximal to the metacarpal-phalangeal junction, under the pad.	Ying-spring point (fire)
HT-9 *Shao Chong* Minor Channel	• Canine: On the medial aspect of the nail bed of the 5th digit of the front foot. • Equine: Halfway between SI-1 and ST-45, 0.5 cun proximal to coronary band.	Jing-well point (wood) Mother point

Small Intestine Meridian (SI): Taiyang; 1 pm – 3 pm; Thoracic limb (begin on distal leg, end on head)

Name	Location	Indications
SI-1 *Shao Ze* Minor Marsh	• Equine: Just cranial to lateral collateral cartilage of forelimb, 0.5 cun proximal to coronary band.	Jing-well point (metal)
SI-3 *Hou Xi* Back Ravine	• Canine: Proximal to the metacarpophalangeal joint on the lateral side of the 5th metacarpal.	Mother point for Deficiency Shu-stream point (wood) Confluent point of GV Meridian.
SI-8 *Xiao Hai* Small Sea	• Canine: On medial side of the elbow between the medial humeral epicondyle and the olecranon. This point is in the ulnar nerve ("funny bone").	Son point for Excess He-sea point (earth)

SI-9 *Jian Zhen* *(Qiang Feng)* Shoulder Hollow	• Canine: Caudal to humerus, in a large depression along the caudal border of the Deltoid muscle at its juncture with the lateral and the long heads of the triceps brachii	
SI-16	• Canine: Dorsal border of the brachiocephalicus muscle at the level of the second cervical vertebral space (C2-C3)	
SI-19 *Ting Gong* Hearing Place	• Canine: Rostral to the tragus (ventral to TH-21 and dorsal to GB-2 and TH-17), at the posterior border of the mandible and slightly dorsal to the condyloid process (a hole with the mouth open in humans). • Equine: At the TMJ, In the indentation of the rostral medial corner of the ear base (indentation very evident when mouth open)	

Bladder Meridian (BL): Taiyang; 3 pm – 5 pm; Pelvic limb (begins on face, ends on distal leg)

Name	Location	Indications
BL-1 *Jing Ming* Bright Eyes	• Canine: 0.1 cun dorsal to the medial canthus of the eye. • Equine: Indentation at medial canthus of eye	
BL-2 *Zan Zhu* Bamboo Gathering	• Canine: In the supraorbital ridge below the medial end of the eyebrow (at the supraorbital notch).	
BL-10 *Tian Zhu* Celestial Pillar	• Canine: 1.5 cun from the dorsal midline of the neck at the level of the junction of C1 and C2 (at the caudal ends of the wings of the atlas. • Equine: In a depression just caudal to the wings of the atlas, 2 cun below the dorsal midline	
BL-11 *Da Zhu* Big Shuttle	• Canine: 1.5 cun lateral to the caudal border of the spinous process of the 1st thoracic vertebrae. The point may be punctured by a needle inserted midway between the spinous process and the medial border of the scapula directing the needle slightly lateral. • Equine: Cranial to the withers, (at level of 2nd thoracic vertebral space), 3 cun lateral to dorsal midline	Influential point for Bone.
BL-12 *Feng Men* Wind Gate	• Canine: 1.5 cun lateral to the caudal border of the dorsal spinous process of the 2nd thoracic vertebrae. • Equine: At highest point of withers (4th thoracic vertebral space), 1 cun lateral to dorsal midline	Influential for wind and trachea

BL-13 *Fei Shu* *(Bo Lan)* Lung's Hollow	• Canine: 1.5 cun lateral to the caudal border of the dorsal spinous process of the 3rd thoracic vertebrae. • Equine: At the 8th intercostal space, 3 cun lateral to the dorsal midline (in the iliocostal muscle groove).	Back-shu (Association) point for Lung
BL-14 *Jue Yin Shu* Pericardium Hollow	• Canine: 1.5 cun lateral to the caudal border of the dorsal spinous process of the 4th thoracic vertebrae. • Equine: At the 9th intercostal space, 3 cun lateral to the dorsal midline (in the iliocostal muscle groove).	Back-shu (Association) point for Pericardium
BL-15 *Xin Shu* Heart's Hollow	• Canine: 1.5 cun lateral to the caudal border of the dorsal spinous process of the 5th thoracic vertebrae. • Equine: At the 10th intercostal space, 3 cun lateral to the dorsal midline (in the iliocostal muscle groove)	Back-shu (Association) point for Heart
BL-16 *Du Shu* Governing Hollow	• Equine: At the 11th intercostal space, 3 cun lateral to the dorsal midline (in the iliocostal muscle groove)	Association point for GV
BL-17 *Ge Shu* *(Gan Zhi Shu)* Diaphragm's Hollow	• Canine: 1.5 cun lateral to the caudal border of the spinous process of the 7th thoracic vertebrae, in the depression caudal to the medial border of the scapula. • Equine: At the 12th intercostal space, 3 cun lateral to the dorsal midline (in the iliocostal muscle groove)	Association point for diaphragm Influential point for Blood.
BL-18 *Gan Shu* Liver's Hollow	• Canine: 1.5 cun lateral to the caudal border of the spinous process of the 10th thoracic vertebrae. • Equine: At the 13th and 14th intercostal spaces (2 points), 3 cun lateral to the dorsal midline (in the iliocostal muscle groove)	Back-shu (Association) point for Liver
BL-19 *Dan Shu* Gall Bladder Hollow	• Canine: 1.5 cun lateral to the caudal border of the spinous process of the 11th thoracic vertebrae. • Equine: At the 15th intercostal space, 3 cun lateral to the dorsal midline (in the iliocostal muscle groove)	Back-shu (Association) point for Gall Bladder
BL-20 *Pi Shu* Spleen's Hollow	• Canine: 1.5 cun lateral to the caudal border of the spinous process of the 12th thoracic vertebrae. • Equine: At the 17th (last) intercostal space, 3 cun lateral to the dorsal midline (in the iliocostal muscle groove)	Back-shu (Association) point for Spleen
BL-21 *Wei Shu* Stomach's Hollow	• Canine: 1.5 cun lateral to the caudal border of the spinous process of the 13th thoracic vertebrae. • Equine: Thoracolumbar junction (T18 - L1), 3 cun lateral to dorsal midline	Back-shu (Association) point for Stomach Promote GI motility, relieve colic pain

BL-22 San Jiao Shu Triple Heater Shu	• Canine: 1.5 cun lateral to the caudal border of the spinous process of the 1st lumbar vertebrae. • Equine: 1st lumbar vertebral space (L1-L2), 3 cun lateral to dorsal midline	Back-shu (Association) point for Triple Heater
BL-23 *Shen Shu* Kidney's Hollow	• Canine: 1.5 cun lateral to the caudal border of the dorsal spinous process of the 2nd lumbar vertebrae. • Equine: 2nd lumbar vertebral space (L2-L3, dorsal to caudal aspect of last rib), 3 cun from dorsal midline	Back-shu (Association) point for Kidney
BL-24 *Qi Hai Shu* Qi Sea Hollow	• Equine: 4th lumbar vertebral space (L4-L5), 3 cun from midline	Sea of Qi
BL-25 *Da Chang Shu* Large Intestine Hollow	• Canine: 1.5 cun lateral to the caudal border of the dorsal spinous process of the 5th lumbar vertebrae. • Equine: 5th lumbar vertebral space (L5-L6, cranial edge of wing of ilium), 3 cun lateral to dorsal midline	Back-shu (Association) point for Large Intestine
BL-26 *Guan Yuan Shu* Source Hollow	• Equine: Lumbosacral space (L6-S1), 3 cun lateral to dorsal midline	Gates of Original / Source Qi
BL-27 *Xiao Chang Shu* Small Intestine Hollow	• Equine: 1st sacral vertebral space (S1-S2), 3 cun lateral to dorsal midline	Association point for Small Intestine
BL-28 *Pang Guang Shu* Bladder's Hollow	• Canine: Lateral to the 2nd sacral foramen in the depression between the medial border of the dorsal iliac spine and the sacrum • Equine: 2nd sacral vertebral space (S2-S3), 3 cun lateral to dorsal midline	Back-shu (Association) point for Bladder
BL-35 *Hui Yang* Meeting of Yang	• Canine: In the crease just lateral to the tail base 0.5 cun lateral from midline.	
BL-36 *Cheng Fu* Support	• Canine: In the middle of the gluteal crease ventral to the tuber ischii. • Equine: In the groove between the biceps femoris and the semitendinosus, 2 cun dorsal to tuber ischii	

BL-37 *Yin Men* Abundance Gate	• Equine: In groove between the biceps femoris and the semitendinosus, at the level of the tuber ischii	
BL-39 *Wei Yang* Yang in the bend	• Canine: On the lateral end of the popliteal crease on the medial border of the biceps femoris tendon. Just lateral to BL-40. • Equine: At the ventral extent of the groove between the biceps femoris and the semitendinosus mm. at the level of the stifle joint	Lower He-sea for Triple Heater Communicating point with the Triple Heater Meridian
BL-40 *Wei Zhong* Bend Middle	• Center: In the center of the popliteal crease. The point is found by directing the needle anteriorly towards the patella. • Equine: Midpoint of the transverse crease of the popliteal fossa.	He-sea point (earth) Master point for caudal back, hips Lower he-sea point for Bladder Use for dysuria, urinary incontinence, hip joint, back problems
BL-41 *Fu Fen* Attached Branch	• Equine: 3 cun lateral to BL-12	Extra Influential point for wind or trachea
BL-42 *Po Hu* Corporeal Soul Door	• Equine: 3 cun from BL-13	Extra association point for lung
BL-43 *Gao Huang* Upper Interior	• Equine: 3 cun from BL-14	Extra association point for Pericardium
BL-44 *Shen Tang* Spirit House	• Equine: 3 cun from BL-15	Extra association point for heart
BL-45 *Yi Xi* Sigh Smile	• Equine: 3 cun from BL-16	Extra association point for GV
BL-46 *Ge Guan* Diaphragm Pass	• Equine: 3 cun from BL-17	Extra association point for diaphragm

BL-47 *Hun Men* Mood Gate	• Equine: 3 cun from BL-18 (2 points)	Extra association point for Liver
BL-48 *Yang Gang* Yang Headrope	• Equine: 3 cun from BL-19	Extra association point for Gall Bladder
BL-49 *Yi She* Mentation Abode	• Equine: 3 cun from BL-20	Extra association point for Spleen
BL-50 *Wei Cang* Stomach Granary	• Equine: 3 cun from BL-21	Extra association point for Stomach Promotes gastrointestinal motility and relieves colic pain
BL-51 *Huang Men* Interior Gate	• Equine: 3 cun from BL-22	Extra association point for Triple Heater
BL-52 *Zhi Shi* Will Chamber	• Canine: 3 cun lateral to the caudal border of the dorsal spinous process of the 2nd lumbar vertebrae at the lateral border of the m. longissimus, lateral to BL 23. • Equine: 3 cun from BL-23	Extra association point for Kidney
BL-54 *Zhi Bian* *(Ba Shan)* Sequential Limit	• Canine: Dorsal to the greater trochanter of the femur. One of the "three bowling-ball points" around the hip joint. • Equine: Midway on a line connecting *Bai Hui* (dorsal midline at lumbosacral space) and the greater trochanter of the femur	Master point for hind legs.
BL-60 *Kun Lun* Mountains	• Canine: In the thin fleshy tissue between the lateral malleolus and the calcaneous level with the tip of the lateral malleolus. The point is opposite (slightly dorsal) to KID-3 • Equine: Between the lateral malleolus of the tibia and the calcaneal tuber (opposite KI-3)	Jing-river point (fire)
BL-62 *Shen Mai* Extending Vessel	• Canine: In the depression directly distal to the lateral malleolus.	Confluent point to Yang-qiao Meridian
BL-67 *Zhi Yin* Terminal Yin	• Canine: On the lateral aspect of the nail bed of the 5th digit of the rear foot. • Equine: Caudolateral ting point	Jing-Well point (metal) Mother point for deficiency

Kidney Meridian (KID): Shaoyin; 5 pm – 7 pm; Pelvic limb (begins on bottom of foot, ends on chest)

Name	Location	Indications
KID-1 *Yang Quan* Gushing Spring	• Canine: Between the 2nd and 3rd metatarsal bones underneath the central pad of the rear foot. • Canine Alternative: Between the 3rd and 4th metatarsal bones underneath the central pad of the rear foot. • This represents one of the four gates where animals touch the earth. It is needled by inserting the needle just proximal to the 3rd and 4th metatarsal bones and directing anteriodistally under the pad toward the webbing between the 3rd and 4th toes. • Equine: In a depression between the bulbs of the heel	Jing-well point (wood) Son point for Excess
KID-3 *Tai Xi* Great Ravine	• Canine: In the thin fleshy tissue between the medial malleolus and calcaneus level with the tip of the medial malleolus. The point is opposite and slightly ventral to BL-60.	Yuan (Source) point for Kidney Shu-stream point (earth)
KID-6 *Zhao Hai* Shining Sea	• Canine: In the depression immediately distal to the medial malleolus.	Confluent point to Yin-qiao Meridian
KID-7 *Fu Liu* Recover Flow	• Canine: 2 cun above the tip of the medial malleolus, anterior to the calcaneal tendon.	Mother point for Deficiency Jing-river point (metal)
KID-27 *Shu Fu* Transport House	• Equine: Between the sternum and first rib over the descending pectoral muscle.	Association point of all association points

Pericardium Meridian (PC): Jueyin; 7 pm – 9 pm; Thoracic limb (begins on chest, ends on distal leg)

Name	Location	Indications
PC-1 *Tian Chi* *(Cheng Deng)* Celestial Pool	• Equine: At the level of the point of the elbow, in the fifth intercostal space.	Confluent point with the GB Channel
PC-3 *Qu Ze* Elbow Marsh	• Canine: In the crease of the elbow just medial to the biceps tendon.	He-sea point (water)

PC-6 *Nei Guan* Inner Pass	• Canine: 3 cun above the transverse crease of the carpus located on the opposite side of the arm from TH-5. The point is located more medially in animals than it is in human beings, although both are located in the center of the palmar side of the arm. • Equine: Proximal and cranial to the border of chestnut	Luo-connecting point to Triple Heater Meridian Master point of chest/cranial abdomen Confluent point to Yin Wei channel.
PC-8 *Lao gong* Palace of Toil	• Canine: Between the 2nd and 3rd metacarpal bones proximal to the metacarpal-phalangeal joint on the medial side of the 3rd metacarpal bone. This point is found underneath the large central pad. • Canine Alternative: Between the 3rd and 4th metacarpal bones proximal to the metacarpal-phalangeal joint on the lateral side of the 3rd metacarpal bone. This point is found underneath the large central pad.	Yang-spring point (fire)
PC-9 *Zhong Chong* Central Hub	• Canine: Point is located on the tip of the 3rd toe. • Canine Alternative: Between the 3rd and 4th metacarpal bone distal to the metacarpophalangeal joint under the central pad. This represents one of the four gates where the energy of the feet touches the ground. Insertion is made by passing a needle through PC-8 and directing it anteriodistal under the pad toward the webbing between the 3rd and 4th toes (similar to KID-1 in the rear foot). • Equine: Between the heel bulbs	Jing-well point (metal) Use for hyperactivity, anhidrosis, superficial tendon problems

Triple Heater Meridian (TH): Shaoyang; 9 pm – 11 pm; Thoracic limb (begin on distal limb, end on face)

Name	Location	Indications
TH-1 *Guan Chong* Passage Hub	• Equine: Just lateral to the cranial midline, ting point	Jing-well point: forelimb joint problem, sore or cracked front heels
TH-3 *Zhong Zhu* Central Island	• Canine: On the dorsum of the forefoot between the 4th and 5th metacarpals in the depression proximal to the metacarpophalangeal joint	Shu-stream point (wood)
TH-5 *Wai Guan* Outer Pass	• Canine: 3 cun above the carpus on the craniolateral aspect of the foreleg in the interosseous space between the radius and ulna. This point is directly opposite PC-6 on the ventromedial aspect of the foreleg (which is the best way to find PC-6).	Luo-connecting point to the Pericardium Meridian Confluent point to Yang-wei Meridian
TH-10 *Tian Jing* Celestial Well	• In a depression on the triceps tendon Just proximal to the olecranon	Son point for Excess He-sea point (earth)

TH-14 *Jian Liao* *(Jian Wai Yu)* Shoulder Seam	• Canine: Caudal and distal to the acromion on the caudal margin of the acromial head of the deltoideus muscle. • Equine: Caudal margin of shoulder joint, at the level of the point of the shoulder	
TH-15 *Tian Liao* *(Bo Jiao)* Celestial Bonehole	• Equine: Depression on dorsal border of scapula at junction of scapula and scapular cartilage	
TH-16 *Tian You* Celestial Window	• Equine: Caudal border of the brachiocephalicus muscle, over the 1st cervical vertebral space	
TH-17 *Yi Feng* Wind Screen	• Canine: Ventral to the ear in the depression between the mandible and the mastoid process.	
TH-21 *Er Men* Ear Gate	• Canine: Rostral to the supratragic notch directly dorsal to SI-19 at the posterior border of the mandible and dorsal to the condyloid process with the mouth open.	
TH-23 *Si Zhu Kong* Silk Bamboo Hole	• Canine: In the depression on the rim of the orbit at the end of the eyebrow were it extended to the lateral canthus. • Equine: Near the lateral canthus of the eye, at the end of the eyebrow	

Gall Bladder Meridian (GB): Shaoyang; 11 pm – 1 am; Pelvic limb (begins on face, ends on distal limb)

Name	Location	Indications
GB-1 *Tong Zi Liao* Pupil Bone-Hole	• Canine: 0.2 cun Lateral to the lateral canthus in the depression over the rim of the orbit. • Equine: One cun caudoventral to the lateral canthus of the eye, over the transverse facial vein	
GB-2 *Ting Hui* Confluence of Hearing	• Canine: Rostral to the intertragic notch directly below SI-19 at the posterior border of the condyloid process of the mandible with the mouth open.	
GB-14 *Yang Bai* Yang White	• Canine: 1 cun above the extended midpoint of the eyebrow (at the end of the visible eyebrow).	

GB-20 *Feng Chi* Wind Pond	• Canine: The point is rostral and medial to the cranial edge of the wings of the atlas in a depression below the occipital bones and medial to the jugular process. • Equine: In the large depression just caudal to the occipital condyle	
GB-21 *Jian Jing* *(Bo Zhong)* Shoulder Well	• Canine: In a groove in the muscle in front of the scapula and Midway between GV-14 and the acromion. • Equine: In a depression located halfway along the cranial edge of the scapula	
GB-24 *Ri Yue* Sun Moon	• Equine: 15th intercostal space, caudodorsal to LIV-14	Alarm point for Gall Bladder
GB-25 *Jing Men* Capital Gate	• Canine: On the lateral side of the abdomen on the lower border of the free end of the 13th rib. • Equine: Caudal border of last rib (18) at the costochondral junction	Front-Mu (Alarm) point for the Kidney
GB-29 *Ju Liao* Squatting Bone-hole	• Canine: Midway between the greater trochanter and the craniodorsal edge of the iliac spine. • Canine Alternative: In a depression just cranial to the greater trochanter on a line between the greater trochanter and the iliac spine (one of the 3 bowling ball point around the head of the femur). • Equine: In a depression midway between wing of ilium and greater trochanter	
GB-30 *Huan Tiao* Circular Jump	• Canine: In a depression midway between the greater trochanter and the tuber ischii (one of the 3 bowling ball points around the head of the femur). • Equine: In a depression, caudoventral margin of greater trochanter	
GB-31 *Feng Shi* Wind Market	• Canine: In the groove between the biceps femoris and the semimembranosus muscles 7 cun above the popliteal crease.	
GB-33 *Yang Guan* Knee Yang Gate	• Canine: In the depression between the insertion of the biceps femoris tendon and the femur in the hollow above the lateral condyle of the femur.	
GB-34 *Yang Ling Quan* Yang Tomb Spring	• Canine: In the depression anterior and distal to the head of the fibula on the lateral side of the rear leg. • Equine: Caudodistal to head of fibula	He-sea point (earth) Influential for ligaments / tendons Lower He Se point for GB Use for vomiting; biliary disorders
GB-39 *Xuan Zhong* Hanging Bell	• Canine: 3 cun above the lateral malleolus in the depression caudal to the posterior border of the fibula near where the lateral saphenous vein crosses. This point is opposite SP-6.	Influential point for Marrow/CSF.

GB-41 *Zu Ling Qi* Near Tears on the Foot	• Canine: In the depression distal to the proximal junction of the 4th and 5th metatarsal bones	Shu-stream point (wood) Confluent point to Dai Meridian
GB-44 *Zu Qiao Yin* Foot Orifice Yin	• Equine: Craniolateral ting point	Jing-well point (metal) Use for hip problems

Liver Meridian (LIV): Jueyin; 1 am – 3 am; Pelvic limb (begins on distal limb, ends on chest)

Name	Location	Indications
LIV-1 *Da Dun* Large Pile	• Equine: Craniomedial ting point	Jing-well point (wood)
LIV-2 *Xing Jian* Moving Between	• Canine: On the medial aspect of the second toe distal to the metatarsophalangeal joint in the webbing • Canine Alternative: On the medial aspect of the 3rd toe distal to the metatarsophalangeal joint in the webbing.	Ying-spring point (fire)
LIV-3 *Tai Chong* Supreme Surge	• Canine: On the medial aspect of the second toe proximal to the metatarsophalangeal joint. • Canine Alternative: On the medial aspect of the third toe proximal to the metatarsophalangeal joint.	Shu-stream point (earth) Yuan-primary (Source) point
LIV-4 *Zhong Feng* Mound Center	• Equine: Cranial aspect of hock, on the saphenous vein, medial to cunean tendon	
LIV-8 *Qu Quan* Crooked Spring	• Canine: On the medial side of the knee above the medial end of the popliteal crease between the medial condyle and the insertion of the semimembranosus and semitendinosus muscles.	He-sea point (water) point
LIV-13 *Zhang Men* Gate of Symbol	• Canine: On the lateral side of the body just below the free end of the 12th rib • Equine: Distal end of 18th rib	Front-Mu (Alarm) point for Spleen Influential for Yin (Zang) organs. Master point for viscera
LIV-14 *Qi Men* Cycle Gate	• Canine: In a depression at the costochondral junction near the mammary line of the 6th intercostal space. • Equine: 14th intercostal space at the level of the elbow	Front-Mu (Alarm) point of Liver

Conception Vessel Meridian (CV): Ventral midline

Name	Location	Indications
CV-1 *Hui Yin* Yin meeting	• Canine: In the depression on the midline halfway between the anus and scrotum or vulva	
CV-3 *Zhong Ji* Central Pole	• Canine: On the ventral midline 4 cun caudal to the umbilicus • Equine: 4 cun caudal to the umbilicus	Front-Mu (Alarm) point of Bladder
CV-4 *Guan Yuan* Origin Pass	• Canine: On the ventral midline 3 cun caudal to the umbilicus. • Equine: 3 cun caudal to umbilicus	Front-Mu (Alarm) point for Small Intestine
CV-5 *Shi Men* Stone Gate	• Canine: On the ventral midline 2 cun caudal to the umbilicus. • Equine: Midway between pubic symphysis and umbilicus	Mu (Alarm) point for Triple Heater
CV-6 *Qi Hai* Sea of Qi	• Canine: On the ventral midline 1.5 cun caudal to the umbilicus.	
CV-12 *Zhong Wan* Middle Stomach	• Canine: On the ventral midline halfway between the umbilicus and the xiphoid process. • Equine: Midway between xiphoid and umbilicus	Influential for Yang (Fu) organs. Mu (Alarm) point for the Stomach Horses do not tolerate needling at this point
CV-14 *Ju Que* Great Palace	• Canine: On the ventral midline halfway between CV-12 and the xiphoid process (1/4 the distance from the xiphoid process towards the umbilicus). • Equine: At the xiphoid	Front-Mu (Alarm) point for Heart
CV-17 *Shan Zhong* Chest Center	• Canine: On the ventral midline in a depression at the level of the fourth intercostal space. • Equine: At the level of the caudal border of elbow	Front-Mu (Alarm) point for PC Influential point for Qi
CV-22 *Tian Tu* Celestial Chimney	• Canine: On the ventral midline at the tip of the manubrium.	

Governing Vessel Meridian (GV): Dorsal Midline

Name	Location	Indications
GV-1 *Chang Qiang* Long Strong	• Canine: In the depression on the dorsal midline halfway between the anus and base of the tail • Equine: Depression between the anus and the ventral aspect of the tail	Lou connecting point for CV Meridian
GV-3 *Yang Guan* Yang pass	• Canine: Variable location. It is the largest Deficiency point located between the dorsal process of L4-L5 or L5-L6 or L6-L7	
GV-4 *Ming Men* Life Gate	• Canine: On the midline, between the dorsal spinous processes of the 2nd and 3rd lumbar vertebrae. • Equine: 2nd lumbar vertebral space at the same level as BL-23	
GV-14 *Da Zhui* Big Vertebra	• Canine: In the depression on the dorsal midline between the C7-T1 dorsal spinous processes (T1 is the first palpable spinous process in the caudal neck level with the greater tubercles of the humerus) • Equine: Depression at the cervicothoracic vertebral space	Master point for fever
GV-17 *Nao Hu* Brain's Door	• Canine: In the depression on the dorsal midline on a line drawn from the caudal (trailing) edge of the ears just in front of the occipital protuberance	
GV-20 *Bai Hui* Hundred Meetings	• Canine: In the depression on the dorsal midline on a line drawn from the tips of the ears level with the center of the ear canals. • Equine: At the highest point of the poll	
GV-21 *Qian Ding* Before the Vertex	• Canine: In the depression on the dorsal midline on a line drawn from the cranial (leading) edge of the ears	
GV-26 *Ren Zhong* Human Center	• Canine: In the depression on the dorsal midline on a line drawn at the ventral limits of the nasal openings where it crossed the philtrum • Equine: Center of upper lip, between the ventral limits of the nostrils	

Classical Points:

Name	Location	Indications
An Shen Pacify Shen	• Halfway between GB-20 and TH-17 caudal to the ear base	Use for calming Shen, otitis, and deafness
Bai Hui Hundred Meetings	• Canine: In the depression on the dorsal midline just caudal to the wings of the ileum in the L7-S1 space. • Equine: On the dorsal midline at the lumbosacral space (L7-S1)	Use for hip, lumbar or pelvic limb disorders, colic, diarrhea, and Yang Deficiency
Ba Jiao Sacral Eight points	• Equine: Four points along the Bladder Meridian, at the first, second, third and fourth spaces between the dorsal spinous processes of the sacrum	Use for pain of the back, hips and hindquarters.
Ba Shan Attach to Mountain	• Canine: Bilaterally at the midpoint between *Bai Hui* and the sciatic tuber • Equine: Midpoint between *Bai Hui* and greater trochanter	Use for arthritis of the hip, sciatic paralysis, and injury of the loin and croup.
Cheng Deng Stirrup	• Equine: 2 cun ventrocaudal to the olecranon	Same as Yan Zhou
Chui Jing Drooping Eye	• Equine: Depression just above eye	Use for keratitis and conjunctivitis. Inject blood for acute eye problems
Da Feng Men Great Wind Gate	• Canine: On the dorsal midline between the cranial rim of the 2 ear bases (½ cun in front of GV-20) • Equine: Just in front of forelock	Use to relieve internal wind (Epilepsy, seizure, tremor, encephalitis, tetanus). Use for sedation by directing the needle towards the tail.
Dan Tian Pelvic Cavity	• Equine: 1.5 cun cranial and ventral to the tuber coxae	Use for infertility and hip arthritis
Da Zhui Great Vertebrae	• Canine: In the dorsal midline between C7 and T1	Use for fever and immune deficiency.
Ding Chuan Stopping Asthma	• Equine: 0.5 cun lateral to GV-14	
Duan Xue Stop Bleeding	• Equine: Three points on the dorsal midline. One is in the 17th thoracic vertebral space, another is in the thoracolumbar vertebral space and the third is in the first lumbar vertebral space	Use for any type of hemorrhage

Er Jian Ear Tip	• Canine: On the convex surface of the ear at the auricular vein on the tip of ear • Equine: Vein at tip of ear	Use for abdominal pain, fever, Wind-Heat, Heat, anhidrosis, heatstroke and colic.
Fei Men Lung Gate	• Equine: On the cranial border of the scapula, 1/3 of the distance from dorsal to ventral	Use for shoulder pain or injury, suprascapular nerve paralysis, lung and upper airway disease.
Fei Pan Lung Hugging	• Equine: On the caudal border of the scapula, 1/3 of the distance from dorsal to ventral	Similar to Fei Men but more for the lower airway and lung
Fen Shui Dividing Water	• Equine: The center of vortex pilus of the upper lip	Use for colic, facial paralysis, and shock
Gang Tui Anus Prolapse	• Canine: 1 cun bilateral to anus	Use to raise Spleen Qi
Gong Zi Shoulder Bow	• Equine: 3 cun from top of scapula, caudal to dorsal spine	Use for shoulder lameness and muscle atrophy and suprascapular nerve paralysis
Guan Yuan Shu Primary Qi Gate	• Canine: In the longissimus muscle groove, caudal to the last rib and cranial to the tip of transverse process of L1 • Equine: On Bladder Meridian, caudal to last rib	Use for diarrhea, poor appetite, abdominal pain, nausea, general weakness, and pain on lateral aspect of stifle and hind limb.
Hua Tuo Jia Ji Hua Tuo's Paravertebral Points	• Canine: 0.5 cun lateral to each vertebra	Use for IVDD
Hou Hai Back Sea	• Canine: In the depression between the anus and the ventral tail base	Use for diarrhea, constipation, rectal paralysis, and rectal prolapse.
Jiu Wei Cervical Nine Points	• Equine: Most cranial point is 1.5 cun caudal to BL-10 and 3.5 cm ventral to the mane, the most caudal point is 3 cun cranial to TH-15 and 5 cm ventral to the mane, the other seven points are located equidistantly between the most cranial and caudal points	Use for neck stiffness
Jiang Ya Ginger Bud	• Equine: Alar cartilage at lateral corner of nostril. Put the needle through the cartilage from lateral to medial and leave in 30 minutes	Use for colic

Liu Feng Six Seams	• Canine: Between the toes	Use for paresis or paralysis
Long Hui Dragon Meeting	• Canine: Central midline between the eyebrows • Equine: Midpoint on a line drawn from the lateral canthus of one eye to the other	Use for seizures and nasal congestion. Similar indications as *Da Feng Men*
Mi Jiao Gan Vagosympathetic Trunk	• Equine: Dorsal to jugular vein, at the junction of the cranial and middle 1/3 of neck	Use for diarrhea and indigestion
Ming Men Life Gate	• Canine: Dorsal midline between L2 and L3	Use for renal failure, lumbar pain, IVDD, diarrhea due to Yang Deficiency.
Qi Hai Shu Sea of Qi	• Equine: Along Bladder Meridian at 16th IC space	Use for weakness, gaseous bowel and to enhance performance
Qian Ti Men Heels of Hoof	• Equine: Two points on each front hoof, at the caudodorsal borders of each heel bulb	Use for laminitis and navicular disease
Qian Jiu Central Bulb	• Equine: On caudal midline of front hoof, proximal to the heel bulbs	Use for laminitis, navicular disease and chronic lameness
Qu Chi Pond on the curve	• Equine: Craniomedial aspect of the hock on the saphenous vein at the level of the dorsomedial talus (tibial tarsal bone)	Use for acute hock injury and chronic arthritis
Si Liao Four Points	• Canine: A group of 4 acupoints 0.5 cun lateral to the sacrum. The cranial point is at the first dorsal sacral foramina. The caudal point is at the second dorsal sacral foramina. The remaining 2 points are equidistantly located between the cranial and caudal points.	Use for lumbosacral pain, hind limb weakness, infertility, and metritis.
Shan Gen Mountain Base	• Canine: On the dorsal midline of boundary between hairy and non-hairy areas.	Use for poor appetite, sinusitis, coma, shock, Wind-Cold, Wind-Heat
Shui Gou Water Passage	• Canine: At the intersection between the dorsal middle 1/3 of the philtrum	Use for coma, shock, fever, bronchitis, Lung Heat, and facial paralysis.

Shen Jiao Kidney Corner	• Equine: 2 cun caudal to *Shen Shu*	Similar uses as *Bai Hui*
Shen Peng Kidney shelf	• Equine: 2 cun cranial to *Shen Shu*	Similar uses as *Bai Hui*
Shen Shu Kidney Hollow	• Equine: 2 cun lateral to Bai Hui	Use for Kidney Qi or Yin Deficiency, renal failure, deafness, urinary incontinence, edema, and back pain.
Shen Tang Kidney Hall	• Equine: 4 cun ventral to skin fold of thigh, on the saphenous vein	Use for acute hip and lumbar injury, laminitis, orchitis and scrotal inflammation
Tai Yang Great Yang	• Canine: In the depression about 1 cun posterior to the lateral canthus • Equine: 2 fingers from lateral canthus on transverse facial vein	Use for facial paralysis, headache, acute eye problems and anhidrosis
Tian Men Gate of Heaven	• Canine: On the dorsal midline between the caudal rim of the two ear bases.	Use for epilepsy, seizure, loss of voice, and dizziness.
Tian Ping Celestial Balance	• Canine: Between T13 and L1 on the dorsal midline.	Use for internal hemorrhage (hematuria, hemafecia) and to prevent minor surgical bleeding.
Tong Guan Passing Pass	• Equine: Veins on ventral surface of tongue, use hemoacupuncture	Use to promote appetite. Offer food immediately after acupuncture
Wei Jian Tail Tip	• Canine: Tip of the tail • Equine: At the tip of the tail, Hemoacupuncture point.	Use for tail paralysis, hind limb weakness, IVDD, anhidrosis, colic, heatstroke and shock
Wei Jie Tail Vertebrae	• Canine: Dorsal midline between Cd 1 and Cd 2	Use for tail paralysis and hind limb weakness.
Wei Duan Tail End	• Equine: At the sacral coccygeal space, 1.5 cun to the midline	Use for hindquarter injury, back pain and hind limb paralysis.
Wei Gen Tail Base	• Equine: On the mid line, in a depression at the first coccygeal vertebral space	Same as *Wei Duan*

Xi Yan Eye of the Knee	• Canine: In the depression below the patella and medial to the patellar ligament. Unrelated to any Meridian (referred to as the "medial eye of the knee" or *Xi Ao*) and ST-35 (Lateral eye of the knee) are both described as the point *Xi Yan*.	Stifle problems, rear limb weakness
Xiong Tang Thoracic vein	• Equine: Cephalic vein, cranial and dorsal to axilla, just at point where leg joins body. A hemoacupuncture point.	Use for acute shoulder and elbow injury, laminitis, anhidrosis and to clear Heat.
Yan Chi Wing of Ilium	• Equine: Midpoint between top of tuber coxa and *Shen Peng*	Use for mare infertility, poor athletic performance and hindquarter pain/arthritis
Yan Zhou Covering elbow	• Equine: In a depression 1.5 cun dorsomedial to the olecranon	Use for elbow joint pain and for sprains, arthritis and swelling
Yang Ling Yang Tomb	• Equine: In a depression 5 cun caudal to the patella	Used for stifle pain and pelvic lameness
Yao Yang Guan Lumbar Yang Gate	• Canine: Dorsal midline between L4 and L5	Use for lumbosacral IVDD and hind limb weakness.
Yin Tang Hall of Impression	• Canine: Midline between the eyebrows. *Yin Tang* is the same as *Long Hui*	Use for nasal congestion or discharge
Ying Xiang Receive Fragrance	• Canine: In the nasal labial groove at the level of the midpoint of the lateral border of the ala nasi.	Use for nasal congestion and facial paralysis Do NOT use Moxa
Yu Tang Jade Hall	• Equine: Hard palate, 0.5 cun lateral to center on 3rd transverse ridge of palate	Use for indigestion and gastrointestinal disorders. For Stomach Heat use hemoacupuncture.
Zhou Shu Elbow association point	• Equine: Between olecranon tuber and lateral epicondyle of humerus	Use for elbow joint pain or injury and arthritis.
Zhong Wan Middle Stomach	• Canine: Midpoint between CV-8 and the xiphoid process	Use for vomiting, food stasis, abdominal distention and diarrhea.

HERBAL FORMULAS

Herbal formulas are found in several forms including powders, capsules and teapills. High doses of powdered herbal medications for horses should be given via nasogastric tube. Lower doses of the powders can be applied as a top dressing on the food for both horses and small animals. Capsules or pills may be used for small animal patients. The general recommendations for administration are as follows:

Equine patients of average body weight

- High dosages via nasogastric tube: Give 200-250 grams once daily for 3 to 5 days.

- Top dressing on food: Give 15-30 grams twice daily for 1 to 2 months.

Small animal patients

- Powder mixed with food: Give ½ gram per 10 to 20 pounds body weight twice daily for 1 to 2 months.

- Capsules or teapills: Give 1 capsule or pill per 10 to 20 pounds body weight twice daily for 1 to 2 months.

Selected herbal formulas are found below by their Pin Yin names. The ingredients are listed by their English common name, Chinese name and scientific name.

An Gong Niu Huang Wan

	Common Name	Pin Yin	Botanical, Latin or Chemical Name
11%	Cattle gallstone	Niu Huang	*Calculus Bovis*
11%	Rhinoceros horn	Xi Jiao	*Rhinoceros unicornis L.*
3%	Musk	She Xiang	*Moschus moschiferus L.*
11%	Coptis root	Huang Lian	*Coptis chinensis Franch*
11%	Scutellaria root	Huang Qin	*Scutellaria baicalensis Georgi*
11%	Gardenia fruit	Zhi Zi	*Gardenia jasminoides Ellis*
11%	Realgar	Xiong Huang	*Arsenic disulfide ore*
3%	Borneol	Bing Pian	*Dryobalanops aromatica Gaertn. f.*
11%	Curcuma root	Yu Jin	*Curcuma aromatica Salisb.*
11%	Cinnabaris*	Zhu Sha	*Red mercuric sulfide*
6%	Pearl	Zhen Zhu	*Magarita; product of Pteria martensii (Dunker)*

* *Zhu Sha* contains the heavy metal mercury. May substitute Oyster *Mu Li*.

Ba Ji San

	Common Name	Pin Yin	Botanical Name
12%	Morinda root	Ba Ji Tian	*Morinda officinalis How*
12%	Cistanche	Rou Cong Rong	*Cistanche deserticola Y.C. Ma.*
12%	Psoralea	Bu Gu Zhi	*Psoralea corylifolia L.*
12%	Fenugreek seed	Hu Lu Ba	*Trigonella foenum-graecum L.*
6%	Cinnamon bark	Rou Gui	*Cinnamomum cassia Presl.*
8%	Nutmeg seed	Rou Dou Kou	*Myristica fragrans Houtt.*
8%	Fennel fruit	Hui Xiang	*Foeniculum vulgare Mill.*
8%	Citrus peel	Chen Pi	*Citrus reticulata Blanco*
8%	Green tangerine peel	Qing Pi	*Citrus reticulata Blanco*
5%	Sichuan chinaberry	Chuan Lian Zi	*Melia toosendan Sieb.*
4%	Areca seed	Bing Lang	*Areca catechu L.*
5%	Akebia stem	Mu Tong	*Akebia trifoliata (Thunb.) Koidz var. australis*

Ba Zhen Tang

	Common Name	Pin Yin	Botanical Name
10%	Ginseng	Ren Shen	*Panax ginseng C. A. Mey.*
15%	White Atractylodes	Bai Zhu	*Atractylodes macrocephala Koidz*
15%	Poria	Fu Ling	*Poria cocos (Schw.) Wolf*
8%	Licorice root	Gan Cao	*Glycyrrhiza uralensis Fisch.*
15%	Prepared rehmannia root	Shu Di Huang	*Rehmannia glutinosa Libosch*
15%	Chinese angelica root	Dang Gui	*Angelica sinensis (Oliv.) Diels*
12%	White peony root	Bai Shao Yao	*Paeonia lactiflora Pall.*
10%	Ligusticum rhizome	Chuan Xiong	*Ligusticum wallichii Franch*

Ba Zheng San

	Common Name	Pin Yin	Botanical or Chemical Name
15%	Dianthus	Qu Mai	*Dianthus chinensis L.*
12%	Gardenia fruit	Zhi Zi	*Gardenia jasminoides Ellis*
7%	Licorice root	Gan Cao	*Glycyrrhiza uralensis Fisch.*
12%	Juncus	Deng Xin Cao	*Juncus effuses L. var. decipiens Buchen.*
12%	Plantago seed	Che Qian Zi	*Plantago asiatica L.*
12%	Rhubarb root	Da Huang	*Rheum palmatum L.*
15%	Talc	Hua Shi	*Hydrous magnesium silicate*
15%	Akebia stem	Mu Tong	*Akebia trifoliata (Thunb.) Koidz var. australis*

Bai He Gu Jin Tang

	Common Name	Pin Yin	Botanical Name
8%	Chinese angelica root	Dang Gui	*Angelica sinensis (Oliv.) Diels*
8%	Tendrilled fritillaria bulb	Chuan Bei Mu	*Fritillaria cirrhosa D. Don*
5%	Licorice root	Gan Cao	*Glycyrrhiza uralensis Fisch.*
13%	Lily bulb	Bai He	*Lillium brownii F.E. Brown var. colchesteri*
13%	Ophiopogon root	Mai Men Dong	*Ophiopogon japonicus Krt-Gawler*
8%	White peony root	Bai Shao Yao	*Paeonia lactiflora Pall.*
8%	Platycodon root	Jie Geng	*Platycodon grandiflorum (Jacq.) A. DC*
16%	Raw rehmannia root	Sheng Di Huang	*Rehmannia glutinosa Libosch*
16%	Prepared rehmannia root	Shu Di Huang	*Rehmannia glutinosa Libosch*
5%	Scrophularia	Xuan Shen	*Scrophularia ningpoensis Hemsl.*

Bai He Gu Jin Tang Modification

	Common Name	Pin Yin	Botanical Name
7%	Chinese angelica root	Dang Gui	*Angelica sinensis (Oliv.) Diels*
10%	White Atractylodes	Bai Zhu	*Atractylodes macrocephala Koidz*
7%	Tendrilled fritillaria bulb	Chuan Bei Mu	*Fritillaria cirrhosa D. Don*
10%	Ginseng	Ren Shen	*Panax ginseng C. A. Mey.*
5%	Licorice root	Gan Cao	*Glycyrrhiza uralensis Fisch.*
10%	Lily bulb	Bai He	*Lillium brownii F.E. Brown var. colchesteri*
10%	Ophiopogon root	Mai Men Dong	*Ophiopogon japonicus Krt-Gawler*
8%	White peony root	Bai Shao Yao	*Paeonia lactiflora Pall.*
8%	Platycodon root	Jie Geng	*Platycodon grandiflorum (Jacq.) A. DC*
10%	Raw rehmannia root	Sheng Di Huang	*Rehmannia glutinosa Libosch*
10%	Prepared rehmannia root	Shu Di Huang	*Rehmannia glutinosa Libosch*
5%	Scrophularia	Xuan Shen	*Scrophularia ningpoensis Hemsl.*

Bai Hu Tang

	Common Name	Pin Yin	Botanical or Chemical Name
20%	Anemarrhena rhizome	Zhi Mu	*Anemarrhena asphodeloides Bunge*
10%	Licorice root	Gan Cao	*Glycyrrhiza uralensis Fisch.*
50%	Gypsum fibrosum	Shi Gao	*Calcium sulphate*
20%	Oryza (rice)	Jing Mi	*Oryza sativa L.*

Bai Zhu San

	Common Name	Pin Yin	Botanical Name or Animal Species
12%	White Atractylodes	Bai Zhu	*Atractylodes macrocephala Koidz*
10%	Pilose asiabell root	Dang Shen	*Codonopsis pilosula (Franch.) Nannf.*
10%	Chinese angelica root	Dang Gui	*Angelica sinensis (Oliv.) Diels*
12%	Prepared rehmannia root	Shu Di Huang	*Rehmannia glutinosa Libosch*
8%	Ligusticum rhizome	Chuan Xiong	*Ligusticum wallichii Franch*
8%	White peony root	Bai Shao Yao	*Paeonia lactiflora Pall.*
10%	Donkey-hide gelatin	E Jiao	*Equus asinus L.*
5%	Citrus peel	Chen Pi	*Citrus reticulata Blanco*
6%	Cardamon fruit	Sha Ren	*Amomum villosum Lour.*
8%	Scutellaria root	Huang Qin	*Scutellaria baicalensis Georgi*
5%	Licorice root	Gan Cao	*Glycyrrhiza uralensis Fisch*
6%	Perilla Leaf	Zi Su Ye	*Perilla frutescens (L.)Britt. Var. crispa*

Bao He Wan

	Common Name	Pin Yin	Botanical or Latin Name
11%	Citrus peel	Chen Pi	*Citrus reticulata Blanco*
11%	Forsythia fruit	Lian Qiao	*Forsythia suspensa (Thunb.) Vahl*
23%	Hawthorn fruit	Shan Zha	*Crataegus pinnatifida Bge var major N.E.Br.*
22%	Medicated leaven	Shen Qu	*Massa Fermentata Medicinalis*
11%	Pinellia tuber	Ban Xia	*Pinellia ternata (Thunb.) Breit*
11%	Poria	Fu Ling	*Poria cocos (Schw.) Wolf*
11%	Radish seed	Lai Fu Zi	*Raphanus sativus L.*

Bao Yuan Tang

	Common Name	Pin Yin	Botanical Name
30%	Astragalus root	Huang Qi	*Astragalus membranaceus (Fisch.) Bge.*
35%	Cinnamon twig	Gui Zhi	*Cinnamomum cassia Presl.*
20%	Ginseng	Ren Shen	*Panax ginseng C. A. Mey.*
15%	Licorice root	Gan Cao	*Glycyrrhiza uralensis Fisch.*

Bi Xie Sheng Shi Tang

	Common Name	Pin Yin	Botanical Name
10%	Black cardamon seed	Yi Zhi Ren	*Alpinia oxyphylla Miq.*
10%	Moutan bark	Mu Dan Pi	*Paeonia suffruticosa Andr.*
10%	Poria	Fu Ling	*Poria cocos (Schw.) Wolf*
10%	Hypoglauca	Bi Xie	*Dioscorea hypoglauca Palib.*
10%	Dictamnus root-bark	Bai Xian Pi	*Dictamnus dasycarphus Turcz.*
10%	Rice paper pith	Tong Cao	*Tetrapanax papyriferus (Hook.) K. Koch*
10%	Gardenia fruit	Zhi Zi	*Gardenia jasminoides Ellis*
10%	Phellodendron bark	Huang Bai	*Phellodendron amourense Rupr.*
10%	Atractylodes rhizome	Cang Zhu	*Atractylodes lancea (Thunb.) DC.*
10%	Alisma tuber	Ze Xie	*Alisma plantago-aquatica L var orientala*

Bing Peng San

	Common Name	Pin Yin	Botanical or Chemical Name
45%	Dehydrated mirabilite	Xuan Ming Fen	*Mirabilitum Purum*
45%	Borax	Peng Sha	*Sodium tetraborate*
5%	Borneol	Bing Pian	*Dryobalanops aromatica Gaertn. f.*
5%	Cinnabaris*	Zhu Sha	*Red mercuric sulfide*

* Warning: *Zhu Sha* contains Mercury. Only use low dosages topically for a short time. Over-dosage or long-term use can cause mercury poisoning.

Bu Fei San

	Common Name	Pin Yin	Botanical Name
15%	Aster root	Zi Wan	*Aster tataricus L. F.*
20%	Astragalus root	Huang Qi	*Astragalus membranaceus (Fisch.) Bge.*
15%	Pilose asiabell root	Dang Shen	*Codonopsis pilosula (Franch.) Nannf.*
15%	Mulberry bark	Sang Bai Pi	*Morus alba L*
20%	Prepared rehmannia root	Shu Di Huang	*Rehmannia glutinosa Libosch*
15%	Schisandra fruit	Wu Wei Zi	*Schisandra chinensis Baill.*

Bu Xin Dan

	Common Name	Pin Yin	Botanical or Chemical Name
8%	Chinese angelica root	Dang Gui	*Angelica sinensis (Oliv) Diels*
8%	Asparagus tuber	Tian Men Dong	*Asparagus cochinchinensis Merr.*
5%	Biota seed	Bai Zi Ren	*Biota orientalis (L.) Endl.*
3%	Cinnabaris*	Zhu Sha	*Red mercuric sulfide*
8%	Pilose asiabell root	Dang Shen	*Codonopsis pilosula (Franch.) Nannf.*
8%	Ophiopogon root	Mai Men Dong	*Ophiopogon japonicus Krt-Gawler*
5%	Platycodon root	Jie Geng	*Platycodon grandiflorum (Jacq.) A. DC*
8%	Polygala root	Yuan Zhi	Polygala tenuifolia Willd.
8%	Poria	Fu Ling	*Poria cocos (Schw.) Wolf*
10%	Raw rehmannia root	Sheng Di Huang	*Rehmannia glutinosa Libosch*
8%	Salvia root	Dan Shen	*Salvia miltiorrhiza Bunge*
8%	Schisandra fruit	Wu Wei Zi	*Schisandra chinensis Baill.*
8%	Scrophularia root	Xuan Shen	*Scrophularia ningpoensis Hemsl.*
5%	Zizyphus seed	Suan Zao Ren	*Zizyphus spinosa Hu*

* Contains the heavy metal mercury. May substitute Oyster *Mu Li.*

Bu Xue Xi Feng San

	Common Name	Pin Yin	Botanical Name or Animal Species
10%	Pilose asiabell root	Dang Shen	*Codonopsis pilosula (Franch.) Nannf.*
10%	White Atractylodes	Bai Zhu	*Atractylodes macrocephala Koidz*
10%	Chinese angelica root	Dang Gui	*Angelica sinensis (Oliv.) Diels*
10%	Prepared rehmannia root	Shu Di Huang	*Rehmannia glutinosa Libosch*
10%	Ligusticum rhizome	Chuan Xiong	*Ligusticum wallichii Franch*
10%	White peony root	Bai Shao Yao	*Paeonia lactiflora Pall.*
12%	Uncaria stem with hooks	Gou Teng	*Uncaria sinensis (Oliv) Havil*
12%	Silkworm	Jiang Can	*Beauveria bassiana infects Bombyx mori L.*
8%	Cicada moulted shell	Chan Tui	*Cryptotympana atrata Fabr.*
8%	Typhonium rhizome	Bai Fu Zi	*Typhonium giganteum Engl.*

Bu Yang Huan Wu Tang

Common Name		Pin Yin	Botanical Name or Animal Species
84%	Baked astragalus root	Huang Qi	*Astragalus membranaceus (Fisch.) Bge.*
5%	Chinese angelica root	Dang Gui	*Angelica sinensis (Oliv.) Diels*
3%	White peony root	Bai Shao Yao	*Paeonia lactiflora Pall.*
2%	Earthworm	Di Long	*Pheretima aspergillum Perrier*
2%	Ligusticum rhizome	Chuan Xiong	*Ligusticum wallichii Franch*
2%	Safflower flower	Hong Hua	*Carthamus tinctorius L.*
2%	Peach kernel	Tao Ren	*Prunus persica (L.) Batsch*

Bu Zhong Yi Qi Tang

Common Name		Pin Yin	Botanical Name
24%	Baked astragalus root	Huang Qi	*Astragalus membranaceus (Fisch.) Bge.*
8%	Baked licorice root	Gan Cao	*Glycyrrhiza uralensis Fisch.*
5%	Bupleurum root	Chai Hu	*Bupleurum chinense DC.*
16%	Chinese angelica root	Dang Gui	*Angelica sinensis (Oliv) Diels*
5%	Cimicifuga rhizome	Sheng Ma	*Cimicifuga foetida L.*
10%	Citrus peel	Chen Pi	*Citrus reticulata Blanco*
16%	Ginseng	Ren Shen	*Panax ginseng C. A. Mey.*
16%	White Atractylodes	Bai Zhu	*Atractylodes macrocephala Koidz*

Cang Zhu Bai Hu Tang

Common Name		Pin Yin	Botanical or Chemical Name
20%	Anemarrhena rhizome	Zhi Mu	*Anemarrhena asphodeloides, Bunge*
10%	Licorice root	Gan Cao	*Glycyrrhiza uralensis Fisch.*
30%	Gypsum fibrosum	Shi Gao	*Calcium sulphate*
20%	Oryza (rice)	Jing Mi	*Oryza sativa L.*
20%	Atractylodes rhizome	Cang Zhu	*Atractylodes lancea (Thunb.) DC.*

Chai Hu Gui Zhi Tang

Common Name		Pin Yin	Botanical Name
15%	Bupleurum root	Chai Hu	*Bupleurum chinense DC.*
15%	Cinnamon twig	Gui Zhi	*Cinnamomum cassia Presl.*
10%	Ginseng	Ren Shen	*Panax ginseng C. A. Mey.*
10%	Licorice root	Gan Cao	*Glycyrrhiza uralensis Fisch.*
10%	Jujube	Da Zao	*Ziziphus jujuba Mill var. inermis (Bge.) Rehd.*
10%	White peony root	Bai Shao Yao	*Paeonia lactiflora Pall.*
10%	Pinellia tuber	Ban Xia	*Pinellia ternata (Thunb.) Breit*
10%	Scutellaria root	Huang Qin	*Scutellaria baicalensis Georgi*
10%	Fresh ginger rhizome	Sheng Jiang	*Zingiber officinale Rosc.*

Chai Hu Shu Gan Wan

Common Name		Pin Yin	Botanical Name
9%	Nut-grass rhizome	Xiang Fu	*Cyperus rotundus L.*
6%	White peony root	Bai Shao Yao	*Paeonia lactiflora Pall.*
6%	Corydalis tuber	Yan Hu Suo	*Corydalis yanhusuo W.T. Wang*
6%	Citrus peel	Chen Pi	*Citrus reticulata Blanco*
6%	Immature bitter orange	Zhi Shi	*Citrus aurantium L.*
6%	Magnolia Bark	Hou Po	*Magnolia officinalis, Rehd. et Wils.*
6%	Moutan bark	Mu Dan Pi	*Paeonia suffruticosa Andr.*
6%	Cardamon fruit	Sha Ren	*Amomum villosum Lour.*
6%	Green tangerine peel	Qing Pi	*Citrus reticutata Blanco*
9%	Bupleurum root	Chai Hu	*Bupleurum chinense DC.*
3%	Licorice root	Gan Cao	*Glycyrrhiza uralensis Fisch.*
7%	Saussurea root	Mu Xiang	*Saussurea lappa Clarke*
6%	Citrus, Buddha's hand	Fo Shou	*Citrus medica L. var. sarcodactylis (Noot.)*
6%	Aquilaria	Chen Xiang	*Aquilaria agallocha Roxb.*
6%	Cardamon fruit	Bai Dou Kou	*Amomum cardamomum L.*
6%	Sandalwood	Tan Xiang	*Santalum album L.*

Chui Bi San

Common Name		Pin Yin	Botanical Name
20%	Sichuan Pepper	Chuan Jiao	*Zanthoxylum bungeanum Maxim.*
20%	Veratrum	Li Lu	*Veratrum nigrum L.*
20%	Dahurian Angelica	Bai Zhi	*Angelica dahurica (Fisch. ex Hoffm.) Benth*
20%	Pinellia tuber	Ban Xia	*Pinellia ternata (Thunb.) Breit*
20%	Gleditsia fruit	Zao Jiao	*Gleditsia sinensis Lam.*

Da Bu Yin Wan

Common Name		Pin Yin	Botanical Name or Animal Species
22%	Anemarrhena rhizome	Zhi Mu	*Anemarrhena asphodeloides, Bunge*
22%	Phellodendron bark	Huang Bai	*Phellodendron amourense, Rupr.*
28%	Prepared rehmannia root	Shu Di Huang	*Rehmannia glutinosa Libosch*
28%	Tortoise plastron	Gui Ban	*Chinemys reevesil (Gray)*

Da Chai Hu Tang

Common Name		Pin Yin	Botanical or Chemical Name
10%	Immature bitter orange	Zhi Shi	*Citrus aurantium L.*
15%	Bupleurum root	Chai Hu	*Bupleurum chinense DC.*
10%	Jujube	Da Zao	*Ziziphus jujuba Mill var. inermis (Bge.) Rehd.*
10%	Mirabilite	Mang Xiao	*Sodium Sulfate*
10%	White peony root	Bai Shao Yao	*Paeonia lactiflora Pall.*
10%	Pinellia tuber	Ban Xia	*Pinellia ternata (Thunb.) Breit*
10%	Rhubarb root	Da Huang	*Rheum palmatum L.*
15%	Scutellaria root	Huang Qin	*Scutellaria baicalensis Georgi*
10%	Fresh ginger rhizome	Sheng Jiang	*Zingiber officinale Rosc.*

Da Cheng Qi Tang

Common Name		Pin Yin	Botanical Name
20%	Immature bitter orange	Zhi Shi	*Citrus aurantium L.*
15%	Magnolia Bark	Hou Po	*Magnolia officinalis, Rehd. et Wils.*
45%	Mirabilite	Mang Xiao	*Sodium Sulfate*
20%	Rhubarb root	Da Huang	*Rheum palmatum L.*

Da Ding Feng Zhu

	Common Name	Pin Yin	Botanical Name or Animal Species
13%	Fresh egg yolk	Ji Zi Huang	*Egg yolk of Gallus gallus domesticus*
7%	Donkey-hide gelatin	E Jiao	*Equus asinus L.*
13%	White peony root	Bai Shao Yao	*Paeonia lactiflora Pall.*
8%	Licorice root	Gan Cao	*Glycyrrhiza uralensis Fisch.*
5%	Schisandra fruit	Wu Wei Zi	*Schisandra chinensis Baill.*
13%	Raw rehmannia root	Sheng Di Huang	*Rehmannia glutinosa Libosch*
13%	Ophiopogon root	Mai Men Dong	*Ophiopogon japonicus Krt-Gawler*
5%	Cannabis	Huo Ma Ren	*Cannabis sativa L.*
9%	Tortoise plastron	Gui Ban	*Chinemys reevesil (Gray)*
5%	Soft-shelled turtle shell	Bie Jia	*Amyda sinensis (Wiegmann)*
9%	Oyster Shell	Mu Li	*Ostrea gigas Thunb.*

Da Xiang Lian San

	Common Name	Pin Yin	Botanical Name
58%	Saussurea root	Mu Xiang	*Saussurea lappa Clarke*
29%	Coptis root	Huang Lian	*Coptis chinensis Franch*
13%	Evodia	Wu Zhu Yu	*Evodia rutaecarpa (Juss.) Benth.*

Dang Gui Bu Xue Tang

	Common Name	Pin Yin	Botanical Name
83%	Baked astragalus root	Huang Qi	*Astragalus membranaceus (Fisch.) Bge.*
17%	Chinese angelica root	Dang Gui	*Angelica sinensis (Oliv.) Diels*

Di Er You

	Common Name	Pin Yin	Botanical or Chemical Name
27.5%	Alum	Bai Fan	*Aluminium potassium sulfate crystals*
0.5%	Borneol	Bing Pian	*Dryobalanops aromatica Gaertn. f.*
72%	Coptis root	Huang Lian	*Coptis chinensis Franch*
1,000 ml	Glycerol	Gan You	*Glycerol*

Di Gu Pi Powder

Common Name		Pin Yin	Botanical Name
8%	Lycium root-bark	Di Gu Pi	*Lycium chinense Mill.*
6%	Moutan bark	Mu Dan Pi	*Paeonia suffruticosa Andr.*
15%	Prepared rehmannia root	Shu Di Huang	*Rehmannia glutinosa Libosch*
10%	Cistanche	Rou Cong Rong	*Cistanche deserticola Y.C. Ma.*
7%	Gentian root	Qin Jiao	*Gentiana macrophylla Pall*
8%	Psoralea	Bu Gu Zhi	*Psoralea corylifolia L.*
8%	Drynaria rhizome	Gu Sui Bu	*Drynaria fortunei (Kunze) J. Sm.*
8%	Eucommia bark	Du Zhong	*Eucommia ulmoides Oliv.*
6%	Alisma tuber	Ze Xie	*Alisma plantago-aquatica L var orientala*
5%	Salvia root	Dan Shen	*Salvia miltiorrhiza Bunge*
7%	Chinese clematis root	Wei Ling Xian	*Clematis chinensis Osbeck*
5%	Chinese angelica root	Dang Gui	*Angelica sinensis (Oliv.) Diels*
7%	Phellodendron bark	Huang Bai	*Phellodendron amourense Rupr.*

Ding Tong San

Common Name		Pin Yin	Botanical Name
33%	Chinese angelica root	Dang Gui	*Angelica sinensis (Oliv.) Diels*
17%	Safflower flower	Hong Hua	*Carthamus tinctorius L.*
17%	Myrrh	Mo Yao	*Commiphora myrrha Engl.*
17%	Frankincense	Ru Xiang	*Boswellia carterii Birdw.*
16%	Dragon's Blood	Xue Jie	*Resin of Daemonorops draco Bl.*

Ding Xian Wan

Common Name		Pin Yin	Botanical Name or Animal Species
6%	Pinellia tuber	Ban Xia	*Pinellia ternata (Thunb.) Breit*
3%	Arisaema with bile	Dan Nan Xing	*Arisaemae cum Felle Bovis*
4%	Citrus peel	Chen Pi	*Citrus reticulata Blanco*
6%	Tendrilled fritillaria bulb	Chuan Bei Mu	*Fritillaria cirrhosa D. Don*
6%	Poria	Fu Ling	*Poria cocos (Schw.) Wolf*
12%	Ophiopogon root	Mai Men Dong	*Ophiopogon japonicus Krt-Gawler*
12%	Salvia root	Dan Shen	*Salvia miltiorrhiza Bunge*
3%	Acorus rhizome	Shi Chang Pu	*Acorus gramineus Soland.*
3%	Dried Scorpion body	Quan Xie	*Buthus martensi Karsch*
3%	Silkworm	Jiang Can	*Beauveria bassiana infects Bombyx mori L.*
6%	Gastrodia tuber	Tian Ma	*Gastrodia elata Bl.*
1%	Cinnabaris*	Zhu Sha	*Red mercuric sulfide*
4%	Polygala root	Yuan Zhi	*Polygala tenuifolia Willd.*
3%	Juncus	Deng Xin Cao	*Juncus effuses L. var. decipiens Buchen.*
6%	Poria	Fu Shen	*Poria Cocos (Schw.) Wolf*
3%	Amber	Hu Po	*Succinum*
2%	Licorice root	Gan Cao	*Glycyrrhiza uralensis Fisch.*
2%	Fresh ginger rhizome	Sheng Jiang	*Zingiber officinale Rosc.*
15%	Bamboo sap	Zhu Li	*Phyllostachys nigra Munro var. henonis*

* Contains the heavy metal mercury. May substitute Oyster *Mu Li.*

Du Huo Ji Sheng Tang

Common Name		Pin Yin	Botanical Name
8%	Pubescent angelica root	Du Huo	*Angelica pubescens Maxim.*
7%	Gentian root	Qin Jiao	*Gentiana macrophylla Pall*
6%	Ledebouriella root	Fang Feng	*Ledebouriella divaricata Hiroe*
3%	Asarum herb	Xi Xin	*Asarum sieboldi Miq.*
7%	Achyranthes	Niu Xi	*Achyranthes bidentata Bl.*
13%	Mulberry mistletoe	Sang Ji Sheng	*Loranthus parasiticus Merr.*
7%	Eucommia bark	Du Zhong	*Eucommia ulmoides Oliv.*
10%	Prepared rehmannia root	Shu Di Huang	*Rehmannia glutinosa Libosch*
7%	Chinese angelica root	Dang Gui	*Angelica sinensis (Oliv.) Diels*
6%	White peony root	Bai Shao Yao	*Paeonia lactiflora Pall.*
6%	Ligusticum rhizome	Chuan Xiong	*Ligusticum wallichii Franch*
4%	Cinnamon bark	Rou Gui	*Cinnamomum cassia Presl.*
6%	Ginseng	Ren Shen	*Panax ginseng C. A. Mey.*
6%	Poria	Fu Ling	*Poria cocos (Schw.) Wolf*
4%	Licorice root	Gan Cao	*Glycyrrhiza uralensis Fisch.*

Er Miao San

	Common Name	Pin Yin	Botanical Name
50%	Phellodendron bark	Huang Bai	*Phellodendron amourense Rupr.*
50%	Atractylodes rhizome	Cang Zhu	*Atractylodes lancea (Thunb.) DC.*

Er Chen Tang

	Common Name	Pin Yin	Botanical Name
30%	Citrus peel	Chen Pi	*Citrus reticulata Blanco*
20%	Licorice root	Gan Cao	*Glycyrrhiza uralensis Fisch.*
20%	Pinellia tuber	Ban Xia	*Pinellia ternata (Thunb.) Breit*
30%	Poria	Fu Ling	*Poria cocos (Schw.) Wolf*

Er Chen Tang Modification

	Common Name	Pin Yin	Botanical Name
8%	Jack-in-the-pulpit rhizome	Tian Nan Xing	*Arisaema consanguineum Schott*
16%	Immature bitter orange	Zhi Shi	*Citrus aurantium L.*
8%	Borneol	Bing Pian	*Dryobalanops aromatica Gaertn. f.*
18%	Citrus peel	Chen Pi	*Citrus reticulata Blanco*
12%	Licorice root	Gan Cao	*Glycyrrhiza uralensis Fisch.*
15%	Pinellia tuber	Ban Xia	*Pinellia ternata (Thunb.) Breit*
15%	Poria	Fu Ling	*Poria cocos (Schw.) Wolf*
8%	Typhonium rhizome	Bai Fu Zi	*Typhonium giganteum Engl.*

Fang Feng Tang

	Common Name	Pin Yin	Botanical Name
18%	Ledebouriella root	Fang Feng	*Ledebouriella divaricata Hiroe*
18%	Schizonepeta	Jing Jie	*Schizonepeta tenuifolia Briq.*
16%	Peppermint	Bo He	*Mentha haplocalyx Briq.*
16%	Phellodendron bark	Huang Bai	*Phellodendron amourense Rupr.*
16%	Sophora root	Ku Shen	*Sophora flavescens Ait.*
16%	Sichuan Pepper	Chuan Jiao	*Zanthoxylum bungeanum Maxim.*

Fang Feng Tong Sheng San

	Common Name	Pin Yin	Botanical or Chemical Name
5%	Chinese angelica root	Dang Gui	*Angelica sinensis (Oliv) Diels*
5%	White atractylodes	Bai Zhu	*Atractylodes macrocephala Koidz*
5%	Talcum	Hua Shi	*Talcum*
5%	Ephedra	Ma Huang	*Ephedra sinica Stapf*
5%	Forsythia fruit	Lian Qiao	*Forsythia suspensa (Thunb.) Vahl*
5%	Gardenia fruit	Zhi Zi	*Gardenia jasminoides Ellis*
5%	Licorice root	Gan Cao	*Glycyrrhiza uralensis Fisch.*
10%	Gypsum fibrosum	Shi Gao	*Calcium sulphate*
8%	Ledebouriella root	Fang Feng	*Ledebouriella divaricata Hiroe*
5%	Ligusticum rhizome	Chuan Xiong	*Ligusticum wallichii Franch*
5%	Peppermint	Bo He	*Mentha haplocalyx Briq.*
5%	Mirabilite	Mang Xiao	*Sodium Sulfate*
5%	White peony root	Bai Shao Yao	*Paeonia lactiflora Pall.*
5%	Platycodon root	Jie Geng	*Platycodon grandiflorum (Jacq.) A. DC*
5%	Rhubarb root	Da Huang	*Rheum palmatum L.*
7%	Schizonepeta	Jing Jie	*Schizonepeta tenuifolia Briq.*
5%	Scutellaria root	Huang Qin	*Scutellaria baicalensis Georgi*
5%	Fresh ginger rhizome	Sheng Jiang	*Zingiber officinale Rosc.*

Gan Mai Da Zao Tang

	Common Name	Pin Yin	Botanical Name
34%	Baked licorice root	Zhi Gan Cao	*Glycyrrhiza uralensis Fisch.*
33%	Wheat grain	Fu Xiao Mai	*Triticum aestivum L.*
33%	Jujube	Da Zao	*Ziziphus jujuba Mill var. inermis (Bge.) Rehd.*

Ge Gen San

	Common Name	Pin Yin	Botanical Name
15%	Pueraria root	Ge Gen	*Pueraria lobata (Willd.) Ohwi.*
10%	White peony root	Bai Shao Yao	*Paeonia lactiflora Pall.*
10%	Millettia	Ji Xue Teng	*Millettia dielsiana Harms.*
10%	Cinnamon twig	Gui Zhi	*Cinnamomum cassia Presl.*
10%	Chinese angelica root	Dang Gui	*Angelica sinensis (Oliv.) Diels*
10%	Ligusticum rhizome	Chuan Xiong	*Ligusticum wallichii Franch*
10%	Chaenomeles fruit	Mu Gua	*Chaenomeles lagenaria (Loisel.) Koidz.*
10%	Chinese clematis root	Wei Ling Xian	*Clematis chinensis Osbeck*
5%	Licorice root	Gan Cao	*Glycyrrhiza uralensis Fisch.*
10%	Notopterygium root	Qiang Huo	*Notopterygium incisum Ting ex HT Chang*

Gui Pi Tang

Common Name		Pin Yin	Botanical Name
12%	Astragalus root	Huang Qi	*Astragalus membranaceus (Fisch.) Bge.*
5%	Baked licorice root	Zhi Gan Cao	*Glycyrrhiza uralensis Fisch.*
10%	Chinese angelica root	Dang Gui	*Angelica sinensis (Oliv) Diels*
8%	Fresh ginger rhizome	Sheng Jiang	*Zingiber officinale Rosc.*
10%	Ginseng	Ren Shen	*Panax ginseng C. A. Mey.*
5%	Jujube	Da Zao	*Ziziphus jujuba Mill var. inermis (Bge.) Rehd.*
10%	Longan aril	Long Yan Rou	*Euphoria longan (Lour.) Steud*
10%	Polygala root	Yuan Zhi	*Polygala tenuifolia, Willd.*
5%	Poria	Fu Ling	*Poria cocos (Schw.) Wolf*
5%	Saussurea root	Mu Xiang	*Saussurea lappa Clarke*
10%	White atractylodes	Bai Zhu	*Atractylodes macrocephala Koidz*
10%	Wild jujube	Suan Zao Ren	*Ziziphus jujube Mill. var. spinosa Hu*

Gui Xing San

Common Name		Pin Yin	Botanical Name
9%	Black cardamon seed	Yi Zhi Ren	*Alpinia oxyphylla Miq.*
8%	Cardamon fruit	Sha Ren	*Amomum villosum Lour.*
8%	Chinese angelica root	Dang Gui	*Angelica sinensis (Oliv) Diels*
10%	White atractylodes	Bai Zhu	*Atractylodes macrocephala Koidz*
9%	Cinnamon bark	Rou Gui	*Cinnamomum cassia Presl.*
10%	Citrus peel	Chen Pi	*Citrus reticulata Blanco*
8%	Green tangerine peel	Qing Pi	*Citrus reticutata Blanco*
10%	Dry ginger	Gan Jiang	*Zingiber officinale Rosc.*
6%	Licorice root	Gan Cao	*Glycyrrhiza uralensis Fisch.*
8%	Magnolia Bark	Hou Po	*Magnolia officinalis Rehd. et Wils.*
8%	Nutmeg seed	Rou Dou Kou	*Myristica fragrans Houtt.*
6%	Schisandra fruit	Wu Wei Zi	*Schisandra chinensis Baill.*

Gui Zhi Tang

Common Name		Pin Yin	Botanical Name
20%	Cinnamon twig	Gui Zhi	*Cinnamomum cassia Presl.*
10%	Licorice root	Gan Cao	*Glycyrrhiza uralensis Fisch.*
25%	Jujube	Da Zao	*Ziziphus jujuba Mill var. inermis (Bge.) Rehd.*
20%	White peony root	Bai Shao Yao	*Paeonia lactiflora Pall.*
25%	Fresh ginger	Sheng Jiang	*Zingiber officinale Rosc.*

Huang Lian Bai Hu Tang

Common Name		Pin Yin	Botanical Name or Chemical Name
20%	Anemarrhena rhizome	Zhi Mu	*Anemarrhena asphodeloides, Bunge*
10%	Licorice root	Gan Cao	*Glycyrrhiza uralensis Fisch.*
30%	Gypsum fibrosum	Shi Gao	*Calcium sulphate*
20%	Oryza (rice)	Jing Mi	*Oryza sativa L.*
23%	Coptis root	Huang Lian	*Coptis chinensis Franch*

Huang Lian Jie Du Tang

Common Name		Pin Yin	Botanical Name
23%	Coptis root	Huang Lian	*Coptis chinensis Franch*
31%	Gardenia fruit	Zhi Zi	*Gardenia jasminoides Ellis*
23%	Phellodendron bark	Huang Bai	*Phellodendron amourense Rupr.*
23%	Scutellaria root	Huang Qin	*Scutellaria baicalensis Georgi*

Hui Xiang San

Common Name		Pin Yin	Botanical Name
8%	Chinese angelica root	Dang Gui	*Angelica sinensis (Oliv) Diels*
3%	Asarum herb	*Xi Xin*	*Asarum sieboldi Miq.*
7%	Cinnamon bark	Rou Gui	*Cinnamomum cassia Presl.*
7%	Citrus peel	Chen Pi	*Citrus reticulata Blanco*
6%	Green tangerine peel	Qing Pi	*Citrus reticutata Blanco*
9%	Fennel fruit	Hui Xiang	*Foeniculum vulgare Mill.*
6%	Ligusticum	Gao Ben	*Ligusticum sinense Oliv.*
7%	Sichuan chinaberry	Chuan Lian Zi	*Melia toosendan Sieb.*
8%	Morinda root	Ba Ji Tian	*Morinda officinalis How*
6%	Nutmeg seed	Rou Dou Kou	*Myristica fragrans Houtt.*
5%	Pharbitis	Qian Niu Zi	*Pharbitis nil (L.) Choisy*
8%	Piper fruit	Bi Cheng Qie	*Piper cubeba L.*
8%	Psoralea	Bu Gu Zi	*Psoralea corylifolia L.*
7%	Fenugreek seed	Hu Lu Ba	*Trigonella foenum-graecum L.*
5%	Akebia stem	Mu Tong	*Akebia trifoliata (Thunb.) Koidz var. australis*

Huo Po Xia Ling Tang

Common Name		Pin Yin	Botanical Name
10%	Agastache	Huo Xiang	*Pogostemon cablin (Blanco) Benth.*
15%	Poria	Fu Ling	*Poria cocos (Schw.) Wolf*
5%	Pinellia tuber	Ban Xia	*Pinellia ternata (Thunb.) Breit*
15%	Apricot seed	Xing Ren	*Prunus armeniaca L.*
20%	Coix seed	*Yi Yi Ren*	*Coix lacrymajobi L var Ma-Yuen (Roman)*
3%	Cardamon fruit	Bai Dou Kou	*Amomum cardamomum L.*
6%	Polyporus	Zhu Ling	*Polyporus umbeliatus (Pers.) Fries*
15%	Prepared soybean	Dan Dou Chi	*Glycine max (L.) Merr*
6%	Alisma tuber	Ze Xie	*Alisma plantago-aquatica L var orientala*
5%	Magnolia bark	Hou Po	*Magnolia officinalis Rehd. et Wils.*

Huo Xue Hua Yu Gao

Common Name		Pin Yin	Botanical Name
11%	Chinese clematis root	Wei Ling Xian	*Clematis chinensis Osbeck*
9%	Frankincense	Ru Xiang	*Boswellia carterii Birdw.*
9%	Myrrh	Mo Yao	*Commiphora myrrha Engl.*
9%	Dragon's Blood	Xue Jie	*Resin of Daemonorops draco Bl.*
9%	Angelica root-end	Dang Gui Wei	*Angelica sinensis (Oliv.) Diels*
9%	Dahurian Angelica	Bai Zhi	*Angelica dahurica (Fisch. ex Hoffm.) Benth*
9%	Corydalis tuber	Yan Hu Suo	*Corydalis yanhusuo W.T. Wang*
9%	Rhubarb root	Da Huang	*Rheum palmatum L.*
9%	Momordica seed	Mu Bie Zi	*Momordica cochinchinensis (Lour.)*
9%	Safflower flower	Hong Hua	*Carthamus tinctorius L.*
9%	Gardenia fruit	Zhi Zi	*Gardenia jasminoides Ellis*

Jin Suo Gu Jing Wan

Common Name		Pin Yin	Botanical Name or Animal Species
25%	Astragalus seed	Sha Yuan Ji Li	*Astragalus complanatus R. Brown*
13%	Dragon bone	Long Gu	*Os Draconis (fossilized bone)*
25%	Euryale seed	Qian Shi	*Euryale ferox Salisb*
12%	Lotus seed	Lian Rou	*Nelumbo nucifera Gaertn.*
12%	Lotus stamen	Lian Xu	*Nelumbo nucifera Gaertn.*
13%	Oyster Shell	Mu Li	*Ostrea gigas Thunb.*

Jing Fang Bai Du San

Common Name		Pin Yin	Botanical Name or Animal Species
10%	Schizonepeta	Jing Jie	*Schizonepeta tenuifolia Briq.*
10%	Ledebouriella root	Fang Feng	*Ledebouriella divaricata Hiroe*
10%	Notopterygium root	Qiang Huo	*Notopterygium incisum Ting ex HT Chang*
10%	Pubescent angelica root	Du Huo	*Angelica pubescens Maxim.*
10%	Peucedanum root	Qian Hu	*Peucedanum praeruptorum Dunn.*
10%	Bupleurum root	Chai Hu	*Bupleurum chinense DC.*
10%	Ripe Bitter Orange fruit	Zhi Ke	*Citrus aurantium L. (Rutaceae)*
10%	Poria	Fu Ling	*Poria cocos (Schw.) Wolf*
10%	Platycodon root	Jie Geng	*Platycodon grandiflorum (Jacq.) A. DC*
10%	Ligusticum rhizome	Chuan Xiong	*Ligusticum wallichii Franch*

Ju Pi San

Common Name		Pin Yin	Botanical Name
12%	Chinese angelica root	Dang Gui	*Angelica sinensis (Oliv) Diels*
12%	Areca seed	Bing Lang	*Areca catechu L.*
7%	Asarum herb	Xi Xin	*Asarum sieboldi Miq.*
10%	Cinnamon bark	Rou Gui	*Cinnamomum cassia Presl.*
14%	Citrus peel	Chen Pi	*Citrus reticulata Blanco*
13%	Green tangerine peel	Qing Pi	*Citrus reticutata Blanco*
12%	Fennel fruit	Hui Xiang	*Foeniculum vulgare Mill.*
12%	Magnolia Bark	Hou Po	*Magnolia officinalis Rehd. et Wils.*
8%	Dahurian Angelica	Bai Zhi	*Angelica dahurica (Fisch. ex Hoffm.) Benth*

Jue Ming San

Common Name		Pin Yin	Botanical Name
11%	Abalone shell	Shi Jue Ming	*Haliotis diversicolor Reeve*
11%	Cassia seed	Jue Ming Zi	*Cassia obtusifolia L.*
7%	Eriocaulon	Gu Jing Cao	*Eriocaulon buergerianum Koern.*
8%	Buddleia flower	Mi Meng Hua	*Buddleia officinalis Maxim.*
9%	Coptis root	Huang Lian	*Coptis chinensis Franch*
9%	Gardenia fruit	Zhi Zi	*Gardenia jasminoides Ellis*
9%	Scutellaria root	Huang Qin	*Scutellaria baicalensis Georgi*
9%	Myrrh	Mo Yao	*Commiphora myrrha Engl.*
9%	Baked astragalus root	Huang Qi	*Astragalus membranaceus (Fisch.) Bge.*
9%	Dioscorea rhizome	Huang Yao Zi	*Dioscorea bulbifera L.*
9%	Stephania	Bai Yao Zi	*Stephania cepharantha Hayata.*

Li Zhong Tang

Common Name		Pin Yin	Botanical Name
25%	White Atractylodes	Bai Zhu	*Atractylodes macrocephala Koidz*
25%	Dry ginger	Gan Jiang	*Zingiber officinale Rosc.*
25%	Ginseng	Ren Shen	*Panax ginseng C. A. Mey.*
25%	Licorice root	Gan Cao	*Glycyrrhiza uralensis Fisch.*

Lian Po Yin

Common Name		Pin Yin	Botanical Name
4%	Coptis root	Huang Lian	*Coptis chinensis Franch*
10%	Magnolia bark	Hou Po	*Magnolia officinalis Rehd. et Wils.*
10%	Gardenia fruit	Zhi Zi	*Gardenia jasminoides Ellis*
10%	Prepared soybean	Dan Dou Chi	*Glycine max (L.) Merr*
3%	Pinellia tuber	Ban Xia	*Pinellia ternata (Thunb.) Breit*
60%	Phragmites rhizome	Lu Gen	*Phragmites communis (L.) Trin.*
3%	Acorus rhizome	Shi Chang Pu	*Acorus gramineus Soland.*

Li Fei San

Common Name		Pin Yin	Botanical Name or Animal Species
8%	Gecko body	Ge Jie	*Gekko gecko L.*
8%	Tendrilled fritillaria bulb	Chuan Bei Mu	*Fritillaria cirrhosa D. Don*
8%	Anemarrhena rhizome	Zhi Mu	*Anemarrhena asphodeloides, Bunge*
8%	Gentian root	Qin Jiao	*Gentiana macrophylla Pall*
8%	Perilla seed	Su Zi	*Perilla frutescens (L.) Britt.*
8%	Lily bulb	Bai He	*Lillium brownii F.E. Brown var. colchesteri*
8%	Chinese yam	Shan Yao	*Dioscorea opposita Thunb.*
8%	Asparagus tuber	Tian Men Dong	*Asparagus cochinchinensis Merr.*
6%	Loquat leaf	Pi Pa Ye	*Eriobotrya japonica (Thunb.) Lindl.*
8%	Stephania	Bai Yao Zi	*Stephania cepharantha Hayata.*
8%	Gardenia fruit	Zhi Zi	*Gardenia jasminoides Ellis*
8%	Trichosanthes root	Gua Lou Gen	*Trichosanthes kirilowii Maxim.*
6%	Cimicifuga rhizome	Sheng Ma	*Cimicifuga foetida L.*

Ling Yang Gou Teng Tang

	Common Name	Pin Yin	Botanical Name
9%	Chrysanthemum flower	Ju Hua	*Chrysanthemum morifolium Ramat*
9%	Tendrilled fritillaria bulb	Chuan Bei Mu	*Fritillaria cirrhosa D. Don*
6%	Licorice root	Gan Cao	*Glycyrrhiza uralensis Fisch.*
7%	Mulberry Leaves	Sang Ye	*Morus alba L.*
7%	White peony root	Bai Shao Yao	*Paeonia lactiflora Pall.*
7%	Poria	Fu Ling	*Poria cocos (Schw.) Wolf*
15%	Raw rehmannia root	Sheng Di Huang	*Rehmannia glutinosa Libosch*
16%	Scrophularia root	Xuan Shen*	*Scrophularia ningpoensis Hemsl*
9%	Uncaria stem with hooks	Gou Teng	*Uncaria sinensis (Oliv) Havil*
15%	Bamboo leaf	Zhu Ye	*Phyllostachys nigra (Lodd.) Munro var. henonis*

* This is a substitute for Antelope horn *Ling Yang Jiao.*

Liu Wei Di Huang Wan

	Common Name	Pin Yin	Botanical Name
12%	Alisma tuber	Ze Xie	*Alisma plantago-aquatica L var orientala*
16%	Cornus	Shan Zhu Yu	*Cornus officinalis Sieb. et Zucc.*
16%	Chinese yam	Shan Yao	*Dioscorea opposita Thunb.*
12%	Moutan bark	Mu Dan Pi	*Paeonia suffruticosa Andr.*
12%	Poria	Fu Ling	*Poria cocos (Schw.) Wolf*
32%	Prepared rehmannia root	Shu Di Huang	*Rehmannia glutinosa Libosch*

Long Dan Xie Gan Tang

	Common Name	Pin Yin	Botanical Name
16%	Alisma tuber	Ze Xie	*Alisma plantago-aquatica L var orientala*
7%	Chinese angelica root	Dang Gui	*Angelica sinensis (Oliv) Diels*
8%	Bupleurum root	Chai Hu	*Bupleurum chinense DC.*
8%	Gardenia fruit	Zhi Zi	*Gardenia jasminoides Ellis*
9%	Gentian root	Long Dan Cao	*Gentiana scabra Bunge*
8%	Licorice root	Gan Cao	*Glycyrrhiza uralensis Fisch.*
12%	Plantago seed	Che Qian Zi	*Plantago asiatica L.*
12%	Raw rehmannia root	Sheng Di Huang	*Rehmannia glutinosa Libosch*
12%	Scutellaria root	Huang Qin	*Scutellaria baicalensis Georgi*
8%	Akebia stem	Mu Tong	*Akebia trifoliata (Thunb.) Koidz var. australis*

Ma Huang Tang

	Common Name	Pin Yin	Botanical Name
35%	Apricot seed	Xing Ren	*Prunus armeniaca L.*
25%	Cinnamon twig	Gui Zhi	*Cinnamomum cassia Presl.*
25%	Ephedra	Ma Huang	*Ephedra sinica Stapf*
15%	Licorice root	Gan Cao	*Glycyrrhiza uralensis Fisch.*

Nei Xiao San

	Common Name	Pin Yin	Botanical Name or Animal Species
15%	Fritillaria bulb	Zhe Bei Mu	*Fritillaria thunbergii Miq.*
19%	Oyster Shell	Mu Li	*Ostrea gigas Thunb.*
10%	Prunella	Xia Ku Cao	*Prunella vulgaris L.*
12%	Scrophularia root	Xuan Shen	*Scrophularia ningpoensis Hemsl*
12%	Trichosanthes root	Tian Hua Fen	*Trichosanthes kirilowii Maxim*
12%	Platycodon root	Jie Geng	*Platycodon grandiflorum (Jacq.) A. DC*
10%	Rhubarb root	Da Huang	*Rheum palmatum L.*
10%	Dahurian Angelica	Bai Zhi	*Angelica dahurica (Fisch. ex Hoffm.) Benth*

Qing Fei San

	Common Name	Pin Yin	Botanical Name
13%	Fritillaria bulb	Zhe Bei Mu	*Fritillaria thunbergii Miq.*
38%	Isatis root	Ban Lang Gen	*Isatis tinctoria L.*
25.50%	Lepidium seed	Ting Li Zi	*Lepidium apetalum Willd.*
10.50%	Licorice root	Gan Cao	*Glycyrrhiza uralensis Fisch.*
13%	Platycodon root	Jie Geng	*Platycodon grandiflorum (Jacq.) A. DC*

Qing Gong Tang

	Common Name	Pin Yin	Botanical Name or Animal Species
15%	Forsythia fruit	Lian Qiao	*Forsythia suspensa (Thunb.) Vahl*
15%	Lotus seed	Lian Zi	*Nelumbo nucifera Gaertn.*
20%	Ophiopogon root	Mai Men Dong	*Ophiopogon japonicus Krt-Gawler*
25%	Scrophularia root	Xuan Shen	*Scrophularia ningpoensis Hemsl*
10%	Water buffalo horn*	Shui Niu Jiao	*Bubalus bubalis L.*
15%	Bamboo stem and leaf	Dan Zhu Ye	*Lophatherum gracile Brongn. var. elatum*

* May substitute Moutan *Mu Dan Pi.*

Qing Hao Bie Jia Tang

Common Name		Pin Yin	Botanical Name or Animal Species
20%	Soft-shelled turtle shell	Bie Jia	*Amyda sinensis (Wiegmann)*
20%	Anemarrhena rhizome	Zhi Mu	*Anemarrhena asphodeloides Bunge*
20%	Sweet wormwood	Qing Hao	*Artemisia apiacea Hance.*
20%	Moutan bark	Mu Dan Pi	*Paeonia suffruticosa Andr.*
20%	Raw rehmannia root	Sheng Di Huang	*Rehmannia glutinosa Libosch*

Qing Qi Hua Tan Tang

Common Name		Pin Yin	Botanical Name or Animal Species
10%	Anemarrhena rhizome	Zhi Mu	*Anemarrhena asphodeloides Bunge*
6%	Citrus peel	Chen Pi	*Citrus reticulata Blanco*
10%	Tendrilled Fritillaria bulb	Chuan Bei Mu	*Fritillaria cirrhosa D. Don*
12%	Gardenia fruit	Zhi Zi	*Gardenia jasminoides Ellis*
4%	Licorice root	Gan Cao	*Glycyrrhiza uralensis Fisch.*
10%	Mulberry root bark	Sang Bai Pi	*Morus alba L.*
10%	Ophiopogon root	Mai Men Dong	*Ophiopogon japonicus Krt-Gawler*
8%	Platycodon root	Jie Geng	*Platycodon grandiflorum (Jacq.) A. DC*
10%	Poria	Fu Ling	*Poria cocos (Schw.) Wolf*
12%	Scutellaria root	Huang Qin	*Scutellaria baicalensis Georgi*
8%	Trichosanthes peel	Gua Lou Pi	*Trichosanthes kirilowii Maxim.*

Qing Ying Tang

Common Name		Pin Yin	Botanical Name or Animal Species
8%	Coptis root	Huang Lian	*Coptis chinensis Franch*
10%	Forsythia fruit	Lian Qiao	*Forsythia suspensa (Thunb.) Vahl*
14%	Honeysuckle flower	Jin Yin Hua	*Lonicera japonica Thunb.*
15%	Ophiopogon root	Mai Men Dong	*Ophiopogon japonicus Krt-Gawler*
20%	Raw rehmannia root	Sheng Di Huang	*Rehmannia glutinosa Libosch*
10%	Salvia root	Dan Shen	*Salvia miltiorrhiza Bunge*
15%	Scrophularia root	Xuan Shen	*Scrophularia ningpoensis Hemsl*
3%	Water buffalo horn*	Shui Niu Jiao	*Bubalus bubalis L.*
5%	Bamboo stem and leaf	Dan Zhu Ye	*Lophatherum gracile Brongn. var. elatum*

* May substitute Moutan *Mu Dan Pi*

Qing Zao Jiu Fei Tang

	Common Name	Pin Yin	Botanical or Latin Name
10%	Apricot seed	Xing Ren	*Prunus armeniaca L.*
10%	Cannabis	Huo Ma Ren	*Cannabis sativa L.*
12%	Donkey-hide gelatin	E Jiao	*Equus asinus L.*
10%	Loquat leaf	Pi Pa Ye	*Eriobotrya japonica (Thunb.) Lindl.*
8%	Ginseng	Ren Shen	*Panax ginseng g C. A. Mey.*
35%	Gypsum fibrosum	Shi Gao	*Calcium sulphate*
15%	Mulberry Leaves	Sang Ye	*Morus alba L.*
15%	Ophiopogon root	Mai Men Dong	*Ophiopogon japonicus Krt-Gawler*

Qu Mai San

	Common Name	Pin Yin	Botanical or Latin Name
9%	Atractylodes rhizome	Cang Zhu	*Atractylodes lancea (Thunb.) DC.*
9%	Bitter orange	Zhi Qiao	*Citrus aurantium L.*
9%	Citrus peel	Chen Pi	*Citrus reticulata Blanco*
9%	Green tangerine peel	Qing Pi	*Citrus reticutata Blanco*
13%	Hawthorn fruit	Shan Zha	*Crataegus pinnatifida Bge. var. major N.E.Br.*
13%	Barley sprouts	Mai Ya	*Hordeum vulgare L.*
5%	Licorice root	Gan Cao	*Glycyrrhiza uralensis Fisch.*
9%	Magnolia Bark	Hou Po	*Magnolia officinalis Rehd. et Wils.*
18%	Medicated leaven	Shen Qu	*Massa Fermentata Medicinalis*
6%	Radish seed	Lai Fu Zi	*Raphanus sativus L.*

Ren Shen Bai Hu Tang

	Common Name	Pin Yin	Botanical or Latin Name
20%	Anemarrhena rhizome	Zhi Mu	*Anemarrhena asphodeloides, Bunge*
10%	Licorice root	Gan Cao	*Glycyrrhiza uralensis Fisch.*
30%	Gypsum fibrosum	Shi Gao	*Calcium sulphate*
20%	Oryza (rice)	Jing Mi	*Oryza sativa L.*
20%	Ginseng	Ren Shen	*Panax ginseng C. A. Mey.*

Ren Shen Ge Jie San

Common Name		Pin Yin	Botanical Name or Animal Species
10%	Anemarrhena Rhizome	Zhi Mu	*Anemarrhena asphodeloides Bunge*
10%	Apricot seed	Xing Ren	*Prunus armeniaca L.*
15%	Fritillaria bulb	Chuan Bei Mu	*Fritillaria cirrhosa D.*
15%	Gecko body	Ge Jie	*Gekko gecko L.*
15%	Ginseng	Ren Shen	*Panax ginseng C. A. Mey.*
10%	Licorice root	Gan Cao	*Glycyrrhiza uralensis Fisch.*
10%	Mulberry root bark	Sang Bai Pi	*Morus alba L.*
15%	Poria	Fu Ling	*Poria cocos (Schw.) Wolf*

Ru Yi Jin Huang San

Common Name		Pin Yin	Botanical Name
12.5%	Rhubarb root	Da Huang	*Rheum palmatum L.*
12.5%	Phellodendron bark	Huang Bai	*Phellodendron amourense Rupr.*
25%	Trichosanthes root	Tian Hua Fen	*Trichosanthes kirilowii Maxim*
12.5%	Turmeric rhizome	Jiang Huang	*Curcuma longa L.*
5%	Jack-in-the-pulpit rhizome	Tian Nan Xing	*Arisaema consanguineum Schott*
12.5%	Dahurian Angelica	Bai Zhi	*Angelica dahurica (Fisch. ex Hoffm.) Benth*
5%	Citrus peel	Chen Pi	*Citrus reticulata Blanco*
5%	Atractylodes rhizome	Cang Zhu	*Atractylodes lancea (Thunb.) DC.*
5%	Magnolia Bark	Hou Po	*Magnolia officinalis Rehd. et Wils.*
5%	Licorice root	Gan Cao	*Glycyrrhiza uralensis Fisch.*

Sang Ju Yin

Common Name		Pin Yin	Botanical Name
19.5%	Mulberry leaves	Sang Ye	*Morus alba L.*
8%	Chrysanthemum flower	Ju Hua	*Chrysanthemum morifolium Ramat*
15.5%	Apricot seed	Xing Ren	*Prunus armeniaca L.*
13%	Forsythia fruit	Lian Qiao	*Forsythia suspensa (Thunb.) Vahl*
6.5%	Peppermint	Bo He	*Mentha haplocalyx Briq.*
15.5%	Platycodon root	Jie Geng	*Platycodon grandiflorum (Jacq.) A. DC*
6.5%	Licorice root	Gan Cao	*Glycyrrhiza uralensis Fisch.*
15.5%	Phragmites rhizome	Lu Gen	*Phragmites communis (L.) Trin.*

Sang Ren Tang Plus

Common Name		Pin Yin	Botanical Name
14%	Mulberry leaves	Sang Ye	Morus alba L.
10%	Apricot seed	Xing Ren	Prunus armeniaca L.
12%	Glehnia root	Sha Shen	Glehnia littoralis F. Schmidt ex Miq.
12%	Fritillaria bulb	Zhe Bei Mu	Fritillaria thunbergii Miq.
10%	Gardenia fruit	Zhi Zi	Gardenia jasminoides Ellis
10%	Prepared soybean	Dan Dou Chi	Glycine max (L.) Merr
12%	Ophiopogon root	Mai Men Dong	Ophiopogon japonicus Krt-Gawler
10%	Stemona	Bai Bu	Stemona japonica Miq
10%	Tussilago flower	Kuan Dong Hua	Tussilago farfara L.

Sang Zhi San

Common Name		Pin Yin	Botanical Name
10%	Morinda root	Ba Ji Tian	Morinda officinalis How
10%	Drynaria rhizome	Gu Sui Bu	Drynaria fortunei (Kunze) J. Sm.
10%	Psoralea	Bu Gu Zhi	Psoralea corylifolia L.
10%	Cinnamon twig	Gui Zhi	Cinnamomum cassia Presl.
10%	Achyranthes	Niu Xi	Achyranthes bidentata Bl.
10%	Pubescent angelica root	Du Huo	Angelica pubescens Maxim.
8%	Chinese clematis root	Wei Ling Xian	Clematis chinensis Osbeck
10%	Eucommia bark	Du Zhong	Eucommia ulmoides Oliv.
8%	Mulberry twig	Sang Zhi	Morus alba L.
7%	Notopterygium root	Qiang Huo	Notopterygium incisum Ting ex HT Chang
7%	Ledebouriella root	Fang Feng	Ledebouriella divaricata Hiroe

Shen Fu Tang

Common Name		Pin Yin	Botanical Name
60%	Aconite (prepared)	Fu Zi	Aconitum carmichaeli Debx.
40%	Ginseng	Ren Shen	Panax ginseng C. A. Mey.

Shen Ling Bai Zhu San

Common Name		Pin Yin	Botanical Name
10%	Cardamon fruit	Sha Ren	*Amomum villosum Lour.*
8%	Baked licorice root	Gan Cao	*Glycyrrhiza uralensis Fisch.*
12%	Chinese yam	Shan Yao	*Dioscorea opposita Thunb.*
8%	Coix seed	*Yi Yi Ren*	*Coix lacrymajobi L var Ma-Yuen (Roman)*
10%	Dolichos seed	*Bian Dou*	*Dolichos lablab L.*
8%	Ginseng	Ren Shen	*Panax ginseng C. A. Mey.*
10%	Lotus seed	Lian Zi	*Nelumbo nucifera Gaertn.*
10%	Platycodon root	Jie Geng	*Platycodon grandiflorum (Jacq.) A. DC*
10%	Poria	Fu Ling	*Poria cocos (Schw.) Wolf*
14%	White Atractylodes	Bai Zhu	*Atractylodes macrocephala Koidz*

Shen Qi Wan

Common Name		Pin Yin	Botanical or Chemical Name
10%	Aconite (prepared)	Fu Zi	*Aconitum carmichaeli Debx.*
10%	Alisma tuber	Ze Xie	*Alisma plantago-aquatica L var orientala*
10%	Cinnamon twig	Gui Zhi	*Cinnamomum cassia Presl.*
12%	Cornus	Shan Zhu Yu	*Cornus officinalis Sieb. et Zucc.*
13%	Chinese yam	Shan Yao	*Dioscorea opposita Thunb.*
10%	Moutan bark	Mu Dan Pi	*Paeonia suffruticosa Andr.*
10%	Poria	Fu Ling	*Poria cocos (Schw.) Wolf*
25%	Prepared rehmannia root	Shu Di Huang	*Rehmannia glutinosa Libosch*

Shen Qi Yin Xu Fang

Common Name		Pin Yin	Botanical Name
9%	Alisma tuber	Ze Xie	*Alisma plantago-aquatica L var orientala*
9%	Baked astragalus root	Huang Qi	*Astragalus membranaceus (Fisch.) Bge.*
10%	Cornus	Shan Zhu Yu	*Cornus officinalis Sieb. et Zucc.*
9%	Cuscuta	Tu Si Zi	*Cuscuta chinensis Lam.*
8%	Chinese yam	Shan Yao	*Dioscorea opposita Thunb.*
8%	Lindera root	Wu Yao	*Lindera strychnifolia (Sieb. Et Zucc.) Villar*
6%	Epimedium	Yin Yang Huo	*Epimedium sagittatum (Sieb. et Zucc.) Maxim*
8%	White peony root	Bai Shao Yao	*Paeonia lactiflora Pall.*
9%	Raw rehmannia root	Sheng Di Huang	*Rehmannia glutinosa Libosch*
12%	Poria	Fu Ling	*Poria cocos (Schw.) Wolf*
12%	Prepared rehmannia root	Shu Di Huang	*Rehmannia glutinosa Libosch*

Sheng Jing San

Common Name	Pin Yin	Botanical or Chemical Name
7% Actinolite	Yang Qi Shi	*Calcium Magnesium Iron Silicate Hydroxide*
7% Chinese angelica root	Dang Gui	*Angelica sinensis (Oliv) Diels*
6% Baked astragalus root	Huang Qi	*Astragalus membranaceus (Fisch.) Bge.*
7% Cistanche	Rou Cong Rong	*Cistanche deserticola Y.C. Ma.*
2% Citrus peel	Chen Pi	*Citrus reticulata Blanco*
5% Pilose asiabell root	Dang Shen	*Codonopsis pilosula (Franch.) Nannf.*
7% Cuscuta	Tu Si Zi	*Cuscuta chinensis Lam.*
7% Cynomorium	Suo Yang	*Cynomorium songaricum Rupr.*
7% Dipsacus root	Xu Duan	*Dipsacus asper Wall.*
6% Epimedium	Yin Yang Huo	*Epimedium sagittatum (Sieb. et Zucc.) Maxim*
5% Lycium fruit	Gou Qi Zi	*Lycium barbarum L.*
5% Ophiopogon root	Mai Men Dong	*Ophiopogon japonicus Krt-Gawler*
5% White peony root	Bai Shao Yao	*Paeonia lactiflora Pall.*
5% Fleeceflower root	He Shou Wu	*Polygonum multiflorum Thunb.*
7% Psoralea Fruit	Bu Gu Zhi	*Psoralea corylifolia L.*
7% Prepared rehmannia root	Shu Di Huang	*Rehmannia glutinosa Libosch*
5% Scrophularia root	Xuan Shen	*Scrophularia ningpoensis Hemsl*

Sheng Tong Zhu Yu Tang

Common Name	Pin Yin	Botanical Name or Animal Species
10% Peach kernel	Tao Ren	*Prunus persica (L.) Batsch*
10% Safflower flower	Hong Hua	*Carthamus tinctorius L.*
5% Gentian root	Qin Jiao	*Gentiana macrophylla Pall*
5% Notopterygium root	Qiang Huo	*Notopterygium incisum Ting ex HT Chang*
10% Myrrh	Mo Yao	*Commiphora myrrha Engl.*
10% Chinese angelica root	Dang Gui	*Angelica sinensis (Oliv) Diels*
10% Flying squirrel feces	Wu Ling Zhi	*Trogopterus xanthipes Milne-Edwards*
5% Nut-grass rhizome	Xiang Fu	*Cyperus rotundus L.*
10% Achyranthes	Niu Xi	*Achyranthes bidentata Bl.*
5% Licorice root	Gan Cao	*Glycyrrhiza uralensis Fisch.*
10% Ligusticum rhizome	Chuan Xiong	*Ligusticum wallichii Franch*
10% Earthworm	Di Long	*Pheretima aspergillum Perrier*

Shi Pi Yin

	Common Name	Pin Yin	Botanical Name
5%	Aconite root (prepared)	Fu Zi	*Aconitum carmichaeli Debx.*
10%	Dry ginger	Gan Jiang	*Zingiber officinale Rosc.*
10%	Tsaoko fruit	Cao Guo	*Amomum tsao-ko Crevost et Lem.*
10%	White atractylodes	Bai Zhu	*Atractylodes macrocephala Koidz*
5%	Licorice root	Gan Cao	*Glycyrrhiza uralensis Fisch.*
5%	Fresh ginger rhizome	Sheng Jiang	*Zingiber officinale Rosc.*
5%	Jujube	Da Zao	*Ziziphus jujuba Mill var. inermis (Bge.) Rehd.*
10%	Magnolia bark	Hou Po	*Magnolia officinalis Rehd. et Wils.*
10%	Poria	Fu Ling	*Poria cocos (Schw.) Wolf*
10%	Saussurea root	Mu Xiang	*Saussurea lappa Clarke*
10%	Areca peel	Da Fu Pi	*Areca catechu L.*
10%	Chaenomeles fruit	Mu Gua	*Chaenomeles lagenaria (Loisel.) Koidz.*

Shi Zao Tang

	Common Name	Pin Yin	Botanical Name
25%	Genkwa flower	Yuan Hua	*Daphne genkwa Sieb. et Zucc.*
25%	Kan-sui root	Gan Sui	*Euphorbia kansui Liou*
25%	Euphorbia	Da Ji	*Euphorbia pekinensis Rupr.*
25%	Jujube	Da Zao	*Ziziphus jujuba Mill var. inermis (Bge.) Rehd.*

Si Jun Zi Tang

	Common Name	Pin Yin	Botanical Name
10%	Ginseng	Ren Shen	*Panax ginseng C. A. Mey.*
40%	White Atractylodes	Bai Zhu	*Atractylodes macrocephala Koidz*
14%	Poria	Fu Ling	*Poria cocos (Schw.) Wolf*
34%	Licorice root	Gan Cao	*Glycyrrhiza uralensis Fisch.*

Si Ni Tang

	Common Name	Pin Yin	Botanical Name
33%	Aconite root (prepared)	Fu Zi	*Aconitum carmichaeli Debx.*
34%	Licorice root	Gan Cao	*Glycyrrhiza uralensis Fisch.*
33%	Dry ginger	Gan Jiang	*Zingiber officinale Rosc.*

Si Sheng Gao

Common Name		Pin Yin	Botanical Name
25%	Pinellia tuber	Ban Xia	Pinellia ternata (Thunb.) Breit
25%	Sichuan aconite root	Chuan Wu	Aconitum carmichaeli Debx.
25%	Wild aconite	Cao Wu	Aconitum kusnezoffii
25%	Jack-in-the-pulpit rhizome	Tian Nan Xing	Arisaema consanguineum Schott

Si Shen Wan

Common Name		Pin Yin	Botanical Name
30%	Psoralea	Bu Gu Zi	Psoralea corylifolia L.
15%	Nutmeg seed	Rou Dou Kou	Myristica fragrans Houtt.
15%	Evodia	Wu Zhu Yu	Evodia rutaecarpa (Juss.) Benth.
10%	Schisandra fruit	Wu Wei Zi	Schisandra chinensis Baill.
15%	Fresh ginger rhizome	Sheng Jiang	Zingiber officinale Rosc.
15%	Jujube	Da Zao	Ziziphus jujuba Mill var. inermis (Bge.) Rehd.

Si Wu Tang

Common Name		Pin Yin	Botanical Name
25%	Chinese angelica root	Dang Gui	Angelica sinensis (Oliv) Diels
15%	Ligusticum root	Chuan Xiong	Ligusticum wallichii Franch.
25%	White peony root	Bai Shao Yao	Paeonia lactiflora Pall.
35%	Prepared rehmannia root	Shu Di Huang	Rehmannia glutinosa Libosch

Su Zi Jiang Qi Tang

Common Name		Pin Yin	Botanical Name
18%	Perilla seed	Su Zi	Perilla frutescens (L.) Britt.
10%	Licorice root	Gan Cao	Glycyrrhiza uralensis Fisch.
18%	Pinellia tuber	Ban Xia	Pinellia ternata (Thunb.) Breit
13%	Chinese angelica root	Dang Gui	Angelica sinensis (Oliv) Diels
13%	Peucedanum root	Qian Hu	Peucedanum praeruptorum Dunn.
10%	Magnolia bark	Hou Po	Magnolia officinalis Rehd. et Wils.
10%	Fresh ginger rhizome	Sheng Jiang	Zingiber officinale Rosc.
8%	Cinnamon bark	Rou Gui	Cinnamomum cassia Presl.

Suo Quan Wan

Common Name		Pin Yin	Botanical Name
50%	Black Cardamon seed	Yi Zhi Ren	*Alpinia oxyphylla Miq.*
50%	Lindera root	Wu Yao	*Lindera strychnifolia (Sieb. Et Zucc.) Villar*

Tao Hong Si Wu Tang

Common Name		Pin Yin	Botanical Name
18%	Chinese angelica root	Dang Gui	*Angelica sinensis (Oliv) Diels*
15%	Ligusticum rhizome	Chuan Xiong	*Ligusticum wallichii Franch*
15%	Red peony root	Chi Shao Yao	*Paeonia lactiflora Pall.*
25%	Raw rehmannia root	Sheng Di Huang	*Rehmannia glutinosa Libosch*
17%	Peach kernel	Tao Ren	*Prunus persica (L.) Batsch*
10%	Safflower flower	Hong Hua	*Carthamus tinctorius L.*

Tian Ma Gou Teng Yin

Common Name		Pin Yin	Botanical Name or Animal Species
9%	Gastrodia tuber	Tian Ma	*Gastrodia elata Bl.*
9%	Uncaria stem with hooks	Gou Teng	*Uncaria sinensis (Oliv) Havil*
10%	Abalone shell	Shi Jue Ming	*Haliotis diversicolor Reeve*
9%	Gardenia fruit	Zhi Zi	*Gardenia jasminoides Ellis*
9%	Scutellaria root	Huang Qin	*Scutellaria baicalensis Georgi*
9%	Chinese motherwort	Yi Mu Cao	*Leonurus heterophyllus Sweet*
9%	Achyranthes	Niu Xi	*Achyranthes bidentata Bl.*
9%	Eucommia bark	Du Zhong	*Eucommia ulmoides Oliv.*
9%	Mulberry mistletoe	Sang Ji Sheng	*Loranthus parasiticus Merr.*
9%	Polygonum vine	Ye Jiao Teng	*Polygonum multiflorum Thunb.*
9%	Poria	Fu Ling	*Poria cocos (Schw.) Wolf*

Tian Ma Plus

Common Name		Pin Yin	Botanical Name or Animal Species
5%	Arisaema with bile	Dan Nan Xing	*Arisaemae cum Felle Bovis*
8%	Silkworm	Jiang Can	*Beauveria bassiana infects Bombyx mori L.*
6%	Cicada moulted shell	Chan Tui	*Cryptotympana atrata Fabr.*
8%	Cornus	Shan Zhu Yu	*Cornus officinalis Sieb. et Zucc.*
8%	Dragon bone	Long Gu	*Os Draconis (fossilized bone)*
7%	Earthworm	Di Long	*Pheretima aspergillum Perrier*
8%	Gastrodia tuber	Tian Ma	*Gastrodia elata Bl.*
3%	Licorice root	Gan Cao	*Glycyrrhiza uralensis Fisch.*
7%	Moutan bark	Mu Dan Pi	*Paeonia suffruticosa Andr.*
8%	Oyster Shell	Mu Li	*Ostrea gigas Thunb.*
5%	Pinellia tuber	Ban Xia	*Pinellia ternata (Thunb.) Breit*
6%	Fleeceflower root	He Shou Wu	*Polygonum multiflorum Thunb.*
8%	Prepared rehmannia root	Shu Di Huang	*Rehmannia glutinosa Libosch*
8%	Uncaria stem with hooks	Gou Teng	*Uncaria sinensis (Oliv) Havil*
5%	Bamboo shavings	Zhu Ru	*Phyllostachys nigra Munro var.henonis*

Tian Ma San

Common Name		Pin Yin	Botanical Name or Animal Species
6%	Cicada moulted shell	Chan Tui	*Cryptotympana atrata*
15%	Pilose asiabell root	Dang Shen	*Codonopsis pilosula (Franch.) Nannf.*
11%	Gastrodia tuber	Tian Ma	*Gastrodia elata Bl.*
5%	Licorice root	Gan Cao	*Glycyrrhiza uralensis Fisch.*
10%	Ledebouriella root	Fang Feng	*Ledebouriella divaricata Hiroe*
10%	Ligusticum rhizome	Chuan Xiong	*Ligusticum wallichii Franch*
7%	Peppermint	Bo He	*Mentha haplocalyx Briq.*
12%	Fleeceflower root	He Shou Wu	*Polygonum multiflorum Thunb.*
14%	Poria	Fu Ling	*Poria cocos (Schw.) Wolf*
10%	Schizonepeta	Jing Jie	*Schizonepeta tenuifolia Briq.*

Wai Feng San

Common Name		Pin Yin	Botanical Name or Animal Species
15%	Schizonepeta	Jing Jie	*Schizonepeta tenuifolia Briq.*
15%	Xanthium	Cang Er Zi	*Xanthium sibiricum Patr. Ex Widd.*
20%	Silkworm	Jiang Can	*Beauveria bassiana infects Bombyx mori L.*
10%	Red peony root	Chi Shao Yao	*Paeonia lactiflora Pall.*
10%	Moutan bark	Mu Dan Pi	*Paeonia suffruticosa Andr.*
15%	Kochia fruit	Di Fu Zi	*Kochia scoparia (L.) Schrad.*
15%	Dictamnus root-bark	Bai Xian Pi	*Dictamnus dasycarphus Turcz.*

Wei Cang He

Common Name		Pin Yin	Botanical Name or Animal Species
11%	Agastache	Huo Xiang	*Pogostemon cablin (Blanco) Benth.*
7%	Processed pinellia tuber	Zhi Ban Xia	*Pinellia ternata (Thunb.) Breit*
9%	Areca seed	Bing Lang	*Areca catechu L.*
9%	Citrus peel	Chen Pi	*Citrus reticulata Blanco*
10%	Lindera root	Wu Yao	*Lindera strychnifolia (Sieb. Et Zucc.) Villar*
9%	Hawthorn fruit	Shan Zha	*Crataegus pinnatifida Bge var major N.E.Br.*
10%	Atractylodes rhizome	Cang Zhu	*Atractylodes lancea (Thunb.) DC.*
9%	Saussurea root	Mu Xiang	*Saussurea lappa Clarke*
8%	Forsythia fruit	Lian Qiao	*Forsythia suspensa (Thunb.) Vahl*
9%	Ripe bitter orange fruit	Zhi Ke	*Citrus aurantium L. (Rutaceae)*
9%	Magnolia bark	Hou Po	*Magnolia officinalis Rehd. et Wils.*

Wei Ling San

Common Name		Pin Yin	Botanical Name
10%	Alisma tuber	Ze Xie	*Alisma plantago-aquatica L var orientala*
20%	Atractylodes rhizome	Cang Zhu	*Atractylodes lancea (Thunb.) DC.*
13%	Cinnamon twig	Gui Zhi	*Cinnamomum cassia Presl.*
12%	Citrus peel	Chen Pi	*Citrus reticulata Blanco*
8%	Licorice root	Gan Cao	*Glycyrrhiza uralensis Fisch.*
15%	Magnolia Bark	Hou Po	*Magnolia officinalis, Rehd. et Wils.*
10%	Polyporus	Zhu Ling	*Polyporus umbeliatus (Pers.) Fries*
12%	Poria	Fu Ling	*Poria cocos (Schw.) Wolf*

Wu Mei Wan

	Common Name	Pin Yin	Botanical or Chemical Name
10%	Aconite (prepared)	Fu Zi	*Aconitum carmichaeli Debx.*
10%	Chinese angelica root	Dang Gui	*Angelica sinensis (Oliv) Diels*
8%	Asarum herb	Xi Xin	*Asarum sieboldi Miq.*
12%	Cinnamon twig	Gui Zhi	*Cinnamomum cassia Presl.*
10%	Coptis root	Huang Lian	*Coptis chinensis Franch*
10%	Ginseng	Ren Shen	*Panax ginseng C. A. Mey.*
20%	Mume	Wu Mei	*Prunus mume Sieb. et Zucc.*
10%	Phellodendron bark	Huang Bai	*Phellodendron amurense Rupr.*
10%	Dry ginger	Gan Jiang	*Zingiber officinale Rosc.*

Xi Jiao Di Huang Tang

	Common Name	Pin Yin	Botanical Name
20%	Moutan bark	Mu Dan Pi	*Paeonia suffruticosa Andr.*
20%	White peony root	Bai Shao Yao	*Paeonia lactiflora Pall.*
45%	Raw rehmannia root	Sheng Di Huang	*Rehmannia glutinosa Libosch*
15%	Imperata rhizome	Bai Mao Gen *	*Imperata cylindrica (L.) P. Beauv.var. major*

* This is a substitute for the Rhinoceros horn *Xi Jiao* of original formula.

Xi Xin San

	Common Name	Pin Yin	Botanical Name
13%	Arctium fruit	Niu Bang Zi	*Arctium lappa L.*
8%	Coptis root	Huang Lian	*Coptis chinensis Franch*
10%	Forsythia fruit	Lian Qiao	*Forsythia suspensa (Thunb.) Vahl*
10%	Gardenia fruit	Zhi Zi	*Gardenia jasminoides Ellis*
10%	Phellodendron bark	Huang Bai	*Phellodendron amurense Rupr.*
7%	Platycodon root	Jie Geng	*Platycodon grandiflorum (Jacq.) A. DC*
9%	Poria	Fu Shen	*Poria Cocos (Schw.) Wolf*
10%	Scutellaria root	Huang Qin	*Scutellaria baicalensis Georgi*
10%	Trichosanthes root	Tian Hua Fen	*Trichosanthes kirilowii Maxim*
8%	Akebia stem	Mu Tong	*Akebia trifoliata (Thunb.) Koidz var. australis*
5%	Dahurian angelica	Bai Zhi	*Angelica dahurica (Fisch ex Hoffm.) Benth.*

Xi Xian Cao San

Common Name		Pin Yin	Botanical Name or Animal Species
20%	Siegesbeckia	Xi Xian Cao	*Siegesbeckia pubescens Makino*
20%	Scutellaria root	Huang Qin	*Scutellaria baicalensis Georgi*
15%	Donkey-hide gelatin	E Jiao	*Equus asinus L.*
15%	Biota branch and leaf	Ce Bai Ye	Biota orientalis *(L.) Endl.*
20%	Raw rehmannia root	Sheng Di Huang	*Rehmannia glutinosa Libosch*
10%	Licorice root	Gan Cao	*Glycyrrhiza uralensis Fisch.*

Xiang Ru San

Common Name		Pin Yin	Botanical Name
10%	Bupleurum root	Chai Hu	*Bupleurum chinense DC.*
10%	Chinese angelica root	Dang Gui	*Angelica sinensis (Oliv.) Diels*
5%	Licorice root	Gan Cao	*Glycyrrhiza uralensis Fisch.*
10%	Scutellaria root	Huang Qin	*Scutellaria baicalensis Georgi*
10%	Coptis root	Huang Lian	*Coptis chinensis Franch*
10%	Forsythia fruit	Lian Qiao	*Forsythia suspensa (Thunb.) Vahl*
12%	Gypsum fibrosum	Shi Gao	*Calcium sulphate*
10%	Trichosanthes root	Tian Hua Fen	*Trichosanthes kirilowii Maxim*
13%	Elsholtzia	Xiang Ru	*Elsholtzia splendens Nakai ex Maekwa*
10%	Gardenia fruit	Zhi Zi	*Gardenia jasminoides Ellis*

Xiao Chai Hu Tang

Common Name		Pin Yin	Botanical Name
25%	Bupleurum root	Chai Hu	*Bupleurum chinense DC.*
15%	Ginseng	Ren Shen	*Panax ginseng C. A. Mey.*
10%	Licorice root	Gan Cao	*Glycyrrhiza uralensis Fisch.*
10%	Jujube	Da Zao	*Ziziphus jujuba Mill var. inermis (Bge.) Rehd.*
15%	Pinellia tuber	Ban Xia	*Pinellia ternate (Thunb.) Breit.*
15%	Scutellaria root	Huang Qin	*Scutellaria baicalensis Georgi*
10%	Dry ginger	Gan Jiang	*Zingiber officinale Rosc.*

Xiao Huang San

Common Name		Pin Yin	Botanical Name or Animal Species
6%	Scutellaria root	Huang Qin	*Scutellaria baicalensis Georgi*
5%	Gardenia fruit	Zhi Zi	*Gardenia jasminoides Ellis*
17%	Artemisia	Yin Chen Hao	*Artemisia capillaris*
5%	Dioscorea stem	Huang Yao Zi	*Dioscorea bulbifera L.*
5%	Anemarrhena rhizome	Zhi Mu	*Anemarrhena asphodeloides, Bunge*
5%	Fritillaria bulb	Zhe Bei Mu	*Fritillaria thunbergii Miq.*
5%	Coptis root	Huang Lian	*Coptis chinensis Franch*
5%	Phellodendron bark	Huang Bai	*Phellodendron amourense Rupr.*
5%	Forsythia fruit	Lian Qiao	*Forsythia suspensa (Thunb.) Vahl*
10%	Rhubarb root	Da Huang	*Rheum palmatum L.*
5%	Curcuma root	Yu Jin	*Curcuma aromatica Salisb.*
5%	Schizonepeta	Jing Jie	*Schizonepeta tenuifolia Briq.*
7%	Ledebouriella root	Fang Feng	*Ledebouriella divaricata Hiroe*
7%	Peppermint	Bo He	*Mentha haplocalyx Briq.*
3%	Cicada moulted shell	Chan Tui	*Cryptotympana atrata Fabr.*
5%	Licorice root	Gan Cao	*Glycyrrhiza uralensis Fisch.*

Xiao Huo Luo Dan

Common Name		Pin Yin	Botanical Name or Animal Species
20%	Sichuan aconite root	Chuan Wu	*Aconitum carmichaeli Debx.*
20%	Wild Aconite root	Cao Wu	*Aconitum kusnezoffii*
20%	Jack-in-the-pulpit rhizome	Tian Nan Xing	*Arisaema consanguineum Schott*
10%	Myrrh	Mo Yao	*Commiphora myrrha Engl.*
10%	Frankincense	Ru Xiang	*Boswellia carterii Birdw.*
20%	Earthworm	Di Long	*Pheretima aspergillum Perrier*

Xiao Qing Long Tang

Common Name		Pin Yin	Botanical Name
13%	Cinnamon twig	Gui Zhi	*Cinnamomum cassia Presl.*
13%	Ephedra	Ma Huang	*Ephedra sinica Stapf*
12%	Licorice root	Gan Cao	*Glycyrrhiza uralensis Fisch.*
13%	Dry ginger	Gan Jiang	*Zingiber officinale Rosc.*
13%	Asarum herb	*Xi Xin*	*Asarum sieboldi Miq.*
13%	Schisandra fruit	Wu Wei Zi	*Schisandra chinensis Baill.*
13%	White peony root	Bai Shao Yao	*Paeonia lactiflora Pall.*
13%	Pinellia tuber	Ban Xia	*Pinellia ternata (Thunb.) Breit*

Xiao Yao San

	Common Name	Pin Yin	Botanical Name
18%	Bupleurum root	Chai Hu	*Bupleurum chinense DC.*
18%	Chinese angelica root	Dang Gui	*Angelica sinensis (Oliv) Diels*
18%	White peony root	Bai Shao Yao	*Paeonia lactiflora Pall.*
18%	White atractylodes	Bai Zhu	*Atractylodes macrocephala Koidz*
18%	Poria	Fu Ling	*Poria cocos (Schw.) Wolf*
10%	Licorice root	Gan Cao	*Glycyrrhiza uralensis Fisch.*

Xue Fu Zhu Yu Tang

	Common Name	Pin Yin	Botanical Name
12%	Achyranthes	Niu Xi	*Achyranthes bidentata Bl.*
12%	Chinese angelica root	Dang Gui	*Angelica sinensis (Oliv) Diels*
8%	Ripe Bitter Orange fruit	Zhi Ke	*Citrus aurantium L. (Rutaceae)*
5%	Bupleurum root	Chai Hu	*Bupleurum chinense DC.*
11%	Safflower flower	Hong Hua	*Carthamus tinctorius L.*
4%	Licorice root	Gan Cao	*Glycyrrhiza uralensis Fisch.*
6%	Ligusticum rhizome	Chuan Xiong	*Ligusticum wallichii Franch*
8%	Red peony root	Chi Shao Yao	*Paeonia lactiflora Pall.*
16%	Peach kernel	Tao Ren	*Prunus persica (L.) Batsch*
6%	Platycodon root	Jie Geng	*Platycodon grandiflorum (Jacq.) A. DC*
12%	Raw rehmannia root	Sheng Di Huang	*Rehmannia glutinosa Libosch*

Yang Wei Tang

	Common Name	Pin Yin	Botanical Name
20%	Dolichos seed	Bian Dou	*Dolichos lablab L.*
20%	Glehnia root	Sha Shen	*Glehnia littoralis F. Schmidt ex Miq.*
10%	Licorice root	Gan Cao	*Glycyrrhiza uralensis Fisch.*
10%	Mulberry Leaves	Sang Ye	*Morus alba L.*
20%	Ophiopogon root	Mai Men Dong	*Ophiopogon japonicus Krt-Gawler*
20%	Polygonatum	Yu Zhu	*Polygonatum odoratum (Mill.) Druce*

Yang Xin Tang

Common Name		Pin Yin	Botanical Name
8%	Chinese angelica root	Dang Gui	*Angelica sinensis (Oliv) Diels*
16%	Astragalus root	Huang Qi	*Astragalus membranaceus (Fisch.) Bge.*
8%	Biota seed	Bai Zi Ren	*Biota orientalis (L.) Endl.*
10%	Cinnamon bark	Rou Gui	*Cinnamomum cassia Presl.*
12%	Pilose asiabell root	Dang Shen	*Codonopsis pilosula (Franch.) Nannf.*
8%	Licorice root	Gan Cao	*Glycyrrhiza uralensis Fisch.*
8%	Ligusticum rhizome	Chuan Xiong	*Ligusticum wallichii Franch*
10%	Polygala root	Yuan Zhi	*Polygala tenuifolia Willd.*
10%	Poria	Fu Ling	*Poria cocos (Schw.) Wolf*
10%	Schisandra fruit	Wu Wei Zi	*Schisandra chinensis Baill.*

Yang Yin Xi Feng San

Common Name		Pin Yin	Botanical Name or Animal Species
11%	White peony root	Bai Shao Yao	*Paeonia lactiflora Pall.*
25%	Prepared rehmannia root	Shu Di Huang	*Rehmannia glutinosa Libosch*
16%	Cornus	Shan Zhu Yu	*Cornus officinalis Sieb. et Zucc.*
8%	Moutan bark	Mu Dan Pi	*Paeonia suffruticosa Andr.*
12%	Uncaria stem with hooks	Gou Teng	*Uncaria sinensis (Oliv) Havil*
12%	Silkworm	Jiang Can	*Beauveria bassiana infects Bombyx mori L.*
8%	Cicada moulted shell	Chan Tui	*Cryptotympana atrata Fabr.*
8%	Typhonium rhizome	Bai Fu Zi	*Typhonium giganteum Engl.*

Yi Yi Ren San

Common Name		Pin Yin	Botanical Name
10%	Coix seed	*Yi Yi Ren*	*Coix lacrymajobi L var Ma-Yuen (Roman)*
10%	Stephania	Han Fang Ji	*Stephania tetrandra S. Moore.*
10%	Pubescent angelica root	Du Huo	*Angelica pubescens Maxim.*
10%	Notopterygium root	Qiang Huo	*Notopterygium incisum Ting ex HT Chang*
10%	Atractylodes rhizome	Cang Zhu	*Atractylodes lancea (Thunb.) DC.*
7%	Ledebouriella root	Fang Feng	*Ledebouriella divaricata Hiroe*
7%	Cinnamon twig	Gui Zhi	*Cinnamomum cassia Presl.*
5%	Sichuan aconite root	Chuan Wu	*Aconitum carmichaeli Debx.*
7%	Ligusticum rhizome	Chuan Xiong	*Ligusticum wallichii Franch*
8%	Chinese angelica root	Dang Gui	*Angelica sinensis (Oliv.) Diels*
8%	Siegesbeckia	Xi Xian Cao	*Siegesbeckia pubescens Makino*
8%	Chinese clematis root	Wei Ling Xian	*Clematis chinensis Osbeck*

Yin Chen San Plus

Common Name		Pin Yin	Botanical or Chemical Name
10%	Alisma tuber	Ze Xie	*Alisma plantago-aquatica L var orientala*
20%	Artemisia	Yin Chen Hao	*Artemisia capillaris*
11%	Coptis root	Huang Lian	*Coptis chinensis Franch*
10%	Gardenia fruit	Zhi Zi	*Gardenia jasminoides Ellis*
12%	Moutan bark	Mu Dan Pi	*Paeonia suffruticosa Andr.*
10%	Red peony root	Chi Shao Yao	*Paeonia lactiflora Pall.*
10%	Polyporus	Zhu Ling	*Polyporus umbeliatus (Pers.) Fries*
10%	Poria	Fu Ling	*Poria cocos (Schw.) Wolf*
12%	Raw rehmannia root	Sheng Di Huang	*Rehmannia glutinosa Libosch*
5%	Rhubarb root	Da Huang	*Rheum palmatum L.*

Yin Qiao San

Common Name		Pin Yin	Botanical Name
9%	Arctium fruit	Niu Bang Zi	*Arctium lappa L.*
15%	Forsythia fruit	Lian Qiao	*Forsythia suspensa (Thunb.) Vahl*
6%	Bamboo stem and leaf	Dan Zhu Ye	*Lophatherum gracile Brongn. var. elatum*
5%	Licorice root	Gan Cao	*Glycyrrhiza uralensis Fisch.*
9%	Peppermint	Bo He	*Mentha haplocalyx Briq.*
18%	Phragmites rhizome	Lu Gen	*Phragmites communis (L.) Trin.*
7%	Platycodon root	Jie Geng	*Platycodon grandiflorum (Jacq.) A. DC*
9%	Prepared Soybean	Dan Dou Chi	*Glycine max (L.) Merr*
7%	Schizonepeta	Jing Jie	*Schizonepeta tenuifolia Briq.*
15%	Honeysuckle flower	Jin Yin Hua	*Lonicera japonica Thunb.*

You Gui Wan

Common Name		Pin Yin	Botanical or Animal Species
5%	Aconite (prepared)	Fu Zi	*Aconitum carmichaeli Debx.*
8%	Lycium fruit	Gou Qi Zi	*Lycium barbarum L.*
10%	Cinnamon twig	Gui Zhi	*Cinnamomum cassia Presl.*
10%	Cornus	Shan Zhu Yu	*Cornus officinalis Sieb. et Zucc.*
10%	Chinese yam	Shan Yao	*Dioscorea opposita Thunb.*
10%	Deer antler gelatin	Lu Jiao Jiao	*Cervus Nippon Temmiinck*
10%	Cuscuta	Tu Si Zi	*Cuscuta chinensis Lam.*
20%	Prepared rehmannia root	Shu Di Huang	*Rehmannia glutinosa Libosch*
10%	Eucommia bark	Du Zhong	*Eucommia ulmoides Oliv.*
7%	Chinese angelica root	Dang Gui	*Angelica sinensis (Oliv.) Diels*

Yue Ju Wan

Common Name		Pin Yin	Botanical or Latin Name
20%	Atractylodes rhizome	Cang Zhu	Atractylodes lancea (Thunb.) DC.
20%	Nut-grass rhizome	Xiang Fu	Cyperus rotundus L.
20%	Ligusticum rhizome	Chuan Xiong	Ligusticum wallichii Franch
20%	Medicated leaven	Shen Qu	Massa Fermentata Medicinalis
11%	Gardenia fruit	Zhi Zi	Gardenia jasminoides Ellis

Yu Jin San

Common Name		Pin Yin	Botanical Name
11%	Coptis root	Huang Lian	Coptis chinensis Franch
16%	Curcuma root	Yu Jin	Curcuma aromatica Salisb.
11%	Gardenia fruit	Zhi Zi	Gardenia jasminoides Ellis
12%	White peony root	Bai Shao Yao	Paeonia lactiflora Pall.
12%	Phellodendron bark	Huang Bai	Phellodendron amurense Rupr.
16%	Rhubarb root	Da Huang	Rheum palmatum L.
11%	Scutellaria root	Huang Qin	Scutellaria baicalensis Georgi.
11%	Terminalia fruit	He Zi	Terminalia chebula Retz.

Yu Nu Jian

Common Name		Pin Yin	Botanical or LatinName
37%	Gypsum fibrosum	Shi Gao	Calcium sulphate
37%	Prepared rehmannia root	Shu Di Huang	Rehmannia glutinosa Libosch
15%	Ophiopogon root	Mai Men Dong	Ophiopogon japonicus Krt-Gawler
11%	Achyranthes	Niu Xi	Achyranthes bidentata Bl.

Yu Ping Feng San

Common Name		Pin Yin	Botanical Name
20%	Baked astragalus root	Huang Qi	Astragalus membranaceus (Fisch.) Bge.
40%	White Atractylodes	Bai Zhu	Atractylodes macrocephala Koidz
40%	Ledebouriella root	Fang Feng	Ledebouriella divaricata Hiroe

Zeng Ye Tang

Common Name		Pin Yin	Botanical Name
40%	Scrophularia root	Xuan Shen	*Scrophularia ningpoensis Hemsl*
30%	Ophiopogon root	Mai Men Dong	*Ophiopogon japonicus Krt-Gawler*
30%	Raw rehmannia root	Sheng Di Huang	*Rehmannia glutinosa Libosch*

Zhen Wu Tang

Common Name		Pin Yin	Botanical Name
8%	Achyranthes	Niu Xi	*Achyranthes bidentata Bl.*
10%	Aconite (prepared)	Fu Zi	*Aconitum carmichaeli Debx.*
10%	Alisma tuber	Ze Xie	*Alisma plantago-aquatica L var orientala*
10%	Cinnamon twig	Gui Zhi	*Cinnamomum cassia Presl.*
10%	Cornus	Shan Zhu Yu	*Cornus officinalis Sieb. et Zucc.*
10%	Chinese yam	Shan Yao	*Dioscorea opposita Thunb.*
10%	Moutan bark	Mu Dan Pi	*Paeonia suffruticosa Andr.*
8%	Plantago seed	Che Qian Zi	*Plantago asiatica L.*
10%	Poria	Fu Ling	*Poria cocos (Schw.) Wolf*
14%	Prepared rehmannia root	Shu Di Huang	*Rehmannia glutinosa Libosch*

Zhen Xin San

Common Name		Pin Yin	Botanical or Chemical Name
3%	Cinnabaris*	Zhu Sha	*Red mercuric sulfide*
11%	Pilose asiabell root	Dang Shen	*Codonopsis pilosula (Franch.) Nannf.*
10%	Coptis root	Huang Lian	*Coptis chinensis Franch*
11%	Curcuma root	Yu Jin	*Curcuma aromatica Salisb.*
6%	Ephedra	Ma Huang	*Ephedra sinica Stapf*
11%	Gardenia fruit	Zhi Zi	*Gardenia jasminoides Ellis*
10%	Ledebouriella root	Fang Feng	*Ledebouriella divaricata Hiroe*
7%	Licorice root	Gan Cao	*Glycyrrhiza uralensis Fisch.*
10%	Polygala root	Yuan Zhi	*Polygala tenuifolia Willd.*
10%	Poria	Fu Ling	*Poria cocos (Schw.) Wolf*
11%	Scutellaria root	Huang Qin	*Scutellaria baicalensis Georgi*

* Contains the heavy metal mercury. May substitute Oyster *Mu Li*.

Zhi Bai Di Huang Wan

Common Name		Pin Yin	Botanical Name
12%	Alisma tuber	Ze Xie	*Alisma plantago-aquatica L var orientala*
12%	Cornus	Shan Zhu Yu	*Cornus officinalis Sieb. et Zucc.*
12%	Chinese yam	Shan Yao	*Dioscorea opposita Thunb.*
12%	Moutan bark	Mu Dan Pi	*Paeonia suffruticosa Andr.*
12%	Poria	Fu Ling	*Poria cocos (Schw.) Wolf*
16%	Prepared rehmannia root	Shu Di Huang	*Rehmannia glutinosa Libosch*
12%	Anemarrhena rhizome	Zhi Mu	*Anemarrhena asphodeloides, Bunge*
12%	Phellodendron bark	Huang Bai	*Phellodendron amourense Rupr.*

Zhi Li Tang

Common Name		Pin Yin	Botanical Name
5%	Coptis root	Huang Lian	*Coptis chinensis Franch*
7%	Scutellaria root	Huang Qin	*Scutellaria baicalensis Georgi*
7%	Phellodendron bark	Huang Bai	*Phellodendron amurense Rupr.*
7%	Baked astragalus root	Huang Qi	*Astragalus membranaceus (Fisch.) Bge.*
5%	Atractylodes rhizome	Cang Zhu	*Atractylodes lancea (Thunb.) DC.*
7%	Chinese yam	Shan Yao	*Dioscorea opposita Thunb.*
7%	Gardenia fruit	Zhi Zi	*Gardenia jasminoides Ellis*
14%	Sanguisorba root	Di Yu	*Sanguisorba officinalis L.*
7%	Pinellia tuber	Ban Xia	*Pinellia ternata (Thunb.) Breit*
7%	Bamboo shavings	Zhu Ru	*Phyllostachys nigra (Lodd.) Munro var.henonis*
5%	Bitter orange	Zhi Qiao	*Citrus aurantium L.*
4%	Chinese angelica root	Dang Gui	*Angelica sinensis (Oliv.) Diels*
4%	Saussurea root	Mu Xiang	*Saussurea lappa Clarke*
7%	White peony root	Bai Shao Yao	*Paeonia lactiflora Pall.*
4%	Licorice root	Gan Cao	*Glycyrrhiza uralensis Fisch.*

Zhi Sou San

Common Name		Pin Yin	Botanical Name
16%	Aster root	Zi Wan	Aster tataricus L. F.
12%	Citrus peel	Chen Pi	Citrus reticulata Blanco
16%	Cynanchum root	Bai Qian	Cynanchum stauntonhi (Decne) Hand-Mazz
8%	Licorice root	Gan Cao	Glycyrrhiza uralensis Fisch.
16%	Platycodon root	Jie Geng	Platycodon grandiflorum (Jacq.) A. DC
16%	Schizonepeta	Jing Jie	Schizonepeta tenuifolia Briq.
16%	Stemona	Bai Bu	Stemona japonica Miq

Zhu Sha San

Common Name		Pin Yin	Botanical or Chemical Name
9%	Cinnabaris*	Zhu Sha	Red mercuric sulfide
35%	Coptis root	Huang Lian	Coptis chinensis Franch
21%	Ginseng	Ren Shen	Panax ginseng C. A. Mey.
35%	Poria	Fu Ling	Poria cocos (Schw.) Wolf

* Contains the heavy metal mercury. May substitute Oyster Mu Li.

REFERENCES

Bensky, Dan and Andrew Gamble. *Chinese Herbal Medicine Materia Medica (Revised Edition)*. Seattle: Eastland Press, 1993.

Bian, Bao. *Quan Ji Tong Xuan Lun (Treatment of Sick Horses)*. Beijing: China Agriculture Press, 1991. (Originally published during Yuan Dynasty, 1206 to 1369 A.D.)

Chen, Youbang, Deng Liangyue, Shi Xueming and Wu Xuezhang. *Chinese Acupuncture Therapeutics*. Beijing: China Science & Technology Press, 1990.

Cheng, Lingfeng. *China Agricultural Encyclopedia-Traditional Chinese Veterinary Medicine*. Beijing: China Agriculture Press, 1991.

Cheng, Xinnong. *Chinese Acupuncture and Moxibustion*. Beijing: Foreign Languages Press, 1987.

Cook, John, comp. *The Book of Positive Quotations*. New York: Gramercy Books, 1993.

Daintith, John, et al., eds. *The Macmillan Dictionary of Quotations*. New Jersey: Chartwell Books, Inc., 1989.

Deng, Tietao, ed. *Traditional Chinese Medical Diagnosis*. Beijing: People's Hygiene Publishing House, 1995. (In Chinese)

Flaws, Bob. *The Secret of Chinese Pulse Diagnosis*. Boulder: Blue Poppy Press, 1995.

Guo, Huaixi. *Ma Niu Tuo Jing Da Quan (The Complete Collection of Diseases of Horses, Cattle and Camels)*. Beijing: China Agriculture Press. (Original publication 1785 A.D.)

Hua, Tuo. *Zhong Cang Jing (The Classic of the Secret Transmission)*. Jiangsu Science and Technology Press, 1985. (Originally published in 198 A.D.)

Huang Di Nei Jing (Yellow Emperor's Classic of Internal Medicine). Beijing: People's Health Press, 1979. (Original publication in Warring States Period, 475 to 221 B.C.)

Jia, Sixie. *Qi Min Yao Shu (Basic Techniques for Farmers)*. Beijing: Science Press, 1958. (Originally published around 533 to 544 A.D.)

Kaptchuk, Ted J. *The Web That Has No Weaver-Understanding Chinese Medicine*. Chicago: Contemporary Books, 2000.

Lao Tsu. *Tao Te Ching*. (Gia-Fu Feng and Jane English, Trans.) New York: Vintage Books, 1972.

Li, Shi. *Si Mu An Ji Ji* (*A Collection of Ways to Care for and Treat Horses*). Beijing: China Agriculture Press, 1959. (Originally published in Tang Dynasty, 618 to 907 A.D.)

Li, Shizhen. *Ben Cao Gang Mu* (*Materia Medica Compendium*). Shenyang: Liaoning Nationality Press, 1999. (Originally published in 1590)

Lin, Yiming and Bai Caoyong. *Traditional Chinese Veterinary Herbal Formulas*. Chengdu: Chengdu Technology University Press, 1995.

Maciocia, Giovanni. *The Foundations of Chinese Medicine*. Edinburgh: Churchill Livingstone, 1998

Ling Shu Jing (*Spiritual Axis*). Beijing: People's Health Press, 1981. (Originally published during Warring States Period, 475 to 221 B.C.)

Ni, Maoshing. *The Yellow Emperor's Classic of Medicine-A New Translation of the Neijing Suwen*. Boston: Shambhala, 1995.

Qiu, Beiran and Chen Hanping. *New Integrated Prescriptions for Chinese Acupuncture and Moxibustion*. Shanghai: Shanghai Science & Technology Press, 1992.

Qiu, Maoliang and Chang Shanchen. *Acupuncture and Moxibustion*. Shanghai: Shanghai Science and Technology Press, 1985.

Qu, Ziming, Xu Fangzhou and Jiang Tiji. *Compendium of Chinese Veterinary Herbal Medicine*. Beijing: China Agricultural Science & Technology Press, 1991.

Su Wen (*Plain Questions*). Beijing: People's Health Press, 1979. (Original publication in the Warring States Period, 475 to 221 B.C.)

Wiseman, Nigel. *English-Chinese Chinese-English Dictionary of Chinese Medicine*. Changsha: Hu Nan Science & Technology Press, 1996.

Wu, Yan and Warren Fischer. *Practical Therapeutics of Traditional Chinese Medicine*. Brookline, Massachusetts: Paradigm Publications, 1997.

Xie, Huisheng. *Traditional Chinese Veterinary Medicine*. Beijing: Beijing Agricultural University Press, 1994.

Xu, Jianqin, Zhang Kejia and Li Chengming. *Recent Development of Traditional Chinese Veterinary Medicine*. China Agricultural University Press, 2001

Yu, Benyuan and Yu Benheng. *Yuan Heng Liao Ma Ji* (*Yuan-Heng's Therapeutic Treatise of Horses*). Beijing: China Agriculture Press, 1963. (Originally published in 1608)

Yu, Chuan. *Chinese Veterinary Acupuncture*. Beijing: China Agriculture Press, 1984.

Yu, Chuan. *Traditional Chinese Veterinary Acupuncture and Moxibustion*. Beijing: China Agriculture Press, 1995.

Yu, Chuan, ed. *Traditional Chinese Veterinary Medicine* (Second Edition). Beijing: China Agricultural Publishing House, 1987. pp.112-116. (In Chinese)

Yu, Chuan and Chang Liqun. *Complete Set of Secret Recipes of Traditional Chinese Veterinary Medicine*. Shanxi: Shanxi Science & Technology Press, 1992 (In Chinese)

Yu, Chuan and Chen Zibin, eds. *Modern Complete Works of Traditional Chinese Veterinary Medicine*. Nanning: Guangxi Sciency and Techonology Press, 2000.

Zhang, Kejia, ed. *Compendium of Traditional Chinese Veterinary Herbal Formulas Encyclopedia*. China Agriculture Press, 1994.

Zhang, Zhongjing. *Shang Han Za Bing Lun* (*Treatise on Cold-Induced Disorders and Miscellaneous Diseases*). Shanghai: Shanghai Science & Technology Press, 1980. (Originally published in 220 A.D.)

INDEX

Five Shu-transportation Points

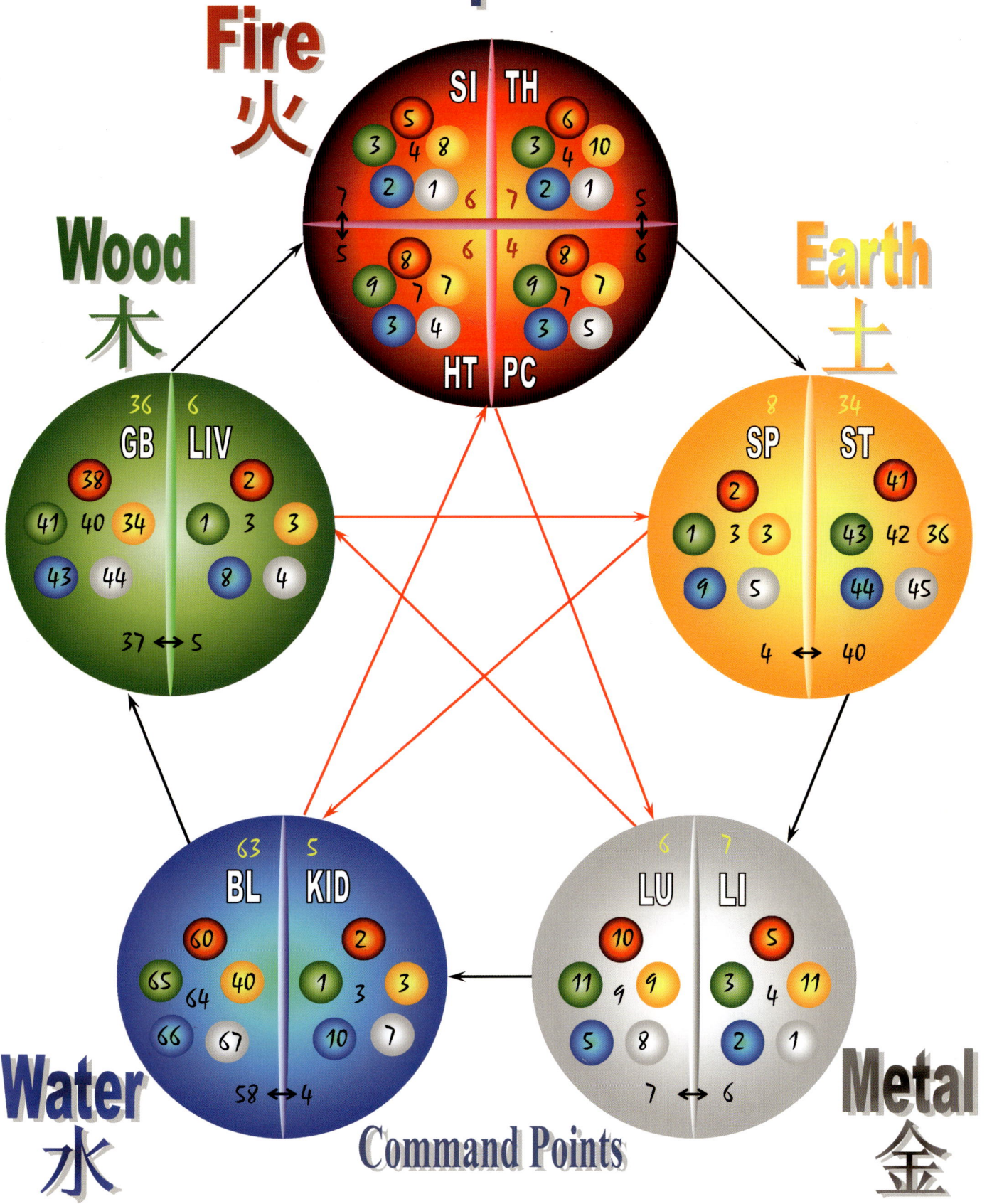

TCVM Pattern Diagnosis-Flow Chart

A Disease

External invasion of Evil Qi
Emotional stress
Dietary imbalance
Traumatic injury

Overwork
Aging
Chronic illness
Genetic deficit

Excess Pattern

- Acute onset
- Young age
- Acute traumatic injury
- Acute infectious disease
- Inflammation
- Loud voice
- Pain/stagnation
- Lump/nodule, Phlegm
- Stink smell
- Hyperactive, or fever
- Tongue: Purple or red
- Pulse: Forceful

Deficiency Pattern

- Chronic course
- Geriatric patient
- Fatigue
- Exercise intolerance
- General weakness
- Coldness or low fever
- Immunodeficiency
- Tongue: Pale or deep red
- Pulse: Deep and Weak

Six Pathogens

- Wind
- Cold
- Heat (Fire)
- Dryness
- Dampness
- Summer Heat

Secondary Pathogens

- Stagnation
  — Qi Stagnation
  — Blood Stagnation
- Phlegm
- Crystal Stone
- Food Stasis

Common Patterns

- Wind-Cold
- Wind-Heat
- Heat in Qi
- Heat in Ying
- Heat in Blood
- Heat-Toxin
- Damp-Heat
- Cold-Damp
- Wind-Cold-Damp
- Summer Heat

Qi Deficiency

- Spleen Qi Deficiency
- Lung Qi Deficiency
- Heart Qi Deficiency
- Kidney Qi Deficiency

Blood Deficiency

- Liver Blood Deficiency
- Heart Blood Deficiency

Yin Deficiency

- Lung Yin Deficiency
- Spleen Yin Deficiency
- Heart Yin Deficiency
- Liver Yin Deficiency
- Kidney Yin Deficiency

Yang Deficiency

- Spleen Yang Deficiency
- Heart Yang Deficiency
- Kidney Yang Deficiency

Differentiation Chart of Excess Patterns

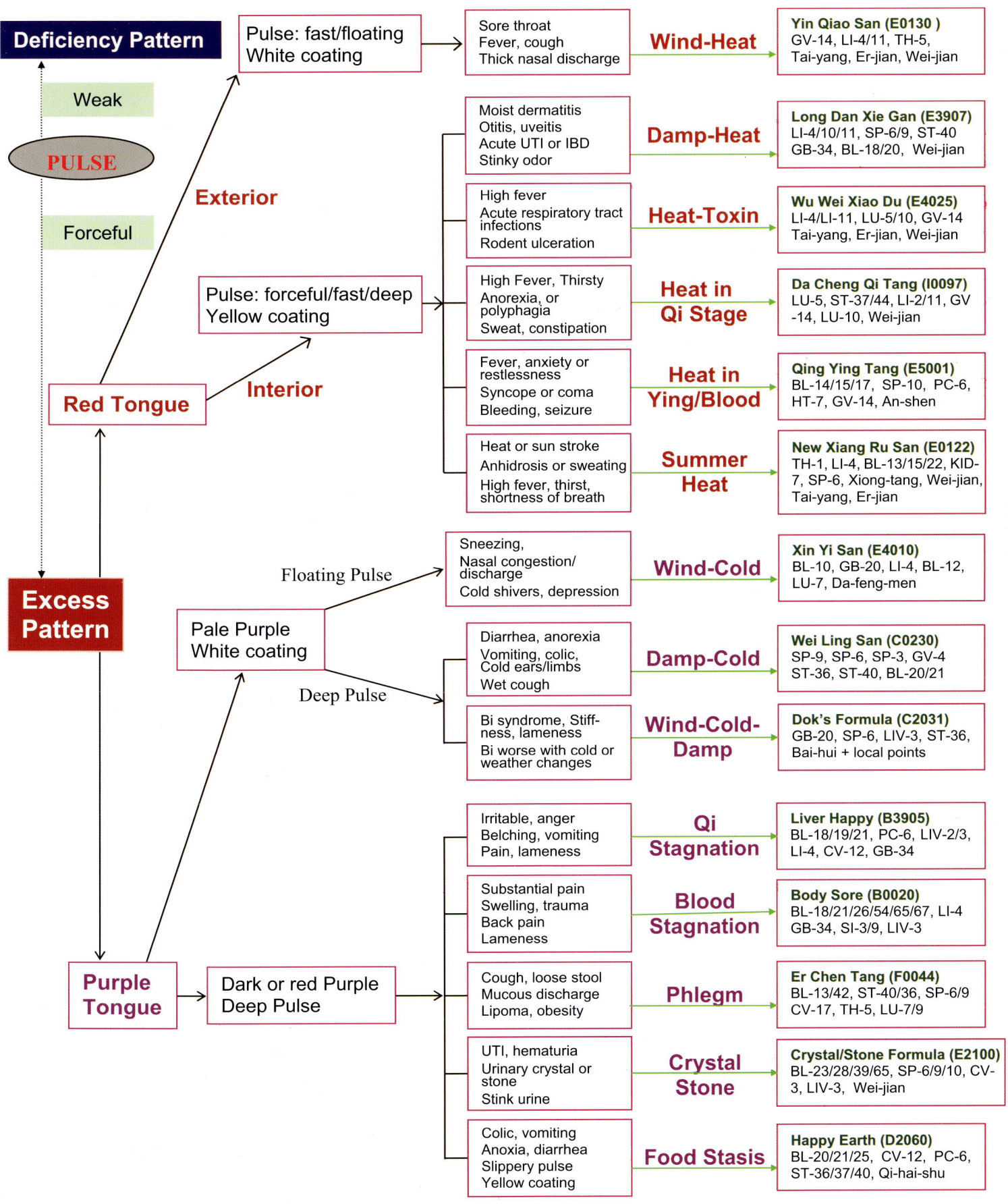

Deficiency Pattern

Weak

PULSE

Forceful

Exterior

Red Tongue

Interior

Excess Pattern

Purple Tongue

Branch	Symptoms	Pattern	Formula / Points
Pulse: fast/floating White coating	Sore throat / Fever, cough / Thick nasal discharge	**Wind-Heat**	**Yin Qiao San (E0130)** GV-14, LI-4/11, TH-5, Tai-yang, Er-jian, Wei-jian
Pulse: forceful/fast/deep Yellow coating	Moist dermatitis / Otitis, uveitis / Acute UTI or IBD / Stinky odor	**Damp-Heat**	**Long Dan Xie Gan (E3907)** LI-4/10/11, SP-6/9, ST-40 GB-34, BL-18/20, Wei-jian
	High fever / Acute respiratory tract infections / Rodent ulceration	**Heat-Toxin**	**Wu Wei Xiao Du (E4025)** LI-4/LI-11, LU-5/10, GV-14 Tai-yang, Er-jian, Wei-jian
	High Fever, Thirsty / Anorexia, or polyphagia / Sweat, constipation	**Heat in Qi Stage**	**Da Cheng Qi Tang (I0097)** LU-5, ST-37/44, LI-2/11, GV-14, LU-10, Wei-jian
	Fever, anxiety or restlessness / Syncope or coma / Bleeding, seizure	**Heat in Ying/Blood**	**Qing Ying Tang (E5001)** BL-14/15/17, SP-10, PC-6, HT-7, GV-14, An-shen
	Heat or sun stroke / Anhidrosis or sweating / High fever, thirst, shortness of breath	**Summer Heat**	**New Xiang Ru San (E0122)** TH-1, LI-4, BL-13/15/22, KID-7, SP-6, Xiong-tang, Wei-jian, Tai-yang, Er-jian
Pale Purple White coating — Floating Pulse	Sneezing, / Nasal congestion/ discharge / Cold shivers, depression	**Wind-Cold**	**Xin Yi San (E4010)** BL-10, GB-20, LI-4, BL-12, LU-7, Da-feng-men
Pale Purple White coating — Deep Pulse	Diarrhea, anorexia / Vomiting, colic, / Cold ears/limbs / Wet cough	**Damp-Cold**	**Wei Ling San (C0230)** SP-9, SP-6, SP-3, GV-4 ST-36, ST-40, BL-20/21
	Bi syndrome, Stiff-ness, lameness / Bi worse with cold or weather changes	**Wind-Cold-Damp**	**Dok's Formula (C2031)** GB-20, SP-6, LIV-3, ST-36, Bai-hui + local points
Dark or red Purple Deep Pulse	Irritable, anger / Belching, vomiting / Pain, lameness	**Qi Stagnation**	**Liver Happy (B3905)** BL-18/19/21, PC-6, LIV-2/3, LI-4, CV-12, GB-34
	Substantial pain / Swelling, trauma / Back pain / Lameness	**Blood Stagnation**	**Body Sore (B0020)** BL-18/21/26/54/65/67, LI-4 GB-34, SI-3/9, LIV-3
	Cough, loose stool / Mucous discharge / Lipoma, obesity	**Phlegm**	**Er Chen Tang (F0044)** BL-13/42, ST-40/36, SP-6/9 CV-17, TH-5, LU-7/9
	UTI, hematuria / Urinary crystal or stone / Stink urine	**Crystal Stone**	**Crystal/Stone Formula (E2100)** BL-23/28/39/65, SP-6/9/10, CV-3, LIV-3, Wei-jian
	Colic, vomiting / Anoxia, diarrhea / Slippery pulse / Yellow coating	**Food Stasis**	**Happy Earth (D2060)** BL-20/21/25, CV-12, PC-6, ST-36/37/40, Qi-hai-shu

Differentiation Chart of Deficiency Patterns

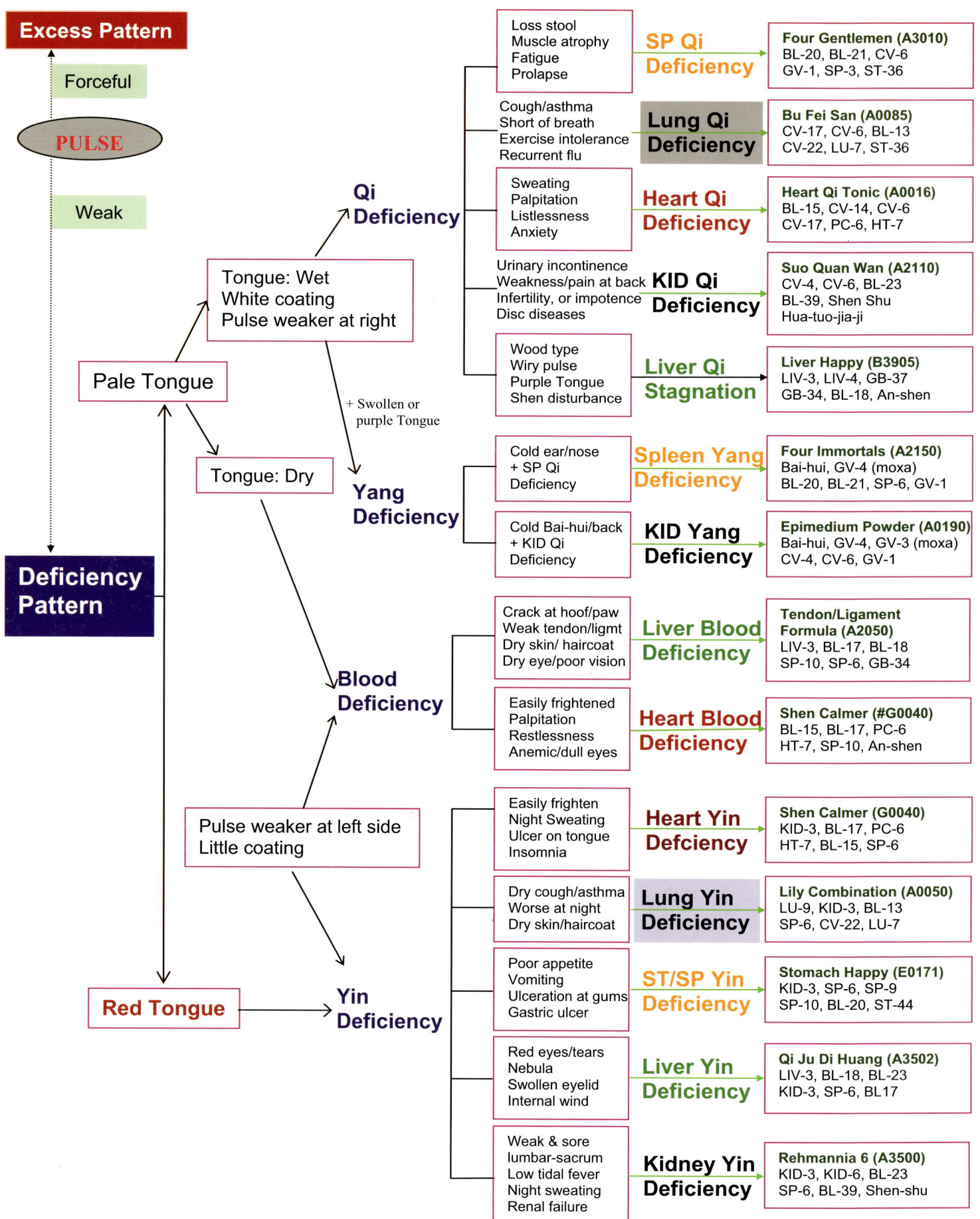

Excess Pattern

Forceful

PULSE

Weak

Deficiency Pattern

Pale Tongue

Tongue: Wet
White coating
Pulse weaker at right

Tongue: Dry

Red Tongue

Pulse weaker at left side
Little coating

Qi Deficiency

+ Swollen or purple Tongue

Yang Deficiency

Blood Deficiency

Yin Deficiency

Loss stool
Muscle atrophy
Fatigue
Prolapse
→ **SP Qi Deficiency** → **Four Gentlemen (A3010)**
BL-20, BL-21, CV-6
GV-1, SP-3, ST-36

Cough/asthma
Short of breath
Exercise intolerance
Recurrent flu
→ **Lung Qi Deficiency** → **Bu Fei San (A0085)**
CV-17, CV-6, BL-13
CV-22, LU-7, ST-36

Sweating
Palpitation
Listlessness
Anxiety
→ **Heart Qi Deficiency** → **Heart Qi Tonic (A0016)**
BL-15, CV-14, CV-6
CV-17, PC-6, HT-7

Urinary incontinence
Weakness/pain at back
Infertility, or impotence
Disc diseases
→ **KID Qi Deficiency** → **Suo Quan Wan (A2110)**
CV-4, CV-6, BL-23
BL-39, Shen Shu
Hua-tuo-jia-ji

Wood type
Wiry pulse
Purple Tongue
Shen disturbance
→ **Liver Qi Stagnation** → **Liver Happy (B3905)**
LIV-3, LIV-4, GB-37
GB-34, BL-18, An-shen

Cold ear/nose
+ SP Qi Deficiency
→ **Spleen Yang Deficiency** → **Four Immortals (A2150)**
Bai-hui, GV-4 (moxa)
BL-20, BL-21, SP-6, GV-1

Cold Bai-hui/back
+ KID Qi Deficiency
→ **KID Yang Deficiency** → **Epimedium Powder (A0190)**
Bai-hui, GV-4, GV-3 (moxa)
CV-4, CV-6, GV-1

Crack at hoof/paw
Weak tendon/ligmt
Dry skin/ haircoat
Dry eye/poor vision
→ **Liver Blood Deficiency** → **Tendon/Ligament Formula (A2050)**
LIV-3, BL-17, BL-18
SP-10, SP-6, GB-34

Easily frightened
Palpitation
Restlessness
Anemic/dull eyes
→ **Heart Blood Deficiency** → **Shen Calmer (#G0040)**
BL-15, BL-17, PC-6
HT-7, SP-10, An-shen

Easily frighten
Night Sweating
Ulcer on tongue
Insomnia
→ **Heart Yin Defciency** → **Shen Calmer (G0040)**
KID-3, BL-17, PC-6
HT-7, BL-15, SP-6

Dry cough/asthma
Worse at night
Dry skin/haircoat
→ **Lung Yin Deficiency** → **Lily Combination (A0050)**
LU-9, KID-3, BL-13
SP-6, CV-22, LU-7

Poor appetite
Vomiting
Ulceration at gums
Gastric ulcer
→ **ST/SP Yin Deficiency** → **Stomach Happy (E0171)**
KID-3, SP-6, SP-9
SP-10, BL-20, ST-44

Red eyes/tears
Nebula
Swollen eyelid
Internal wind
→ **Liver Yin Deficiency** → **Qi Ju Di Huang (A3502)**
LIV-3, BL-18, BL-23
KID-3, SP-6, BL17

Weak & sore
lumbar-sacrum
Low tidal fever
Night sweating
Renal failure
→ **Kidney Yin Deficiency** → **Rehmannia 6 (A3500)**
KID-3, KID-6, BL-23
SP-6, BL-39, Shen-shu